Handbook of
Veterinary Neurology

Handbook of
Veterinary Neurology

Second Edition

John E. Oliver, Jr., D.V.M., M.S., Ph.D.
Professor
Department of Small Animal Medicine
College of Veterinary Medicine
University of Georgia
Athens, Georgia

Diplomate
American College of Veterinary Internal Medicine,
Neurology

Michael D. Lorenz, D.V.M.
Dean
College of Veterinary Medicine
Kansas State University
Manhattan, Kansas

Diplomate
American College of Veterinary Internal Medicine,
Internal Medicine

W.B. SAUNDERS COMPANY
A Division of Harcourt Brace & Company
Philadelphia / London / Toronto / Montreal / Sydney / Tokyo

W.B. SAUNDERS COMPANY
A Division of
Harcourt Brace & Company

The Curtis Center
Independence Square West
Philadelphia, Pennsylvania 19106

Library of Congress Cataloging-in-Publication Data

Oliver, John E. (John Eoff),
Handbook of veterinary neurology / John E. Oliver, Jr., Michael D. Lorenz.—2nd ed.
p. cm.
Rev. ed. of: Handbook of veterinary neurologic diagnosis. 1983.
ISBN 0-7216-6968-9
1. Veterinary neurology—Handbooks, manuals, etc. 2. Nervous system—Diseases—Diagnosis—Handbooks, manuals, etc. I. Lorenz, Michael D. II. Oliver, John E. (John Eoff), 1933– Handbook of veterinary neurologic diagnosis. III. Title.
SF895.044 1993
636.089'680475—dc20 92-22000

HANDBOOK OF VETERINARY NEUROLOGY ISBN 0-7216-6968-9

Printed in the United States of America

Last digit is the print number: 9 8 7 6 5 4 3 2

To our families, who gave us the time
To our teachers, who showed us the way
To our colleagues, who kept us honest
And, most of all, to our students, who made it worthwhile

Preface

The second edition of the *Handbook of Veterinary Neurologic Diagnosis* has been renamed *Handbook of Veterinary Neurology* to reflect the scope of coverage. Surgical techniques are not described, but medical therapy and recommendations for surgery are included. Large animal diseases receive more attention in this edition. The format of the chapters has not changed, but there is extensive revision of all segments. Many of the algorithms and tables have been simplified and cross references to the text added. Because of the explosive growth of clinical neurology, many new diseases are included.

The introductory chapter including a brief description of neuropathology was deleted, since the information is readily available in general pathology books. The tables listing diseases affecting specific breeds have been expanded as an Appendix. The chapters on history and neurologic examination are combined into one chapter. The chapter on disorders of behavior was deleted because there are several books on behavioral problems in animals. We have added chapters on Disorders of Involuntary Movement and on Pain.

A special thanks to all the readers of the first edition who took the time to give us so much positive feedback. We hope you like this one even better.

John E. Oliver, Jr.
Michael D. Lorenz

Contents

I Fundamentals

I

Fundamentals

1

Neurologic History and Examination

The objectives in the management of a patient with a problem that may be related to the nervous system are (1) to determine that the problem is caused by a lesion in the nervous system, (2) to localize the lesion in the nervous system, (3) to estimate the extent of the lesion in the nervous system, (4) to determine the cause or the pathologic process, or both, and (5) to estimate the prognosis with no treatment or with various alternative methods of treatment.

Many diseases are ill-defined and may be accompanied by a complex combination of clinical signs and laboratory data. Diagnosis of these diseases may seem impossible. L. L. Weed has demonstrated the value of starting the diagnostic process by independently listing and analyzing all of the patient's problems.[1] A minimum set of data (minimum data base) is necessary in order to solve any medical problem. The minimum data base may be modified because of risk, cost, or accessibility, as balanced against the severity of the disease. Priorities should be established for collecting data that evaluate the most probable causes of a problem. Tests for rare diseases and those that are dangerous are reserved until last.

Weed's problem-oriented system is eminently suited for neurologic diagnosis. The steps necessary for the management of a neurologic problem are listed in Table 1–1.

Minimum Data Base

The initial evaluation of a patient, including a history and a physical examination, usually will provide evidence that a neurologic problem is present (Table 1–2). Some problems are difficult to classify, for example, syncope versus convulsions or weakness (loss of muscle strength) versus paresis (loss of neural control). The initial physical examination of every patient should include a screening neurologic examination designed to detect the presence of any neurologic abnormality. It is described later in this chapter under Neurologic Examination.

The minimum data base recommended for an animal with a neurologic problem is listed in Table 1–3. Chemistry panels are usually available at less cost than individual tests, so selection of tests is usually not necessary. Otherwise, the selection of chemistry profiles should be based on the problems presented. Additions to the data base are recommended for specific problems.

Problem List

A problem list is formulated from information obtained from the minimum data base. For each problem a diagnostic plan is formulated. A diagnostic plan for a neurologic problem includes the following steps: (1) The level of the lesion is localized with a neurologic examination. Confirmation of the lesion may require survey or contrast radiography. (2) The extent of the lesion is estimated both longitudinally and transversely. The neurologic examination provides most of this information, but ancillary diagnostic procedures may be of assistance. (3) The cause of the pathologic process is deter-

TABLE 1–1 Plan for Neurologic Diagnosis

Collect minimum data base
Identify problems
Identify one or more problems related to nervous system
Localize level of lesion
Estimate extent of lesion within that level
Determine cause or pathology
Determine prognosis with and without therapy

Modified with permission from Oliver JE Jr: Localization of lesions in the nervous system. Hoerlein BF (ed): Canine Neurology, 3rd ed. Philadelphia, WB Saunders, 1978.

mined. The history is most useful for establishing the class of disease (neoplasia, infectious disease, trauma, and so forth). Laboratory, radiographic, or electrophysiologic tests are usually required to substantiate the diagnosis. From this information, the clinician can establish a prognosis with and without appropriate therapy, based on information available about the disease (see Table 1–1).

This chapter describes the history and neurologic examination.

TABLE 1–3 Minimum Data Base: Neurologic Problem

History
Physical examination
Neurologic examination
Clinical pathology
CBC
Urinalysis
Chemistry profile
BUN levels
ALT levels
Calcium levels
Alkaline phosphatase levels
Fasting blood glucose levels
Total serum protein levels
Albumin levels

Modified with permission from Oliver JE Jr: Localization of lesions in the nervous system. In Hoerlein BF (ed): Canine Neurology, 3rd ed. Philadelphia, WB Saunders, 1978.

Taking the History

Traditionally, the history was taken by the veterinarian. Paraprofessional personnel were not expected to obtain information other than the signalment (species, breed, age, sex, and so

TABLE 1–2 Clinical Problems in the Nervous System

Problem	*Localization*
Usually of CNS Origin	
Convulsions	Cerebrum, diencephalon
Altered mental status	Cerebrum, limbic system
Stupor or coma	Brain stem reticular formation
Abnormal behavior	Limbic system
Paresis, paralysis	See Tables 2–2, 2–3, and 2–4
Proprioceptive deficit	Similar to UMN – see Tables 2–2, 2–3, and 2–4
Ataxia	
Head tilt, nystagmus	Vestibular system
Intention tremor, dysmetria	Cerebellum
Proprioceptive deficit, no head involvement	Spinal cord
Hypesthesia, analgesia	See Figures 1–32 to 1–35; CN V
Possibly of CNS Origin	
Syncope	Usually cardiovascular, metabolic
Weakness	See Figure 2–7 and Table 2–3; metabolic or muscular
Lameness	Orthopedic – see Table 2–1
Pain, hyperesthesia	
Generalized	Thalamus, meningitis
Localized	See Figures 1–32 to 1–35; CN V
Blindness	
Pupils normal	Occipital cortex (contralateral)
Pupils abnormal	See Chapter 12
Hearing deficit	
No vestibular signs	Cochlea
Vestibular signs	CN VIII, labyrinth
Anosmia	Nasal passages, CN I
Visceral dysfunction	See Chapter 3

Modified with permission from Oliver JE Jr: Localization of lesions in the nervous system. In Hoerlein BF (ed): Canine Neurology, 3rd ed. Philadelphia, WB Saunders, 1978.

forth). The development of the concept of a *defined data base* in conjunction with a problem-oriented medical record system has provided the impetus for change.[1] If one establishes a minimum base of necessary information about every patient, or about every patient with a certain problem, then one can obtain that information in a number of ways.

Owner-Supplied History

A basic history can be obtained by use of a well-designed questionnaire. The receptionist gives the questionnaire to the client, who completes it in the reception area. A paraprofessional (veterinary technician, nurse) can assist the client in answering difficult questions. The general medical history is available for review by the veterinarian, who notes significant items that may need further clarification. Problem-specific owner histories can be used to supplement the general history.

Role of the Veterinarian

The most important parts of the history should be reviewed with the client by the veterinarian. Misinterpretation of terminology, of a course of events, or of clinical signs occurs frequently. The veterinarian may need to rephrase questions several times before receiving a meaningful answer.

The manner in which a question is phrased is important. Questions that imply negligence or ignorance on the part of the client may lead to defensive answers. Questions that suggest a correct answer may lead the client to interpret events incorrectly. All questions should be framed so that the answer "I don't know" is an acceptable alternative; otherwise, the client may hypothesize rather than relate facts.[2]

Neurologic History

Signalment

The species, breed, age, and sex of the patient may provide important clues to the diagnosis. Although very few diagnoses can be positively ruled in or out on the basis of the signalment, many diseases are more or less likely to occur among certain groups of animals.

The prevalence of some diseases varies greatly among species and breeds. Many infectious diseases are species-specific, such as canine distemper, feline infectious peritonitis, and scrapie of sheep. Known inherited diseases must be considered, especially in cases involving young animals. Appendix 1 lists many of the diseases with a species or breed predilection. Infectious diseases are listed in Chapter 16.

Young animals are more likely to have congenital and inherited disorders and infectious diseases. Older animals are likely to have degenerative and neoplastic diseases. Although these criteria are not absolute, the probability is much greater that an 8-year-old brachycephalic dog will have a neoplasm of the central nervous system (CNS) rather than a congenital anomaly. In the preliminary assessment, and sometimes in the final assessment, a diagnosis is an ordering of probabilities.

Sign-Time Graph

Construction of a sign-time graph is useful for evaluating the course of a disease (Fig. 1–1). The sign-time graph plots the severity of clinical signs (on the vertical axis) against time (on the horizontal axis). A complete history will allow the clinician to construct a graph that has no major gaps.[3]

The sign-time graph is not usually drawn and entered on the case record. Rather, it is a useful tool for the clinician to construct mentally.

The time of onset of some problems may be very exact (e.g., an automobile accident), or it may be very difficult to determine, as in the case of neoplastic disease. The first time the client recognized a problem must be taken as the starting point. Sometimes seemingly unrelated episodes may be the earliest signs and will be recognized as such only as the complete history unfolds. For example, an animal with degenerative spinal cord disease may have been observed to stumble or may have had difficulty with stairs some time before clear manifestations of paresis were evident.

The course of the disease as revealed by the sign-time graph provides important information about the cause of the disease (see Fig. 1–1). Slowly progressive diseases with an unrelenting course are immediately distinguished from acute diseases. The first step in making an etiologic diagnosis is classifying the problem as acute or chronic and progressive or nonprogressive. With this information, the problem logically falls into a group of diseases (Figs. 1–1 and 1–2, Table 1–4). The neurologic examination can further narrow the choice of diseases by indicating whether the problem is focal or diffuse (see Fig. 1–2). After a general etiologic or pathologic diagnosis is considered, the diagnostic plan can be established so that one can rule in or out each of the probable causes (see diagnostic methods in Chap. 4).

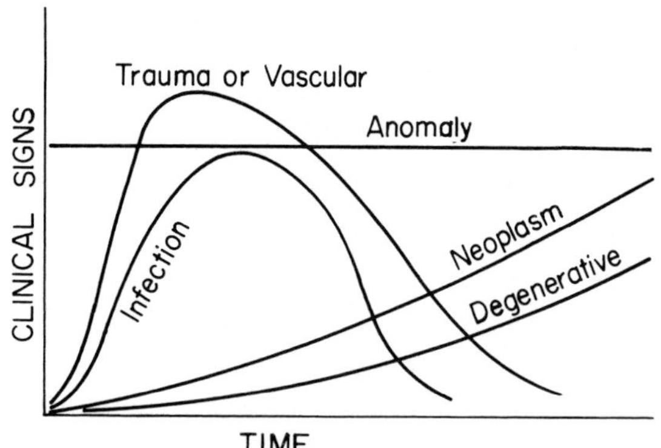

Figure 1–1 Sign-time graph of neurologic diseases. Progression of metabolic, nutritional, and toxic diseases is variable, depending on the cause.

Neurologic Signs

Signs that are likely to be associated with an abnormality of the nervous system are listed in Table 1–2.

Seizures always indicate a problem in the brain, although the problem may be secondary to a metabolic or toxic condition. Differentiation between seizures and syncope may be difficult and may require wording the questions carefully and interpreting the answers even more carefully.

Stupor and coma are manifestations of abnormal cerebral or brain stem function. Behavioral changes may be caused by primary brain abnormalities or may be secondary to environmental factors.

Paresis and paralysis, signs of primary motor dysfunction, are caused by a neurologic abnormality. Lameness of musculoskeletal origin is differentiated from these signs by the neurologic examination.

Sensory deficits, such as loss of proprioception or hypesthesia (decreased sensation), are always a result of an abnormality in the nervous system.

Pain may be related to neural lesions. The client's observations may be helpful in localizing the animal's pain. A careful physical and neurologic examination is essential in order to verify the signs.

Visual deficits may be caused by an abnormality of the eye or of the nervous system. An ocular and neurologic examination is necessary in order to make a diagnosis. Historical information may be deceptive in the case of visual abnormalities. Animals in their normal surroundings may function normally even though they may be completely blind.

Deficits in hearing usually are not recognized unless they are bilateral. Bilateral hearing loss is usually caused by abnormalities of the inner ear; brain lesions causing deafness are rare.

Loss of the sense of smell (anosmia) is rarely recognized, except in working dogs. Inappe-

TABLE 1–4 Checklist for Differential Diagnosis

	Category of Disease	*Examples*
D	Degenerative	Primary degeneration Storage disease Demyelinating diseases Neuronopathies Intervertebral disk disease Spondylosis Spondylopathies
A	Anomalous	Congenital defects
M	Metabolic	Nervous system disorders secondary to an abnormality of other organ systems (e.g., hypoglycemia, uremia)
N	Neoplastic	All tumors
	Nutritional	All nutritional problems
I	Idiopathic	Epilepsy Facial paralysis Vestibular syndrome
	Immune	Myasthenia gravis (acquired) Polyradiculoradiculoneuritis
	Inflammatory	Infectious diseases
T	Traumatic	Physical injury
	Toxic	Exposure to all toxic agents (may include tetanus and botulism)
V	Vascular	Infarcts Hemorrhage

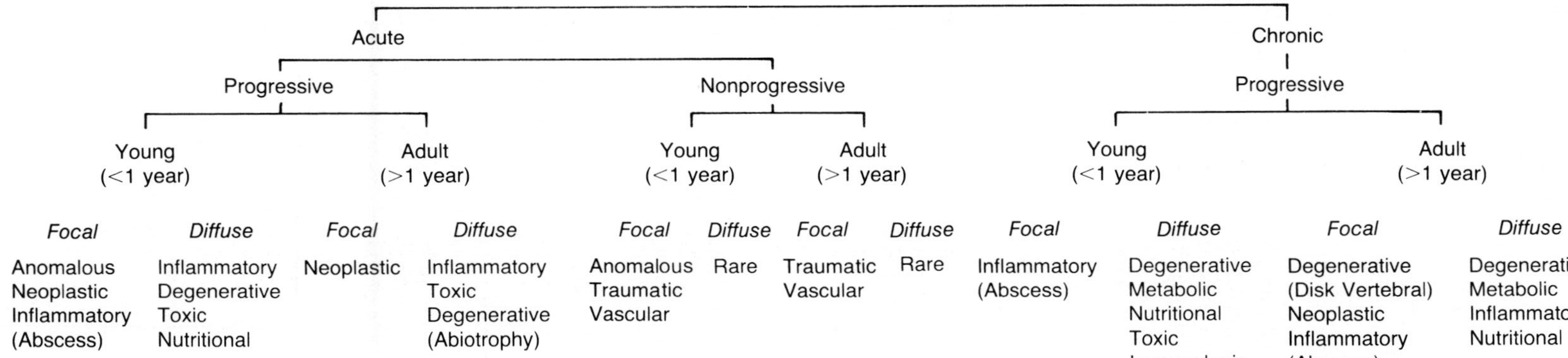

Figure 1–2 Classification of neurologic diseases, in approximate order of frequency.

tence occasionally may be associated with anosmia.

Prognosis

Providing the owner with a reasonably accurate prognosis is an essential part of clinical neurology. The prognosis is influenced by many variables. The major variables are the location, the extent, and the cause of the lesion.

The clinical course of the problem affords significant insight into the prognosis. A slowly progressive disease carries a much poorer prognosis than one that has passed its peak of severity and is improving (see Fig. 1–1). Degenerative and neoplastic diseases will appear on the sign-time graph as progressive diseases.

Clinical signs are also valuable clues to prognosis. Spinal cord compression produces signs that vary with increasing compression (Fig. 1–3). The signs are not related to the location of the tracts in the spinal cord but do correlate with the size of the fibers. When compressed, large fibers lose function before small fibers do. Functional recovery is possible until pain sensation is lost. An animal with no response to a painful stimulus has a very low probability of recovery. Animals that do recover frequently have severe motor deficits.

The duration of the lesion is also a significant factor in prognosis because nervous tissue tolerates injury for only a short time. Spinal cord compression has been studied more thoroughly than most CNS injuries. Spinal cord compression severe enough to abolish voluntary motor function but not severe enough to abolish the response to a painful stimulus is associated with a reasonably good prognosis for recovery if decompression is achieved within 5 to 7 days. The longer the duration of compression, however, the slower is the recovery. If decompression is delayed for more than 7 days, the probability of recovery is not significantly different, regardless of whether decompression is indeed accomplished. Compression that abolishes pain sensation for 2 to 4 hours is associated with a very poor prognosis.

The location and character of the lesion are also important. An infarction of the spinal cord can vary from mild to severe. Equally severe lesions have different prognoses, depending on the location. For example, an infarct primarily affecting gray matter at the L1 segment, with intact sensation to the pelvic limbs, has a reasonably good prognosis. The same degree of injury at the L5 segment is likely to produce permanent dysfunction because of destruction of the motor neurons supplying the femoral nerve.

The prognoses of the many disorders affecting the nervous system are discussed throughout the text.

The Neurologic Examination

In the neurologic examination, the clinician systematically evaluates the functional integrity of the various components of the nervous system. The examination can be conveniently divided into the following parts: observation; palpation; examination of postural reactions, spinal reflexes, and cranial nerve responses; and sensory evaluation (Table 1–5). In every complete physical examination, each of these categories is investigated in order to assess any problem possibly related to the nervous system. An abbreviated neurologic examination might include the items marked with an asterisk in Table 1–5. Positive findings on any of these tests indicate the need for a more complete neurologic examination. Neurologic responses of neonatal dogs are outlined in Table 1–6.

The neurologic examination is usually described as a complicated process wholly sepa-

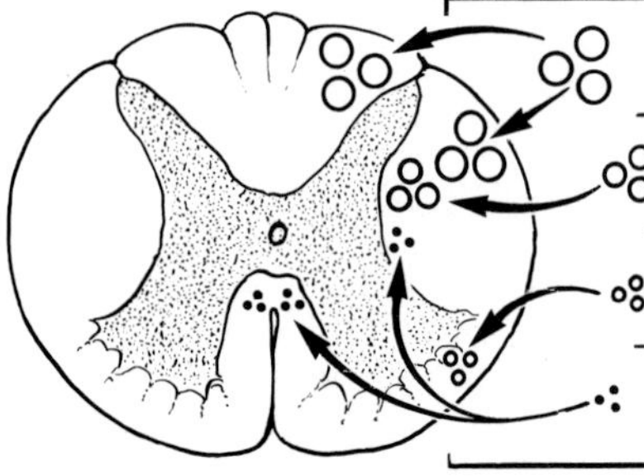

Fiber Size	Function	Signs with Increasing Compression	Prognosis
	Proprioception	Proprioceptive Deficits	Good
	Voluntary Motor	Paresis, Paralysis	Fair
	Superficial Pain	Loss of Cutaneous Sensation	Fair
	Deep Pain	Loss of Deep Pain	Poor

Figure 1–3 Progression of signs in spinal cord compression.

TABLE 1–5 Neurologic Examination

I. *Observation**
  Mental status
  Posture
  Movement
II. *Palpation**
  Integument
  Muscles
  Skeleton
III. *Postural Reactions*
  Proprioceptive positioning*
  Wheelbarrowing
  Hopping*
  Extensor postural thrust
  Hemistanding and hemiwalking
  Placing (tactile)
  Placing (visual)
  Sway test
  Tonic neck
IV. *Spinal Reflexes*
  Myotatic
    Pelvic limb
      Quadriceps femoris muscle*
      Cranial tibial muscle
      Gastrocnemius muscle
    Thoracic limb
      Extensor carpi radialis muscle
      Triceps brachii muscle
      Biceps brachii muscle
  Flexor*
  Extensor thrust
  Perineal*
  Crossed extensor
  Extensor toe
V. *Cranial Nerves*
  Olfactory
  Optic*
  Oculomotor*
  Trochlear
  Trigeminal*
  Abducent*
  Facial*
  Vestibulocochlear*
  Glossopharyngeal*
  Vagus*
  Accessory
  Hypoglossal*
VI. *Sensation*
  Touch
  Hyperesthesia*
  Superficial pain*
  Deep pain†

* Included in a screening examination.
† If superficial pain is absent.

rate from the physical examination. In reality, much of the neurologic examination is done as a routine part of the physical examination. The examiner need only be aware of what is being observed. The addition of a few extra steps completes the examination. A brief description of integration of the neurologic examination with the physical examination in a small animal patient is presented as an example. This is followed by detailed discussion of each of the components. The process of completing the neurologic examination varies, depending on the examiner's routine in a physical examination.

The Efficient Neurologic Examination

1. Observation: Completed while taking the history.

2. Palpation: Usually done very early in a physical examination.

3. Postural reactions: Require special tests. Hopping and proprioceptive positioning of each leg are usually all that are necessary. Proprioceptive positioning can be done during palpation: when the examiner's hand reaches the foot, the foot is knuckled under and the response observed.

4. Spinal reflexes: Require special tests. Quadriceps (knee jerk), extensor carpi radialis, and flexion reflexes are adequate. If gait and postural reactions are normal, spinal reflexes are usually normal.

5. Cranial nerves: Can be examined very easily during the general physical examination when the head is examined. While observing the head, the examiner notes symmetry of the face (CN VII) and symmetry of eye position and pupils (CN III, IV, and VI). A menacing gesture is made at each eye, provoking a blink (CN II and VII). The medial and lateral canthus is touched on each eye, provoking a blink (CN V—ophthalmic and maxillary branches; CN VII). The examiner turns the head side to side, observing vestibular eye movements (CN III, IV, VI, and VIII), then shines a light in each eye, observing the pupillary light reflex (CN II and III). The nose and lower jaw are touched or pinched, eliciting facial or behavioral movements (CN V—maxillary and mandibular; CN VII). The temporal and masseter muscles are palpated and the mouth opened, with the examiner noting jaw tone (CN V—mandibular). With the patient's mouth open, while assessing mucous membranes and tonsils, the examiner notes symmetry of the larynx and pharynx and touches the pharynx, causing a gag reflex (CN IX and X). The examiner observes symmetry of the tongue and, as the mouth is closed, rubs the nose; most animals will lick, illustrating symmetry of tongue movements (CN XII). During palpation of the animal the trapezius and brachiocephalicus muscles were observed for atrophy (CN XI). The only cranial nerve not tested was CN I—olfactory, which can be assessed by an aversive response to alcohol. It is not tested unless there is some suspicion of forebrain deficit.

TABLE 1–6 Neurologic Evaluation of the Neonatal Dog

	Response		
	Strong (Age, days)	Weak, Variable (Age, days)	Absent or Adultlike (Age, days)
Motor Responses			
Crossed extensor reflex	1–16	16–18	18+ (absent)
Magnus reflex	1–17	17–21	21+ (absent)
Neck extension posture	Flexion, 1–4	Hyperextension, 4–21	Normotonia, 21+
Forelimb placing	4+	2–4	0–2 (absent)
Hind limb placing	8+	6–8	0–6 (absent)
Forelimb supporting	10+	6–19	0–6 (absent)
Hind limb supporting	15+	11–15	0–11 (absent)
Standing on all fours	21+	18–21	1–18 (absent)
Body righting (cutaneous)	1+	0–1	–
Sensory Responses			
Rooting reflex	0–14	14–25	25+ (absent)
Nociceptive withdrawal reflex	0–19	19–23	23+ (adult-like)
Panniculus reflex	0–19	19–25	25+ (adult-like)
Reflex urination	0–22	22–25	25+ (absent)
Visual and Auditory Responses			
Blinking response to light	16+	4–16	0–4 (absent)
Visual orientation	25+	20–25	0–20 (absent)
Auditory startle reflex	24+	15–24	0–15 (absent)
Sound orientation	25+	18–25	0–18

Modified with permission from Fox MW: The clinical behavior of the neonatal dog. J Am Vet Med Assoc 143:1331–1335, 1963.

This assessment of cranial nerves adds less than 2 minutes to the usual examination of the head.

6. Sensory examination: Hyperesthesia may have been detected during palpation. Response to pain can be assessed during flexion reflex testing and cranial nerve evaluation. Areas of suspicion are pursued last to avoid upsetting the animal early in the examination. Testing for deep pain is done only if the animal is not responsive to superficial stimulation.

The complete neurologic examination adds only a minimum amount of time to the total physical examination.

Components of the Neurologic Examination

Observation

During every physical examination, the veterinarian should observe the animal's *mental status, posture*, and *movement*. The animal should be allowed to move around the examination room or in an open area while the history is being taken.[4–6]

Mental Status

Technique. The examiner can obtain a general impression of the animal's level of consciousness and behavior by observing its response to environmental stimuli or to people. Natural variations, such as the aggressive curiosity of puppies, the indifference of older hounds, and the withdrawal of cats, must be recognized as normal behavior. Overt aggression and fear-biting usually can be recognized.

Anatomy and Physiology. Consciousness is a function of the cerebral cortex and the brain stem. Sensory stimuli from the body, such as touch, temperature, and pain, and from outside the body, such as sight, sound, and odors, provide input to the reticular formation. Consciousness is maintained by diffuse projections of the reticular formation to the cerebral cortex (Fig. 1–4). This arousal system is termed the *reticular activating system*.[7] A common cause of decreased levels of consciousness is a disruption of the pathways between the reticular formation and the cerebral cortex. The limbic system, consisting of portions of the cerebrum and diencephalon, constitutes the substrate for behavior.

Assessment. An animal's mental status may be recorded as alert, depressed, stuporous, or comatose, depending on its level of conciousness (see Chap. 13). Behavioral changes may include aggression, fear, withdrawal, and disorientation. Other signs related to abnormal behavior include yawning, head pressing, compulsive walking, circling, and "stargazing."

Depression in an animal is characterized by a conscious but inactive state. The animal is rela-

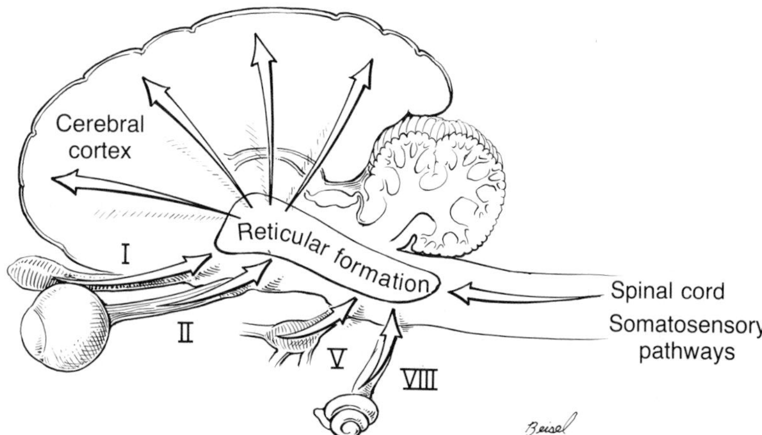

Figure 1–4 The ascending reticular activating system in the brain stem receives sensory information from the spinal cord and the cranial nerves. It projects, through thalamic relays, diffusely to the cerebral cortex, thus maintaining consciousness.

tively unresponsive to the environment and tends to sleep when undisturbed. Depression may be caused by systemic problems, such as fever, anemia, or metabolic disorders. When associated with primary brain problems, depression usually indicates diffuse cerebral cortex disease.

Stupor is exemplified by an animal that tends to sleep when undisturbed. Innocuous stimuli such as touch or noise may not cause arousal, but a painful stimulus will cause the animal to awaken. Stupor usually is associated with partial disconnection of the reticular formation and the cerebral cortex, as in diffuse cerebral edema with compression of the brain stem.

Coma is a state of deep unconsciousness. The animal cannot be aroused even with painful stimuli, although simple reflexes may be intact. For example, pinching the foot will produce a flexor reflex but will not cause arousal. Coma indicates complete disconnection of the reticular formation and the cerebral cortex. The most common cause in small animals is acute head injury with hemorrhage in the pons and the midbrain.[8] Animals that are unable to stand because of spinal cord dysfunction are alert.

Behavioral disorders are often functional, that is, related to environment and training. Primary brain disease, however, also can cause alterations in behavior. It is indicative of a cerebral or diencephalic lesion.

Posture

Technique. Abnormalities in posture may be noticed while the history is being recorded and the animal is free to move about. Further observations may necessitate moving the animal to different positions so that its ability to regain normal posture can be evaluated.

Anatomy and Physiology. Normal posture is maintained by coordinated motor responses to sensory inputs from receptors in the limbs and body, vision, and the vestibular system to the CNS. Vestibular receptors sense alterations in the position of the animal's head in relation to gravity, and detect motion. Sensory information is processed through the brain stem, cerebellum, and cerebrum. The cerebellum and vestibular system are especially important. The integrated output through motor pathways to the muscles of the neck, trunk, and limbs maintains normal posture. All domestic animals can maintain an erect posture shortly after birth; however, they vary in their ability to stand and walk.

Assessment

HEAD The most frequent abnormality in the posture of the head is a tilt or a twist to one side (Fig. 1–5). Intermittent head tilt, especially if associated with rubbing of the ear, may be due to otitis externa or ear mites. A continuous head tilt with resistance to straightening of the head by the examiner is almost always a manifestation of an abnormality in the vestibular

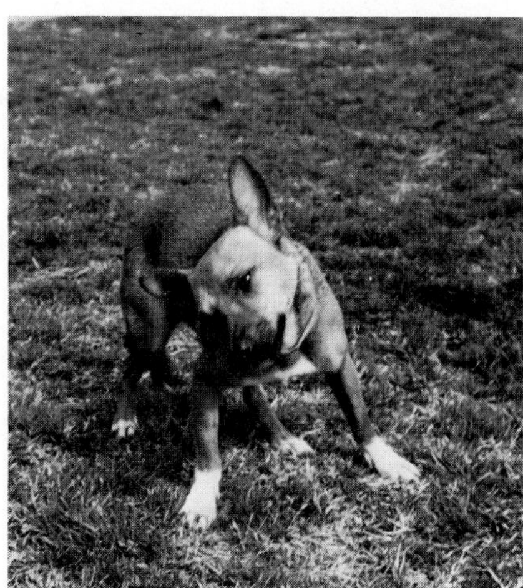

Figure 1–5 A dog with a head tilt and a broad-based stance, typical of vestibular disease.

system (see Chap. 11). Signs may range from tilting of the head (roll) or twisting of the head and neck (yaw) to twisting and rolling of the head, neck, and body. A yaw may indicate brain stem or cerebral disease; a roll is usually vestibular in origin. Both must be differentiated from spasms of cervical muscles from spinal cord or nerve root disease.

The head and neck may be held in a fixed position when there is cervical pain. Dogs with caudal cervical pain and weakness of the thoracic limb often arch their back and put their nose to the ground, apparently in an effort to keep weight off the thoracic limbs.

TRUNK Abnormal posture of the trunk may be associated with congenital or acquired lesions of the vertebrae or abnormal muscle tone from brain or spinal cord lesions. Deviations in spinal contour consist of (1) *scoliosis*—lateral deviation, (2) *lordosis*—ventral deviation (swayback), and (3) *kyphosis*—dorsal deviation.

LIMBS Abnormal posture of the limbs includes improper positioning and increased or decreased extensor tone. A *wide-based stance* is common to all forms of ataxia, including cerebellar and vestibular ataxia and abnormal conscious proprioception (see Chap. 9). It may also be seen in cases of generalized weakness. Proprioceptive deficits or lower motor neuron (LMN) or upper motor neuron (UMN) lesions may cause the animal to stand with a foot knuckled over (see Chap. 2). Uneven distribution of weight on the limbs may provide a clue to weakness or pain. Animals will try to carry most of their weight on the thoracic limbs when the pelvic limbs are weak or painful, and most of their weight on the pelvic limbs when the thoracic limbs are affected.

Decreased tone in limb muscles is often associated with LMN lesions and will cause abnormal posture. The limbs will be positioned passively, often with the toes knuckled.

Decerebrate rigidity is characterized by extension of all four limbs and the trunk. It is caused by a lesion in the rostral brain stem (midbrain or pons). Opisthotonos may be associated with decerebrate rigidity if the rostral lobes of the cerebellum are damaged. Opisthotonos is dorsiflexion of the head and the neck.

Decerebellate rigidity is similar, but the pelvic limbs are usually flexed. It is seen only in association with an acute lesion of the cerebellum.

Increased tone in the extensor muscles is a sign of UMN disease (see Chap. 4). Partial lesions may produce an exaggerated straightness in the stifle and hock joints. Decerebrate rigidity is an extreme form of increased extensor tone. Increased tone in the forelimbs with flaccid paralysis of the hind limbs is called the Schiff-Sherrington phenomenon and is associated with spinal cord lesions between T2 and L4. Increased tone in both extensors and flexors is seen in tetanus and strychnine poisoning.

Movement

The animal should be observed for abnormal movements while resting and at gait. Careful observation is important as movement may be the most significant part of the neurologic examination, especially in large animals, where postural reaction testing is more difficult.

Gait

Technique. The gait should be observed with the animal on a surface that offers adequate traction (carpet, synthetic turf, grass). Gaits vary among species and breeds, and the examiner must be knowledgeable of these differences. Some breeds of dogs have been selectively developed for characteristic gaits. Because of this breeding, neurologic diseases may have been genetically selected. The gait should be observed from the side and while the animal is moving toward and away from the examiner. Each limb should be evaluated while the animal is walking and trotting. The animal should be turned in wide and tight circles and should be backed up. Large animals are walked up and down a slope and with the head and neck extended.[9] The examiner may exaggerate minimal abnormalities in gait by blindfolding the animal.

Anatomy and Physiology. The neural organization of gait and posture is complex, involving all levels of the nervous system. Limbs are maintained in extension for supporting weight by spinal cord reflexes. Stepping movements also are programmed at the spinal level (Fig. 1–6). Organization of the stepping movement for locomotion occurs at the brain stem level in the reticular formation. Cerebellar regulation of this system makes locomotion smooth and coordinated. Vestibular input maintains balance. Cerebral cortical input to the system is necessary for voluntary control and fine coordination, especially of learned movements.[10–12]

An animal with a cerebral cortex lesion will be able to walk but will not have the precision of movement of a healthy animal. Postural reactions will be grossly abnormal. Severe rostral brain stem lesions (of the midbrain and the pons) cause decerebrate rigidity, because the voluntary motor pathways that inhibit extensor muscle activity are lost. The substrate for loco-

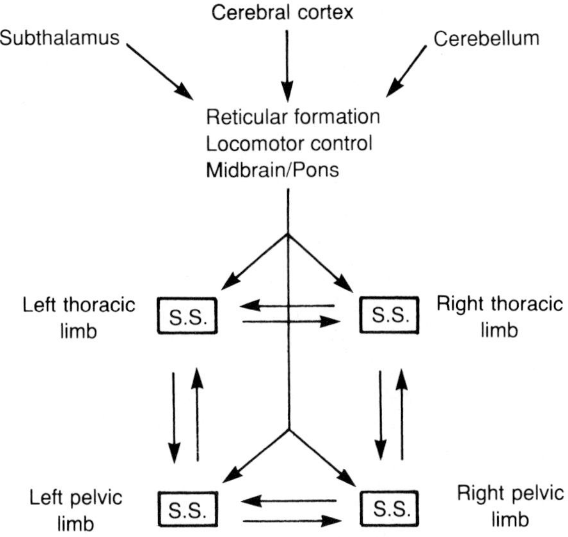

Figure 1–6 Schematic diagram of automatic control of locomotion. Spinal stepping reflexes are controlled by the brain stem centers for locomotion. Voluntary control is imposed from the cerebral cortex. The cerebellum and other areas coordinate the movements.

motion is still present and may be seen in animals with chronic lesions, but it is usually masked by the increased extensor tone. Lesions in the pons or the medulla will abolish integrated locomotion. Acute lesions of the cerebellum produce rigidity, whereas chronic lesions produce ataxia and an uncoordinated gait.

Assessment. Abnormalities of gait may include proprioceptive deficits, paresis, circling, ataxia, and dysmetria.

Proprioception, or position sense, is the ability to recognize the location of the limbs in relation to the rest of the body. A deficit appears as a misplacement or a knuckling of the foot that may not occur with every step. The proprioceptive pathways in the spinal cord are in the dorsal and dorsolateral columns and project to both the cerebellum (unconscious) and the cerebral cortex (conscious) (see the section on sensation in this chapter).

Paresis is a deficit of voluntary movements. Affected limbs will have inadequate or absent voluntary motion, which may be described as *monoparesis*—paresis of one limb; *paraparesis*—paresis of both pelvic limbs; *tetraparesis* or *quadriparesis*—paresis of all four limbs; or *hemiparesis*—paresis of the thoracic and the pelvic limb on the same side.

The suffix *plegia* may be used to denote complete loss of voluntary movements and is used by some authors to indicate both motor and sensory loss. In this text, *paresis* indicates partial deficit of motor function, whereas *paralysis* (*-plegia*) indicates a complete loss of voluntary movements. In general, the only difference in the two is the severity of the lesion; the localization is the same.

Paresis is caused by disruption of the voluntary motor pathways, which extend from the cerebral cortex through the brain stem to the lateral columns of the spinal cord. They continue to synapse on the LMN in each spinal cord segment that innervates the muscles. Paresis may be of the UMN or the LMN type (see Chaps. 2 and 6–8).

A neurologic disease may cause an animal to *circle*. Circling may vary from a tendency to drift in wide circles to forced spinning in a tight circle. Circling usually is not a localizing sign, except that tight circles usually are caused by caudal brain stem lesions. The direction of the circling is usually toward the side of the lesion, but there are exceptions, especially in lesions rostral to the midbrain. Twisting or head tilt associated with circling usually indicates involvement of the vestibular system (see Chaps. 2 and 9).

Ataxia is lack of coordination without spasticity, paresis, or involuntary movements, although each of these conditions may be seen in association with ataxia. Truncal ataxia is characterized by poorly controlled swaying of the body. The movement of the limbs is uncoordinated. The feet may be crossed or placed too far apart. Ataxia can be exaggerated by elevating the head or walking the animal on a slope. Ataxia may be caused by lesions of the cerebellum, the vestibular system, or the proprioceptive pathways (see Chap. 9).

Dysmetria is characterized by movements that are too long (hypermetria) or too short (hypometria). "Goose-stepping" is the most common sign of dysmetria. The stride may be abruptly stopped, forcing the animal to lurch from side to side. Dysmetria of the head and the neck may be most apparent when the animal tries to drink or eat and overshoots or undershoots the target. Dysmetria usually is caused by cerebellar or cerebellar pathway lesions and may be associated with ataxia and intention tremors (see Chap. 9).

Involuntary Abnormal Movement

Technique. Abnormal movements may occur while the animal is at rest or when it is moving, and may be intermittent or continuous. The most frequently recognized movement disorders are tremors and myoclonus.

Assessment. A *tremor* is produced by alternating contractions of opposing groups of muscles. The oscillatory movements are small and rapid. Tremors from neurologic causes must be differentiated from those induced by fatigue, fear, chilling, drug reactions, or primary muscle disease (see Chap. 11).

An *intention tremor* is one that is more pronounced when movements are initiated. It is an important sign of cerebellar disease. A *continuous tremor* usually is associated with an abnormality of the motor system.

Myoclonus is a coarse jerking of muscle groups. Myoclonus associated with canine distemper encephalomyelitis is usually a rhythmic jerking of one muscle group, such as the flexors of the elbow or the temporal muscle. The myoclonus of distemper has been called chorea; however, chorea more accurately describes irregular, purposeless movements that are brief and that often vary from one part of the body to the other. Two forms of myoclonus may be seen in the dog. In acute encephalitis, the lesion is probably related to destruction of areas in the basal nuclei. The more common chronic form is related to the interneurons or the LMN at the segmental level.[13] *Cataplexy* is a sudden, complete loss of muscle tone that causes the animal to fall limp. It is usually seen in association with narcolepsy (see Chap. 14). *Athetosis* is a "pill-rolling" movement of the hands in people with Parkinson's disease. A similar movement disorder has been produced in cats with lesions of the basal nuclei, but has not been described in clinical patients.

Palpation

Technique. After the mental status, posture, and gait of the animal have been assessed, the physical examination is initiated. Careful inspection and palpation of the musculoskeletal systems and of the integument may be performed at one time or on a regional basis in conjunction with other parts of the examination. Comparison of one side with the other for symmetry is best done as one step in the examination.[14]

Assessment

INTEGUMENT Although the skin is not often involved in neurologic disease, careful inspection may reveal clues to the diagnosis. Scars may indicate previous trauma. Worn nails may be associated with paresis or with proprioceptive deficits. Coat and eye color may be related to a hereditary abnormality. For example, blue eyes and a white coat is associated with deafness in cats. A myelomeningocele may be palpated as it attaches to the skin in the lumbosacral region. The temperature of the extremities may be significantly lowered with arterial occlusion. Dermatomyositis is an inflammatory disease of the skin and muscle of collie and Shetland sheepdogs. There are cutaneous lesions of the face, lips, ears, and over bony prominences.

SKELETON Careful palpation of the skeletal system may reveal *masses, deviation of normal contour, abnormal motion,* or *crepitation.* Tumors involving the skull or the spinal column may be palpable as a mass. The spinous processes of the vertebrae should be palpated for irregularities of contour. Deviations may indicate a luxation, a fracture, or a congenital anomaly. Depressed or elevated skull fractures often can be palpated, especially in animals with minimal temporal muscle mass. Open fontanelles and suture lines in the skull may indicate hydrocephalus. Abnormal motion or crepitation may be detected in fractures and luxations. When spinal luxations or fractures are suspected, manipulation should not be attempted, because additional displacement may cause serious spinal cord damage. Peripheral nerve injuries may be associated with fractures of the long bones.

MUSCLES Muscles are evaluated for *size, tone,* and *strength.* All of the muscles should be systematically palpated, starting with the head, extending down the neck and the trunk, and continuing down each limb.

Changes in muscle size may be apparent from observation as well as from palpation. Loss of muscle mass (atrophy) is the most frequent finding. Atrophy may indicate LMN disease or disuse. Criteria for differentiating the two are presented in Chapter 2. Localized muscle atrophy, which usually accompanies LMN disease, is an important localizing sign.

Muscle tonus is maintained through the spinal stretch (myotatic) reflex. Alterations in tone, either increased or decreased, can be detected by palpation and passive manipulation of the limb. Increased tone of the extensor muscles, a common finding in UMN disease, manifests as an increased resistance to passive flexion of the limb (see Chap. 2 for an interpretation).

Muscle strength is difficult to evaluate even in the most cooperative patients. The extensor muscles can be evaluated during postural reactions, such as hopping, in which the animal must support all of its weight on one limb (see the section on hopping in this chapter). The flexor muscles can be evaluated by comparing the relative strength of pull during a flexor reflex (see the section on the flexor reflex in this chapter). Loss of muscle strength is usually a sign of LMN disease.

Postural Reactions

The complex responses that maintain an animal's normal, upright position are known as postural reactions. If an animal's weight is shifted from one side to the other, from front to rear, or from rear to front, the increased load on the supporting limb or limbs requires increased tone in the extensor muscles to keep the limb from collapsing. Part of the alteration in tone is accomplished through spinal reflexes, but in order for the changes to be smooth and coordinated, the sensory and motor systems of the brain must be involved.

Abnormalities of complex reactions, such as the hopping reaction, do not provide precise localizing information, because lesions in any one of several areas of the nervous system may affect the reaction. The assessment of postural reactions, however, is an important part of the neurologic examination. Minimal deficits in the function of a key component, such as the cerebral cortex, may cause significant alterations in postural reactions that are not detected when one observes the gait.

The following postural reactions are listed in a sequence found to be convenient for performing an examination. In an initial screening examination, the reactions marked with an asterisk in Table 1–5 should be tested. If they are normal, it is unlikely that abnormalities will be found in the other reactions.

Proprioceptive Positioning Reaction

Technique. Proprioception is the ability of the animal to recognize the location of its limbs without visual information. Although proprioception is a sensory function, the tests described in this section require motor reactions, so it has been included as a postural reaction.[15]

The simplest method of evaluation entails flexing the foot so that the dorsal surface is on the floor (Fig. 1–7). The animal should immediately return the foot to a normal position. Most animals will not allow weight bearing to occur in the abnormal position. Another method is to place the foot on a sheet of cardboard and slowly slide the cardboard laterally. As the limb reaches an abnormal position, the animal should reposition it for normal weight bearing. The first test is the most sensitive for proprioception in the distal extremity, whereas the second test is more likely to detect abnormalities in the proximal portion of the limb. In either method, the examiner should test each foot separately.

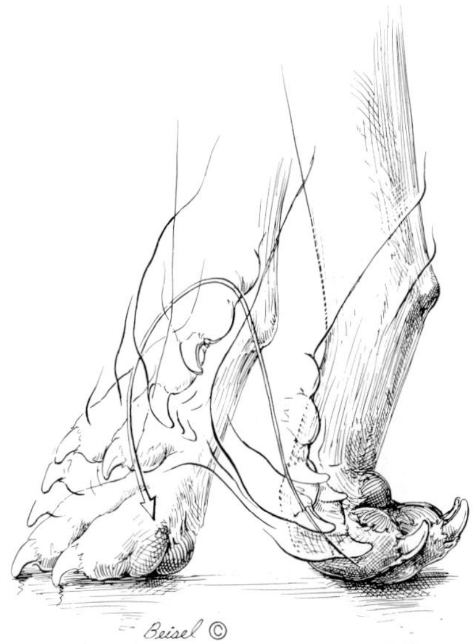

Figure 1–7 Proprioceptive positioning response. Conscious proprioceptive function is tested by placing the dorsal surface of the animal's foot on the floor. The animal should immediately replace it to the normal position. (From Green CE, Oliver JE: Neurologic examination. In Ettinger SJ (ed): Textbook of Veterinary Internal Medicine, 2nd ed. Philadelphia, WB Saunders Co., 1982. Used by permission.)

Anatomy and Physiology. Proprioceptive information is carried in the dorsal columns and the spinomedullothalamic tract in the dorsolateral fasciculus of the spinal cord, through the brain stem, to the sensorimotor cortex (Fig. 1–8). The motor response is initiated by the cerebral cortex and is transmitted to the LMN in the spinal cord (see the section on sensation in this chapter).

Assessment. Because the proprioceptive pathways are very sensitive to compression, abnormalities in proprioceptive positioning may occur before motor dysfunction can be detected (see Chap. 2). The response will be abnormal if there is significant paresis, but other postural reactions, such as hopping, are also affected. Proprioceptive positioning is less useful in large animals because many will not respond. Observation of abnormal postioning of the limbs at rest may be interpreted similarly.[9]

Wheelbarrowing Reaction

Technique. The animal is supported under the abdomen with all of the weight on the thoracic limbs (Fig. 1–9). The normal animal can walk forward and sideways with coordinated movements of both thoracic limbs. The examiner should not lift the pelvic limbs so high that the animal's posture is grossly abnormal. If

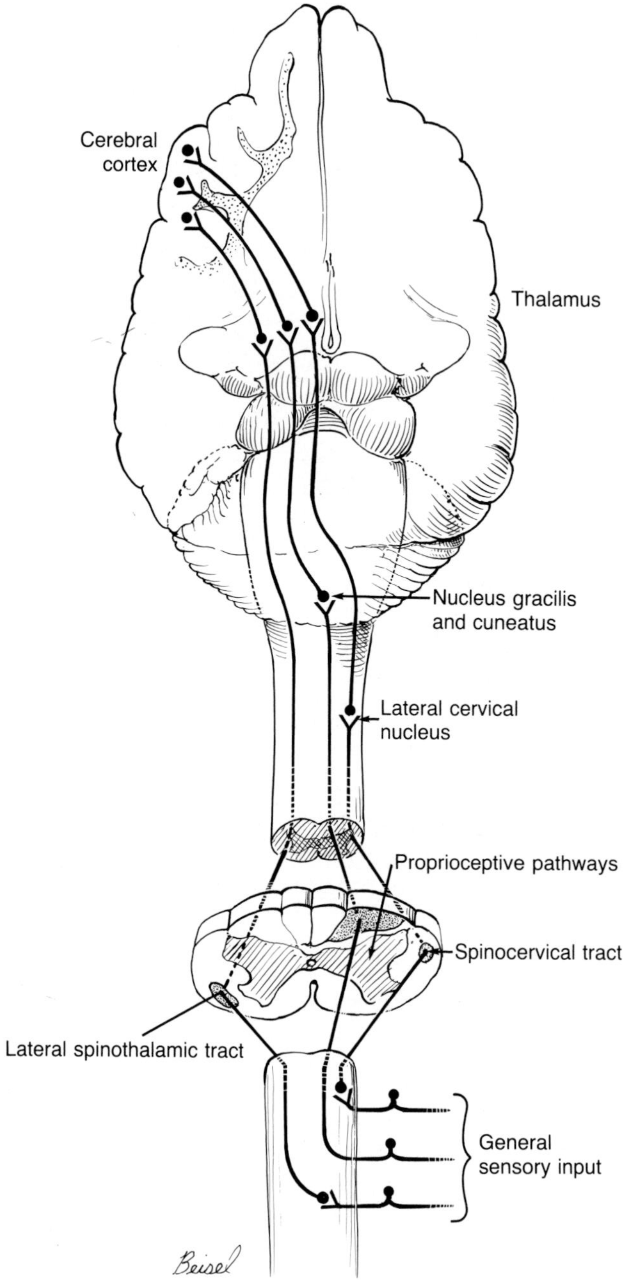

Figure 1–8 Somatic sensory innervation is transmitted to the brain through several pathways. Proprioception is a function of the spinomedullothalamic pathway (near the spinocervical tract) for the pelvic limbs and of the fasciculus cuneatus of the dorsal columns for the thoracic limbs. Pain is transmitted by several tracts (see also Fig. 1–33), including the spinothalamic, spinocervical, and spinoreticular tracts and the dorsal columns.

movements appear normal, the maneuver is repeated with the head lifted and the neck extended. This position prevents visual compensation, making the animal mostly dependent on proprioceptive information. A tonic neck reaction, which causes slightly increased extensor tone in the forelimbs, is also elicited. When the neck is extended, subtle abnormalities of the thoracic limbs may be seen in animals that otherwise appear normal.

Assessment. Weakness in the thoracic limbs may be detected when the wheelbarrowing reaction is tested, because the animal is forced to carry most of its weight on two limbs while standing on only one limb while moving.

Slow initiation of movement may be a sign of proprioceptive deficit or of paresis that is caused by a lesion of the cervical spinal cord, the brain stem, or the cerebral cortex. Exaggerated movements (dysmetria) may indicate an abnormality of the cervical spinal cord, the lower brain stem, or the cerebellum.

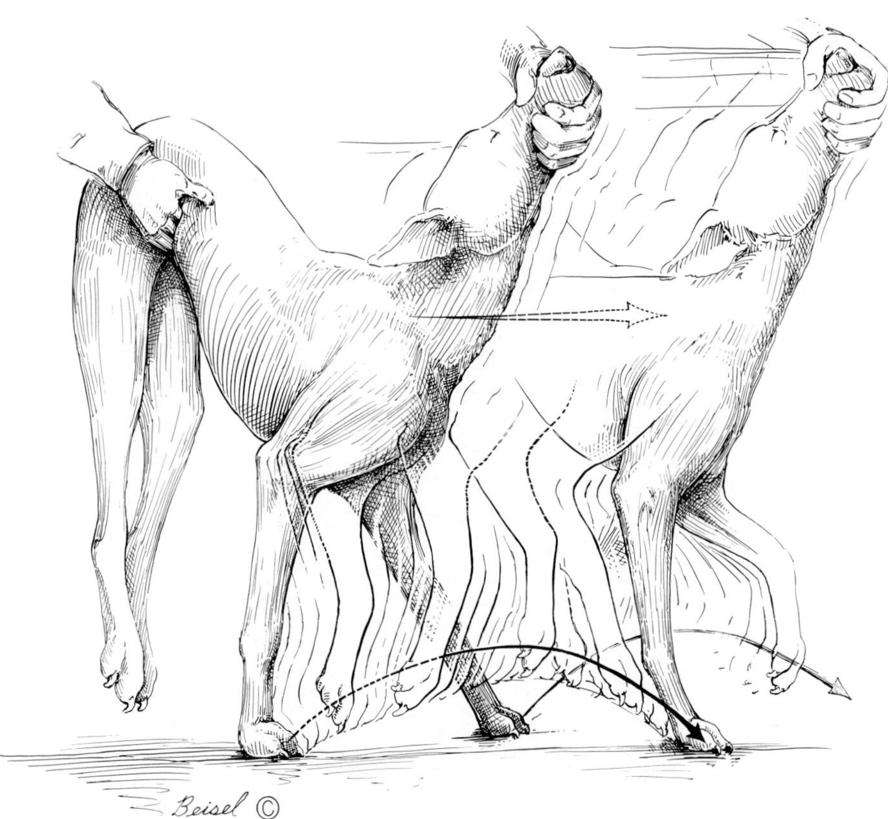

Figure 1–9 Wheelbarrowing with the neck extended. Wheelbarrowing is performed with the pelvic limbs elevated. The body should be in a position as close to normal as possible. The head may be elevated to accentuate abnormalities, as illustrated here. (From Greene CE, Oliver JE: Neurologic examination. In Ettinger SJ (ed): Textbook of Veterinary Internal Medicine, 2nd ed. Philadelphia, WB Saunders Co., 1982. Used by permission.)

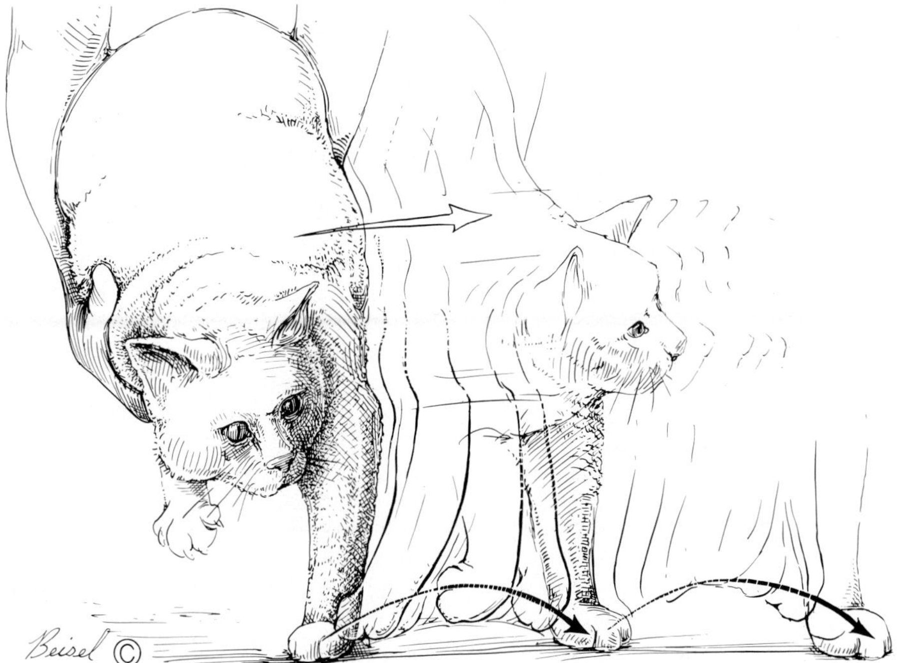

Figure 1–10 The hopping reaction. The normal animal responds to hopping by quickly replacing the limb under the body as it moves laterally. Large animals can be tested by picking up one limb and pushing the body laterally. (From Greene CE, Oliver JE: Neurologic examination. In Ettinger SJ (ed): Textbook of Veterinary Internal Medicine, 2nd ed. Philadelphia, WB Saunders Co., 1982. Used by permission.)

Hopping Reaction

Technique. The hopping reaction of the thoracic limbs is tested with the animal in the position for wheelbarrowing, with one thoracic limb lifted from the ground (Fig. 1–10). The entire weight of the animal is supported on one limb, and the patient is moved forward, laterally, and medially. Medial hopping is much more difficult, and more subtle abnormalities may be detected with this maneuver. Hopping of the pelvic limbs is assessed similarly, following the extensor postural thrust reaction. Large animals, such as giant-breed dogs, horses, and cows can be tested by lifting one limb and shifting the weight of the animal so that it hops on the opposite limb. Alternatively, the animal can be pulled by the tail or pushed laterally to elicit movements similar to the hopping reaction.

Assessment. The hopping reaction is more sensitive than the wheelbarrowing reaction for detecting minor deficits. Poor initiation of the hopping reaction suggests sensory (proprioceptive) deficits, whereas poor follow-through suggests a motor system abnormality (paresis). Asymmetry is easily seen and helps to lateralize lesions.

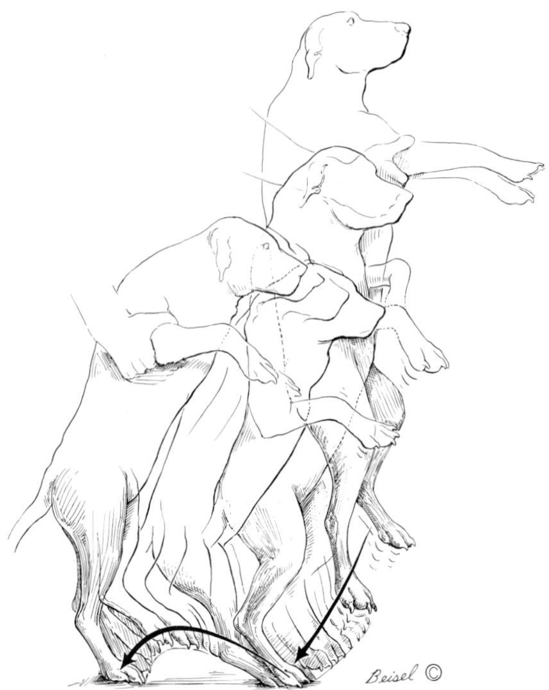

Figure 1–11 The extensor postural thrust reaction. The animal responds by stepping backward when its feet make contact with the floor. (From Greene CE, Oliver JE: Neurologic Examination. In Ettinger SJ (ed): Textbook of Veterinary Internal Medicine, 2nd ed. Philadelphia, WB Saunders Co., 1982. Used by permission.)

Extensor Postural Thrust Reaction

Technique. The extensor postural thrust is elicited by supporting the animal by the thorax caudal to the thoracic limb and lowering the pelvic limbs to the floor (Fig. 1–11). When the limbs touch the floor, they should move caudally in a symmetric walking movement in order for a position of support to be achieved. As the animal is lowered to the floor, it will extend the limbs, anticipating contact. This is a vestibular reaction and may be lacking or uncoordinated with lesions of the vestibular system.

Assessment. Asymmetric weakness, lack of coordination, and dysmetria can be seen in the extensor postural thrust reaction as in the wheelbarrowing reaction.

Hemistanding and Hemiwalking Reactions

Technique. The front and rear limbs on one side are lifted from the ground so that all of the animal's weight is supported by the opposite limbs. Forward and lateral walking movements are then evaluated.

Assessment. Abnormal signs may be seen in hemistanding and hemiwalking as in the other postural reactions. They are most useful in animals with cerebral cortex lesions. These animals have relatively normal gaits but have deficits of postural reactions in both the front and the rear limbs contralateral to the side of the lesion.

Placing Reaction

Technique. Placing is evaluated first without vision (tactile placing) and then with vision (visual placing). The examiner supports the animal under the thorax and covers its eyes with one hand or with a blindfold. The thoracic limbs are brought in contact with the edge of a table at or below the carpus (Fig. 1–12). The normal response is immediate placement of the feet on the table surface in a position that will support weight. Care must be taken not to restrict the movement of either limb. When one limb is consistently slower to respond, the animal should be held in the examiner's other hand to ensure that its movements are not being restricted.

Visual placing is tested by allowing the animal to see the table surface. Normal animals reach for the surface before the carpus touches the table. Peripheral visual fields can be tested by making a lateral approach to the table. The

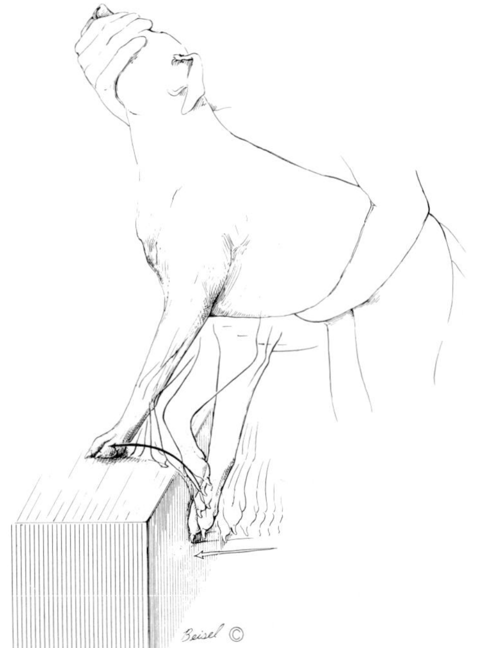

Figure 1–12 The tactile placing reaction is elicited with the animal's eyes covered. When the carpus makes contact with the edge of the surface, the animal should immediately place its foot on the surface. Similar responses can be elicited from large animals by leading them over a curb or up steps. (From Greene CE, Oliver JE: Neurologic examination. In Ettinger SJ (ed): Textbook of Veterinary Internal Medicine, 2nd ed. Philadelphia, WB Saunders Co., 1982. Used by permission.)

veterinarian can evaluate giant-breed dogs and large animals such as horses and cows by leading them over a curb or a step, with and without vision. Some dogs and cats that are accustomed to being held may ignore the table. These animals usually will respond if they are held in a less secure or less comfortable position away from the body of the examiner.

Anatomy and Physiology. Tactile placing requires touch receptors in the skin, sensory pathways through the spinal cord and the brain stem to the cerebral cortex, and motor pathways from the cerebral cortex to the LMN of the forelimbs. Visual placing requires normal visual pathways to the cerebral cortex, communication from the visual cortex to the motor cortex, and motor pathways to the LMN of the forelimbs.[16]

Assessment. A lesion of any portion of the pathway may cause a deficit in the placing reaction. Normal tactile placing with absent visual placing indicates a lesion of the visual pathways. Normal visual placing with abnormal tactile placing suggests a sensory pathway lesion. Cortical lesions will produce a deficit in the contralateral limb. Lesions below the midbrain usually will produce ipsilateral deficits.

Tonic Neck Reaction

Technique. With the animal in a normal standing position, the head is elevated and the neck is extended. The normal reaction is a slight extension of the thoracic limb and a slight flexion of the pelvic limbs. Lowering the head causes the thoracic limbs to flex and the pelvic limbs to extend. Turning the head to the side causes a slight extension of the ipsilateral thoracic limb and a slight flexion of the contralateral thoracic limb. It is easy to remember the normal reactions if one considers the usual movements of an animal. For example, a cat about to jump onto a table extends the head and the neck, extends the front limbs, and flexes the rear limbs. A dog crawling under a bed lowers the head and the neck and flexes the front limbs as it extends the rear limbs for propulsion. A horse making a sharp turn leads with the head and the neck, plants the ipsilateral limb in extension, and flexes the contralateral limb to take a step.[17]

Tonic eye reactions also may be observed. They will be discussed with CN III, CN IV, and CN VI in the section on cranial nerves.

Assessment. The tonic neck reactions are initiated by receptors in the cranial cervical area and are mediated by brain stem reactions. The responses are subtle in normal animals and often are inhibited volitionally through cortical control.

Abnormalities in sensory (proprioception) or motor systems may produce abnormal reactions. Lesions in the cerebellum cause exaggerated tonic neck reactions.

Spinal Reflexes

Examination of the spinal reflexes tests the integrity of the sensory and motor components of the reflex arc and the influence of descending motor pathways on the reflex. Three kinds of responses may be seen. *Absence* or *depression* of a reflex indicates complete or partial loss of either sensory or motor (LMN) components of the reflex. A *normal response* indicates that both sensory and motor components are intact. An *exaggerated response* indicates an abnormality in the motor pathways (UMN) that normally have an inhibitory influence on the reflex, or a deficit of the opposing muscles, if paresis is also present.

The examination should be performed with the animal in lateral recumbency. Muscle tone, previously evaluated with the animal in a standing position, should be tested again at this time. The pelvic limbs are evaluated first. Passive manipulation of the limb assesses the degree of muscle tone, especially in the extensor muscles. Spreading the toes with slight pressure on the foot pads will elicit the extensor thrust reflex. The myotatic (stretch) reflexes then are evaluated. Routinely, only the knee jerk (quadriceps) reflex is tested. The cranial tibial and gastrocnemius muscles can also be evaluated, but these reflexes are more difficult to elicit and quantify. Next, the flexor reflex is tested by gently pinching the toes. To maintain the cooperation of the patient, the examiner should apply the mildest stimulus that will elicit a response. If flexion is induced by touching the foot, there is no need to crush the toe with a hemostat! The perineal reflex is a contraction of the anal sphincter in response to a touch, a pinprick, or a pinch in the perineal area. There may be flexion of the tail simultaneously.

The most predictable myotatic reflex in the thoracic limb is elicited when the extensor carpi radialis muscle (tendons over the carpus in large animals) is struck, producing a slight extension of the carpus. The triceps and biceps reflexes are difficult to elicit and evaluate in many normal animals.

After examining the limbs on one side, the veterinarian turns the animal and examines the opposite limbs.

Myotatic (Stretch) Reflexes

Quadriceps (Knee Jerk, Patellar) Reflex

Technique. With the animal in lateral recumbency, the leg is supported under the femur with the left hand (by a right-handed examiner), and the stifle is flexed slightly (Fig. 1–13). The patellar ligament is struck crisply with the plexor. The response is a single, quick extension of the stifle.[18] The plexor is recommended for performing myotatic reflex testing, but other instruments, such as bandage scissors, may be used. Nose tongs or similar heavy instruments are useful for testing large animals. The examiner should use the same type of instruments in each examination to obtain consistent results.

Anatomy and Physiology. The myotatic or stretch reflexes are basic to the regulation of posture and movement. The reflex arc is a simple, two-neuron (monosynaptic) pathway. The

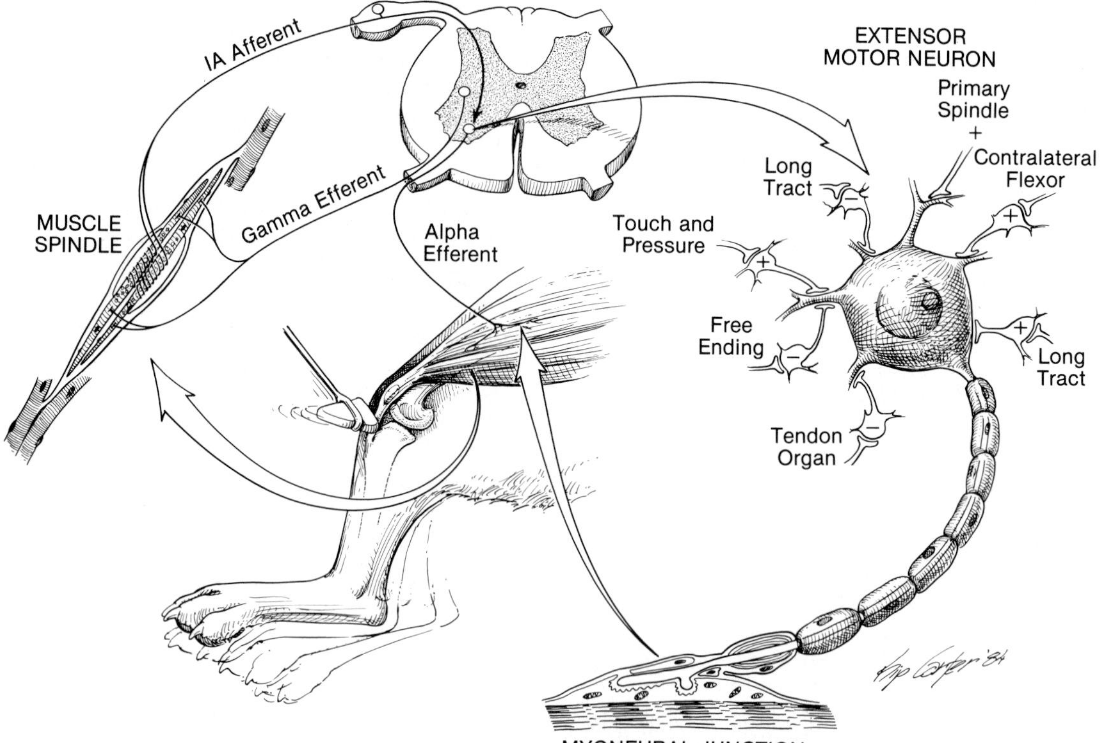

Figure 1–13 Myotactic (stretch) reflex. Percussion of the tendon or muscle stretches the muscle spindle. IA afferent fibers are activated and synapse directly on motor neurons of the muscle. The motor neuron discharges when a threshold level of excitation is reached. The level of excitation of the motor neuron is related to synapses from a variety of sources, as illustrated. The impulse travels down the axon (alpha efferent) to the neuromuscular junction, causing a release of acetylcholine. Acetylcholine binds to receptors on the muscle, causing depolarization and contraction of the muscle. Gamma motor neurons maintain tension on the muscle spindle regardless of the state of contraction of the muscle. (From Oliver JE, Hoerlein BF, Mayhew IG: Veterinary Neurology. Philadelphia, WB Saunders Co., 1987. Used by permission.)

sensory neuron has a receptor in the muscle spindle and its cell body in the dorsal root ganglion. The motor neurons have their cell bodies in the ventral horn of the gray matter of the spinal cord. The axons form the motor components of peripheral nerves that end on the muscle (the neuromuscular junction) (see Fig. 1–13).

The muscle spindle is the stretch receptor of the muscle. The spindle has three to five striated muscle fibers (intrafusal muscle) at each end, with a nonstriated portion in the middle (see Fig. 1–13). The spindles are located in the belly of the skeletal muscle (extrafusal muscle). These sensory fibers are large and have a spiral ending, called the primary ending, around the nonstriated portion of each fiber. Small sensory fibers have secondary endings. Primary endings are of greatest importance in phasic responses (e.g., knee jerk), whereas secondary endings respond primarily to tonic activation (e.g., extensor thrust). The small intrafusal muscle fibers of the spindle are innervated by small (gamma) motor neurons.

Stretching a muscle depolarizes the nerve endings of the spindle, producing a burst of impulses in the sensory fibers. The sensory fibers monosynaptically activate the large (alpha) motor neuron in the spinal cord. The alpha motor neuron discharges impulses through its axon, causing a contraction of the extrafusal muscle fibers of the same muscle. Thus, a sudden stretch of the muscle causes a reflex muscle contraction, as seen in the knee jerk reflex. A more tonic stretch of the muscle causes a slower discharge of sensory activity and a slower, more steady muscle contraction.

Contraction of the extrafusal muscle fibers causes relaxation of the intrafusal fibers, because they are parallel. Loss of tension on the intrafusal fibers stops the sensory input from the spindle. To prevent this situation from occurring, gamma motor fibers adjust the length of the intrafusal fibers. Thus, tension is maintained on the spindle through the range of motion of the limb.

Gamma motor neuron activation of the intrafusal fibers also can stretch the primary spindle endings directly and thus can elicit a response indirectly in the alpha motor neuron. Alpha and gamma motor neurons are facilitated or inhibited by a variety of segmental and long spinal pathways. The output of the motor neurons is a summation of their facilitatory and inhibitory inputs. For example, the quadriceps motor neuron responds to a sudden stretch by a quick contraction (knee jerk) but can be blocked by voluntary inhibition (see Fig. 1–13).

The spindle sensory fibers also facilitate interneurons in the spinal cord, which in turn inhibit motor neurons of antagonistic muscles. This activity is called *reciprocal innervation*. For example, spindle sensory fibers from the quadriceps muscle inhibit antagonistic flexor motor neurons, allowing the limb to extend. Spindle sensory fibers also contribute collaterals to ascending pathways, which provide information to the brain regarding activity in the muscles.

Assessment. The quadriceps reflex is the most reliably interpreted myotatic reflex. The reflex should be recorded as absent (0), depressed (+1), normal (+2), exaggerated (+3), or exaggerated with clonus (+4). Normal responses vary widely among species and among breeds within a species. In large dogs, the response is less brisk than in small dogs. The examiner should become familiar with these natural variations.

Absence (0) of a myotatic reflex indicates a lesion of the sensory or motor component of the reflex arc—an LMN or segmental sign (see Chap. 2). Loss of the reflex in one muscle group suggests a peripheral nerve lesion, i.e., of the femoral nerve. Bilateral loss of the reflex suggests a segmental spinal cord lesion affecting the motor neurons to both limbs located in spinal cord segments L4–L6 in the dog. Differentiation between peripheral nerve and spinal cord lesions may require assessment of the sensory examination and the presence or absence of other neurologic signs.

Depression (+1) of the reflex has the same significance as absence of the reflex, except that the lesion is incomplete. Depression of the reflex is more common with spinal cord lesions in cases in which some, but not all, of the segments (L4–L6) are affected. Other reflexes also must be tested, because generalized depression of reflexes may be seen in polyneuropathies or in abnormalities of the neuromuscular junction (botulism, tick paralysis).

Exaggerated reflexes (+3,+4) and increased tone result from loss of descending inhibitory pathways. The voluntary motor pathways are facilitatory to flexor muscles and inhibitory to extensor muscles. Damage to these pathways will release the myotatic reflex, causing an exaggerated reflex and increased extensor tone. Clonus (+4) is a repetitive contraction and relaxation of the muscle in response to a single stimulus. Clonus often is seen with chronic (weeks to months) loss of descending inhibitory pathways. Clonus has the same localizing significance as exaggerated reflexes. Bilateral exaggerated reflexes most often are associated with damage to descending inhibitory pathways ros-

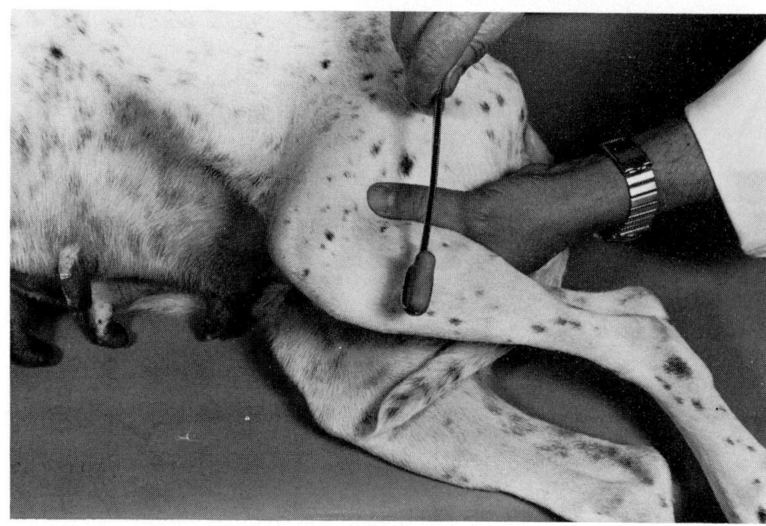

Figure 1–14 The cranial tibial reflex is elicited with the animal in lateral recumbency, with both stifle and hock slightly flexed. The cranial tibial muscle is percussed just below the stifle.

tral to the level of the reflex. UMN injury causing exaggerated myotatic reflexes should also cause paresis. If gait and postural reactions are normal, then the "exaggerated reflex" is likely to be examiner error or normal for the individual.

Cranial Tibial Reflex

Technique. With the animal in lateral recumbency, the examiner tests the cranial tibial reflex. The cranial tibial reflex usually is not tested unless the quadriceps reflex is abnormal or if a lesion of the sciatic nerve is suspected. The belly of the cranial tibial muscle is struck with the plexor just below the proximal end of the tibia (Fig. 1–14). The response is flexion of the hock.

Anatomy and Physiology. The cranial tibial muscle is a flexor of the hock and is innervated by the peroneal branch of the sciatic nerve (with origin in the L6–L7 segments of the spinal cord in the dog).

Assessment. For the inexperienced, the cranial tibial reflex is difficult to elicit in a normal animal. Absent or decreased reflexes should be interpreted with caution. Exaggerated reflexes indicate a lesion above the spinal cord segments that are responsible for the reflex (L6–L7).

Gastrocnemius Reflex

Technique. The gastrocnemius reflex is tested after the cranial tibial reflex. The tendon of the gastrocnemius muscle is struck with the plexor just above the tibial tarsal bone (Fig. 1–15). Slight flexion of the hock is necessary in order for some tension of the muscle to be

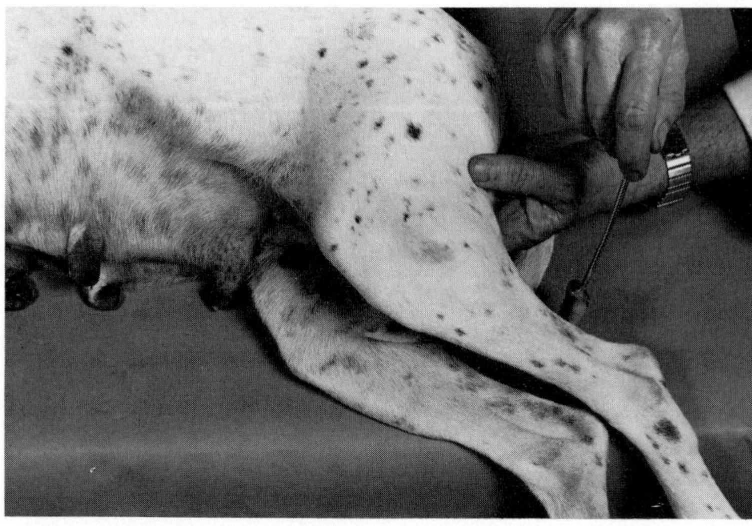

Figure 1–15 The gastrocnemius reflex is elicited with the animal in the same position as for testing of the cranial tibial reflex. The tendon of the gastrocnemius muscle is percussed proximal to the tarsus.

maintained. The response is extension of the hock.

Anatomy and Physiology. The gastrocnemius is primarily an extensor of the hock and is innervated by the tibial branch of the sciatic nerve (with origin in the L7–S1 segments of the spinal cord in the dog).

Assessment. The gastrocnemius reflex is interpreted in the same manner as the cranial tibial reflex, but is even less reliable.

Extensor Carpi Radialis Reflex

Technique. The animal is in lateral recumbency while the reflexes of the thoracic limb are evaluated. The limb is supported under the elbow, with flexion of the elbow and the carpus maintained. The extensor carpi radialis muscle is struck with the plexor just distal to the elbow (Fig. 1–16). The response is a slight extension of the carpus. The carpus must be flexed and the digits must not touch the floor or the other limb, or the reflex will be mechanically inhibited.[17] The extensor tendons crossing the carpal joint are struck in large animals.

Anatomy and Physiology. The extensor carpi radialis is an extensor of the carpus and is innervated by the radial nerve (with origin in the C7, C8, and T1 segments of the spinal cord in the dog).

Assessment. The extensor carpi radialis reflex is more difficult to elicit than the quadriceps reflex but usually can be recognized in dogs. Absent or decreased reflexes should be evaluated with caution. Strong reflexes are usually exaggerated (+3) and indicate a lesion above C7.

Triceps Reflex

Technique. The animal is held in the same position as for the extensor carpi radialis reflex. The triceps brachii muscle is struck with the plexor just proximal to the olecranon (Fig. 1–17). The response is a slight extension of the elbow. The elbow must be maintained in flexion in order for a response to be elicited.

Anatomy and Physiology. The triceps brachii muscle extends the elbow and is essential for weight bearing in the forelimb. Innervation is through the radial nerve (with the origin from spinal cord segments C7–T1 in the dog).

Assessment. The triceps reflex is difficult to elicit in the normal animal. Absent or decreased reflexes should not be interpreted as abnormal. Lesions of the radial nerve can be recognized by a loss of muscle tone and an inability to support weight. Exaggerated reflexes are interpreted in the same way as for the extensor carpi radialis reflex.

Biceps Reflex

Technique. The index or middle finger of the examiner's hand that is holding the animal's elbow is placed on the biceps and the brachialis tendons cranial and proximal to the elbow. The elbow is slightly extended, and the finger is struck with the plexor (Fig. 1–18). The response is a slight flexion of the elbow. Movement of the animal's elbow must not be blocked by the examiner's restraining hand.

Anatomy and Physiology. The biceps brachii and brachialis muscles are flexors of the elbow. They are innervated by the musculocutaneous

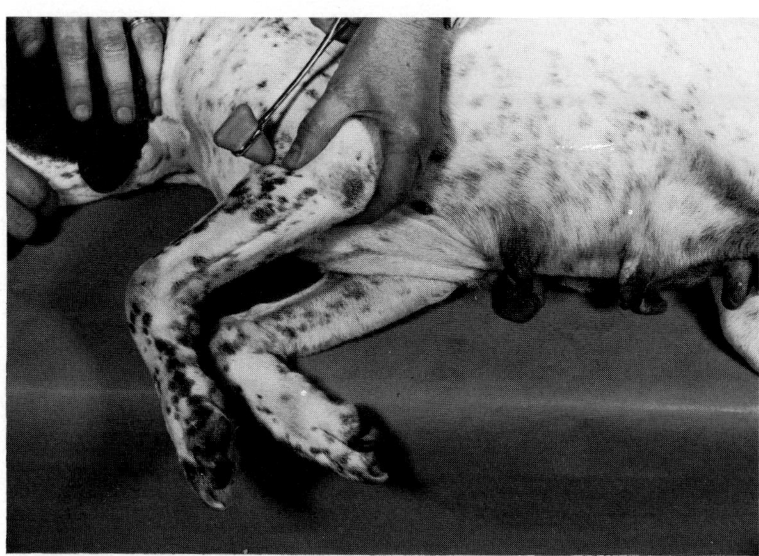

Figure 1–16 The extensor carpi radialis reflex is the most reliable myotactic reflex in the thoracic limb. With the animal in lateral recumbency and the elbow and carpus flexed, the extensor muscle group is percussed distal to the elbow. The digital extensor tendons can be percussed at the carpus in large animals.

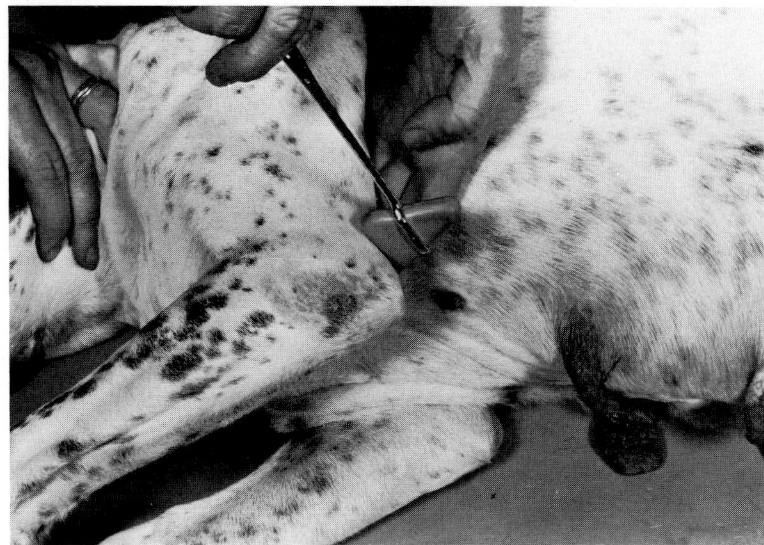

Figure 1–17 The triceps reflex is elicited with the animal in the same position as for the extensor carpi radialis reflex. The triceps tendon is percussed proximal to the elbow.

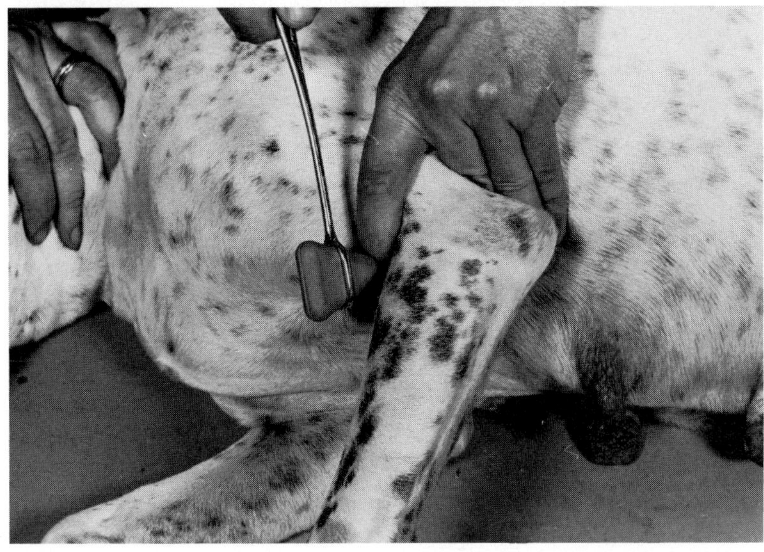

Figure 1–18 The biceps reflex is elicited with the elbow slightly extended. The examiner's finger is placed on the biceps tendon proximal to the elbow, and the finger is percussed.

nerve (which originates from spinal cord segments C6–C8 in the dog).

Assessment. The biceps reflex is difficult to elicit in the normal animal. Absent or decreased reflexes should not be interpreted as abnormal. Flexion of the elbow on the flexor reflex provides a better assessment of the musculocutaneous nerve. An exaggerated (+3) reflex is indicative of a lesion above C6.

Flexor (Pedal, Withdrawal) Reflexes

Pelvic Limb

Technique. The animal is maintained in lateral recumbency, the same position as that for examination of the myotatic reflexes. A noxious stimulus is applied to the foot. The normal response is a flexion of the entire limb, including the hip, the stifle, and the hock (Fig. 1–19). The least noxious stimulus possible should be used. If an animal flexes the limb when the digit is touched, there is no need to crush the digit. If a response is not easily elicited, a hemostat should be used to squeeze across a digit. Pressure should not be so great as to injure the skin. Both medial and lateral digits should be tested on each limb. The limb should be in a slightly extended position when the stimulus is applied in order to allow the limb to flex. The opposite limb also should be free to extend.[19]

Anatomy and Physiology. The flexor reflex is less stereotyped than the myotatic reflex. The response involves all of the flexor muscles of

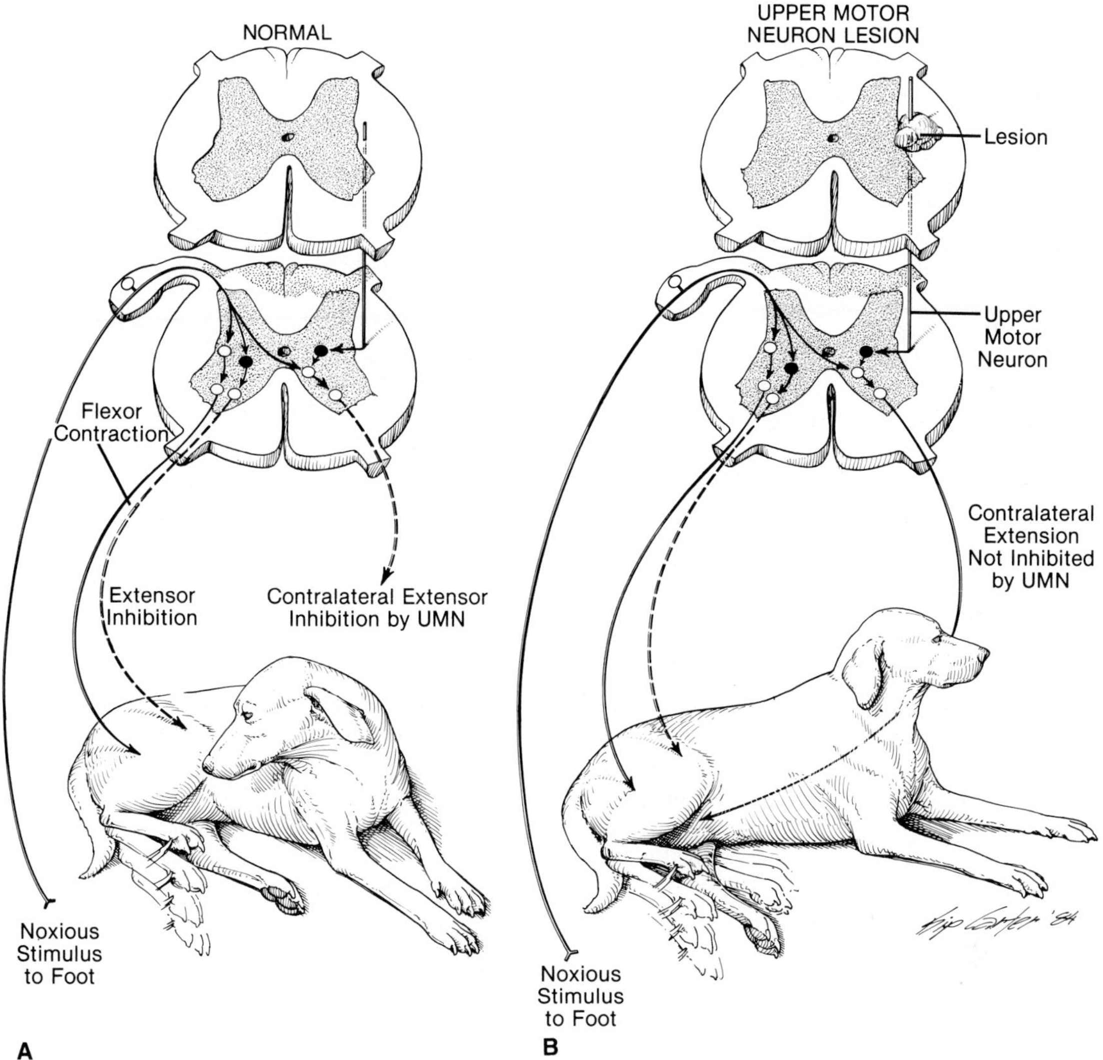

Figure 1–19 Flexor and crossed extension reflexes. *A*. The animal is positioned in lateral recumbency and a noxious stimulus is applied to a digit. The limb is immediately withdrawn. Sensory fibers enter the spinal cord through the dorsal root to synapse on interneurons. Flexor motor neurons are activated, causing flexion of the limb. Simultaneously, inhibitory interneurons cause relaxation of the antagonistic extensor muscles. Other interneurons cross the spinal cord to activate contralateral extensor muscles—the crossed extensor reflex. *B*. The crossed extensor reflex is inhibited unless there has been damage to UMN systems. Sensory fibers also project to the brain, causing a conscious awareness of pain and subsequently a behavioral reaction (*A*). The reflex is not dependent on a behavioral reaction. The behavioral reaction may be absent if sensory pathways are damaged. (From Oliver JE, Hoerlein BF, Mayhew IG: Veterinary Neurology. Philadelphia, WB Saunders Co., 1987. Used by permission.)

the limb and thus requires activation of motor neurons in several spinal cord segments (see Fig. 1–19).

The receptors for the flexor reflex are primarily free nerve endings in the skin and other tissues that respond to noxious stimuli such as pressure, heat, or cold. A stimulus that produces a sensory discharge in these nerves ascends to the spinal cord through the dorsal root. The sensory nerves from the digits of the pelvic limbs are primarily branches of the sciatic nerve, the superficial peroneal nerve on the dorsal surface, and the tibial nerve on the plantar surface. The sciatic nerve originates from spinal cord segments L6–S1. The medial digit is partially innervated by the saphenous nerve, a branch of the femoral nerve that originates from spinal cord segments L4–L6. Interneurons are activated at these segments and at adjacent segments both rostrally and caudally. The interneurons activate sciatic motor neurons, which stimulate flexor muscle contraction (see Fig. 1–19). The net result is a withdrawal of the limb from the painful stimulus. Inhibitory interneurons to the extensor motor neurons also are activated, resulting in decreased activity in the extensor muscles. Relaxation of the extensor muscles and contraction of the flexor muscles allow complete flexion of the limb.

The flexor reflex is a spinal reflex and does not require any activation of the brain. If an animal steps on a sharp piece of glass, it immediately withdraws the foot before consciously perceiving pain. If the spinal cord is completely transected above the segments that are responsible for the reflex, the reflex is present even though the animal has no conscious perception of pain.

Assessment. The pelvic limb flexor reflex primarily involves spinal cord segments L6–S1 and the sciatic nerve. Absence (0) or depression (+1) of the reflex indicates a lesion of these segments or nerves. Unilateral absence of the reflex is more likely the result of a peripheral nerve lesion, whereas bilateral absence or depression of the reflex is more likely the result of a spinal cord lesion. A normal (+2) flexor reflex indicates that the segments and the nerves are functional. An exaggerated (+3) flexor reflex rarely is seen with acute lesions of descending pathways. Chronic and severe descending pathway lesions may cause exaggeration of the reflex. This exaggeration is manifested as a sustained withdrawal after release of the stimulus. A *mass reflex* (+4) occasionally is seen as a sustained flexion of both pelvic limbs in response to a stimulus applied to only one limb. Exaggerated flexor reflexes usually reflect chronicity rather than severity of the lesion.

The crossed extensor reflex and the conscious perception of pain also are evaluated while the flexor reflex is performed, but these assessments will be discussed later.

Thoracic Limb

Technique. The thoracic limb flexor reflex is tested in the same manner as the pelvic limb flexor reflex. Cranial and palmar surfaces and medial and lateral digits should be tested.

Anatomy and Physiology. Branches of the radial nerve innervate the cranial surface of the foot and arise from spinal cord segments C7–T1. The medial palmar surface is innervated by the ulnar and median nerves, which originate from spinal cord segments C8–T1. The lateral palmar surface and most of the lateral digit are innervated by branches of the ulnar nerve. The organization of the flexor reflex of the thoracic limb is similar to that previously described for the pelvic limb. Flexor muscles of the thoracic limb are innervated by the axillary, musculocutaneous, median, and ulnar nerves and by parts of the radial nerve. These nerves originate from spinal cord segments C6–T1, with small contributions from C5 and T2 in some animals.

Assessment. Depressed reflexes indicate a lesion of the C6–T1 segments of the spinal cord or of the peripheral nerves. Exaggerated reflexes indicate a lesion cranial to C6.

Extensor Thrust Reflex

Technique. The reflex may be elicited with the animal in lateral recumbency (the same position as that for the myotatic reflex) or with the animal suspended by the shoulders with the rear limbs hanging free (Fig. 1–20). The toes are

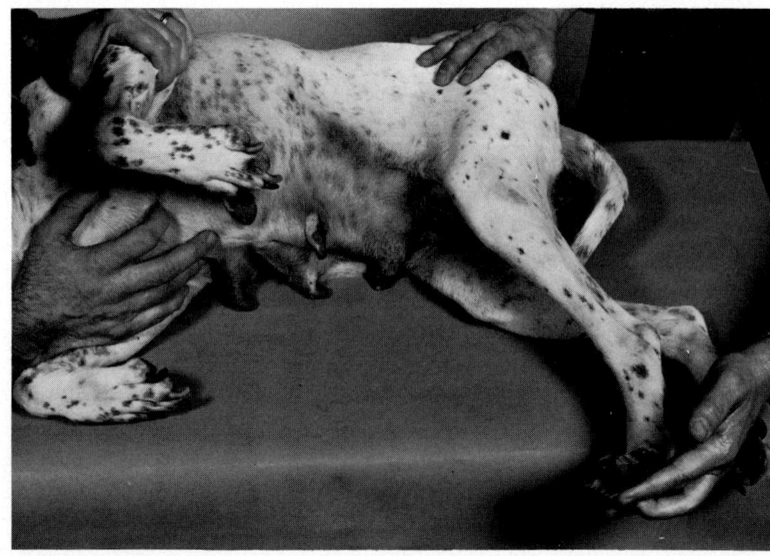

Figure 1–20 The extensor thrust reflex is elicited by spreading the phalanges.

spread, and slight pressure is applied between the pads. The response is a rigid extension of the limb.[20]

Anatomy and Physiology. The extensor thrust reflex is initiated by a stretching of the spindles in the interosseous muscles of the foot.[16] Simultaneously, the cutaneous sensory receptors are stimulated. The extensors predominate, forcing the limb into rigid extension. The sensory fibers are in the sciatic nerve (spinal cord segments L6–S1), and the response involves both femoral and sciatic nerves (spinal cord segments L4–S1). Excessive stimulation of the flexor reflex sensory fibers (e.g., with a noxious stimulus) will cause the flexor reflex to predominate, and withdrawal will occur.

The extensor thrust reflex is important for maintaining posture and is a component of more complex reactions, such as hopping.[17]

Assessment. The extensor thrust reflex is difficult to elicit in normal animals, especially when they are in lateral recumbency. Elicitation of the reflex generally indicates a lesion cranial to L4.

Perineal (Bulbocavernosus, Anal) Reflex

Technique. The perineal reflex is elicited by light stimulation of the perineum with a forceps. Painful stimuli usually are not necessary. The response is a contraction of the anal sphincter muscle and a flexion of the tail (Fig. 1–21). One can obtain a similar response by squeezing the penis or the vulva (bulbocavernosus reflex). If the anal sphincter appears weak or if the response is questionable, the examiner can insert a gloved digit into the anus. Minimal responses often can be felt in this manner.

Anatomy and Physiology. Sensory innervation occurs through the pudendal nerve and spinal cord segments S1–S2 (sometimes S3) in the dog and the cat. Motor innervation of the anal sphincter also occurs through the pudendal nerve. Tail flexion is mediated through the caudal nerves. The organization of the reflex is similar to that of the flexor reflex.

Assessment. The perineal reflex is the best indication of the functional integrity of the sacral spinal cord segments and the sacral nerve roots. Evaluation of this reflex is especially important in animals with urinary bladder dysfunction (see Chap. 3). Absence (0) or depression (+1) of the reflex indicates a sacral spinal cord lesion or a pudendal nerve lesion.

Crossed Extensor Reflex

Technique. The crossed extensor reflex may be observed when the flexor reflex is elicited. The response is an extension of the limb opposite the stimulated limb.[19]

Anatomy and Physiology. The crossed extensor reflex is a part of the normal supporting mechanism of the animal. The weight of an animal in a standing position is evenly distributed among the limbs. If one leg is flexed, increased support is required of the opposite limb. The flexor reflex sensory fibers send collaterals to interneurons on the opposite side of the spinal cord, which excite extensor motor neurons (see Fig. 1–19).

Assessment. The crossed extensor reflex generally is considered an abnormal reflex except in the standing position. In the normal recumbent animal the extension response is inhibited

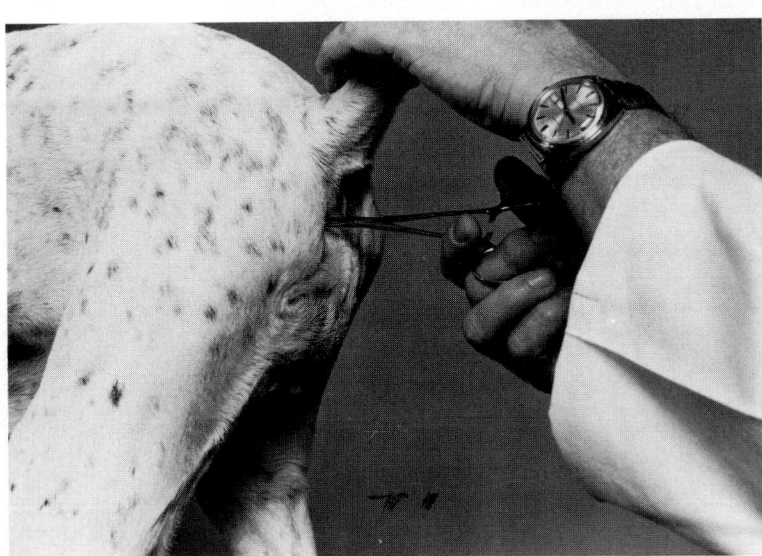

Figure 1–21 The perineal reflex is a contraction of the anal sphincter and a ventral flexion of the tail in response to tactile stimulation of the perineum.

through descending pathways. Crossed extensor reflexes result from lesions in descending pathways, a sign of UMN disease. The crossed extensor reflex has been considered evidence of a severe spinal cord lesion. It is not a reliable indicator of the severity of the lesion, however. Animals that are still ambulatory may have crossed extensor reflexes, especially when the lesion is in the cervical spinal cord or the brain stem.

Extensor Toe (Babinski) Reflex

Technique. The animal is positioned in lateral recumbency (the same position as that for the myotatic reflex). The rear limb is held above the hock, with the hock and the digits slightly flexed. The handle of the plexor or a forceps is used to stroke the limb on the caudolateral surface from the hock to the digits (Fig. 1–22). The normal animal will exhibit no response or a slight flexion of the digits. The abnormal response is an extension and a fanning of the digits.[21]

Anatomy and Physiology. The extensor toe reflex has been compared with the Babinski reflex in human beings.[22] The two reflexes are not strictly analogous, because the Babinski reflex includes elevation and fanning of the large toe, which is not present in domestic animals. The Babinski reflex is reported to be a sign of pyramidal tract damage in human beings. The extensor toe reflex has been produced by lesions in the brain stem[22] and has been seen clinically in dogs with hypertonic pelvic limb paresis.[21] Acute experimental lesions of the sensorimotor cortex, the dorsal columns, the lateral columns, or the ventral columns of the spinal cord have not produced an extensor toe reflex. Some investigators have considered this reflex to be an abnormal form of the flexor reflex.

Assessment. The extensor toe reflex has been observed in dogs with paralysis of the pelvic limbs associated with extensor hypertonus and exaggerated myotatic reflexes. In most cases clinical signs have been present for longer than 3 weeks. The reflex should be interpreted in the same manner as other exaggerated reflexes.

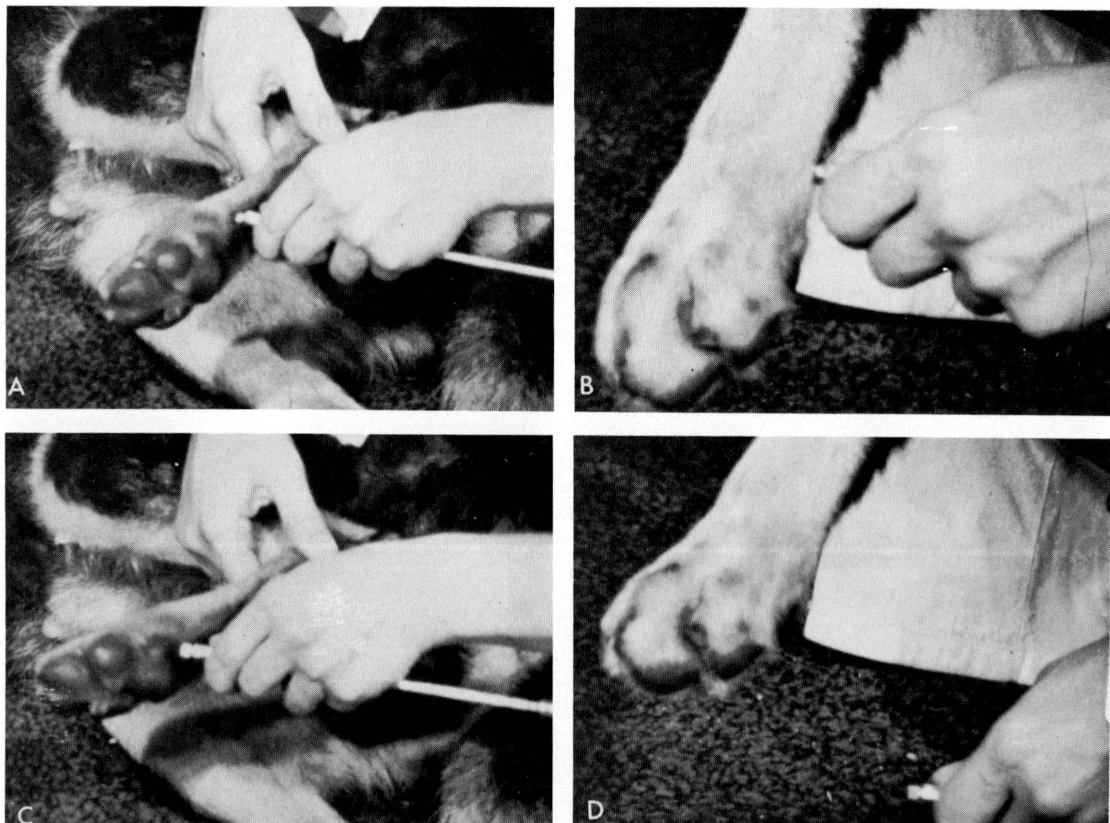

Figure 1–22 The extensor toe response (Babinski's reflex). The toes of the pelvic limbs are in the normal position. The instrument is moving down the metatarsus from the hock toward the digits (*A* and *B*). The digits extend and fan apart as the instrument completes the sweep (*C* and *D*). (Frames from a motion picture.) (From Kneller SK, Oliver JE, Lewis RE: Differential diagnosis of progressive caudal paresis in an aged German shepherd dog. J Am Anim Hosp Assoc 11:414–417, 1975. Used by permission.)

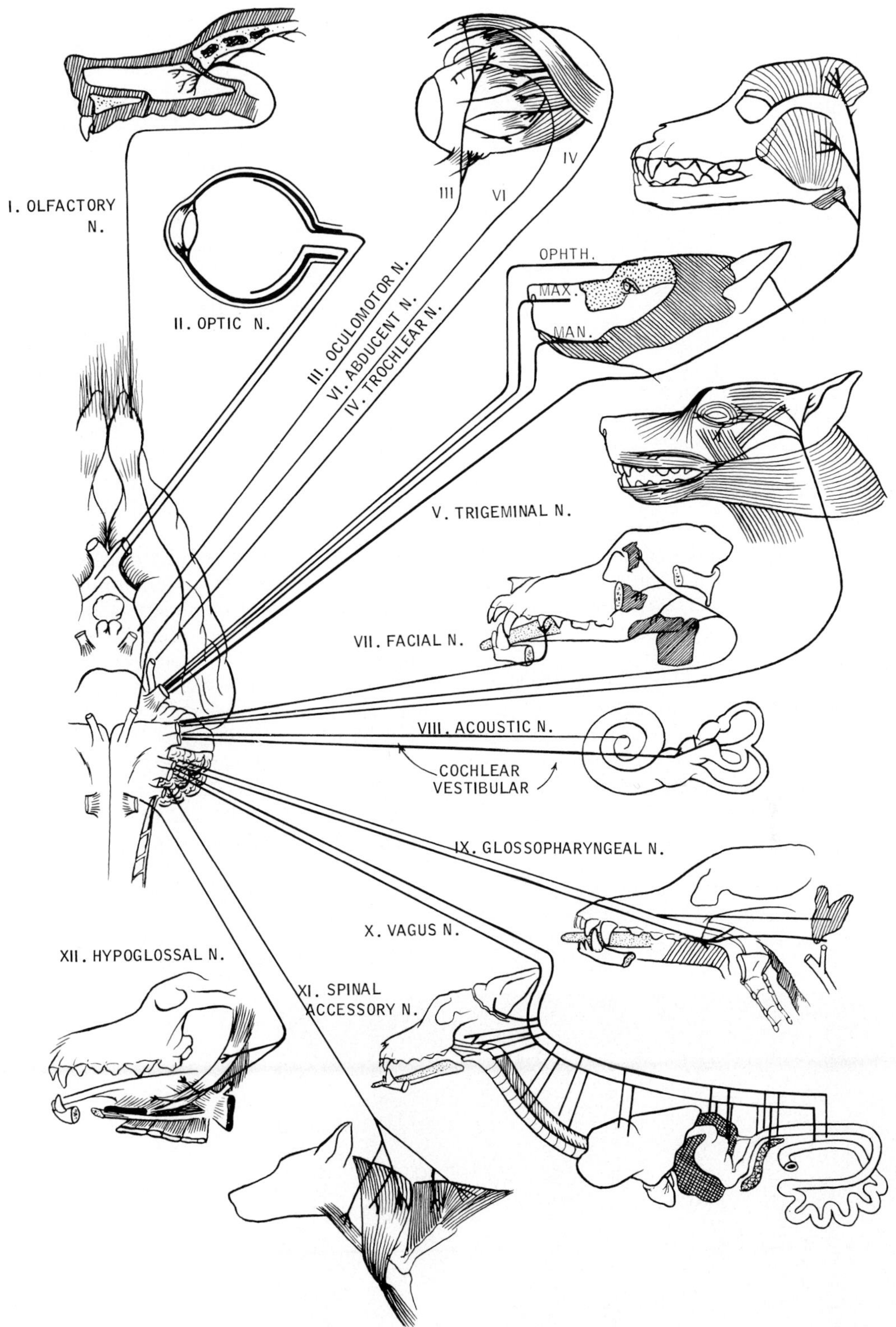

Figure 1–23 The origin and distribution of the cranial nerves in the dog. (From Hoerlein BF: Canine Neurology, 3rd ed. Philadelphia, WB Saunders Co., 1978. Used by permission.)

Cranial Nerves

Examination of the cranial nerves is an important part of the neurologic examination, especially when disease of the brain is suspected. An abnormality of a cranial nerve constitutes evidence of a specific, localized area of disease not provided by postural reactions. The cranial nerve examination is not difficult, and the most frequently affected cranial nerves can be evaluated quickly (Fig. 1–23). The general outline of the cranial nerve examination was discussed under The Efficient Neurologic Examination at the beginning of this chapter.

The detection of any abnormalities on the screening examination may be followed by a more complete examination to define the abnormality further.

Olfactory Nerve (CN I)

The olfactory nerve is the sensory path for the conscious perception of smell.

Technique. A behavioral response to a pleasurable or a noxious odor, either inferred from the history or assessed by direct testing, may be used (Fig. 1–24). Alcohol, cloves, xylol, benzol, or cat food containing fish appear to stimulate the olfactory nerves. Irritating substances such as ammonia or tobacco smoke cannot be used because they stimulate the endings of the trigeminal nerve in the nasal mucosa.

Anatomy and Physiology. Chemoreceptors in the nasal mucosa give rise to axons, which pass through the cribriform plate to the synapse in the olfactory bulb. Axons from the olfactory bulb course through the olfactory tract to the ipsilateral olfactory cortex. Behavioral reactions to smell are controlled by connections to the limbic system.[7]

Assessment. Deficiencies in the sense of smell are difficult to evaluate. Rhinitis is the most common cause of anosmia (loss of olfaction). Tumors of the nasal passages and diseases of the cribriform plate also must be considered. Only rarely are structural lesions such as tumors of importance. Olfaction is also impaired by inflammatory disease such as canine distemper or parainfluenza virus infection.[23]

Optic Nerve (CN II)

The optic nerve is the sensory path for vision and pupillary light reflexes (see Figs. 12–1 and 12–2).

Technique. The optic nerve is tested in conjunction with the oculomotor nerve (CN III), which provides the motor pathway for the pupillary light reflex, and the facial nerve, which provides the motor pathway for the blink reflex. Vision may be assessed by observation of the animal's movements in unfamiliar surroundings, avoidance of obstacles, and following of moving objects. More objective evaluation requires three tests. The examiner elicits the menace reaction by making a threatening gesture with the hand at one eye. The normal response is a blink and, sometimes, an aversive movement of the head (Fig. 1–25). The visual placing reaction (see the section on postural reactions) is an excellent method of assessing vision. The examiner induces the pupillary light reflex by shining a light in each eye and observing for pupillary constriction in both eyes.

Anatomy and Physiology. See Chapter 12.

Assessment. See Chapter 12.

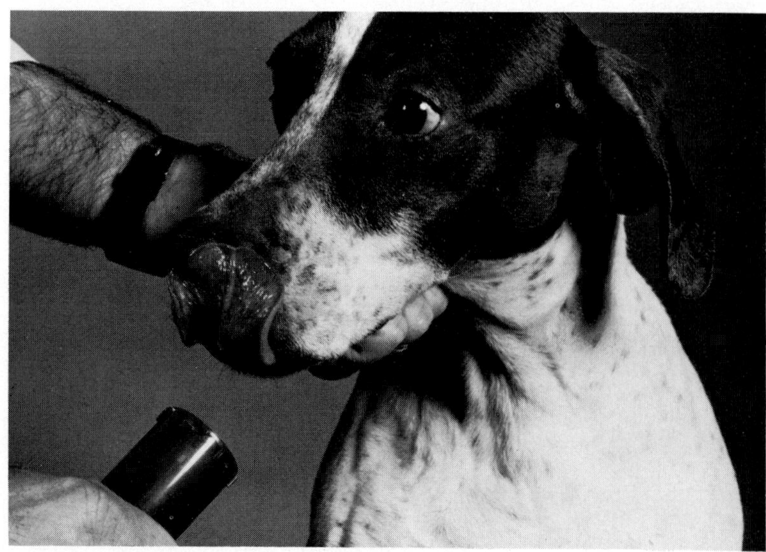

Figure 1–24 Noxious odors that are nonirritating will cause an aversion, or licking reaction.

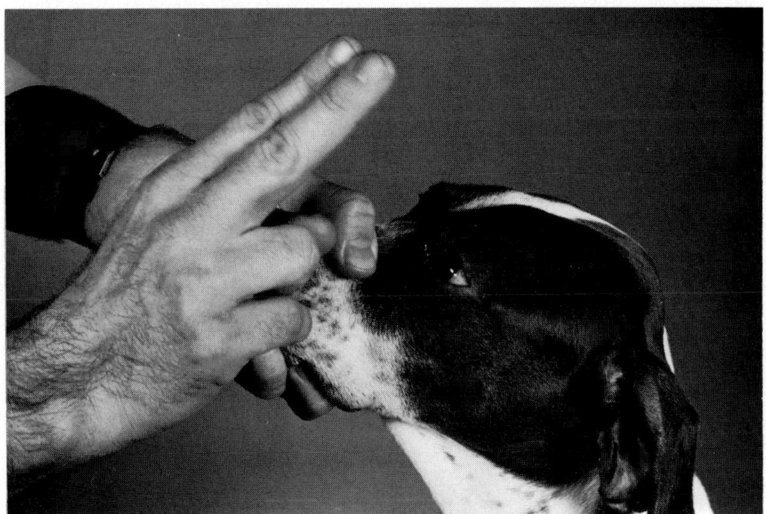

Figure 1–25 The menace reaction is elicited by making a threatening gesture at the eye, which should result in a blink. The examiner must avoid creating wind currents or touching the hairs around the eye, which will cause a palpebral reflex. The sensory pathway is in the optic nerve and the visual pathway. The motor pathway is in the facial nerve.

Oculomotor Nerve (CN III)

The oculomotor nerve contains the parasympathetic motor fibers for pupillary constriction and is the motor pathway for the following extraocular muscles: dorsal, medial and ventral recti, and ventral oblique. It is also the motor pathway for the levator palpebrae muscle of the upper lid (see Fig. 12–4).

Technique. The examiner tests the pupillary light reflex by shining a light in the animal's eye and observing for pupillary constriction in both eyes. One can assess eye movement by observing the eyes as the animal looks in various directions voluntarily or in response to movements in the peripheral fields of vision. A more direct method is to elicit vestibular eye movements (normal nystagmus) by moving the head laterally (Fig. 1–26). The fast beat of the nystagmus will be in the direction of the head movement. The eyes should move in coordination with each other (conjugate movements). One can easily test the rectus muscles by this method. A drooping upper lid (ptosis) is indicative of paresis of the levator palpebrae muscle. Lesions of the oculomotor nerve cause a fixed ventrolateral deviation (strabismus) of the eye and a dilated pupil. In cattle, the eye usually remains horizontal regardless of the head position. The function of each of the extraocular muscles can be assessed in the same manner if the examiner bears this difference in mind. The functions of the extraocular muscles of large animals have not been directly established, but it is assumed that they are similar to the functions of the corresponding muscles in other species.

Anatomy and Physiology. See Chapter 12.

Assessment. See Chapter 12.

Trochlear Nerve (CN IV)

The trochlear nerve is the motor pathway to the dorsal oblique muscle of the eye.

Technique. The trochlear nerve is difficult to assess. Lesions may cause a lateral rotation of the eye, which can be seen most clearly in animals with a horizontal pupil (cow) or a vertical pupil (cat) or by ophthalmoscopic examination of the dorsal retinal vein (see Fig. 12–4). There is a slight deficit in dorsomedial gaze.

Anatomy and Physiology. See Chapter 12.

Assessment. See Chapter 12.

Trigeminal Nerve (CN V)

The trigeminal nerve is the motor pathway to the muscles of mastication and the sensory pathway to the face.

Technique. The motor branch of the trigeminal nerve is in the mandibular nerve and innervates the masseter, temporal, rostral digastric, pterygoid, and mylohyoid muscles.[7] Bilateral paralysis produces a dropped jaw that cannot be closed voluntarily. Unilateral lesions may cause decreased jaw tone. Atrophy of the temporal and masseter muscles is recognized by careful palpation approximately 1 week after the onset of paralysis. Sensation should be tested over the distribution of all three branches—ophthalmic, maxillary, and mandibular. A touch of the skin may be an adequate stimulus in some animals, whereas a gentle pinch with a forceps may be needed in others. The palpebral reflex is a blink response to a touch at the medial canthus of the eye, which tests the ophthalmic branch (see Fig. 1–27). Touching the lateral canthus tests the maxillary branch. The blink response is dependent on innervation of the

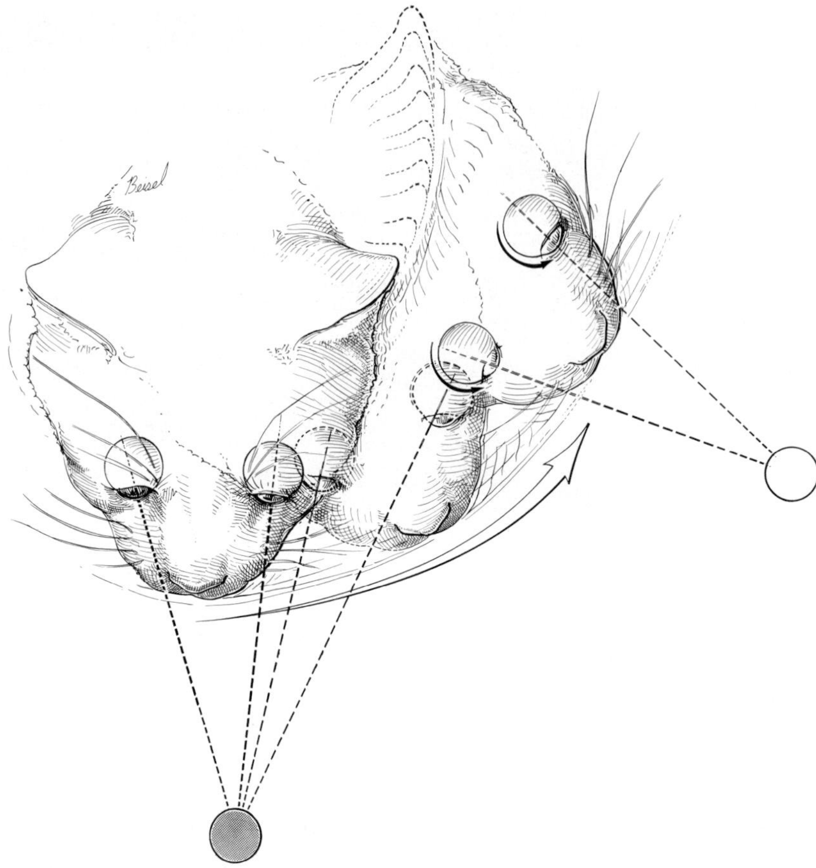

Figure 1–26 Vestibular eye movements are elicited by turning the animal's head from side to side. The eyes will lag behind the head movement and then will rotate to return to the center of the palpebral fissure. Both visual (opticokinetic nystagmus) and vestibular pathways are active in this response, but vestibular pathways predominate and will produce these movements in the absence of vision.

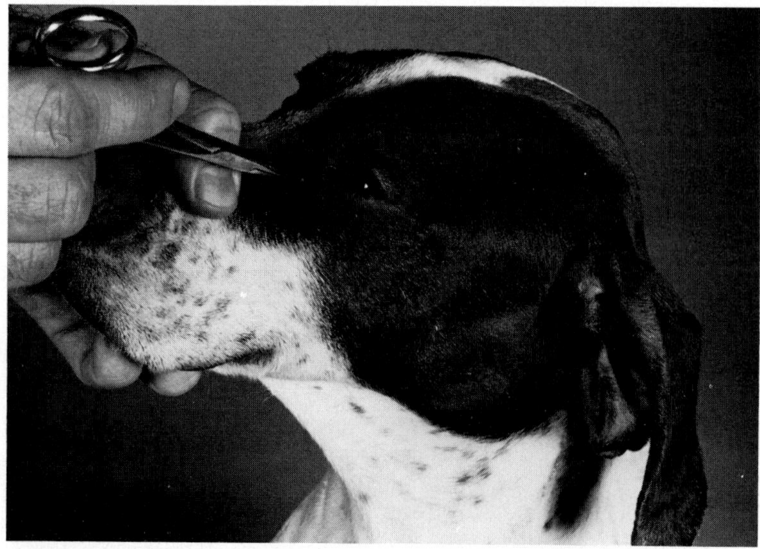

Figure 1–27 The palpebral reflex is checked by touching the eyelid and observing for a blink. The sensory pathway is in the trigeminal nerve; the motor pathway is in the facial nerve.

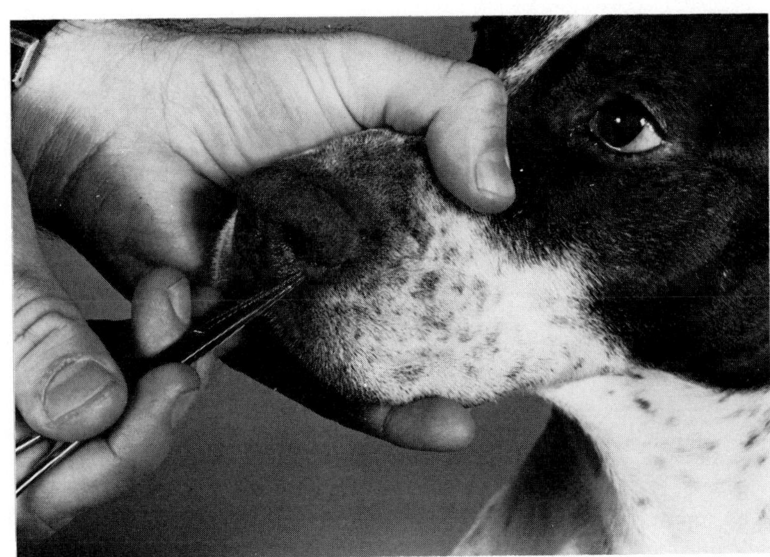

Figure 1–28 Tactile stimulation on the head rostral to the ears tests the sensory branches of the trigeminal nerve. The reactions may be behavioral or reflex. Even depressed or stoic animals will respond to stimulation of the nasal mucosa.

muscles by the facial nerve. Stimulation of the nasal mucosa tests the maxillary branch and should elicit a response even in depressed or stoic animals (see Fig. 1–28). Pinching the jaw tests the mandibular branch.

Anatomy and Physiology. See Chapter 10.

Assessment. See Chapter 10.

Abducent Nerve (CN VI)

The abducent nerve innervates the lateral rectus and the retractor bulbi muscles.

Technique. Eye movements are tested by the method described for the oculomotor nerve. The retractor bulbi muscles can be tested with a palpebral or a corneal reflex. Normally, the globe is retracted, allowing extrusion of the third eyelid. Lesions of the abducent nerve cause a loss of lateral (abducted) gaze and medial strabismus combined with inability to retract the globe (see Fig. 12–4).

Anatomy and Physiology. See Chapter 12.

Assessment. See Chapter 12.

Facial Nerve (CN VII)

The facial nerve is the motor pathway to the muscles of facial expression and the sensory pathway for taste to the palate and the rostral two thirds of the tongue.

Technique. Asymmetry of the face usually is seen in cases of facial paralysis. The lips, the eyelids, and the ears may droop. The nose may be slightly deviated to the normal side, and the nostril may not flare on inhalation. The palpebral fissure may be slightly widened and will fail to close when a palpebral or a corneal reflex is attempted (see Fig. 1–27). Pinching the lip will produce a behavioral response, but the lip may not retract. The examiner can test the animal's sense of taste by moistening a cotton-tipped applicator stick with atropine and touching it to the rostral part of the tongue. The affected side is tested first. Normal dogs will react immediately to the bitter taste. Delayed reactions may occur as the atropine spreads to normal areas of the tongue.

Anatomy and Physiology. See Chapter 10.

Assessment. See Chapter 10.

Vestibulocochlear Nerve (CN VIII)

The vestibulocochlear nerve has two branches: the cochlear division, which mediates hearing, and the vestibular division, which provides information about the orientation of the head with respect to gravity.

Technique

COCHLEAR DIVISION Most tests for hearing are dependent upon behavioral reactions to sound and therefore are subject to misinterpretation. There is no good test for unilateral deficits other than those involving electrophysiologic systems. Crude tests involve startling the animal with a loud noise (clap, whistle). Similar responses may be monitored on an electroencephalogram (EEG) or by observation or direct measurement of the respiratory cycle. Human audiometry equipment can also be adapted for animal use. The most precise measurement involves the use of a signal-averaging computer, which measures electrical activity of the brain stem in response to auditory stimuli (brain stem auditory-evoked response—BAER). BAER not only detects auditory deficits, but also may indicate the location of the lesion (see Chap. 4).

VESTIBULAR DIVISION Abnormalities of the vestibular system produce several characteristic signs. Most vestibular lesions are unilateral except in congenital anomalies and, occasionally, in inflammatory diseases. Unilateral vestibular disease usually produces ataxia, nystagmus, and a head tilt to the side of the lesion.[6]

The head tilt should be apparent on observation (see Fig. 1–5). The examiner can accentuate the head tilt by removing visual compensation or by removing tactile proprioception. Ataxia (an uncoordinated, staggering gait) usually is accompanied by a broad-based stance and a tendency to fall or to circle to the side of the lesion.

Nystagmus should be observed with the head held in varying positions. The direction of the fast component is noted (for example, left horizontal nystagmus). Forced deviation of the globe (strabismus) also may be seen when the head is elevated or lowered. Typically the ipsilateral eye will deviate ventrally when the head is elevated (in small animals). Producing eye movements by moving the animal's head from side to side (see the section on CN III) also tests the vestibular system (see Fig. 1–26). Vestibular lesions may alter the direction or may abolish the response. In some cases, the eyes will not move together (dysconjugate movement).

Postrotatory nystagmus may help evaluate vestibular disease. As an animal is rotated rapidly, physiologic nystagmus is induced. When rotation is stopped, nystagmus (postrotatory) occurs in the opposite direction and is observed for a short time. The receptors opposite the direction of rotation are stimulated more than the ipsilateral receptors, because they are farther from the axis of rotation. Unilateral lesions will produce a difference in the rate and duration of postrotatory nystagmus when the animal is tested in both directions. The test is performed in the following manner: The animal is held by an assistant, who rapidly turns 360 degrees ten times and then stops. The examiner counts the beats of nystagmus. After several minutes, the test is repeated in the opposite direction. Normal animals will have three to four beats of nystagmus, with the fast phase opposite the direction of rotation. Peripheral lesions usually depress the response when the animal is rotated away from the side of the lesion. Central lesions may depress or prolong the response.

The caloric test is a specific test for vestibular function. This test has the advantage of assessing each side independently. It is difficult to perform in many animals, however, and may be unreliable if the patient is uncooperative. Negative responses occur in many normal animals. The examiner performs the test by holding the animal's head securely in one position, irrigating the ear canal with ice water, and observing for nystagmus. A rubber ear syringe should be used for the irrigation. Usually, 50 to 100 ml of cold water is adequate, and the infusion takes approximately 3 minutes. The test should not be performed if the tympanic membrane is ruptured or if the ear canal is plugged. Nystagmus is induced, with the fast phase away from the side being tested. Warm water also will produce the same effect, except that the nystagmus will be in the opposite direction. The use of warm water is even less reliable. If the animal resists and shakes its head, the response usually is abolished. The test is useful for the evaluation of brain stem function in comatose animals, but has been replaced by brain stem auditory-evoked response testing at most institutions.

Anatomy and Physiology. See Chapter 9.

Assessment. See Chapters 2 and 9.

Glossopharyngeal Nerve (CN IX) and Vagus Nerve (CN X)

Cranial nerves IX and X will be considered together because of their common origin and their common intracranial pathway. The glossopharyngeal nerve is the motor pathway to the muscles of the pharynx, along with some fibers from the vagus nerve. The glossopharyngeal nerve also supplies parasympathetic motor fibers to the zygomatic and parotid salivary glands. It is sensory to the caudal one third of the tongue and the pharyngeal mucosa, including the sensation of taste. The vagus nerve is the motor pathway to the pharynx, the larynx, and the palate, and supplies parasympathetic motor fibers to the viscera of the body, except for the pelvic viscera (which are innervated by sacral parasympathetic nerves). Gastric abnormalities are common in vagus nerve problems in ruminants. The vagus nerve is the sensory pathway to the caudal pharynx, the larynx, and the viscera of the body.

Technique. Taste can be evaluated by the method described for evaluating CN VII, although it is more difficult to make an accurate assessment of the caudal part of the tongue. The simplest test for function is to observe the palate and the larynx for asymmetry and to elicit a gag or a swallowing response by inserting a tongue depressor to the pharynx. Stertorous breathing may be observed with laryngeal paralysis. Endoscopic observation of the larynx is useful in the horse. The laryngeal adductor response (slap test) is performed during endoscopic observation. The skin caudal to the dorsal part of the scapula is slapped gently with the hand during expiration. The normal response is brief adduction of the contralateral arytenoid cartilage.[9] Historical evidence of an inability to swallow may be suggestive of an abnormality in CN IX and X. The clinician should be cautious when examining animals with swallowing problems, since dysphagia is one of the signs of rabies.

Anatomy and Physiology. See Chapter 10.

Assessment. See Chapter 10.

Accessory Nerve

The accessory nerve is the motor pathway to the trapezius muscle and parts of the sternocephalicus and brachiocephalicus muscles.

Technique. The detection of an abnormality in an accessory nerve injury may be difficult, except by careful palpation for atrophy of the affected muscles. Passive movement of the head and the neck may demonstrate a loss of resistance to lateral movements in a contralateral direction.

Anatomy and Physiology. The accessory nerve arises from fibers in the ventral roots of C1–C7 spinal cord segments and from the medulla. The fibers course cranially as the spinal root of the accessory nerve, which lies between the dorsal and the ventral spinal nerve roots. It emerges from the skull by way of the tympano-occipital fissure. It then courses caudally in the neck to innervate the trapezius and portions of the sternocephalicus and brachiocephalicus muscles. These muscles elevate and advance the limb and fix the neck laterally.[7]

Assessment. Lesions of the accessory nerve either are rare or are rarely recognized. An injury to the nerve in the spinal canal or the cranium probably would be masked by other, more severe signs of paresis. The course of the nerve in the neck is well-protected by muscle but could be damaged by deep penetrating wounds, injections, or contusion. Atrophy of the affected muscles would be the most obvious sign of injury. Electromyography (EMG) may be necessary for diagnosis. Lesions in the vertebral canal should produce other signs of spinal cord dysfunction.

Hypoglossal Nerve

The hypoglossal nerve is the motor pathway to the intrinsic and extrinsic muscles of the tongue and the geniohyoideus muscle.

Technique. The muscles of the tongue protrude and retract it. Each side is innervated independently. Tongue protrusion is tested by wetting the animal's nose and observing the animal's ability to extend its tongue forward (Fig. 1–29). The strength of retraction can be tested by grasping the tongue with a gauze sponge. Atrophy can be observed if a lesion has been present for 5 to 7 days.

Anatomy and Physiology. See Chapter 10.

Assessment. See Chapter 10.

Sensation

The sensory examination provides information relative to the anatomic location and severity of the lesion. At this point in the neurologic examination, sensation has been tested by assessment of the cranial nerves, the spinal reflexes,

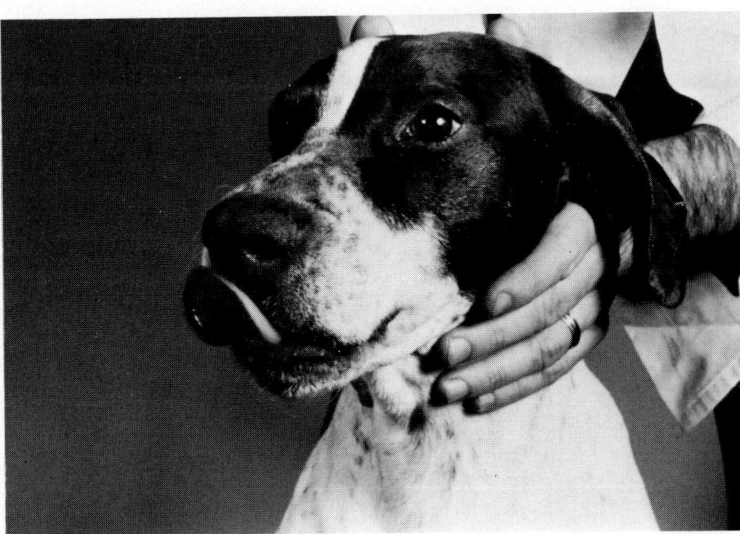

Figure 1–29 Most animals can be induced to lick if their noses are moistened. The tongue should be extended without forced deviation to the side.

and proprioceptive positioning. Sensory modalities still to be tested include touch, superficial pain, and deep pain from the limbs and the trunk.

Technique. The evaluation of sensation begins caudally and progresses cranially. The severity of the stimulus is increased from light touch to a deep palpation. If no response occurs, a light pinch is applied with a hemostat. Harder squeezing with the hemostat may be necessary in some cases. A significant behavioral response at any step indicates the presence of sensation, and more severe stimuli are not needed once sensation has been established. If a dog turns and snaps when its toe is touched, there is no need to squeeze the toe with a hemostat![24]

During palpation of the animal, areas of increased sensitivity (hyperesthesia) are noted. The rear limbs are palpated first, followed by the vertebral column. Beginning with L7 and progressing cranially, the examiner squeezes the transverse processes. Alternatively, one can press each spinous process firmly. While palpating the spine, it is useful for the examiner to place the other hand on the animal's abdomen in order to detect increased tension in the abdominal muscles as sensitive areas are palpated (Fig. 1–30). Localized areas of hyperesthesia are detected in this manner.

The area of hyperesthesia may be defined more precisely by gently pinching the skin with a hemostat. Again, this test should be performed systematically, in a caudal to cranial direction (Fig. 1–31). Two responses may be observed: a twitch of the skin (the cutaneous or panniculus reflex) or a behavioral response, such as a display of anxiety, an attempt to escape, a turning of the head, or a vocalization. When evaluating spinal cord disorders, the examiner tests the skin just lateral to the midline. The test is repeated on a line lateral to the site of the first evaluation and then is repeated on the opposite side. The cranial and caudal margins of a hyperesthetic area can be determined bilaterally. Spinal cord or nerve root lesions produce an area of hyperesthesia, or a transition from decreased to normal sensation, in a pattern conforming to the dermatomal distribution of the nerves (Fig. 1–32). Testing of cutaneous sensation of the neck is unreliable for localizing cervical lesions. Manipulation of the head and the neck and deep palpation of the cervical vertebrae are more useful for localizing pain in this area.

A noxious stimulus that elicits any behavioral response is adequate for determining the presence of deep pain. When a response is difficult to elicit, a hemostat is used to squeeze a digit. *Withdrawal of the limb is not a behaviorial response* (see the section on the flexor reflex in this chapter).

Anatomy and Physiology. Newer concepts emphasize the integration and interaction of all sensory systems and the effect of descending pathways that modify sensation. The concepts presented in this section are in general agreement with current research and are adequate for the clinical interpretation of sensory signs (see also Chap. 15).[25–27]

Sensory fibers from the skin, the muscles, the joints, and the viscera enter the spinal cord at each segment by way of the dorsal nerve root. Fibers that innervate the skin are arranged in regular patterns called *dermatomes* (see Fig. 1–

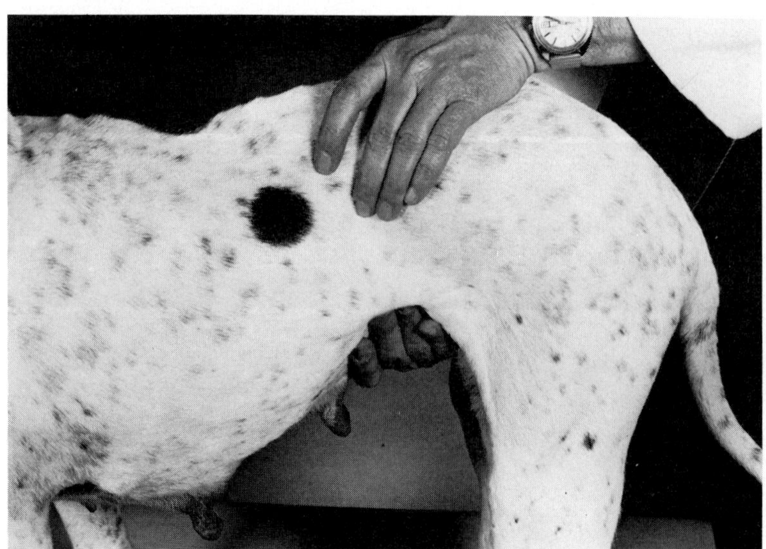

Figure 1–30 Deep palpation may elicit areas of hyperesthesia. Minimal response may be detected by simultaneously palpating adjacent areas for changes in muscle tone (guarding reaction).

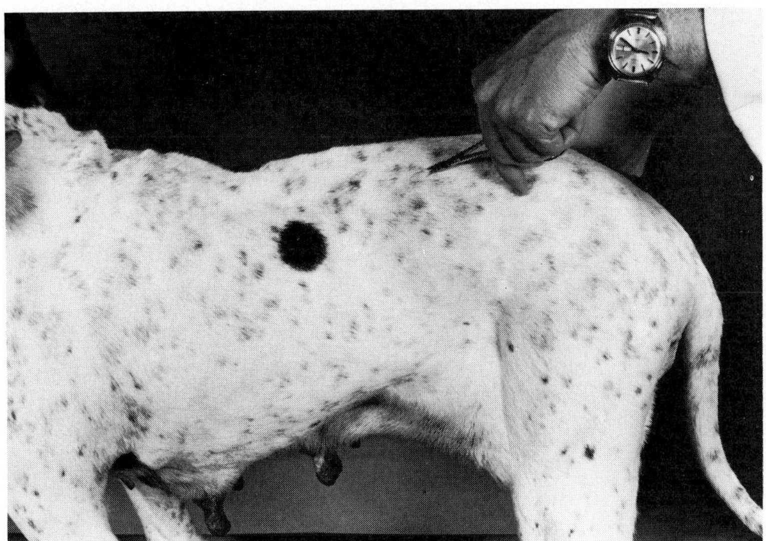

Figure 1–31 Gentle pricking or pinching of the skin can be used to outline the area of hyperesthesia more precisely. Both behavioral reactions and the cutaneous reflex may be elicited. The skin should be stimulated dorsally and laterally in order for the examiner to develop a map of abnormal reactions.

32). A dermatome is the area of skin innervated by one spinal nerve root. Because of overlap, each strip of skin has some innervation from three segments.[28–32]

Proprioceptive fibers entering the spinal cord may ascend in the dorsal columns and the spinomedullothalamic tract to relay information to nuclei in the medulla (see Fig. 1–8). Other fibers synapse on neurons in the dorsal horn of the gray matter. The neurons then send axons cranially along one of several named pathways, both ipsilaterally and contralaterally. The primary functions of these pathways include unconscious proprioception and sensitivity to touch, temperature, and superficial pain.[25]

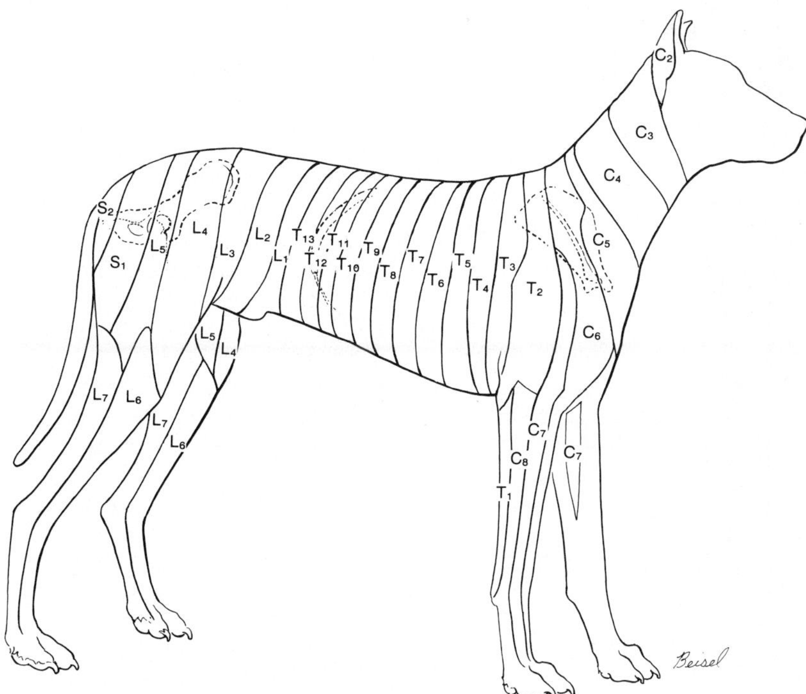

Figure 1–32 Dermatomes of the dog. This illustration represents the results of several studies. Dermatomes vary among individuals, and overlapping innervation of approximately three segments is present in most areas. The distribution to thoracic limbs is tentative. (From Oliver JE, Hoerlein BF, and Mayhew IG: Veterinary Neurology. Philadelphia, WB Saunders Co., 1987. Used by permission.)

The deep pain pathway (spinoreticular and propriospinal tracts) is interrupted at three- to five-segment intervals to synapse on neurons in the spinal cord gray matter. These neurons give rise to axons, which rejoin the pathway on the same side or on the opposite side. The deep pain system is bilateral and multisynaptic and is composed of small diameter fibers (Fig. 1–33).[26]

The *cutaneous or panniculus reflex* is a twitch of the cutaneous muscle in response to a cutaneous stimulus. The sensory nerves from the skin enter by way of the dorsal root. The ascending pathway is probably the same as that for superficial pain. The synapse occurs at the C8, T1 segments with motor neurons of the lateral thoracic nerve that innervates the cutaneous trunci muscle (Fig. 1–34).[7]

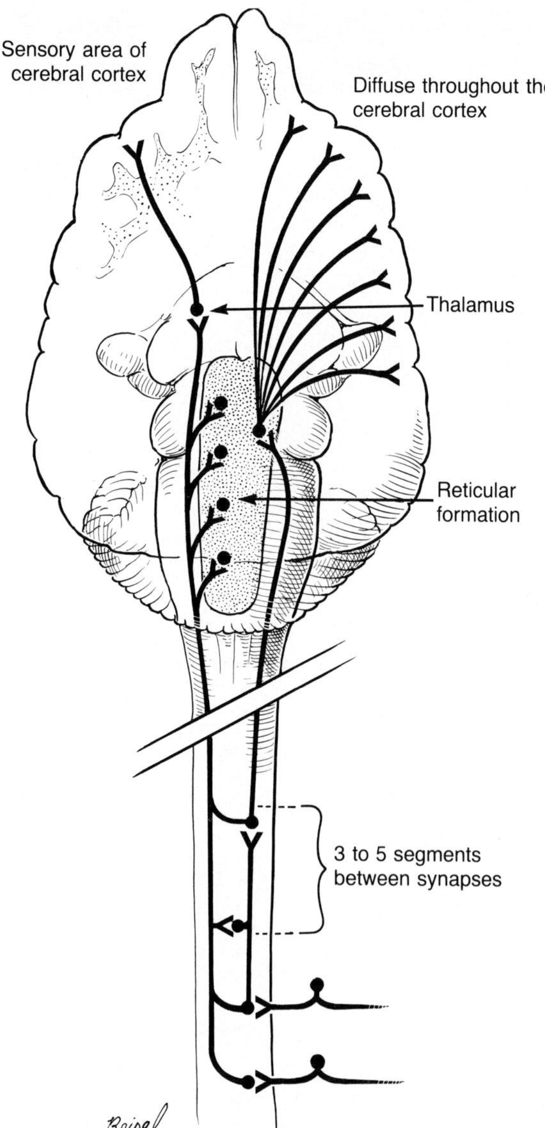

Figure 1–33 The pain pathway in animals is bilateral and multisynaptic (see also Fig. 1–8). The deep pain pathway apparently has synapses every three to five segments, with projections continuing cranially on both sides of the spinal cord.

Assessment. Alterations in a sensory modality are described as absent (0), decreased (+1), normal (+2), or increased (hyperesthesia, +3). Absent or decreased sensation indicates damage to a sensory nerve or a pathway. Increased sensitivity may indicate irritation of a nerve or, more commonly, irritation of adjacent structures (e.g., disk herniation with irritation of meninges).

The cutaneous reflex is most prominent in the "saddle" area of the trunk. It cannot be elicited from stimulation over the sacrum or the neck. The response is absent caudal to the level of a lesion that disrupts the superficial pain pathway. For example, a compression of spinal cord segment L1 results in a normal panniculus response when stimulation is applied to the T13 dermatome but no response caudal to that point.

When alterations in touch, superficial pain, or areas of hyperesthesia are found, the pattern of abnormality is carefully mapped. The pattern generally conforms to one of three possibilities: (1) Transverse spinal cord lesions cause an abnormality in all areas caudal to the lesion. The line of demarcation between normal and abnormal areas follows the pattern of a dermatome (see Fig. 1–32). (2) Hyperesthesia, reflecting an irritation at a spinal cord segment or a nerve root, follows the distribution of one or more dermatomes (usually no more than three). (3) Lesions of a peripheral nerve produce a pattern of abnormality conforming to the distribution of that peripheral nerve (Fig. 1–35). One of these three patterns localizes the lesion to a peripheral nerve (e.g., sciatic nerve, radial nerve) or to a spinal cord segment (accurate to within three segments, e.g., L1–L3).

The presence or absence of sensation provides an important assessment of the extent of neural damage, especially in compressive lesions. When nerves are compressed, large nerve fibers are the first to lose function. With greater compression, small nerve fibers may be affected. In the spinal cord, loss of function develops in the following sequence: (1) loss of proprioception, (2) loss of voluntary motor function, (3) loss of superficial pain sensation, (4) loss of deep pain sensation (see Fig. 1–3). Therefore, an animal with a spinal cord compression that has lost proprioception and voluntary motor function (paralyzed) but still has superficial and deep pain sensation has less spinal cord damage than one that has lost all

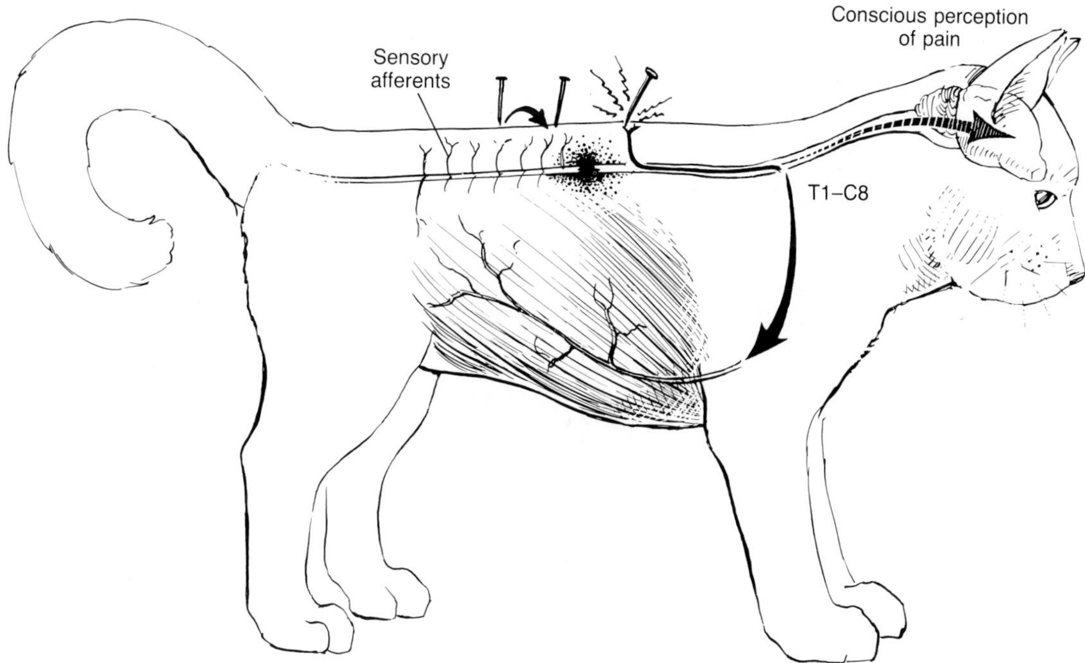

Figure 1–34 The cutaneous (panniculus) reflex is the contraction of cutaneous trunci muscle, producing a skin twitch from stimulation of cutaneous sensory fibers. (From Greene CE, Oliver JE: Neurologic examination. In Ettinger SJ (ed): Textbook of Veterinary Internal Medicine, 2nd ed. Philadelphia, WB Saunders Co., 1982. Used by permission.)

four functions. A loss of deep pain sensation indicates a severely damaged spinal cord and a poor prognosis.

CASE HISTORIES

The following case histories are presented for two purposes. First, they provide examples of the kinds of histories obtained in cases involving neurologic problems and demonstrate the process used in evaluating this information. Second, they can be used to gauge one's understanding of the material in this chapter. After reading the history, but before reading the neurologic examination, draw a sign-time graph and list the most probable categories of disease. Then read the results of the neurologic examination and decide what is normal and abnormal. Try to assess the findings in relation to the anatomic components of each test. Learning to assess the findings of the neurologic examination requires practice. Practice with immediate feedback from an experienced examiner is best but is not always possible. The cases presented here are designed to illustrate the kinds of abnormalities that may be present in the various reactions and reflexes and to assist the reader in making decisions regarding normality or abnormality. Later chapters will include the complete findings in the cases, and a final diagnosis. In this chapter, make only a sign-time graph, establish a list of rule-outs, and evaluate the findings of the neurologic examination.

Case History 1A

Signalment

Canine, West Highland white terrier, female, 6 years old.

History

There are no significant previous medical problems, and vaccinations are current. The dog was found lying down in the fenced-in backyard 4 days earlier. She was unable to walk, although some apparently voluntary movements were noticed in the left thoracic and pelvic limbs. The owners do not believe that conditions have changed since they first found the dog. They do not think the dog is in any pain. Appetite and eliminations are normal, and the dog seems alert and responsive.

Physical Examination

No abnormalities are found other than those detected on the neurologic examination.

Neurologic Examination

The dog is bright, alert, and responsive. She is unable to walk. When placed in a standing position, she falls to the right. Proprioceptive positioning is good in the left thoracic limb, slightly delayed in the left pelvic limb, and absent in the limbs on the right. The hopping reactions appear good in the left thoracic limb, with quick initiation of movement and accurate placement of the limb to support weight. The left pelvic limb has a slow initiation of

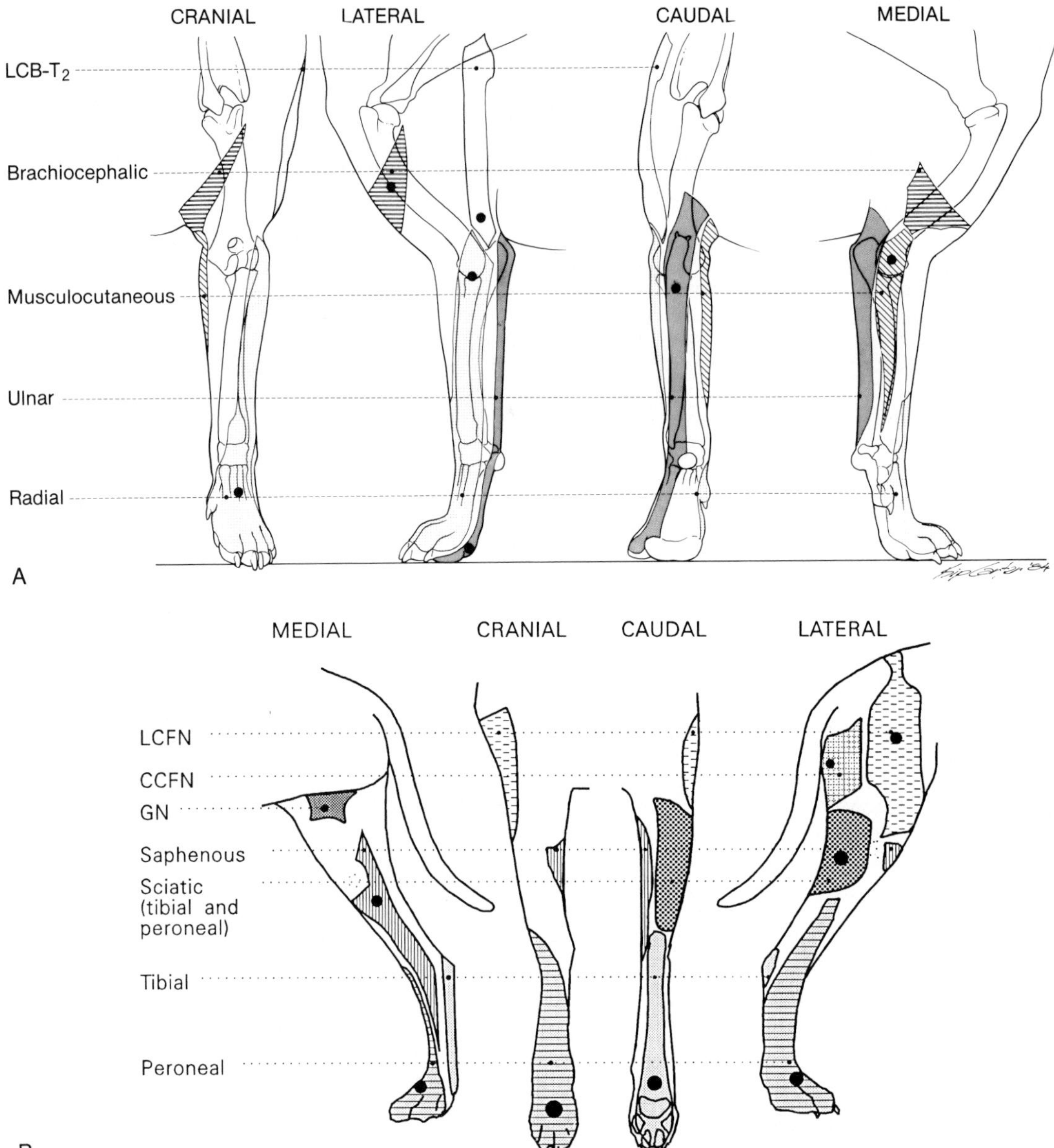

Figure 1–35 *A*. Cutaneous innervation of the left thoracic limb of the dog. Autonomous zones, innervated by only one nerve, are shown, along with recommended sites for testing for sensation (dots). The median nerve does not have an autonomous zone. LCB-T_2, lateral cutaneous branch of the second thoracic nerve. *B*. Cutaneous innervation of the right pelvic limb of the dog. Autonomous zones and testing sites are shown as in *A*. LCFN, lateral cutaneous femoral nerve L3, L4 (L5). CCFN, caudal cutaneous femoral nerve (L7), S1–S2. GN, genitofemoral nerve L(2), L3–L4. (*A* based on Kitchell RL, et al: Electrophysiological studies of cutaneous nerves of the thoracic limb of the dog. Am J Vet Res 41:61, 1980, and Bailey CS, Kitchell RL: Clinical evaluation of the cutaneous innervation of the canine thoracic limb. J Am Anim Hosp Assoc 20:939, 1984. *B* based on Haghighi SS, et al: Electrophysiologic studies of cutaneous innervation of the pelvic limb of male dogs. Am J Vet Res 52:352, 1991, and Bailey CS, Kitchell RL: Cutaneous sensory testing in the dog. J Vet Intern Med 1:128, 1987.)

movement, but the limb is accurately placed. The right limbs do not initiate movement at all. The tactile and visual placing reactions are prompt and accurate in the left thoracic limb, somewhat delayed and inconsistent in the left pelvic limb, and absent in the right limbs. The quadriceps reflex is a single, brisk response, and withdrawal is present when the toes in the left pelvic limb are touched. The extensor carpi radialis reflex is small but present in the left thoracic limb. Attempts to elicit a triceps or a biceps reflex in the left thoracic limb are unsuccessful, but withdrawal is strong with a weak pinch of the digits. The quadriceps reflex is slightly more brisk in the right pelvic limb than in the left pelvic limb. Withdrawal is strong. The extensor carpi radialis reflex is small but present.

Withdrawal is weak compared with the response of the left thoracic limb. The biceps and triceps reflexes cannot be elicited. The cranial nerves are normal. Sensation is present, except that pinching the skin of the right thoracic limb produces no reaction, and pinching a digit on this limb requires considerably more force to produce a behavioral response than does pinching a digit on the other limbs.

Case History 1B

Signalment

Canine, German shepherd, female, 7 years old.

History

The dog has hip dysplasia, which was first diagnosed at 1 year of age. There are no other medical problems, and vaccinations are current. The owners noticed the dog having difficulty with the pelvic limbs approximately 6 months ago. At first she just stumbled a bit on the steps or slipped on the kitchen floor. The problem has progressed slowly, and now she can no longer go up steps. They have noticed that she has some swaying of the rear quarters when she walks. Occasionally she will stumble and fall, even on good footing. They are not aware of any pain. Appetite and eliminations are normal.

Physical Examination

There are no significant physical abnormalities other than neurologic dysfunction.

Neurologic Examination

The dog is alert and responsive. She has some difficulty in getting up, especially on a slick surface. When she walks on the grass, there is some swaying of the rear quarters from side to side. Occasionally she knuckles one of the pelvic limbs and stumbles but does not fall. The pelvic limbs cross at times, but generally they are set wide apart. The thoracic limbs seem normal, but she carries much of her weight on them. The hopping and proprioceptive positioning reactions are good in the thoracic limbs. Hopping on the pelvic limbs is poor. When the dog's weight is shifted laterally, there is a long delay before the leg is moved. When she shifts the leg, it is not moved far enough to support her weight adequately, so that after approximately two hops she falls over. When the digits are knuckled over, she stands in that position without attempting to replace them in a normal position. Both pelvic limbs have similar reactions.

The spinal reflexes are considered normal in the thoracic limbs. The quadriceps reflex is more brisk in the left pelvic limb than in the right. The flexor reflexes are present in both pelvic limbs. The cranial nerves are normal. There are no areas of hyperesthesia on deep palpation of the limb and trunk. The panniculus reflex is present, beginning at approximately L7. The dog immediately reacts to a pinching of the skin of the pelvic limbs in all areas.

Case History 1C

Signalment

Feline, domestic short hair, female, 3 months old.

History

The kitten has always seemed more clumsy than the others in the litter. There were four kittens: one was born dead, and the other two seem normal. This kitten had some difficulty nursing but has grown well and is alert and active. She has a peculiar prancing gait and trembles at times. The owners do not think the condition is getting worse. If anything, the kitten is able to get around somewhat better than when she first started walking.

Physical Examination

No abnormalities are found other than those detected on the neurologic examination.

Neurologic Examination

The kitten is alert and eager to play. The gait is characterized by jerky, exaggerated steps and a swaying of the body. The limbs are picked up rapidly and slapped on the floor. At times, it appears that she stops the step before reaching the floor and lurches to one side. She tries to grab a piece of string with the thoracic limbs but is seldom successful. A head tremor is noticed at times. All postural reactions can be performed, but the movements are exaggerated. Initiation of hopping is slightly delayed, and the response is often too far or too short for proper support of weight. Proprioceptive positioning is present, but the foot is often placed more laterally than expected.

Myotatic reflexes are difficult to test because the kitten is so excited. Flexor reflexes are present in all four limbs.

The menace reaction is absent in both eyes, although the kitten can follow movements of objects, such as a piece of string. At times there is a slight side-to-side oscillation of the eyes. There do not appear to be fast and slow components to the eye movements. The pupillary light reflexes and the palpebral reflex are normal.

There is no hyperesthesia, and the kitten feels a weak pinch of the skin on all four limbs. The panniculus reflex is present, starting at approximately S1.

Case History 1D

Signalment

Feline, Siamese, male, 2 years old.

History

The right eye has seemed irritated for the past 2 months. Uveitis was diagnosed by another veterinarian, but treatment gave only temporary relief. The cat now seems to be lame in the right forelimb. The owners report a trembling of the head when the cat eats. In the last two days, the cat has seemed depressed and has refused to eat. There were no other problems in the past, and vaccinations are current.

Physical Examination

An ophthalmic examination confirms the diagnosis of anterior uveitis in the right eye. The cat is slightly depressed. No other abnormalities are found other than those detected on the neurologic examination.

Neurologic Examination

The cat is slightly depressed but responsive. The left thoracic limb knuckles over when he walks. A tremor of the head is evident when the cat is active, but it tends to disappear when he is at rest. Palpation reveals atrophy of the triceps and all of the muscles below the elbow of the left thoracic limb. The postural reactions are normal on the right side. The hopping reaction is poor (+1) in the left thoracic limb and absent (0) in the left pelvic limb. The proprioceptive positioning reaction is absent in both limbs on the left side. The extensor carpi radialis and flexor reflexes are absent in the left thoracic limb. The quadriceps reflex is exaggerated (+3) in the left pelvic limb as compared with the right pelvic limb. The flexion reflex is present and of approximately the same strength in the left pelvic limb as in the right pelvic limb. Perineal reflexes are present. The cranial nerves are normal, except for miosis of the left eye, which presumably is related to the uveitis. There are no areas of hyperesthesia, and sensation is intact, including superficial and deep pain sensation in the left thoracic limb.

Case History 1E

Signalment

Canine, Yorkshire terrier, male, 8 months old.

History

The dog has been vaccinated in your clinic. Although he has had a reasonably good appetite, he has always been thin and small. Recently the dog has had episodes of abnormal behavior. He paces continuously and resents being held. At times he stops and just stands and stares straight ahead. If someone tries to pick him up at these times, he appears startled. The episodes usually last for 2 to 3 hours, but on occasion he has seemed abnormal for an entire day. The owners cannot recall any days in the past 3 weeks when the dog did not have an "attack."

Physical Examination

The dog is very thin but otherwise normal.

Neurologic Examination

At the time of the initial examination, the dog is normal. Because of the history and the suspicion of metabolic disease, the dog is hospitalized for further evaluation. Food is withheld for 12 hours, blood and urine are collected for laboratory examination, and the dog is given a meal of cat food. Six hours later, the dog is reexamined. At this time he seems depressed. Although his gait seems relatively normal, he walks continually around the room. Limb movement is somewhat jerky, and he occasionally bumps into a chair or a table. Postural reactions are present, but they all appear to be somewhat slow in all limbs. The dog becomes agitated during these reactions. If he is restrained on the table, he becomes quiet and almost goes to sleep. The spinal reflexes are normal. The menace response is present at times but is not consistent. Other cranial nerve responses are normal. The dog's reaction to painful stimuli is somewhat slow but present.

Construct a sign-time graph, a list of rule-outs (general categories of diseases), and interpret the neurologic examination before reviewing the assessments.

Assessment 1A

History. This dog's problem is tetraparesis with an acute onset and no progression. There are two primary groups of diseases that fit: trauma and vascular lesions. Inflammatory (infectious) diseases may have an acute onset, but they are usually progressive. Intervertebral disk problems usually have a slower onset unless they are associated with trauma.

Rule-outs:

1. vascular lesion,
2. trauma, and
3. inflammation (low probability).

Asking additional questions regarding possible sources of trauma proved unrewarding.

Neurologic Examination. The dog's mental status suggests that the cerebrum, the diencephalon, and the rostral brain stem are relatively normal. The dog cannot support weight and cannot move the right limbs voluntarily, indicating hemiparesis. Is the problem strictly unilateral? This question is answered by assessing postural reactions. The right side is obviously abnormal. The left thoracic limb has normal postural reactions, but there is some delay in initiating the hopping reaction in the left pelvic limb. Is that finding abnormal? The answer is maybe. If the hopping reaction is only slightly delayed, you should be cautious in calling it abnormal. Most dogs do not hop as well on the pelvic limbs as on the thoracic limbs. Placing reactions also are difficult to assess in the pelvic limbs. Proprioceptive positioning is more reliable, and this reaction is normal in the left pelvic limb. The extensor postural thrust reaction also can be helpful. In this dog, it appears to be somewhat slow in initiation. We assessed the postural reactions as absent on the right, normal in the left thoracic limb, and questionable in the left pelvic limb.

The quadriceps reflex in the left pelvic limb is brisk but not abnormal for this breed. Smaller dogs have relatively brisk reflexes. The significant finding is that the right quadriceps reflex is stronger than the left. Comparing the two sides gives the examiner a built-in control. We assessed the left quadriceps reflex as normal (+2) and the right as exaggerated (+3). Withdrawals (flexor reflex) are present and strong in both pelvic limbs. The extensor carpi radialis reflex is small, but present and approximately equal, in both thoracic limbs. This reflex is rarely strong and usually is abnormal if it is strong. The triceps and biceps reflexes are absent in both thoracic limbs. Is this finding abnormal? Not in our assessment. These reflexes are so difficult to elicit that we rarely use them. The flexor reflex is markedly weaker on the right than on the left. This is the most significant finding. Either the sensory or motor neurons (or both) of the reflex are damaged. The sensory examination is useful for deciding which neuron type is involved.

Sensation, both superficial and deep, is normal, except in the right thoracic limb. No response is obtained to pinching or to pinprick of the skin distal to the elbow. The rostral, caudal, medial, and lateral surfaces are similar. The dog does respond to a forceful pinch of the digits. The mapping of the distribution of sensory deficits is important for differentiating peripheral nerve lesions from spinal cord lesions.

The localization of the lesion in this case will be discussed at the end of Chapter 2.

Assessment 1B

History. The dog's problems are pelvic limb paresis and ataxia with a chronic onset and a progressive course. A number of diseases can be chronic and progressive (see Fig. 1–2). When the neurologic examination is performed, it is important to establish whether the disease is focal or diffuse. With the information we have, we would include degenerative diseases, neoplasia, and inflammation as the primary rule-outs. Metabolic and nutritional diseases are more likely to affect the whole animal.

Rule-outs:

1. degenerative diseases,
2. neoplasia, and
3. inflammation.

Neurologic Examination. The gait can be described as pelvic limb ataxia and paresis. The swaying movements of the rear quarters indicate some loss of function in paraspinal muscles. The hopping reactions are indicative of both sensory and motor deficits. The slow initiation of the reaction usually means that proprioception is poor. This finding is also confirmed by the complete absence of proprioceptive positioning. The inadequate movement of the limb as the weight is shifted indicates some paresis and loss of motor function. This dog also has some asymmetry in the quadriceps reflex, with the left slightly more brisk than the right. The dog's cranial nerves and sensation are considered normal.

The localization of the lesion in this case will be discussed at the end of Chapter 2.

Assessment 1C

History. The history suggests that the problem is ataxia and tremors of the entire body with onset at birth and no progression. The onset suggests an anomaly or a birth injury. Either of these problems could be nonprogressive. Most of the other diseases affecting neonates, such as degenerative or inflammatory diseases, are progressive.

Rule-outs:

1. anomaly and
2. trauma.

Neurologic Examination. The gait can be described as trunkal ataxia with dysmetria of all four limbs. There is no paresis at gait or on postural reactions. Dysmetria is caused by a loss of coordination between the initiation and the follow-through of a movement. The movement overshoots or undershoots its target. The head tremor was most apparent when the kitten initiated a movement and disappeared at rest. This is an intention tremor. Postural reactions can be difficult to induce when an animal is uncoordinated, but it is important to determine the presence of any paresis. Spinal reflexes also may be difficult to elicit, especially in a young, excited animal. Flexor reflexes can always be tested. The absent menace reaction ordinarily indicates an abnormality in the visual pathways (afferent) or in the facial nerve (efferent). The animal can see and can follow moving objects, however, and the palpebral reflex is intact.

The localization of the lesion will be discussed at the end of Chapter 2.

Assessment 1D

History. The cat has ocular disease, trembling of the head, lameness of the right thoracic limb, and depression. The disease is chronic and progressive. Chronic progressive diseases include degenerative, metabolic, neoplastic, inflammatory, and nutritional diseases. If the neurologic examination substantiates that the signs are multifocal in origin, as the history suggests, then metabolic and nutritional diseases would be much lower on the list.

Rule-outs:

1. inflammatory disease,
2. neoplastic disease, and
3. degenerative disease.

Neurologic Examination. The slight depression and the head tremor suggest that this cat has brain disease, although it is possible that these findings are merely manifestations of generalized disease. The lameness of the left thoracic limb suggests a more focal abnormality. The postural reactions confirm the diagnosis of an abnormality in this limb and in the left pelvic limb; therefore, this is a hemiparesis. The spinal reflexes are absent in the left thoracic limb and present (flexion) to exaggerated (quadriceps reflex) in the left pelvic limb. Atrophy of the muscles of the left thoracic limb is also significant. You should immediately wonder whether the atrophy is a result of disuse or denervation. The history does not give a clear indication of the duration of the lameness. (Disuse atrophy is slow, whereas denervation atrophy is rapid.) Note, however, that the triceps and the muscles below the elbow are atrophied, but the flexors of the elbow and the scapular muscles are not. This finding is strongly indicative of denervation rather than disuse. The sensory examination indicates that the afferent nerves of the limb are intact. With a peripheral nerve lesion, one would expect both motor and sensory loss. Atrophy, loss of reflexes, and intact sensation indicate a lesion in the ventral spinal nerve roots or the motor neurons in the spinal cord. The postural reaction deficits in the pelvic limb on the same side indicate spinal cord disease.

Localization of the lesions will be discussed at the end of Chapter 2.

Assessment 1E

History. The problem is primarily an abnormality in mental status. The neurologic examination is needed to determine if other abnormalities are present. The onset is chronic and the course progressive, but the entire syndrome is episodic. Episodic disorders other than seizures are usually metabolic in origin. Toxicities can wax and wane with exposure, but this phenomenon is rare. Structural disorders such as degeneration, neoplasia, and inflammation may be accompanied by signs that wax and wane, but are rarely associated with periods of normal activity.

Rule-outs:

1. metabolic disorder and
2. toxic disorder.

Neurologic Examination. In addition to being depressed, the dog makes inappropriate responses. He becomes agitated during postural reaction testing but then dozes off when restrained on the table. The menace reaction is not always present. A sharp tap on the eyelid (palpebral reflex) followed by a menacing gesture almost always elicits a response. Menacing gestures at other times may not produce a reaction. This finding is suggestive of inattention rather than loss of vision and may be seen in animals that are severely depressed, disoriented, or demented. The reaction to painful stimuli is interpreted similarly.

The localization of the lesion will be discussed at the end of Chapter 2.

Further questioning regarding the timing of the episodes with feeding revealed that the dog was fed morning and evening. The usual diet was canned dog food. The episodes usually occurred 2 to 4 hours after feeding. This situation is typical of hepatic encephalopathy (see Chap. 13).

REFERENCES

1. Weed LL: Medical Records, Medical Education and Patient Care. Chicago, Year Book Medical Publishers, 1971.
2. Osborne CA, Low DG: The medical history redefined: Idealism vs. realism. Proc AAHA 207–213, 1976.
3. Oliver JE: Neurologic examinations: Taking the history. Vet Med Small Anim Clin 67:433–434, 1972.
4. Oliver JE: Neurologic examinations: Observations on mental status. Vet Med Small Anim Clin 67:654–659, 1972.
5. Oliver JE: Neurologic examinations: Observations on posture. Vet Med Small Anim Clin 67:882–884, 1972.
6. Oliver JE: Neurologic examinations: Observations on movement. Vet Med Small Anim Clin 67:1105–1106, 1972.
7. de Lahunta A: Veterinary Neuroanatomy and Clinical Neurology, 2nd ed. Philadelphia, WB Saunders, 1983.
8. Oliver JE, Hoerlein BF, Mayhew IG: Veterinary Neurology. Philadelphia, WB Saunders, 1987.
9. Mayhew IG: Large Animal Neurology: A Handbook for Veterinary Clinicians. Philadelphia, Lea & Febiger, 1989.
10. Grillner S: Neurobiological bases of rhythmic motor acts in vertebrates. Science 228:143–149, 1985.
11. Grillner S: Locomotion in vertebrates: Central mechanisms and reflex interaction. Physiol Rev 55:247–304, 1975.
12. Willis JB: On the interaction between spinal locomotor generators in quadripeds. Brain Res Rev 2:171–204, 1980.
13. Breazile JE, Blaugh BS, Nail N: Experimental study of canine distemper myoclonus. Am J Vet Res 27:1375–1379, 1966.
14. Oliver JE: Neurologic examinations: Palpation and inspection. Vet Med Small Anim Clin 67:1327–1328, 1972.
15. Oliver JE: Neurologic examinations—sensation: Proprioception and touch. Vet Med Small Anim Clin 67: 295–298, 1972.
16. Holliday TA: The origins of the neurological examination: The postural and attitudinal, placing and righting reactions. In: Proceedings of the Seventh Annual Veterinary Medical Forum, San Diego, 1989, pp 980–983.
17. Roberts TDM: Neurophysiology of Postural Mechanisms. New York, Plenum Press, 1967.
18. Thor KB, Morgan C, Nadelhaft I, Houston M, De Groat W: Organization of afferent and efferent pathways in the pudendal nerve of the female cat. J Comp Neurol 288:263–279, 1989.
19. Oliver JE: Neurologic examinations: Flexion and crossed extension reflexes. Vet Med Small Anim Clin 68:383–385, 1973.
20. Oliver JE: Neurologic examinations—spinal reflexes: Extensor thrust reflex. Vet Med Small Anim Clin 68:763, 1973.
21. Kneller S, Oliver J, Lewis R: Differential diagnosis of progressive caudal paresis in an aged German shepherd dog. J Am Anim Hosp Assoc 11:414–417, 1975.
22. Hoff H, Breckenridge C: Observations on the mammalian reflex prototype of the sign of Babinski. Brain 79:155–167, 1966.
23. Myers LJ, Nusbaum KE, Swango LJ, Hanrahan LN, Sartin E: Dysfunction of sense of smell caused by canine parainfluenza virus infection in dogs. Am J Vet Res 49:188–190, 1988.
24. Oliver JE: Neurologic examinations—sensation: Pain. Vet Med Small Anim Clin 69:607–610, 1974.
25. Willis WD, Coggeshall RE: Sensory Mechanisms of the Spinal Cord, 2nd ed. New York, Plenum Press, 1991.

26. Willis WD, Jr: The Pain System: The Neural Basis of Nociceptive Transmission in the Mammalian Nervous System. Basel, S Karger, 1985.
27. Willis W, Chung J: Central mechanisms of pain. J Am Vet Med Assoc 191:1200–1202, 1987.
28. Kirk E: The dermatomes of the sheep. J Comp Neurol 134:353–370, 1968.
29. Bailey C, Kitchell R, Haghighi S, Johnson R: Cutaneous innervation of the thorax and abdomen of the dog. Am J Vet Res 45:1689–1698, 1984.
30. Fletcher T, Kitchell R: The lumbar, sacral and coccygeal tactile dermatomes of the dog. J Comp Neurol 128:171–180, 1966.
31. Kirk E, Kitchell R, Johnson R: Neurophysiologic maps of cutaneous innervation of the hind limb of sheep. Am J Vet Res 48:1485–1492, 1987.
32. Hekmatpanah J: Organization of tactile dermatomes, C1 through L4, in cat. J Neurophysiol 24:129–140, 1961.

2

Localization of Lesions in the Nervous System

Functional Organization of the Nervous System

Comprehensive knowledge of the anatomy and physiology of the nervous system is very useful in clinical neurology; however, the majority of neurologic problems in clinical practice can be diagnosed and managed through knowledge of the principles of neural organization. This section provides a review and summary of the principles introduced in Chapter 1.[1]

Motor System

Lower Motor Neuron

Definition. The lower motor neuron (LMN) is an efferent neuron connecting the central nervous system (CNS) to an effector (muscle or gland). Any activity of the nervous system ultimately is expressed through LMNs. LMNs are located in all spinal cord segments in the intermediate and ventral horns of the gray matter and in cranial nerve nuclei (CN III–VII, IX–XII) in the brain stem. The axons extending from these cells form the peripheral spinal and cranial nerves (Fig. 2–1).

The nervous system is arranged in a segmental fashion. A spinal cord segment is demarcated by a pair of spinal nerves. Each spinal nerve has a dorsal (sensory) and a ventral (motor) root (Fig. 2–2). The segmentation of the brain is less uniform, but anatomically and functionally distinct sections can be identified (Fig. 2–3). The muscle or group of muscles innervated by one spinal nerve is called a *myotome*. Myotomes are arranged segmentally in the paraspinal muscles but are more irregular in the limbs. Dysfunction of specific muscle is localizing to a spinal nerve or a ventral root (Fig. 2–4).

Signs of LMN *Lesions.* Lesions of the LMN, whether of the cell body or the axon, produce a characteristic group of clinical signs, summarized in Table 2–1. Signs of LMN lesions are easily recognized on neurologic examination. Paralysis, loss of tone, and loss of reflexes occur immediately after the neuron is damaged. Proper interpretation of LMN signs allows the clinician to accurately localize lesions to a peripheral nerve, a nerve root, or a motor neuron within the brain or the spinal cord.

Most muscles are innervated by nerves that originate in more than one spinal cord segment. For example, the quadriceps muscle is innervated by neurons originating in segments L4–L6. Loss of one segment or one root causes partial loss of the innervation of the muscle. The clinical sign is paresis, but not paralysis, of the affected muscles. The reflexes may be depressed. Lesions of peripheral nerves are more likely to cause severe loss of function, and all muscles innervated by the nerve are affected. The reflexes are usually absent in this case (see Fig. 2–4).

Upper Motor Neuron

Definition. *Upper motor neuron* (UMN) is a collective term for motor systems in the brain that control lower motor neurons. The UMN systems are responsible for the initiation and maintenance of normal movements and for the maintenance of tone in the extensor muscles to support the body against gravity. The cell bodies are located in the cerebral cortex, the basal nu-

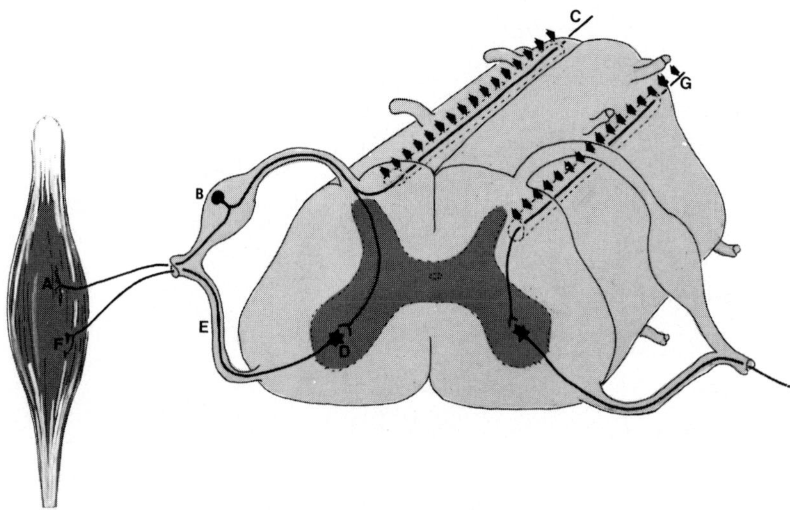

Figure 2–1 Components of the spinal reflex. *A*, muscle spindle; *B*, dorsal root ganglion; *C*, ascending sensory pathway in the dorsal column; *D*, ventral horn motor neuron (LMN); *E*, ventral (motor) root; *F*, neuromuscular junction; *G*, descending motor pathway in the lateral column (UMN). The dorsal and ventral roots join to form the peripheral nerve. (From Oliver JE: Neurologic examination. VM/SAC 68:151–154, 1973. Used by permission.)

clei, and the brain stem. The pathways include primary corticospinal and multisynaptic systems from most parts of the brain (Fig. 2–5; see also discussion under Gait in Chap. 1).

Signs of UMN *Lesions.* UMN lesions produce a characteristic set of clinical signs caudal to the level of the injury. These signs are summarized in Table 2–1 and are compared with signs of LMN lesions. The primary sign of motor dysfunction is paresis. With UMN disease, the paresis or paralysis is associated with increased extensor tone and normal or exaggerated reflexes. Abnormal reflexes (e.g., a crossed extensor reflex) may be seen in some cases. Loss of descending inhibition on the LMN produces these findings. UMN signs are more common than LMN signs in clinical patients. Because lesions at many different levels of the CNS may produce UMN signs, localization of a lesion to a specific segment usually is not possible when only UMN signs are considered. Proper interpretation of UMN signs and other associated signs, however, allows one to localize a lesion to a region. For example, UMN paresis of the pelvic limbs indicates a lesion cranial to L4. If the lesion were at L4–S2, there would be LMN paresis. If the thoracic limbs are normal, the lesion must be caudal to T2. Therefore, pelvic limb paresis (UMN) with normal thoracic limbs indicates a lesion between T3 and L3.

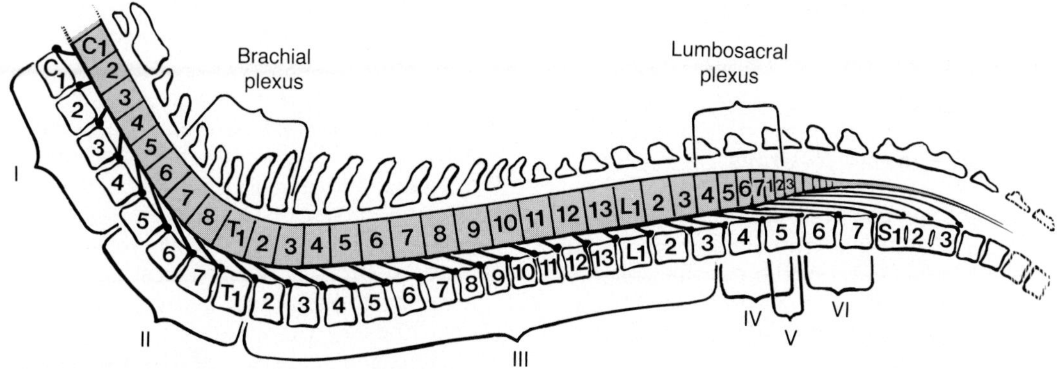

Figure 2–2 The spinal cord has a segmental arrangement; each segment has a pair of spinal nerves. The approximate relationship of spinal cord segments and vertebrae in the dog is illustrated here. Regions of the spinal cord that give rise to characteristic clinical signs when damaged are labeled. *I*, C1–C5, upper motor neuron (UMN) to all limbs; *II*, C6–T2, lower motor neuron (LMN) to thoracic, UMN to pelvic limbs; *III*, T3–L3, normal thoracic, UMN to pelvic limbs; *IV*, L4–S2, normal thoracic, LMN to pelvic limbs; *V*, S1–S3, partial LMN to pelvic limbs, absent perineal reflex, atonic bladder; *VI*, caudal nerves, atonic tail.

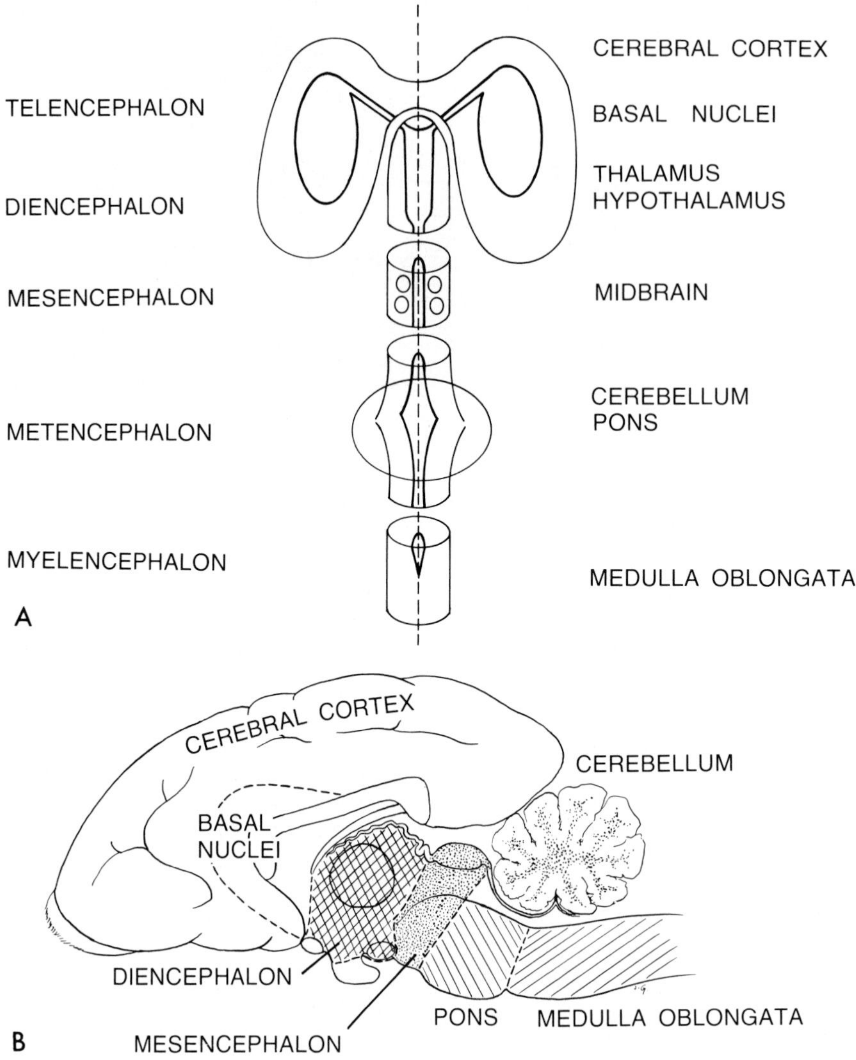

Figure 2–3 Segmental organization of the brain. Five major regions are significant clinically: the cerebrum, including the cerebral cortex, cerebral white matter, and the basal nuclei; the diencephalon, including the thalamus and the hypothalamus; the brain stem, including the midbrain, the pons, and the medulla oblongata; the vestibular system, including the labyrinth (peripheral) and the vestibular nuclei (central) in the rostral medulla; and the cerebellum. (From Hoerlein BF: Canine Neurology, 3rd ed. Philadelphia, WB Saunders Co., 1978. Used by permission.)

Sensory System

Segmental Sensory Neurons

Definition. Sensory neurons are located in the ganglia of the dorsal roots along the spinal cord (see Fig. 2–1) and in the ganglia of some cranial nerves. Exceptions are the special sensory pathways (olfaction, vision, hearing, balance).

The area of skin innervated by one spinal nerve is called a *dermatome*. Dermatomes also are arranged in regular segmental fashion, except for some variation in the limbs (see Fig. 1–32). Alterations in the sensation of a dermatome can be used to localize a lesion to a spinal nerve or a dorsal root. The area of skin innervated by the sensory neurons of a named peripheral nerve have a different distribution (see Fig. 1–35), allowing localization of lesions of peripheral nerves.

Signs of Sensory Neuron Lesions. Lesions of the sensory neurons also produce characteristic clinical signs. Segmental sensory signs include (1) anesthesia (complete lesion), (2) hypesthesia (decreased sensation, partial lesion), (3) hyperesthesia (increased sensation of pain, irritative lesion), and (4) loss of reflexes. Increased or decreased sensation of a dermatome can be mapped by pinching the skin. Mapping the distribution of sensory loss is accurate to within three spinal cord segments (see Chap. 1). Similarly, the alteration of sensitivity in the distribution of a named peripheral nerve localizes the lesion accurately.

Long Tract Sensory Pathways

Definition. Sensory pathways of clinical significance include those responsible for proprioception (position sense) and pain. Sensory neurons from the body are located in the dorsal root ganglia and synapse in the gray matter of the spinal cord (see Fig. 2–1). Proprioceptive pathways are located in the dorsal and dorsolateral portions of the spinal cord. They project to the cerebral cortex and the cerebellum by relays in the brain stem and thalamus. Superficial pain pathways (for perception of discrete pain in the skin, e.g., a pinprick) are located primarily in the ventrolateral (primate) or dorsolateral (cat) portion of the spinal cord, with a relay in the thalamus.[2] The pathway primarily projects to the contralateral cerebral cortex for conscious recognition of pain. The deep pain pathway (for perception of severe pain in the bones, the joints, or the viscera, e.g., a crushing pain) is a bilateral, multisynaptic system that projects to the reticular formation, the thalamus, and the cerebral cortex.[3,4]

Signs of Long Tract Sensory Lesions. The signs of sensory long tract lesions are valuable for the formulation of a prognosis of CNS disorders and for localization. Spinal cord lesions frequently cause decreased sensation caudal to the level of the lesion. Proprioceptive deficits usually are the first signs observed with compressive lesions of the spinal cord. Abnormal positioning of the feet and ataxia may be present before there is any significant loss of voluntary motor activity. Superficial pain sensation (the conscious perception of a pinprick) and voluntary motor activity often are lost at the same time. Deep pain sensation (perception of a strong pinch of a bone or a joint) is the last neurologic function to be lost during spinal cord compression.[5] The level of a spinal cord lesion can be determined if a level of hypesthesia or anesthesia can be detected.

Localization of Lesions

Localization to a Region of the Spinal Cord or the Brain

UMN and LMN Signs

The examination of the motor system should allow the clinician to localize the lesion to one of five levels of the spinal cord or to the brain (see Figs. 2–2 and 2–3). The thoracic and pelvic limbs should be classified as normal or as exhibiting LMN or UMN signs (see Table 2–1). Briefly, LMN signs are paresis, a loss of reflexes, and a loss of tone. UMN signs are a loss of voluntary motor activity (paresis), an increase in tone, and an exaggeration of reflexes. Note that in both cases, paresis (paralysis) is the primary finding. The status of the reflexes distinguishes between the two. The examiner can localize a lesion to a region of the spinal cord or the brain by using these findings and the material presented in Figure 2–6. Figure 2–6 is an algorithm that explains the logic of the diagnosis. For example, paresis in the pelvic limbs with normal thoracic limbs indicates that the brain and spinal cord as far caudal as T2 are functioning. Therefore, there is a lesion caudal to T2. To determine if the lesion is in the T3–L3 or L4–S2 segments, the reflexes of the pelvic limb must be evaluated. If they are normal or exaggerated, the L4–S2 segments must be functioning and the lesion is between T3 and L3. If the reflexes are decreased or absent, the lesion is in the L4–S2 segments. Paresis or paralysis of all four limbs indicates a lesion cranial to T3. Reflexes are tested in all four limbs. Normal or exaggerated reflexes of all limbs indicates a lesion above C6. Other findings are used to localize the lesion further. In this case, one should examine the cranial nerves in order to rule out brain stem disease. The sensory examination is reviewed for possible signs related to the neck (i.e., C1–C5).

Using only the information related to LMN and UMN signs of the limbs, the examiner can localize the lesion to one of the following regions: (1) the brain, (2) C1–C5, (3) C6–T2—brachial plexus (thoracic limb), (4) T3–L3, (5) L4–S2—lumbosacral plexus (pelvic limb), or (6) S3–Cd5. Case histories at the end of the chapter can be used to test the reader's understanding of this concept.

Proprioception

For the purpose of localization, abnormalities of proprioception are interpreted in the same way as UMN signs. For example, loss of proprioception in the pelvic limbs with normal thoracic limbs indicates a lesion in the region of T3–L3 (Table 2–1). Spinal nerve or peripheral nerve lesions may cause a loss of proprioceptive positioning, but the LMN signs are obvious.

Localization to a Segmental Level of the Spinal Cord

LMN Signs

If LMN signs are present in the limbs, the examiner can localize the lesion further by identifying

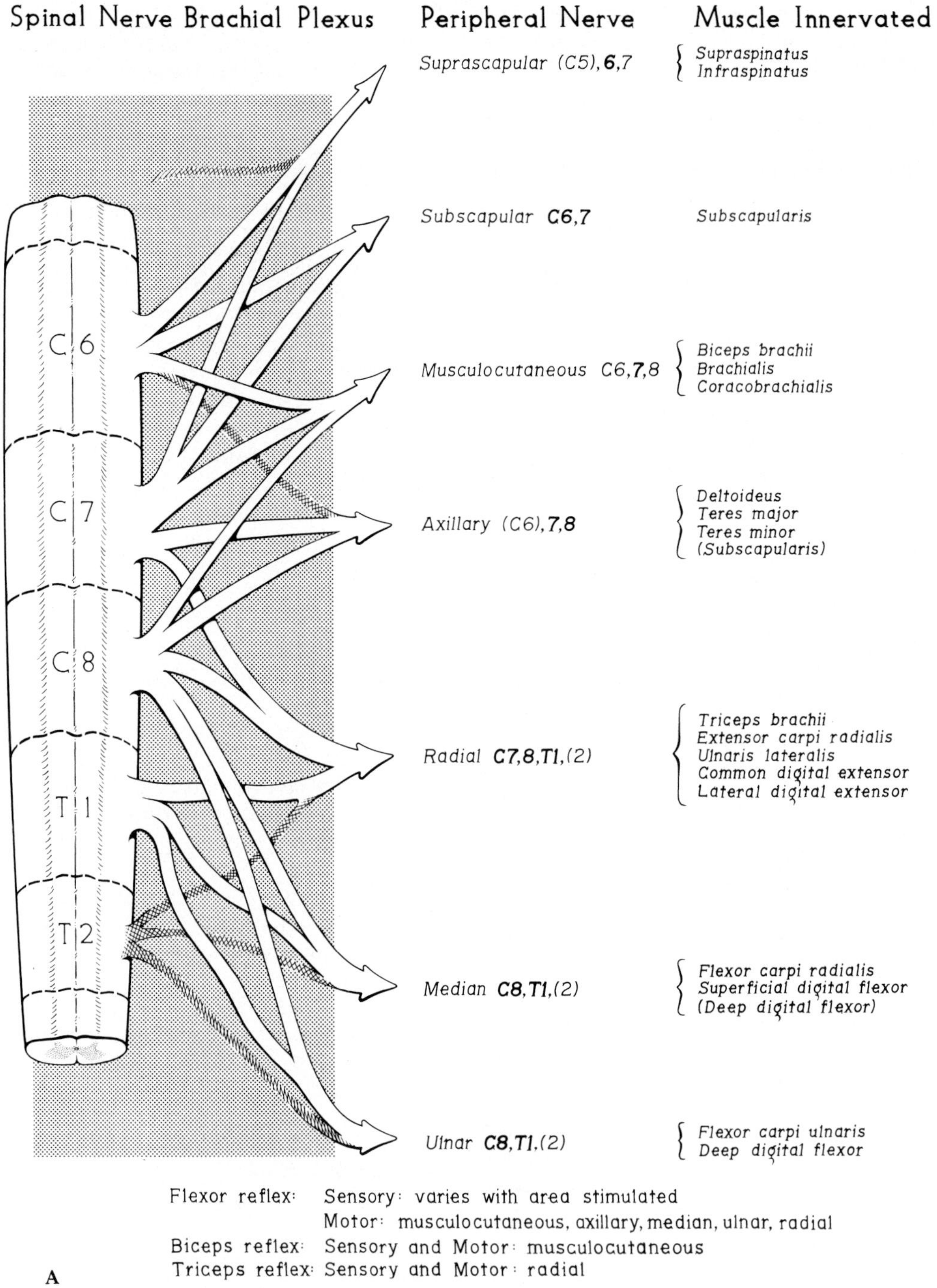

Spinal Nerve Brachial Plexus	Peripheral Nerve	Muscle Innervated
	Suprascapular (C5), **6**,7	Supraspinatus Infraspinatus
	Subscapular **C6,7**	Subscapularis
C6	Musculocutaneous C6,**7**,8	Biceps brachii Brachialis Coracobrachialis
C7	Axillary (C6),**7,8**	Deltoideus Teres major Teres minor (Subscapularis)
C8	Radial **C7,8,T1**,(2)	Triceps brachii Extensor carpi radialis Ulnaris lateralis Common digital extensor Lateral digital extensor
T1	Median **C8,T1**,(2)	Flexor carpi radialis Superficial digital flexor (Deep digital flexor)
T2	Ulnar **C8,T1**,(2)	Flexor carpi ulnaris Deep digital flexor

Flexor reflex: Sensory: varies with area stimulated
Motor: musculocutaneous, axillary, median, ulnar, radial
Biceps reflex: Sensory and Motor: musculocutaneous
Triceps reflex: Sensory and Motor: radial

A

Figure 2–4 *A*. Segmental innervation from cervical intumescence of thoracic limb muscles in the dog. *B*. Segmental innervation from lumbosacral intumescence of pelvic limb muscles in the dog. (From de Lahunta A: Veterinary Neuroanatomy and Clinical Neurology. Philadelphia, WB Saunders Co., 1977. Used by permission.)

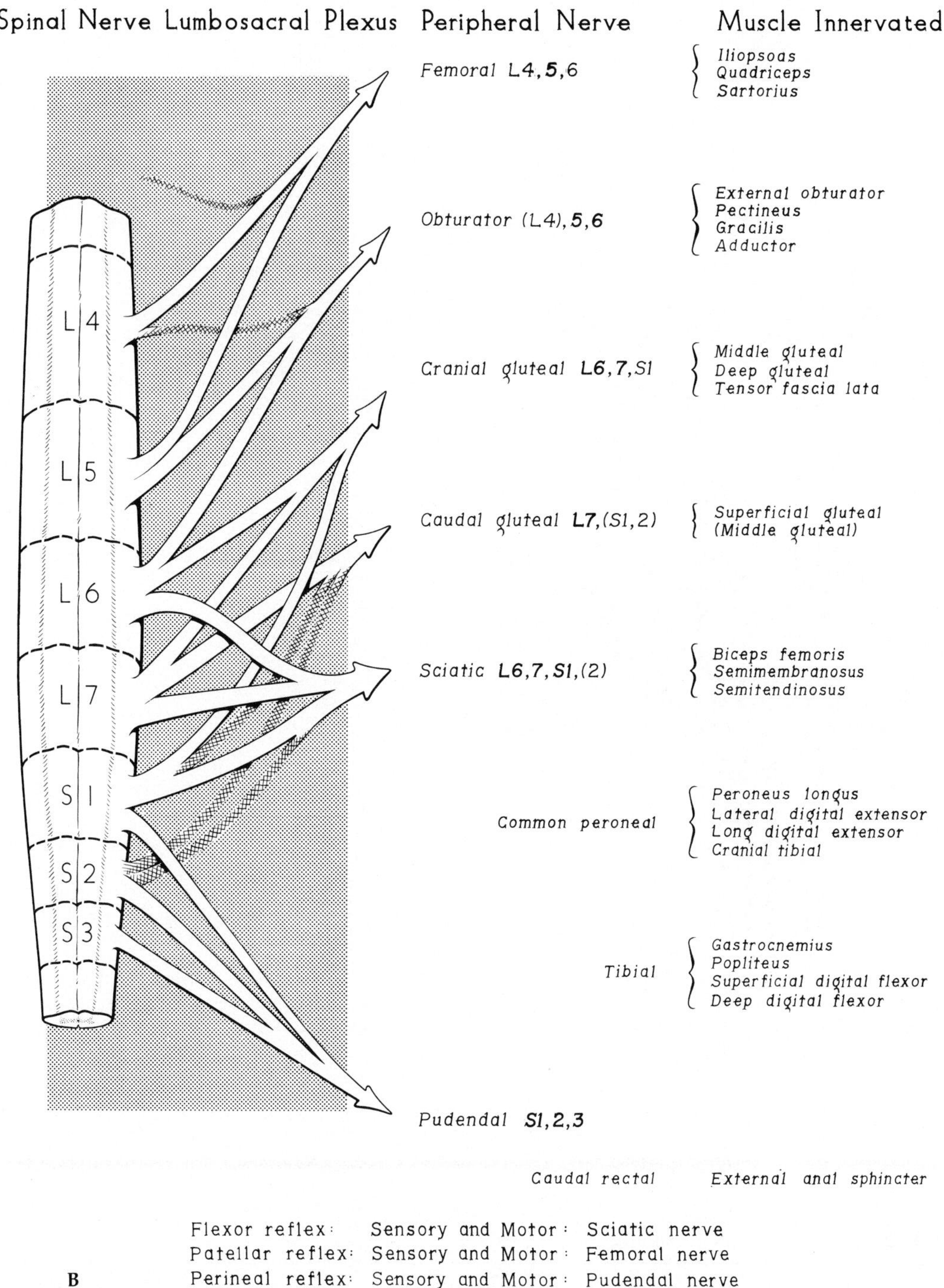
Spinal Nerve
Lumbosacral Plexus
Peripheral Nerve
Muscle Innervated
L4
L5
L6
L7
S1
S2
S3
Femoral L4, 5, 6
Iliopsoas
Quadriceps
Sartorius
Obturator (L4), 5, 6
External obturator
Pectineus
Gracilis
Adductor
Cranial gluteal L6, 7, S1
Middle gluteal
Deep gluteal
Tensor fascia lata
Caudal gluteal L7, (S1, 2)
Superficial gluteal
(Middle gluteal)
Sciatic L6, 7, S1, (2)
Biceps femoris
Semimembranosus
Semitendinosus
Common peroneal
Peroneus longus
Lateral digital extensor
Long digital extensor
Cranial tibial
Tibial
Gastrocnemius
Popliteus
Superficial digital flexor
Deep digital flexor
Pudendal S1, 2, 3
Caudal rectal
External anal sphincter
Flexor reflex: Sensory and Motor: Sciatic nerve
Patellar reflex: Sensory and Motor: Femoral nerve
Perineal reflex: Sensory and Motor: Pudendal nerve

B

Figure 2–4 See legend on opposite page

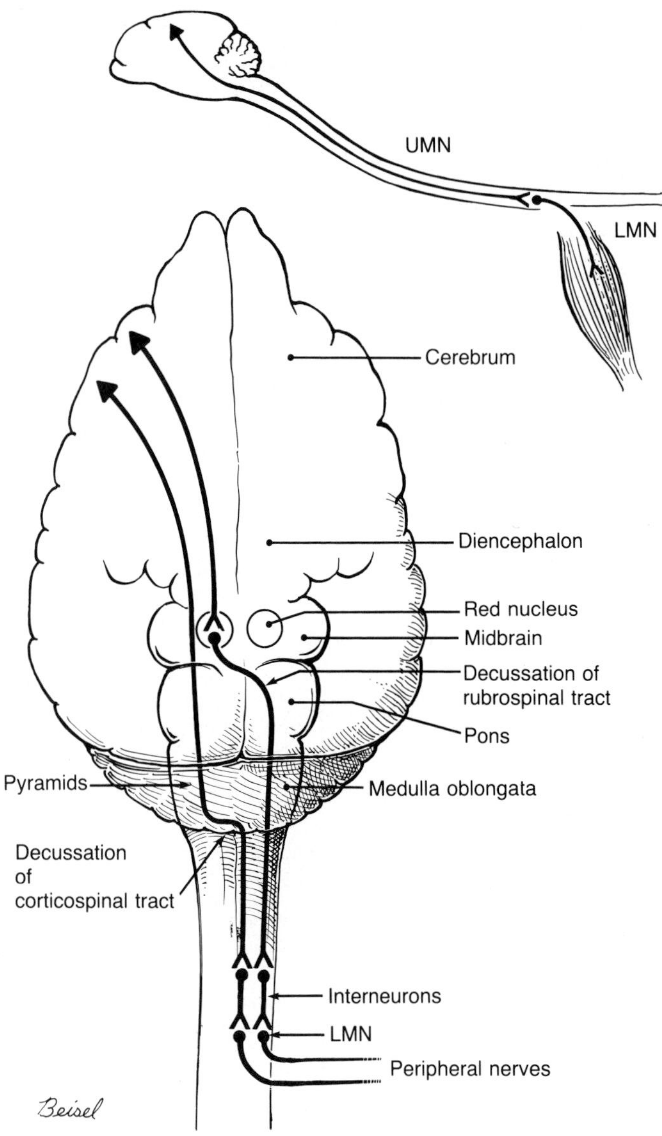

Figure 2–5 Neurons in the cerebral cortex and the brain stem send axons to the lower motor neurons (LMN) in the brain stem and the spinal cord. The upper motor neurons (UMN) provide voluntary control of movement. Two of the major voluntary motor pathways, the corticospinal (pyramidal) pathway and the corticorubrospinal pathway, are illustrated.

TABLE 2–1 Summary of LMN and UMN Signs

	LMN: Segmental Signs	***UMN: Long Tract Signs***
Motor function	Paralysis – loss of muscle power, flaccidity	Paresis to paralysis – loss of voluntary movements
Reflexes	Hyporeflexia to areflexia	Normal to hyperreflexia (especially myotatic reflexes)
Muscle atrophy	Early and severe: neurogenic; contracture after several weeks	Late and mild: disuse
Muscle tone	Decreased	Normal to increased
Electromyographic changes	Abnormal potentials (fibrillation, positive sharp waves) after 5 to 7 days	No changes
Associated sensory signs	Anesthesia of innervated area (dermatome); paresthesia or hyperesthesia of adjacent areas	Decreased proprioception, decreased perception of superficial and deep pain

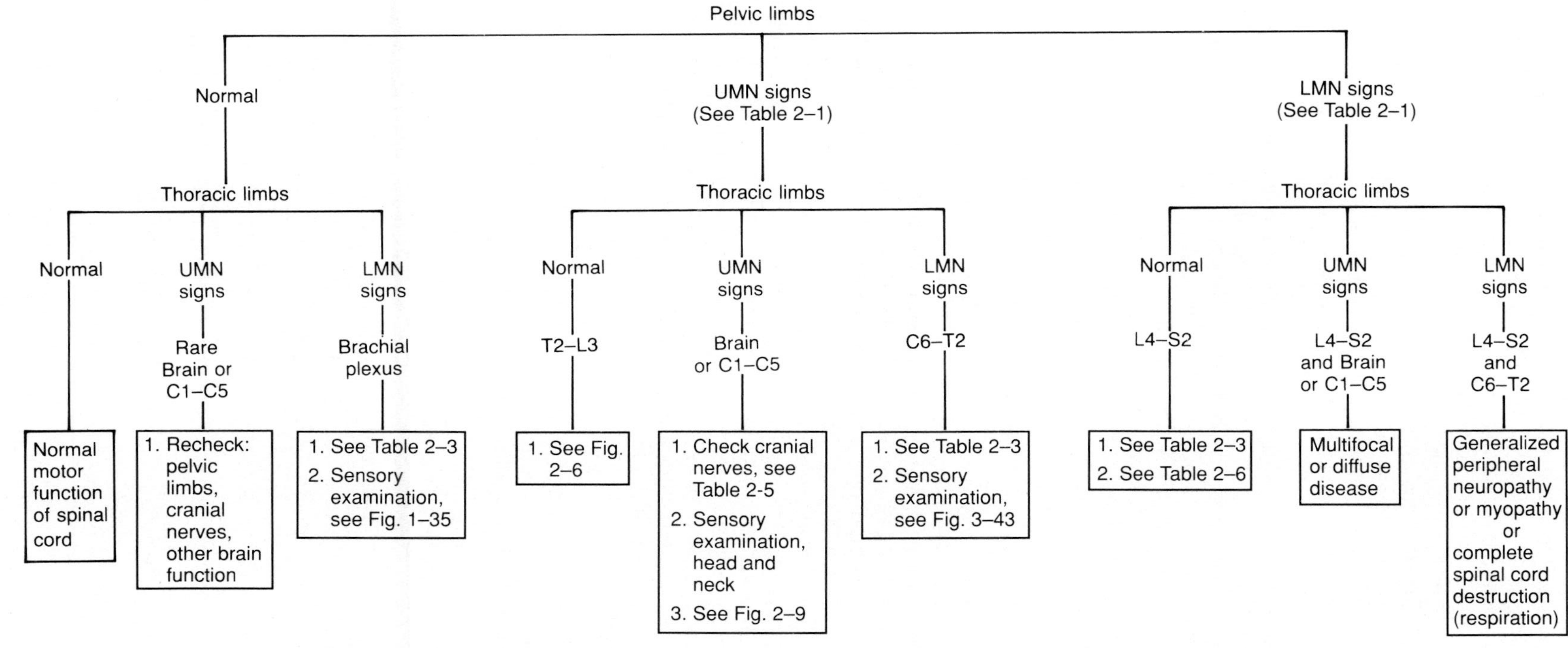

Figure 2–6 Localization of lesions based on motor function. *UMN*, upper motor neuron; *LMN*, lower motor neuron; *C*, cervical; *T*, thoracic; *L*, lumbar; *S*, sacral spinal cord segments. (From Hoerlein BF: Canine Neurology, 3rd ed. Philadelphia, WB Saunders Co., 1978. Used by permission.)

the affected muscles. Table 2–2 lists spinal cord segments (roots) and peripheral nerves for the most commonly tested reflexes. It is possible to localize within two to four segments or to a peripheral nerve if LMN signs are present. Spinal cord segments do not correlate directly with vertebral levels. When the examiner has determined the spinal cord level, Figure 2–2 can be referred to for an estimation of the vertebral level.

Peripheral nerve lesions usually cause monoparesis (paresis of one limb) because the most common lesions are the result of injury to a limb. Localization of lesions in monoparesis will be reviewed in Chapter 6. The primary exception is generalized peripheral neuropathies, which affect all of the limbs. These conditions will be discussed in Chapter 8.

Pain

Hyperesthesia (increased sensitivity) is a very useful localizing sign and may be present when there is little or no motor deficit. The animal's limbs and trunk, especially the vertebral column, are palpated and manipulated while the examiner observes for signs of pain. Obvious reactions may include resistance to movement and tensing of the muscles. If the clinician places one hand on the animal's abdomen while squeezing each vertebral segment with the other hand, increased tension of the abdominal muscles may be felt as painful areas are palpated. The skin is pinched with a hemostat after palpation is completed. A fold of skin is grasped gently with the hemostat and then the skin is pinched lightly so that no significant behavioral reaction is elicited from normal areas. Pinching areas of hyperesthesia will elicit an exaggerated skin twitch or a behavioral response.

The superficial pain examination should be performed in a caudal to cranial direction, because areas caudal to a lesion usually have decreased skin sensation. A level of normal or increased sensation can be ascertained by this method. If a spinal lesion is present, the sensory level should have the conformation of a dermatome (see Fig. 1–32). Peripheral nerves have a different pattern of sensory distribution (see Fig. 1–35).

The cutaneous (panniculus) reflex is elicited with a hemostat in the same manner as that just described for detecting hyperesthesia. Cutaneous sensation enters the spinal cord at each segment (dermatomes) and ascends to the brachial plexus (C8–T1) to the *lateral thoracic* nerve, which innervates the cutaneous trunci (panniculus carnosus) muscle. Contraction of the cutaneous muscle causes a skin twitch. A segmental lesion will block the ascending afferent stimulus, abolishing the reflex. Pinching the skin in a caudal to cranial direction will identify the first level at which the reflex can be elicited. This segment is normal, and the lesion will be one segment caudal to this level. The superficial pain pathways must be blocked in order to abolish the reflex. Normally the cutaneous reflex is most apparent in the thoracolumbar (saddle) area. A minimal response is obtained from a stimulus applied to the sacral or caudal regions, and no response is obtained from a stimulus applied to the cervical region. Cervical pain is assessed by manipulation of the neck and deep palpation of the vertebrae. Although it may be difficult to define the location of the pain precisely, it usually is possible to determine whether it is in the rostral, middle, or cau-

TABLE 2–2 Spinal Reflexes

Reflex	*Muscle(s)*	*Peripheral Nerve*	*Spinal Cord Segments**
Myotatic (stretch)	Biceps brachii	Musculocutaneous	(C6), C7–C8, (T1)
	Triceps brachii	Radial	C7–C8, T1, (T2)
	Extensor carpi radialis	Radial	C7–C8, T1, (T2)
	Quadriceps	Femoral	(L3), L4–L5, (L6)
	Cranial tibial	Peroneal (sciatic)	L6–L7, S1
	Gastrocnemius	Tibial (sciatic)	L6–L7, S1
Flexor (withdrawal)	Thoracic limb	Radial, ulnar, median, musculocutaneous	C6–T2
	Pelvic limb	Sciatic	L6–S1, (S2)
Perineal	Anal Sphincter	Pudendal	S1–S2, (S3)

Modified with permission from Oliver JE Jr: Localization of lesions in the nervous system. In Hoerlein BF: Canine Neurology, 3rd ed. Philadelphia, WB Saunders Co., 1978.

* Parentheses indicate segments that sometimes contribute to a nerve.

TABLE 2–3 Signs of Lesions in the Spinal Cord

Site of Lesion	Sign
Cd1–Cd5	LMN—tail
S1–S3	UMN—tail
Pelvic plexus	LMN—anal sphincter, bladder
Pudendal nerve	
L4–S2	UMN—tail
Lumbosacral plexus	LMN—hind limbs
	UMN or LMN—bladder, sphincters
T3–L3	UMN—hind limbs, bladder, sphincter
	LMN—segmental spinal muscles
C6–T2	UMN—hind limbs, bladder
Brachial plexus	LMN—forelimbs
C1–C6 or brain	UMN—all four limbs, bladder

dal cervical segments by performing palpation carefully and gently.

Hypesthesia (decreased sensation) and anesthesia (no sensation) also are useful localizing signs. Single nerve root lesions usually will not produce a clinically detectable area of decreased sensation because of the overlapping pattern of cutaneous innervation (see Fig. 1–32). Multiple nerve roots may be involved in some lesions, especially in the area of the cauda equina. Lesions of the spinal cord may result in decreased perception of pain caudal to the lesion. Determining the level of decreased sensation was discussed previously, and the prognostic implications of the loss of sensation will be discussed later. The motor examination localizes the lesion to one of six regions of the spinal cord or to the brain (Table 2–3). A carefully performed sensory examination will localize the lesion to within three segments of the spinal cord or to a peripheral nerve. For additional details on pain, see Chapter 15.

Localization in the Brain

If the lesion has been localized to the brain, the next step is to determine what part of the brain is involved. Localization to one of five regions of the brain or to the peripheral vestibular apparatus (labyrinth) is made on the basis of clinical signs (Table 2–4).

TABLE 2–4 Signs of Lesions in the Brain

	Mental Status	Posture	Movement	Postural Reactions	Cranial Nerves
Cerebral cortex	Abnormal behavior, depression, seizures	Normal	Gait normal to slight hemiparesis (contralateral)	Deficits (contralateral)	Normal (vision may be impaired on contralateral side)
Diencephalon (thalamus and hypothalamus)	Abnormal behavior, depression (endocrine and autonomic)	Normal	Gait normal to hemiparesis or tetraparesis	Deficits (contralateral)	CN II
Brain stem (midbrain, pons, medulla)	Depression, stupor, coma	Normal, turning, falling	Hemiparesis to tetraparesis, ataxia	Deficits (ipsi- or contralateral)	CN III–XII
Vestibular, central (medulla)	Depression	Head tilt, falling	Hemiparesis, (usually ipsilateral), ataxia	Deficits (ipsilateral or contralateral)	CN VIII, may also affect CN V and VII; nystagmus
Vestibular, peripheral (labyrinth)	Normal	Head tilt	Normal to ataxia	Normal, although may be awkward	CN VIII, sometimes CN VII; Horner's syndrome, nystagmus
Cerebellum	Normal	Normal	Tremors, dysmetria, ataxia	Normal to dysmetria	Normal, may be menace reaction deficit or nystagmus

Brain Stem

For our purposes, the functional brain stem includes the midbrain, pons, and medulla oblongata. Lesions of the brain stem will produce UMN signs in all four limbs (tetraparesis) or in the thoracic and pelvic limbs on one side (hemiparesis). The paresis or paralysis produced by brain stem lesions is obvious both in the gait and in postural reactions. Cerebral lesions affect postural reactions with minimal change in gait. Abnormal posture, especially of the head and the neck, may be seen.

Cranial nerve signs (CN III–XII) are present in larger brain stem lesions and provide important localizing signs (LMN or sensory) (Fig. 2–7). The evaluation of cranial nerves is outlined in Table 2–5 (see also Chaps. 1, 10, and 12).

Cranial nerve signs are ipsilateral to the lesion, whereas motor signs may be ipsilateral or contralateral, depending on the level and the pathways involved. The animal's mental status may be altered, especially in lesions of the midbrain and the pons, which disrupt the reticular activating system. Signs vary from depression to coma (see Chap. 13).

Diencephalon

Diencephalic lesions (lesions of the thalamus or hypothalamus) may produce UMN signs in all four limbs (tetraparesis) or in the thoracic and pelvic limbs on one side (hemiparesis), depending on the extent of the lesion. The gait is not severely affected (similar to cerebral lesions), but postural reaction deficits are obvious. CN II (optic) may be affected in diencephalic lesions. Space-occupying lesions (e.g., tumors, abscesses) of the diencephalon also may affect CN III, IV, and VI (see Table 2–5). Cranial nerve signs are *ipsilateral* to the lesion, whereas motor signs are *contralateral* to the lesion.

The most characteristic signs of diencephalic lesions are related to abnormal function of the hypothalamus and its connections with the pituitary gland. The hypothalamus is the control center for the autonomic nervous system and most of the endocrine system. If the hypothalamus is not affected, it is difficult to distinguish diencephalic from cerebral lesions.

All sensory pathways of the body, with the exception of those serving olfaction, relay in the diencephalon en route to the cerebral cortex. Clinical signs of lesions in these systems usually are not localizing. A rare generalized hyperesthesia has been described as a result of an abnormality in the relay nuclei of the pain pathways. Large lesions in the diencephalon may produce alterations in the level of consciousness (stupor, coma) because of interference with the reticular activating system (see Chap. 13).

Vestibular System

Vestibular signs may be the result of central (brain stem) or peripheral (labyrinth) disease. It is important to differentiate central disease from peripheral disease because of the differences in treatment and prognosis. Signs of vestibular disease include falling, rolling, tilting of the head, circling, nystagmus, positional strabismus (deviation of one eye in certain positions of the head), and an asymmetric ataxia (Figs. 2–8 and 2–9).

Peripheral lesions involve the labyrinth in the petrosal bone. Middle ear lesions (bulla ossea) usually produce a head tilt with no other signs. Horizontal or rotatory nystagmus may be seen occasionally. Inner ear disease, which actually involves the receptors and the vestibular nerve, usually produces one or more of the signs listed earlier in addition to the head tilt. In either case, the head tilt is ipsilateral to the lesion. Horner's sign (miosis, ptosis, enophthalmos) of the ipsilateral eye may be present with either middle or inner ear disease in the dog and cat, because the sympathetic nerves pass through the middle ear in proximity to the petrosal bone. CN VII (facial) may be affected in inner ear disease as it courses through the petrosal bone, in contact with the vestibulocochlear nerve (CN VIII). The primary characteristics of peripheral vestibular disease are an asymmetric ataxia without deficits in postural reactions and a horizontal, or rotatory, nystagmus that does not change direction with different head positions. The quick phase of the nystagmus is away from the side of the lesion.

Any signs of brain stem disease in association with vestibular signs indicate that central involvement is present. The most frequent differentiating feature is a deficit in postural reactions. Peripheral vestibular disease does not cause paresis or loss of proprioception, whereas central disease frequently does. Postural reactions must be evaluated critically, because an animal with peripheral vestibular disease has deficits in equilibrium, which make the performance of tests such as hopping awkward. An evaluation of proprioceptive positioning is an excellent method for discrimination. Alterations in mental status or deficits in CN V and CN VI also are indicative of central disease (see Fig. 2–8).

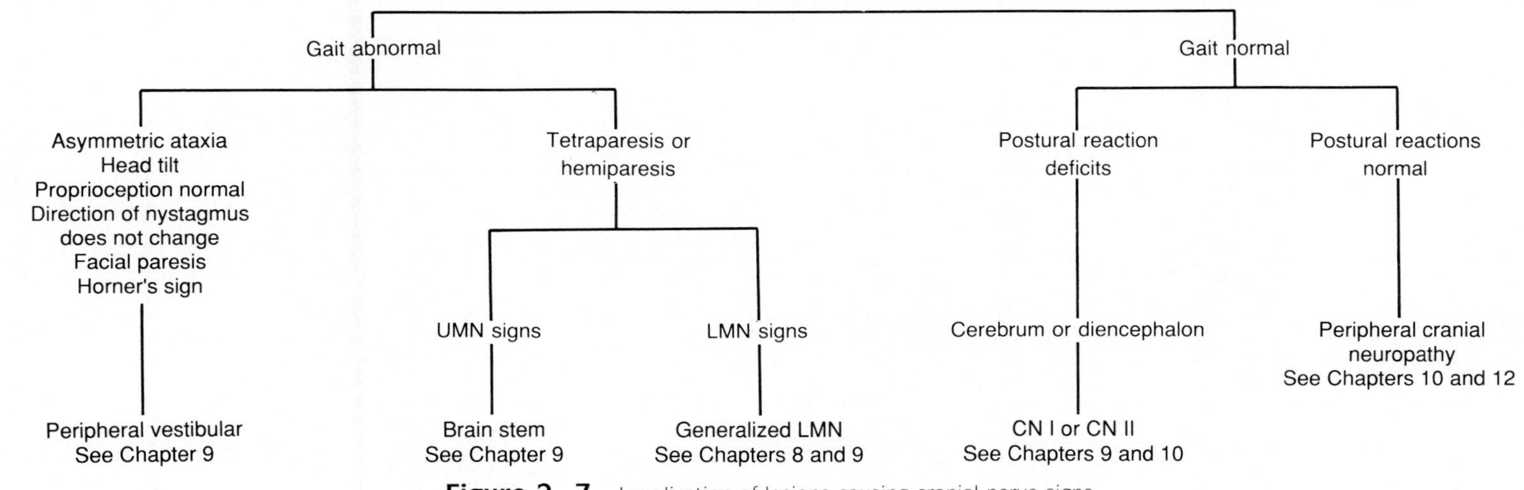

Figure 2–7 Localization of lesions causing cranial nerve signs.

TABLE 2–5 Cranial Nerves

Number and Name	Origin or Termination in Brain	Course	Function	Test	Normal Response	Abnormal Response	Occurrence
CN I Olfactory	Pyriform cortex	Nasal mucosa, cribriform plate, olfactory bulbs, olfactory tract, olfactory stria, pyriform cortex	Sense of smell	Smelling of nonirritating volatile substances (alcohol, food)	Behavioral reaction; aversion or interest	No reaction	Rare: nasal tumors and infections (evaluation difficult)
CN II Optic	Lateral geniculate nucleus (vision), pretectal nucleus (pupillary reflex)	Retina, optic nerve, optic tract, lateral geniculate nucleus, optic radiation, visual cortex or optic tract, pretectal nucleus, parasympathetic nucleus of CN III, oculomotor nerve	Vision, pupillary light reflexes	Menace reaction, obstacle test and behavior, placing reaction, following movement, pupillary light reflex, ophthalmoscopy	Blinks, avoids obstacles and responds to visual cues, placing good, follows objects, pupillary light reflexes present, retina normal	No blink, poor avoidance of obstacles, no visual placing, direct pupillary light reflex absent, retina or optic disk may be abnormal	Optic neuritis, neoplasia, orbital trauma, orbital abscess
CN III Oculomotor	Midbrain, tegmentum (level of rostral colliculus)	Nucleus ventral to mesencephalic aqueduct, exits ventral to midbrain between cerebral peduncles, courses through tentorial notch, runs in cavernous sinus with CN IV and CN VI, exits orbital fissure	Constriction of pupil; ciliary muscle for accommodation reaction of lens; extraocular muscles: dorsal, ventral, and medial rectus, ventral oblique	Pupillary size, pupillary light reflex, eye position, eye movement	Pupils symmetric, pupils constrict to light, eyes centered in palpebral fissure, eyes move in all directions	Mydriasis, ipsilateral, no direct pupil response, ventrolateral strabismus, no movement except laterally (CN VI)	Orbital lesions, tentorial herniation, midbrain lesion
CN IV Trochlear	Midbrain, tegmentum (level of caudal colliculus)	Nucleus ventral to mesencephalic aqueduct, exits dorsal to tectum, caudal to caudal colliculus, contralateral to origin, courses along ridge of petrosal bone, follows course of CN III	Dorsal oblique muscle, rotates dorsal portion of eye medioventrally	Eye position, eye movements	Eye centered in palpebral fissure, eyes move in all directions	Normal; rotation may be detected in animal with elliptical pupil or by position of vessels ophthalmoscopically	Rare, difficult to evaluate; reported in polioencephalomalacia of cattle, but eyes move
CN V Trigeminal (ophthalmic nerve, maxillary nerve, mandibular nerve)	*Motor nucleus:* Pons *Sensory nucleus:* Pons, medulla, C1 spinal cord segment	*Motor:* Pons, exits at cerebellopontine angle, trigeminal canal of petrosal bone, oval foramen, mandibular nerve *Sensory:* Same except trigeminal ganglion in trigeminal canal; ophthalmic, maxillary and mandibular nerves	*Motor:* Muscles of mastication *Sensory:* Face rostral to ears	*Motor:* Ability to close mouth, jaw tone *Sensory:* Palpebral reflex, pinch face, touch nasal mucosa	Closed mouth, good jaw tone; no atrophy of temporal or masseter muscles; palpebral reflex present; behavioral response to noxious stimulus	Jaw hangs open (bilateral), poor jaw tone, atrophy, loss of palpebral reflex or behavioral response to noxious stimulus (check all three branches)	Idiopathic mandibular paralysis, trigeminal neuritis, cerebellopontine angle tumors, rabies, trauma
CN VI Abducent	Medulla (rostral and dorsal)	Medulla, lateral to pyramid, courses ventral to brain stem to join CN III and IV	Lateral rectus and retractor muscles; lateral movement of eye, retraction of globe	Eye position, eye movement	Eye centered in palpebral fissure, eye moves laterally and retracts	Medial strabismus, lack of lateral eye movements or retraction	Orbital trauma, orbital abscess, brain stem disease

CN VII Facial	Medulla (rostral and ventrolateral)	*Motor:* Axons leave nucleus, loop around abducent nucleus, and exit ventrolateral medulla ventral to CN VIII to internal acoustic meatus, facial canal in petrosal bone, and stylomastoid foramen to muscles of face *Taste:* Solitary nucleus and tract, medulla follows course of trigeminal nerve	Muscles of facial expression and taste, rostral two thirds of tongue	Facial symmetry, palpebral reflex, ear movements *Taste:* Atropine applied to rostral two thirds of tongue with cotton swabs	Face symmetric; normal movements of lips, ears, eyelids; palpebral reflex present; ears move in response to stimulation *Taste:* Aversive reaction immediately	Asymmetry of face, ptosis, lip drops, deviation of nasal philtrum, palpebral reflex absent (check CN V), ears do not move *Taste:* No reaction until mouth is closed and material reaches caudal portion of tongue	Idiopathic facial paralysis, polyneuropathies, inner ear infections, brain stem lesions
CN VIII Vestibulocochlear	Vestibular nuclei – medulla; cochlear nuclei – medulla	Inner ear, petrosal bone, internal acoustic meatus, cerebellomedullary angle, medulla	Equilibrium, hearing	*Vestibular:* Posture and gait, eye movements, rotatory and caloric tests *Hearing:* Startle response, electrophysiology (EEG alerting, brain stem evoked response)	*Vestibular:* Normal posture and gait, oculocephalic responses normal, brief postrotatory nystagmus and caloric-induced nystagmus *Hearing:* Startled reaction to handclap, evoked response present	*Vestibular:* Head tilt, head twist, circling, spontaneous nystagmus, prolonged or absent postrotatory nystagmus, abnormal or absent caloric response *Hearing:* Poor startle reaction, no evoked response	Otitis media and otitis interna, idiopathic vestibular disease, polyneuropathy, brain stem disease
CN IX Glossopharyngeal	Medulla (caudal)	*Sensory:* Solitary tract and nucleus *Motor:* Parasympathetic, ambiguus nucleus exit together along lateral surface of medulla, exit through jugular foramen	Sensory and motor to pharynx and palate, parasympathetic to zygomatic and parotid salivary glands (in CN V); sensory to carotid body and sinus	Gag reflex	Swallowing	Poor gag reflex, dysphagia	Rare
CN X Vagus	Medulla (caudal)	Same as CN IX	Sensory and motor to pharynx and larynx, thoracic and abdominal viscera	Gag reflex, laryngeal reflex, slap test, oculocardiac reflex	Swallowing, coughing, bradycardia	Poor gag reflex, dysphagia, inspiratory dyspnea, no retraction of laryngeal folds	Rare, except in laryngeal paralysis (idiopathic); polyneuropathy
CN XI Accessory	Medulla (caudal) and cervical spinal cord	Ambiguus nucleus of medulla and cervical gray matter, axons run rostrally from cervical cord to join cranial roots, exit jugular foramen	Trapezius and parts of sternocephalicus and brachiocephalicus muscles	Palpate for atrophy of muscles; EMG	Normal muscles	Atrophied muscles, denervation	Rare
CN XII Hypoglossal	Medulla (caudal)	Axons exit medulla lateral to pyramid, hypoglossal canal to tongue	Movements of tongue	Protrusion of tongue (wet nose), retraction of tongue	Tongue protrudes symmetrically and can lick in both directions, strong withdrawal of tongue	Tongue deviates to side of lesion, atrophy, weak withdrawal	Brain stem disease, polyneuropathy

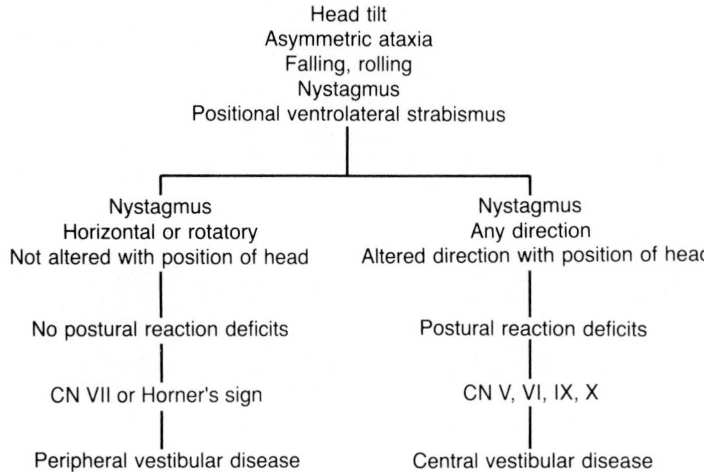

Figure 2–8 Algorithm for differentiating central and peripheral vestibular diseases.

Lesions near the caudal cerebellar peduncle may produce what has been called a paradoxical vestibular syndrome. The signs are usually similar to those of central vestibular disease except that the direction of the head tilt is contralateral to the side of the lesion.[6]

Bilateral vestibular disease, which is usually peripheral, produces a more symmetric ataxia. The animal walks with the limbs flexed and spread apart to maintain balance. The head often sways from side to side. There is no nystagmus, and vestibular eye movements are usually absent.[7]

Cerebellum

The cerebellum coordinates movements. It controls the rate and range of movements without actually initiating motor activity. Cerebellar lesions may be unilateral or bilateral, depending on the etiology. Characteristic signs include ataxia, a wide-based stance, dysmetria, and an intention tremor with little weakness. An involvement of the head differentiates cerebellar lesions from spinal tract lesions, which may produce similar signs in the limbs. For example, dysmetria usually is recognized as a severe head drop when the head is elevated and suddenly released. The animal may stick its nose too far into its water dish when drinking or may even hit the edge of the dish. Intention tremors are uncoordinated movements that become much worse as the animal initiates an activity such as eating or drinking (see Fig. 2–9).[8]

Nystagmus may occur in cerebellar disease, but it is usually more of a tremor of the globe than the slow-quick (jerk) movements associated with vestibular disease. Cerebellar nystagmus is most pronounced as the animal shifts its gaze and fixates on a new field (an intention tremor).

Acute injury to the cerebellum causes a different clinical picture, typically extensor hypertonus in the thoracic limbs, flexion in the pelvic limbs and opisthotonos.[6] Isolated cerebellar trauma is unusual because of the protected location of the cerebellum. These signs are most pronounced when combined with brain stem lesions at the level of the midbrain or the pons.

Lesions of the flocculonodular lobes of the cerebellum produce signs similar to those of vestibular disease, including a loss of equilibrium, nystagmus, and a tendency to fall (see Chap. 9).

Diffuse cerebellar lesions may cause the menace reaction to be absent even if vision is normal.

Cerebrum

Cerebral lesions (including the cerebral hemispheres and basal nuclei) usually cause alterations in behavior or mental status, seizures, loss of vision with intact pupils, and a mild hemiparesis with deficits in postural reactions. Only one or two of these signs may be present, because the cerebrum is a relatively large structure with well-localized functional areas. Signs are generally contralateral to the lesion.

Behavioral changes usually reflect a lesion of the limbic system or the frontal lobe of the cortex. Frontal lobe lesions often cause a disinhibition that results in excessive pacing. Compulsive pacing may continue until the animal walks into a corner and stands with its head pressed against the obstruction. If the lesion is unilateral or asymmetric, the animal may circle. Circling in an animal with a cerebral lesion is usually to the same side as the lesion and tends to be in large circles. The gait is reasonably normal, although obstacles may not be perceived. Circling is not a localizing sign because it can

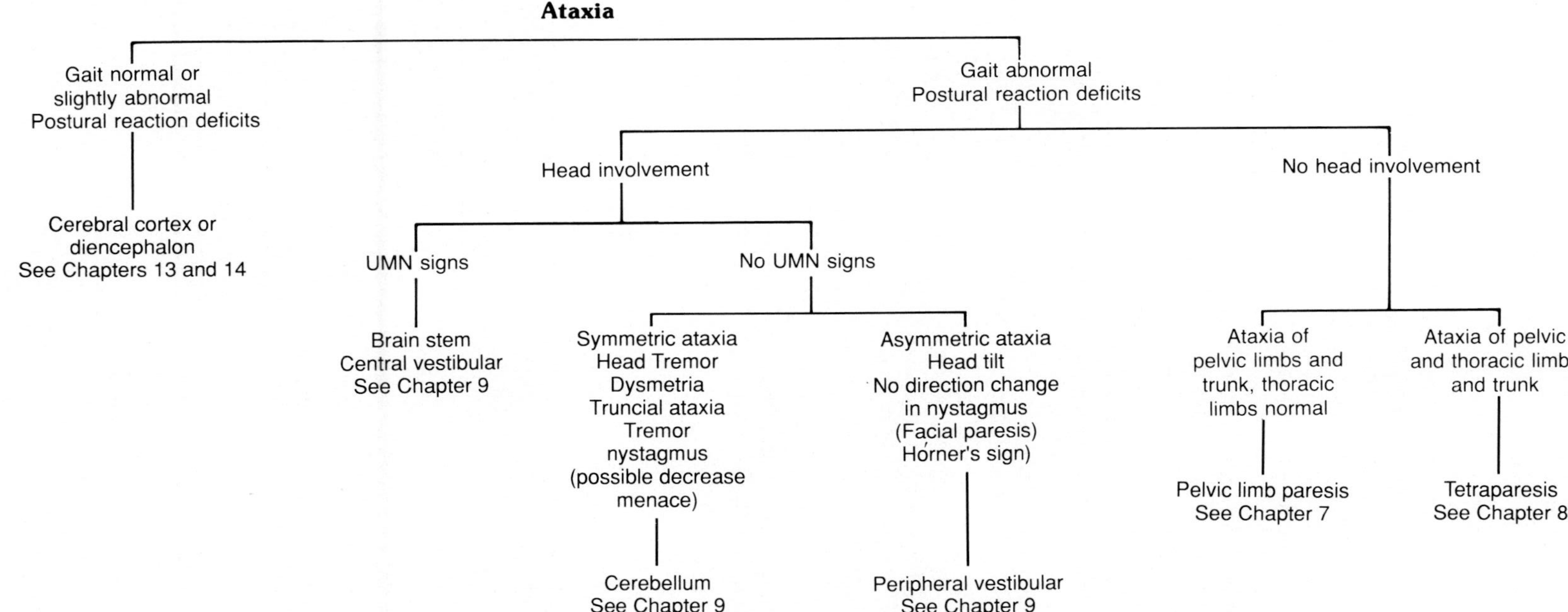

Figure 2–9 Algorithm for the diagnosis of ataxia based on gait, head involvement, and motor function of the limbs.

be caused by lesions in many areas of the brain.

Depression, stupor, and coma represent decreasing levels of consciousness caused by a separation of the cerebral cortex from the reticular activating system of the brain stem. Severe depression usually is caused by brain stem lesions (see Chap. 13). Conscious visual perception requires intact visual pathways to the occipital lobes of the cerebral cortex. Occipital cortical lesions will cause blindness with intact pupillary reflexes (see Chap. 12).

The sensorimotor cortex is important for voluntary motor activity but is not necessary for relatively normal gait and posture. Animals with lesions in this area can stand, walk, and run with minimal deficits. The animal's ability for fine discrimination is lost, however, and it is unable to avoid obstacles smoothly or to perform fine maneuvers such as walking on the steps of a ladder. Markedly abnormal postural reactions are found.

Localization to one of the five regions of the brain is usually adequate for a clinical diagnosis. Cranial nerve signs provide positive evidence for precise localization within the brain stem.

Clinical signs referable to several parts of the nervous system indicate diffuse or multifocal disease, such as infection, metabolic disorder, or malignant neoplasia (see Chap. 16).

CASE HISTORIES

You now should be able to localize the lesion in the cases presented in Chapter 1. The signalment and pertinent neurologic abnormalities will be repeated. Make your assessment before reading ours.

Case History 2A

Signalment

Canine, West Highland white terrier, female, 6 years old.

History

The dog was found lying down in the backyard 4 days earlier. The owners describe some voluntary movements in the left thoracic and pelvic limbs. The condition has not changed since its onset. No pain is observed. Appetite and eliminations are normal (see Case History 1A, Chap. 1).

Physical Examination

Nothing significant was found on the physical examination other than the neurologic observations.

*Neurologic Examination**

(See Case History 1A, Chap. 1.)

A. Observation
   1. Mental status: Alert.
   2. Posture: Recumbent; falls to right when placed on feet.
   3. Gait: None.

B. Palpation: No abnormalities.

C. Postural Reactions

Left	Reactions	Right
+1	Proprioceptive positioning PL	0
+2	TL	0
NE	Wheelbarrowing	NE
+1	Hopping, PL	0
+2	Hopping, TL	0
NE	Extensor postural thrust	NE
NE	Hemistand-hemiwalk	NE
NE	Tonic neck	NE
+1	Placing, tactile PL	0
+2	TL	0
+1	Placing, visual PL	0
+2	TL	0

D. Spinal Reflexes

Left	Reflex Spinal segment	Right
2	Quadriceps L4–L6	+3
+2	Extensor carpi radialis C7–T1	+2
NE	Triceps C7–T1	NE
+2	Flexion, PL L5–S1	+2
+2	Flexion, TL C6–T1	+1
0	Crossed extensor	0
+2	Perineal S1–S2	+2

* *Key*: 0 = absent, +1 = decreased, +2 = normal, +3 = exaggerated, +4 = very exaggerated or clonus, PL = pelvic limb, TL = thoracic limb, NE = not evaluated.

E. Cranial Nerves

Left	Nerve + Function	Right
	CN II—vision	
+2	Menace	+2
+2	CN II, III—pupil size	+2
+2	Stim. left eye	+2
+2	Stim. right eye	+2
+2	CN II fundus	+2
+2	CN III, IV, VI	+2
+2	Strabismus	+2
+2	Nystagmus	+2
+2	CN V—sensation	+2
+2	CN V—mastication	+2
+2	CN VII—facial muscles	+2
+2	Palpebral	+2
+2	CN IX, X—swallowing	+2
+2	CN XII—tongue	+2

F. Sensation: Location.
Hyperesthesia: None.
Superficial pain: Decreased in right thoracic limb.
Deep pain: Decreased in right thoracic limb.

Complete sections G and H before reviewing Case Summary.

G. Assessment (Anatomic diagnosis and estimation of prognosis)

H. Plan (Diagnostic)

Rule-outs *Procedure*
1.
2.
3.
4.

Case History 2B

Signalment

Canine, German shepherd, female, 7 years old.

History

The animal has had hip dysplasia since 1 year of age. Stumbling on the pelvic limbs started 6 months ago and progressed slowly. The dog cannot go up steps and falls even with good footing. There is no evidence of pain (see Case History 1B, Chap. 1).

Physical Examination

Nothing significant was found on the physical examination, other than neurologic abnormalities.

*Neurologic Examination**

(See Case History 1B, Chap. 1.)

A. Observation
1. Mental status: Alert.
2. Posture: Difficulty getting up; wide-based stance.
3. Gait: Truncal ataxia, stumbles; crosses legs, knuckles toes of pelvic limbs.

B. Palpation: Normal.

C. Postural Reactions

Left	Reactions	Right
	Proprioceptive positioning	
0	PL	0
+2	TL	+2
NE	Wheelbarrowing	NE
+1	Hopping, PL	+1
+2	Hopping, TL	+2
NE	Extensor postural thrust	NE
NE	Hemistand-hemiwalk	NE
NE	Tonic neck	NE
	Placing, tactile	
NE	PL	NE
NE	TL	NE
	Placing, visual	
NE	PL	NE
NE	TL	NE

D. Spinal Reflexes

Left	Reflex	Right
	Spinal segment	
	Quadriceps	
+3	L4–L6	+2
	Extensor carpi radialis	
+2	C7–T1	+2
	Triceps	
NE	C7–T1	NE
	Flexion, PL	
+2	L5–S1	+2
	Flexion, TL	
+2	C6–T1	+2
0	Crossed extensor	0
	Perineal	
+2	S1–S2	+2

* *Key*: 0 = absent, +1 = decreased, +2 = normal, +3 = exaggerated, +4 = very exaggerated or clonus, PL = pelvic limb, TL = thoracic limb, NE = not evaluated.

E. Cranial Nerves

Left	Nerve + Function	Right
+2	CN II – vision Menace	+2
+2	CN II, III – pupil size	+2
+2	Stim. left eye	+2
+2	Stim. right eye	+2
+2	CN II – fundus	+2
+2 +2 +2	CN III, IV, VI Strabismus Nystagmus	+2 +2 +2
+2	CN V – sensation	+2
+2	CN V – mastication	+2
+2 +2	CN VII – facial muscles Palpebral	+2 +2
+2	CN IX, X – swallowing	+2
+2	CN XII – tongue	+2

F. Sensation: Location
Hyperesthesia: No.
Superficial pain: +2
Deep pain: +2

Complete sections G and H before reviewing Case Summary.

G. Assessment (Anatomic diagnosis and estimation of prognosis)

H. Plan (Diagnostic)

Rule-outs *Procedure*
1.
2.
3.
4.

Case History 2C

Signalment

Feline, domestic short hair, female, 3 months old.

History

The kitten has been clumsy since birth. It was one of four in the litter: one was born dead, the other two are normal. The kitten has a peculiar prancing gait and trembles at times. It seems to be getting around better now (see Case History 1C, Chap. 1).

Physical Examination

Normal.

*Neurologic Examination**

(See Case History 1C, Chap. 1.)

A. Observation
1. Mental status: Alert.
2. Posture: Slightly wide-based stance. Head tremor that disappears at rest.
3. Gait: Ataxia, dysmetria of all four limbs.

B. Palpation: Normal.

C. Postural Reactions

Left	Reactions	Right
+2	Proprioceptive positioning PL	+2
+2	TL	+2
NE	Wheelbarrowing	NE
+3	Hopping, PL	+3
+3	Hopping, TL	+3
NE	Extensor postural thrust	NE
NE	Hemistand-hemiwalk	NE
NE	Tonic neck	NE
NE	Placing, tactile PL	NE
NE	TL	NE
NE	Placing, visual PL	NE
NE	TL	NE

D. Spinal Reflexes

Left	Reflex	Right
NE	Spinal segment Quadriceps L4–L6	NE
NE	Extensor carpi radialis C7–T1	NE
NE	Triceps C7–T1	NE
+2	Flexion, PL L5–S1	+2
+2	Flexion, TL C6–T1	+2
0	Crossed extensor	0
+2	Perineal S1–S2	+2

E. Cranial Nerves

Left	Nerve + Function	Right
0	CN II – vision Menace	0
+2	CN II, III – pupil size	+2
+2	Stim. left eye	+2
+2	Stim. right eye	+2

* *Key*: 0 = absent, +1 = decreased, +2 = normal, +3 = exaggerated, +4 = very exaggerated or clonus, PL = pelvic limb, TL = thoracic limb, NE = not evaluated.

+2	CN II—fundus	+2
+2	CN III, IV, VI	+2
+2 Pendular	Strabismus Nystagmus	+2 Pendular
+2	CN V—sensation	+2
+2	CN V—mastication	+2
+2 +2	CN VII—facial muscles Palpebral	+2 +2
+2	CN IX, X—swallowing	+2
+2	CN XII—tongue	+2

F. Sensation: Location.
 Hyperesthesia: No.
 Superficial pain: +2.
 Deep pain: +2.

Complete sections G and H before reviewing Case Summary.

G. Assessment (Anatomic diagnosis and estimation of prognosis)

H. Plan (Diagnostic)

Rule-outs *Procedure*

1.
2.
3.
4.

Case History 2D

Signalment

Feline, Siamese, male, 2 years old.

History

Uveitis has been present in the right eye for 2 months. The cat is lame in the right thoracic limb, and its head trembles when the cat eats. The animal has been depressed for 2 days (see Case History 1D, Chap. 1).

Physical Examination

Physical examination reveals anterior uveitis in the right eye. The remaining findings are normal, except for those pertaining to neurologic status.

*Neurologic Examination**

(See Case History 1D, Chap. 1.)

A. Observation
 1. Mental status: Depressed.
 2. Posture: Head tremor that disappears when the animal is at rest.
 3. Gait: Knuckles left thoracic limb.

B. Palpation: Atrophy of triceps and muscles distal to elbow, left thoracic limb.

* *Key*: 0 = absent, +1 = decreased, +2 = normal, +3 = exaggerated, +4 = very exaggerated or clonus, PL = pelvic limb, TL = thoracic limb, NE = not evaluated.

C. Postural Reactions

Left	Reactions	Right
0	Proprioceptive positioning PL	+2
0	TL	+2
NE	Wheelbarrowing	NE
0	Hopping, PL	+2
+1	Hopping, TL	+2
0	Extensor postural thrust	+2
NE	Hemistand-hemiwalk	NE
NE	Tonic neck	NE
NE	Placing, tactile PL	NE
NE	TL	NE
NE	Placing, visual PL	NE
NE	TL	NE

D. Spinal Reflexes

Left	Reflex	Right
+3	Spinal segment Quadriceps L4–L6	+2
0	Extensor carpi radialis C7–T1	+2
NE	Triceps C7–T1	NE
+2	Flexion, PL L5–S1	+2
0	Flexion, TL C6–T1	+2
0	Crossed extensor	0
+2	Perineal S1–S2	+2

E. Cranial Nerves

Left	Nerve + Function	Right
+2	CN II—vision Menace	+2
+2	Miosis CN II, III—pupil size	+2
+2	Stim. left eye	+2
+2	Stim. right eye	+2
+2	CN II—fundus	+2
+2 +2 +2	CN III, IV, VI Strabismus Nystagmus	+2 +2 +2

+2	CN V—sensation	+2
+2	CN V—mastication	+2
+2 +2	CN VII—facial muscles Palpebral	+2 +2
+2	CN IX, X—swallowing	+2
+2	CN XII—tongue	+2

F. Sensation: Location.
   Hyperesthesia: No.
   Superficial pain: +2.
   Deep pain: +2.

Complete sections G and H before reviewing Case Summary.

G. Assessment (Anatomic diagnosis and estimation of prognosis)

H. Plan (Diagnostic)

Rule-outs *Procedure*

1.
2.
3.
4.

Case History 2E

Signalment

Canine, Yorkshire terrier, male, 8 months old.

History

The animal has always been small and thin. Episodes of abnormal behavior have occurred recently. The dog paces, is restless, and resents being held. These episodes typically last 2 to 3 hours, occasionally for a whole day, and have occurred every day for the past 3 weeks (see Case History 1E, Chap. 1).

Physical Examination

On physical examination the dog appears thin. Other findings are normal, except for those pertaining to neurologic status.

*Neurologic Examination**

A. Observation
   1. Mental status: Normal, alert; depressed during day.
   2. Posture: Normal.
   3. Gait: Paces. Sometimes bumps into table.

B. Palpation

C. Postural Reactions

Left	Reactions	Right
+1	Proprioceptive positioning PL	+1
+1	TL	+1
+1	Wheelbarrowing	+1
+1	Hopping, PL	+1
+1	Hopping, TL	+1
+1	Extensor postural thrust	+1
NE	Hemistand-hemiwalk	NE
NE	Tonic neck	NE
+1	Placing, tactile PL	+1
+1	TL	+1
+1	Placing, visual PL	+1
+1	TL	+1

D. Spinal Reflexes

Left	Reflex Spinal segment	Right
+2	Quadriceps L4–L6	+2
+2	Extensor carpi radialis C7–T1	+2
+2	Triceps C7-T1	+2
+2	Flexion, PL L5–S1	+2
+2	Flexion, TL C6–T1	+2
+2	Crossed extensor	+2
+2	Perineal S1–S2	+2

E. Cranial Nerves

Left	Nerve + Function	Right
+2	CN II—vision Menace	+2
+2	CN II, III—pupil size	+2
+2	Stim. left eye	+2
+2	Stim. right eye	+2
+2	CN II—fundus	+2
+2 +2 +2	CN III, IV, VI Strabismus Nystagmus	+2 +2 +2
+2	CN V—sensation	+2
+2	CN V—mastication	+2
+2 +2	CN VII—facial muscles Palpebral	+2 +2
+2	CN IX, X—swallowing	+2
+2	CN XII—tongue	+2

* *Key*: 0 = absent, +1 = decreased, +2 = normal, +3 = exaggerated, +4 = very exaggerated or clonus, PL = pelvic limb, TL = thoracic limb, NE = not evaluated.

F. Sensation: Location.
  Hyperesthesia: No.
  Superficial pain: +2.
  Deep pain: +2.
Complete sections G and H before reviewing Case Summary.
G. Assessment (Anatomic diagnosis and estimation of prognosis)
H. Plan (Diagnostic)

Rule-outs *Procedure*
1.
2.
3.
4.

The following abbreviated cases are presented to give you additional practice in localizing lesions. Use Table 2–2 or 2–5 or Figure 2–7 if necessary. The findings on the neurologic examination are all that you need in order to localize the lesion.

Case History 2F

Signalment

Canine, Dachshund, male, 2 years old.

*Neurologic Examination**

A. Observation
  1. Mental status: Normal.
  2. Posture: Cannot stand.
  3. Gait: Moves thoracic limbs but not pelvic limbs.
B. Palpation: Normal.
C. Postural Reactions

Left	Reactions	Right
0	Proprioceptive positioning PL	0
+2	TL	+2
+2	Wheelbarrowing	+2
0	Hopping, PL	0
+2	Hopping, TL	+2
0	Extensor postural thrust	0
NE	Hemistand-hemiwalk	NE
NE	Tonic neck	NE
0	Placing, tactile PL	0
+2	TL	+2
0	Placing, visual PL	0
+2	TL	+2

* *Key*: 0 = absent, +1 = decreased, +2 = normal, +3 = exaggerated, +4 = very exaggerated or clonus, PL = pelvic limb, TL = thoracic limb, NE = not evaluated.

D. Spinal Reflexes

Left	Reflex Spinal segment	Right
0	Quadriceps L4–L6	0
+2	Extensor carpi radialis C7–T1	+2
+2	Triceps C7–T1	+2
0	Flexion, PL L5–S1	0
+2	Flexion, TL C6–T1	+2
0	Crossed extensor	0
0	Perineal S1–S2	0

E. Cranial nerves: All normal.
F. Sensation: Location.
  Hyperesthesia: No.
  Superficial pain: NE.
  Deep pain: NE.
Complete sections G and H before reviewing Case Summary.
G. Assessment (Anatomic diagnosis and estimation of prognosis)
H. Plan (Diagnostic)

Rule-outs *Procedure*
1.
2.
3.
4.

Case History 2G

Signalment

Feline, domestic, male, 6 years old.

*Neurologic Examination**

A. Observation
  1. Mental status: Normal.
  2. Posture: Recumbent.
  3. Gait: The cat has slight voluntary movements of limbs but cannot walk.
B. Palpation: Normal.
C. Postural Reactions

Left	Reactions	Right
0	Proprioceptive positioning PL	0
0	TL	0

* *Key*: 0 = absent, +1 = decreased, +2 = normal, +3 = exaggerated, +4 = very exaggerated or clonus, PL = pelvic limb, TL = thoracic limb, NE = not evaluated.

0	Wheelbarrowing	0
0	Hopping, PL	0
0	Hopping, TL	0
0	Extensor postural thrust	0
0	Hemistand-hemiwalk	0
0	Tonic neck	0
0	Placing, tactile PL	0
0	TL	0
0	Placing, visual PL	0
0	TL	0

D. Spinal Reflexes

Left	Reflex	Right
	Spinal segment	
+3	Quadriceps L4–L6	+3
+2	Extensor carpi radialis C7–T1	+2
+2	Triceps C7–T1	+2
+2	Flexion, PL L5–S1	+2
+2	Flexion, TL C6–T1	+2 +2
0	Crossed extensor	0
+2	Perineal S1–S2	+2

E. Cranial nerves: All normal.
F. Sensation: Location.
   Hyperesthesia: No.
   Superficial pain: +2.
   Deep pain: +2.

Complete sections G and H before reviewing Case Summary.

G. Assessment (Anatomic diagnosis and estimation of prognosis)
H. Plan (Diagnostic)

Rule-outs — *Procedure*

1.
2.
3.
4.

Case History 2H

Signalment

Equine, Quarter horse, male, 2 years old.

*Neurologic Examination**

A. Observation
   1. Mental status: Alert.
   2. Posture: Normal.
   3. Gait: Knuckles pelvic limbs, sways trunk. Difficulty in backing: will fall.
B. Palpation: Normal.
C. Postural Reactions

Left	Reactions	Right
+1	Proprioceptive positioning PL	+1
+2	TL	+2
NE	Wheelbarrowing	NE
+1	Hopping, PL	+1
+2	Hopping, TL	+2
NE	Extensor postural thrust	NE
NE	Hemistand-hemiwalk	NE
NE	Tonic neck	NE
0	Placing, tactile (curb) PL	0
+2	TL	+2
NE	Placing, visual PL	NE
NE	TL	NE

D. Spinal Reflexes

Left	Reflex	Right
	Spinal segment	
+3	Quadriceps L4–L6	+3
+2	Extensor carpi radialis C7–T1	+2
NE	Triceps C7–T1	NE
+2	Flexion, PL L5–S1	+2
+2	Flexion, TL C6–T1	+2
0	Crossed extensor	0
+2	Perineal S1–S2	+2

* *Key*: 0 = absent, +1 = decreased, +2 = normal, +3 = exaggerated, +4 = very exaggerated or clonus, PL = pelvic limb, TL = thoracic limb, NE = not evaluated.

E. Cranial nerves: All normal.
F. Sensation: Location.
   Hyperesthesia: No.
   Superficial pain: +2.
   Deep pain: +2.
Complete sections G and H before reviewing Case Summary.
G. Assessment (Anatomic diagnosis and estimation of prognosis)
H. Plan (Diagnostic)

Rule-outs	*Procedure*
1.	
2.	
3.	
4.	

Case History 2I

Signalment

Canine, cocker spaniel, female, 8 years old.

*Neurologic Examination**

A. Observation
   1. Mental status: Normal.
   2. Posture: Head tilt to right.
   3. Gait: Tends to circle to the right. Disoriented when picked up for assessment of postural reactions.
B. Palpation: Normal.
C. Postural Reactions

Left	Reactions	Right
+2	Proprioceptive positioning PL	+2
+2	TL	+2
NE	Wheelbarrowing	NE
+2	Hopping, PL	+2
+2	Hopping, TL	+2
+2	Extensor postural thrust	+2
NE	Hemistand-hemiwalk	NE
NE	Tonic neck	NE
+2	Placing, tactile PL	+2
+2	TL	+2
+2	Placing, visual PL	+2
+2	TL	+2

D. Spinal Reflexes: All normal.

E. Cranial Nerves

Left	Nerve + Function	Right
+2	CN II – vision Menace	0
+2	CN II, III – pupil size	+2
+2	Stim. left eye	+2
+2	Stim. right eye	+2
+2	CN II – fundus	+2
	CN III, IV, VI	
No	Strabismus	No
Fast left	Nystagmus	Horizontal
+2	CN V – sensation	+2
+2	CN V – mastication	+2
+2	CN VII – facial muscles	Drooping
+2	Palpebral	0
+2	CN IX, X – swallowing	+2
+2	CN XII – tongue	+2

F. Sensation: Location.
   Hyperesthesia: No.
   Superficial pain: +2.
   Deep pain: +2.
Complete sessions G and H before reviewing Case Summary.
G. Assessment (Anatomic diagnosis and estimation of prognosis)
H. Plan (Diagnostic)

Rule-outs	*Procedure*
1.	
2.	
3.	
4.	

* *Key*: 0 = absent, +1 = decreased, +2 = normal, +3 = exaggerated, +4 = very exaggerated or clonus, PL = pelvic limb, TL = thoracic limb, NE = not evaluated.

Case History 2J

Signalment

Bovine, Jersey, female, 6 months old.

*Neurologic Examination**

A. Observation
   1. Mental status: Coma.
   2. Posture: Recumbent; increased extensor tone in all four limbs.
   3. Gait: None.
B. Palpation: Normal.
C. Postural Reactions: Recumbent, none possible.

* *Key*: 0 = absent, +1 = decreased, +2 = normal, +3 = exaggerated, +4 = very exaggerated or clonus, PL = pelvic limb, TL = thoracic limb, NE = not evaluated.

D. Spinal Reflexes

Left	Reflex	Right
+3	Spinal segment Quadriceps L4–L6	+3
+3	Extensor carpi radialis C7–T1	+3
NE	Triceps C7–T1	NE
Slow; extensor hypertonus	Flexion, PL L5–S1	Slow; extensor hypertonus
Slow; extensor hypertonus	Flexion, TL C6–T1	Slow; extensor hypertonus
0	Crossed extensor	0
+2	Perineal S1–S2	+2

Cranial Nerves

Left	Nerve + Function	Right
0	CN II – vision Menace	0
Midposition	CN II, III – pupil size	Midposition
0	Stim. left eye	0
0	Stim. right eye	0
+2	CN II – fundus	+2
No eye movements 0	CN III, IV, VI Strabismus Nystagmus	No eye movements 0
0	CN V – sensation	0
+2	CN V – mastication	+2
+2 +2	CN VII – facial muscles Palpebral	+2 +2
+1	CN IX, X – swallowing	+1
+2	CN XII – tongue	+2

F. Sensation: Location.
Hyperesthesia: No.
Superficial pain: Not conscious.
Deep pain: Not conscious.

Complete sections G and H before reviewing Case Summary.

G. Assessment (Anatomic diagnosis and estimation of prognosis)

H. Plan (Diagnostic)

Rule-outs	*Procedure*
1.	
2.	
3.	
4.	

Assessment 2A

Postural reactions are abnormal in both limbs on the right side and, possibly, slow in the left pelvic limb. This finding is not characteristic of peripheral nerve lesions, which ordinarily are restricted to one limb or affect all four limbs (generalized polyneuropathy). Because both pelvic and thoracic limbs are affected, the lesion must be rostral to T2. The right pelvic limb has an exaggerated quadriceps reflex, a UMN sign. Would the interpretation be different if the reflex were normal? No; it would not matter. Reflexes may be normal or exaggerated with UMN disease. The weak or absent myotatic reflexes in the thoracic limbs should not be considered diagnostic. They frequently are difficult to elicit. If there were a good response on one side and none on the other, you might be more confident in diagnosing an abnormality. The weak flexion reflex in the right thoracic limb is abnormal, however. This finding is a sign of sensory or motor deficit at the segmental level – an LMN sign. From this observation, you should assess the lesion as between C6 and T2 on the right side. The sensory examination confirms the assessment of a decrease in sensation in the right thoracic limb. Can the lesion be in the peripheral nerves of the brachial plexus? Not unless there is more than one lesion – remember the abnormalities of the right pelvic limb. One lesion in the C6–T2 spinal cord segments could account for both thoracic and pelvic limb abnormalities. A gray matter lesion affecting sensory and motor neurons to the brachial plexus and a white matter lesion affecting the proprioceptive and UMN pathways to the pelvic limb account for all the signs. Why is pain sensation still present in the pelvic limbs? The pain pathways are bilateral, and this lesion is unilateral. If the lesion were bilateral, both pelvic limbs would have severe postural reaction deficits. The slow initiation of hopping in the left pelvic limb may be caused by a partial loss of the proprioceptive pathways to that side. This hypothesis cannot be substantiated by proprioceptive positioning tests. Is the spinal cord lesion the only lesion? The animal's mental status and cranial nerves are normal, and there are no other signs that cannot be explained by the lesion. Always assume that there is one lesion unless there is evidence to the contrary.

Localization: Spinal cord, C6–T2, right side.
Rule-outs (see Chap. 1):
1. vascular lesion,
2. trauma, and
3. inflammation (low probability).

The plan for a definitive diagnosis will be discussed at the end of Chapter 4.

Assessment 2B

Pelvic limb ataxia and paresis suggest a lesion caudal to T2. The postural reactions and the spinal reflexes confirm that the thoracic limbs are not affected. The spinal reflexes are normal or exaggerated in the pelvic limbs, indicating that the lesion is cranial to L4. Therefore, the lesion should be between T3 and L3. The sensory examination does not provide any definitive evidence for a more specific localization. The animal's mental status and the reactions of the cranial nerves and the thoracic limbs do not suggest that there is more than one lesion.

Localization: Spinal cord, T3–L3, symmetric.
Rule-outs (see Chap. 1):
1. degenerative disease,
2. neoplasia, and
3. inflammation.

The plan for a definitive diagnosis will be discussed at the end of Chapter 4.

Assessment 2C

Ataxia, dysmetria, and tremor are signs of cerebellar disease. Paresis is not associated with cerebellar disease, so it is important to be sure that there is no loss of voluntary movements. Brain stem or spinal cord disease may mimic some of the signs of cerebellar dysfunction. In this case, the head is affected, and there is a head tremor, an absent menace reaction, and pendular nystagmus, indicating brain disease. There is neither paresis nor proprioceptive deficits, although the postural reactions are not normal. The abnormality of the postural reactions is also a sign of ataxia and dysmetria. The absence of the menace reaction with an intact palpebral reflex (CN V and VII) and good vision is indicative of cerebellar disease. The nystagmus, which does not have a fast and slow component, is similar in origin to the intention tremor of the head. All of the signs are compatible with cerebellar disease, and there are no signs that cannot be explained by the presence of this lesion.

Localization: Cerebellum.
Rule-outs (see Chap. 1):
1. anomaly and
2. trauma.

The plan for a definitive diagnosis will be discussed at the end of Chapter 4.

Assessment 2D

The animal's mental status and head tremor should immediately signal brain disease. Depression can be caused by a lesion in almost any part of the brain except the cerebellum, or it could be merely a manifestation of a generalized illness. The head tremor suggests cerebellar involvement. If the depression is caused by a brain lesion, there is more than one lesion. The postural reactions indicate a left hemiparesis. Hemiparesis is caused by brain disease more often than by spinal cord disease. Because we are thorough, we assess the spinal reflexes, even though the cat appears to have brain disease, and we find that they are absent in the left thoracic limb. This situation cannot be caused by brain disease. Absent reflexes with intact sensation are not an indication of peripheral nerve disease (with the exception of polyneuropathies), so the lesion must be in the ventral roots or the spinal cord gray matter. The pelvic limb has a UMN paresis, indicating that the spinal cord is involved. Where is the lesion? We have signs localizing it to the left C6–T2 spinal cord, the cerebellum, and, possibly, other brain structures (depression). In addition, there is an inflammatory lesion of the eye. Therefore, the problem is a multifocal or a systemic disease. The signs cannot be explained by one lesion.

Localization: Multifocal or systemic disease, left C6–T2 spinal cord, cerebellum; cerebrum or brain stem.
Rule-outs (see Chap. 1):
1. inflammation,
2. neoplasia, and
3. degenerative disease.

The plan for a definitive diagnosis will be discussed at the end of Chapter 4.

Assessment 2E

The primary abnormality is in the animal's mental status. The dog's mood fluctuates between depression and agitation. He does not always make appropriate responses. The slowness of the postural reactions must be interpreted cautiously in view of the dog's mental status. Severely depressed animals may not be cooperative when postural reaction tests are performed. Compulsive walking is usually a sign of prefrontal cerebral cortex disease. In severe forms of the disease, the animal will walk until it bumps into a corner and will stand pressing its head against the wall. The dog's neurologic signs suggest cerebral disease.

Localization: Cerebrum.
Rule-outs (see Chap. 2):
1. metabolic disease and
2. toxic disease.

Assessment 2F

Normal thoracic limbs, LMN signs in the pelvic limbs.

Localization: L4–S3.

Assessment 2G

UMN signs in all four limbs; normal brain.

Localization: C1–C5.

Assessment 2H

Normal thoracic limbs, UMN signs in the pelvic limbs.

Localization: T3–L3.

Assessment 2I

The head tilt and the nystagmus indicate an abnormality of the vestibular system. The lack of paresis or proprioceptive deficits and the horizontal nystagmus that does not change are characteristic of peripheral vestibular lesions.

The lip and palpebral reflexes indicate involvement of the facial nerve (CN VII). CN VII and CN VIII are both affected in the labyrinth.

Assessment 2J

Coma, decerebrate posture, tetraparesis, and cranial nerve signs indicate involvement of the brain stem. The menace reaction is absent because of the coma and disconnection of the cortex from CN VII.

The pupils indicate a loss of both sympathetic and parasympathetic input and involvement of the midbrain. The eye movements indicate involvement of the core brain stem (medial longitudinal fasciculus). The lesion is in the midbrain (see Chap. 13).

Localization to the brain stem is adequate for the formulation of a clinical diagnosis.

REFERENCES

1. Oliver JE: Localization of lesions in the nervous system. In Hoerlein BF (ed): Canine Neurology, 3rd ed. Philadelphia, WB Saunders, 1978, pp 71–102.
2. Willis W, Chung J: Central mechanisms of pain. J Am Vet Med Assoc 191:1200–1202, 1987.
3. Breazile JE, Kitchell RL: A study of fiber systems within the spinal cord of the domestic pig that subserve pain. J Comp Neurol 133:373–382, 1968.
4. Kennard MA: The course of ascending fibers in the spinal cord of the cat essential to the recognition of painful stimuli. J Comp Neurol 100:511–524, 1954.
5. Tarlov IM: Spinal cord compression: Mechanism of paralysis and treatment. Springfield, IL, Charles C Thomas, 1957.
6. Holliday T: Clinical signs of acute and chronic experimental lesions of the cerebellum. Vet Sci Commun 3:259–278, 1980.
7. Holliday TA: Clinical signs caused by experimental lesions in the vestibular system. In: Proceedings of the Eighth Annual Veterinary Medical Forum. Washington, DC, 1990, pp 1025–1028.
8. Kornegay JN: Ataxia of the head and limbs: Cerebellar diseases in dogs and cats. Prog Vet Neurol 1:255–274, 1990.

3

Disorders of Micturition

Abnormal visceral function may reflect a pathologic change in the nervous system; however, the importance of nervous control of the viscera is often overlooked.

The classic view of the autonomic nervous system as one with discrete boundaries is giving way to a concept of a more integrated system with no limits. For example, conventional theory held that the autonomic system controlled functions that the individual could not modify voluntarily. It has been proved, however, that one can regulate blood pressure, heart rate, micturition, and many other autonomic activities. In conventional theory, the sympathetic (adrenergic) system functions as an antagonist to the parasympathetic (cholinergic) system. This simplistic view, which separates the autonomic system from the somatic system, does not explain well-defined somatovisceral and viscerosomatic reflexes.

Problems associated with micturition are common in neurologic disorders. Other visceral dysfunctions traditionally have been the concern of cardiologists or internists and are discussed in books on cardiology and internal medicine. This chapter reviews the anatomy, the physiology, and the clinical syndromes of micturition.

Anatomy and Physiology of Micturition

Micturition is the reaction that ultimately will occur if a bladder is gradually distended, leading to the coordinated expulsion of its contents.[1] The micturition reflex is a complex integration of parasympathetic, sympathetic, and somatic pathways extending from the sacral segments of the spinal cord to the cerebral cortex. The components of the micturition reflex will be discussed in functional groups before a complete description of the micturition reflex is presented.

The Detrusor Reflex

The primary component of micturition is the detrusor (the muscle of the urinary bladder) reflex. As the bladder fills with urine, there is a very slight increase in bladder pressure with each increase in volume, until the limit of elasticity of the smooth muscle is reached. The sensory nerve endings in the bladder wall are tension recorders and are arranged in series with the muscle fibers. As the bladder nears its capacity, these nerves begin to discharge. The sensory fibers from the bladder are located in the pelvic nerve and originate from the sacral segments of the spinal cord (Fig. 3–1).[2,3] The sensory discharge ascends in the spinal cord to the pontine reticular formation in the brain stem. Integration occurs at this level, eventually giving rise to a motor discharge down the spinal cord to the preganglionic parasympathetic neurons in the intermediate horn of the sacral segments. The preganglionic parasympathetic nerves are located in segments S1–S3 in the cat and the dog.[2,3] They have not been located precisely in other species, but gross dissections indicate they are in the sacral segments. The preganglionic neurons discharge and activate postganglionic neurons, which are located in the pelvic ganglia, along the course of the pelvic nerves, and in the wall of the bladder. Some integration of activity apparently takes place in

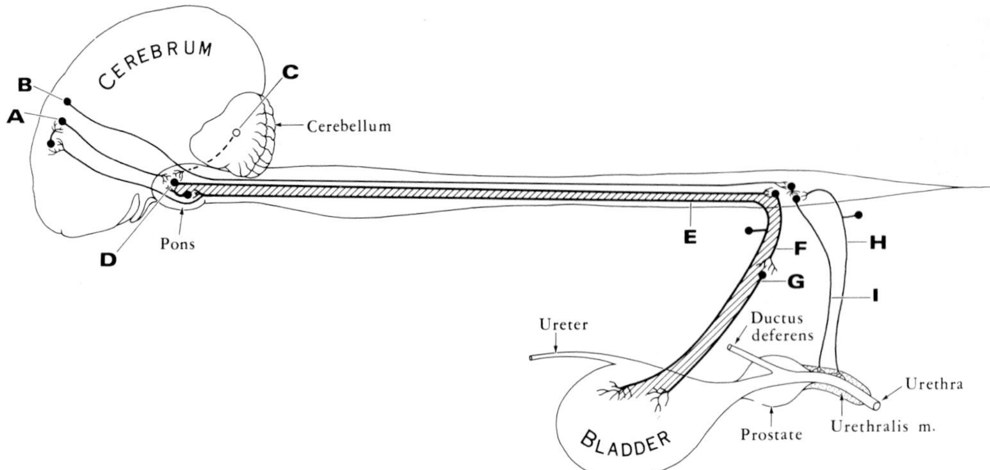

Figure 3–1 Anatomic organization of micturition. *A*. Cortical neurons for voluntary control of micturition. *B*. Cortical neurons for voluntary control of sphincters. *C*. Cerebellar neurons that have an inhibitory influence on micturition. *D*. Pontine reticular neurons that are necessary for the detrusor reflex. *E*. Afferent (sensory) pathway for the detrusor reflex. *F*. Preganglionic pelvic (parasympathetic) neuron to the detrusor. *G*. Postganglionic pelvic (parasympathetic) neuron to the detrusor. *H*. Afferent (sensory) neuron from the urethral spincter, pudendal nerve. *I*. Efferent (motor) neuron to the urethral sphincter, pudendal nerve. (From Oliver JE Jr, Osborne CA: Neurogenic urinary incontinence. In Kirk RW (ed): Current Veterinary Therapy, VII. Philadelphia, WB Saunders Co., 1980, pp 1122–1127. Used by permission.)

the ganglia. Ultimately, the postganglionic neurons synapse on detrusor muscle fibers and cause a contraction—the detrusor reflex (Fig. 3–2, line A).

Integration in the brain stem is necessary in order for the detrusor reflex to be coordinated and sustained long enough for bladder evacuation. Complete lesions of any portion of this pathway will abolish the detrusor reflex.

Voluntary Control of the Detrusor Reflex

The sensory pathway to the brain stem that signals distention of the bladder also sends collaterals to the cerebral cortex (see Fig. 3–1). Integration at the cortical level allows voluntary initiation (e.g., in territorial marking) or inhibition (e.g., in house training) of micturition. The precise location of the control center of cerebral

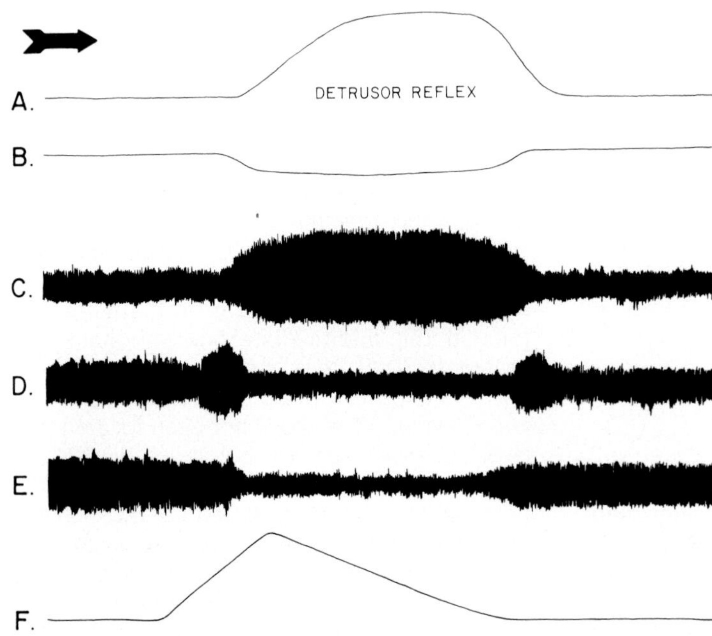

Figure 3–2 Schematic representation of sequential pressure and neural changes during micturition (not drawn to scale). *A*. Intravesical pressure. *B*. Urethral pressure. *C*. Pelvic nerve. *D*. Hypogastric nerve. *E*. Pudendal nerve. *F*. Bladder volume. (Modified with permission from Jonas U, Tanagho EA: Studies on vesicourethral reflexes. Invest Urol 12:357–373, 1975; and Bradley WE, Teague CT: Hypogastric and pelvic nerve activity during the micturition reflex. J Urol 101:438–440, 1969.)

cortex is not clear. Stimulation and evoked-response studies indicate that several areas of the cortex influence the detrusor reflex.[4] Lesions of the cerebral cortex may cause a loss of voluntary control of micturition and may reduce the capacity of the bladder.[5] For example, animals with cerebral tumors may start voiding in the house for no apparent reason.

Cerebellar Inhibition of the Detrusor Reflex

The cerebellum can inhibit the detrusor reflex (see Fig. 3–1). Stimulation of the fastigial nucleus abolishes detrusor reflex contraction.[6]

Lesions of the cerebellum, such as cerebellar hypoplasia, may produce increased frequency of voiding with a reduced bladder capacity.[1]

The Urethral Sphincter

The muscle surrounding the urethra contains muscle spindles that discharge in response to stretch, as do other skeletal muscles. Sensory discharges ascend in the pudendal nerves to the sacral segments. The pudendal urethral motor neurons are located in segments L7–S3 in the dog and the cat, although they are found primarily in S1 and S2 in both species.[2,7] Monosynaptic activation of the motor neurons is transmitted back down the pudendal nerve to the muscle (see Fig. 3–1). Afferent discharge through the pelvic nerves also activates the pudendal nerve. These pathways produce urethral contraction in response to a sudden stretch, maintaining continence during a cough, a sneeze, and so forth.

Voluntary control of the urethral sphincter is provided by cortical pathways to the sacral segments (see Fig. 3–1).

Lesions of the sacral segments or the pudendal nerve will cause a hypotonic paralysis of the sphincter. Cortical or spinal lesions may abolish voluntary control of the sphincter and may produce increased sphincter tone, which increases outflow resistance.[8] Typically, T3–L3 lesions of the spinal cord abolish the long-routed detrusor reflex and cause increased tone in the sphincter.

Sympathetic Innervation

The detrusor reflex is mediated through the parasympathetic nervous system (sacral). The skeletal muscle in the urethral sphincter is innervated by somatic nerves. Sympathetic nerves found in the pelvic plexus, the pelvic ganglia, and the urinary bladder serve to enhance the storage function of micturition.

The preganglionic sympathetic neurons to the bladder are located in the lumbar spinal cord (L2–L5 in the cat, L1–L4 in the dog).[2,3] The fibers course through the caudal mesenteric ganglion and the hypogastric nerve to the bladder and the pelvic plexus. Both alpha- and beta-adrenergic (sympathetic postganglionic) synapses have been found on neurons in the pelvic ganglia, in the bladder wall, and on the detrusor muscle, especially in the area of the trigone.[9]

Pharmacologic studies have demonstrated that alpha-adrenergic receptors are located primarily in the region of the trigone, the bladder neck, and proximal urethra, causing contraction of the smooth muscle. Beta-adrenergic receptors are found in all parts of the bladder and cause relaxation of smooth muscle. The presence of adrenergic synapses on cholinergic ganglion cells suggests that the sympathetic pathways can also modulate the activity of the parasympathetic pathway, but this effect has not been demonstrated in naturally occurring sympathetic firing.[8] Adrenergic innervation of the bladder neck and the trigone has been demonstrated to have major significance in the prevention of retrograde ejaculation.

Lesions of the sympathetic pathways apparently do not have a major effect on micturition; however, there is increasing acceptance of the theory that the sympathetic pathways play an important role in animals and in human beings with lesions of the parasympathetic pathways.[9–11] Patients with neurogenic bladder dysfunction complicated by a narrowing of the bladder neck or spasms of the urethra may be helped by alpha-adrenergic blockade.[9]

Sensory Pathways from the Bladder

Sensory fibers originating in the bladder run in both the pelvic and the hypogastric nerves. Stretch receptors in the bladder wall give rise to fibers that run through the pelvic nerve into the sacral spinal cord (S1–S3 in the cat and the dog) and ascend to the pontine reticular formation to initiate the detrusor reflex. Sensory fibers in the hypogastric nerve reach the spinal cord at the lumbar segments (L2–L5 in the cat, L1–L4 in the dog).[2,3] Afferent fibers from both pelvic and hypogastric nerves reach the cerebral cortex in the cat, while only hypogastric neural activity is relayed to the cortex in the dog.[12] The hypogastric fibers respond to overdistention of the bladder. Activation of these fibers is perceived as pain.[13] It is possible for a lesion of the lower lumbar or sacral spinal cord to abolish micturition, although the animal will still be able to perceive overdistention of the bladder as a painful sensation mediated through the hypogastric nerve.

Motor Innervation of the Detrusor Muscle

Each motor nerve in the bladder wall innervates many muscle cells, although not all muscle cells have direct innervation. The neuromuscular junction is characterized by a varicosity of the axon containing synaptic vesicles, a thinning of the Schwann cell layer, and a close apposition to specialized areas of the detrusor muscle fibers. Excitation of the innervated muscle cell (pacemaker cell) initiates a spread of excitation and contraction through adjacent cells by means of "tight junctions."[8] It also has been hypothesized that the spread of excitation occurs by diffusion of a neurotransmitter in the extracellular space to adjacent detrusor muscle fibers.

Disruption of tight junctions between muscle fibers may occur when the bladder is overdistended (e.g., in obstruction of the urethra). If tight junctions are disrupted, the wave of excitation cannot spread, and a flaccid bladder will result. Reconnection of the junction will occur in 1 to 2 weeks if the distention is relieved early enough. If the bladder remains distended too long or if infection is present, fibrosis develops between the cells, preventing restoration of function.

Reflex Integration

The micturition reflex involves a coordinated and sustained contraction of the detrusor muscle and relaxation of the urethra. Pelvic nerve sensory neurons that produce the detrusor reflex also send collaterals to inhibitory interneurons in the sacral spinal cord.[13] The inhibitory interneurons synapse on the pudendal motor neurons, which are also in the sacral segments, to reduce motor activity in the pudendal nerves and the periurethral striated muscle (see Fig. 3–2, line B and record E). As the detrusor contracts, the urethra relaxes, allowing urine to pass. If the long pathways are intact, voluntary activation of the pudendal neurons by the corticospinal pathways can override this effect and block micturition. Lesions of the long tracts or at the segmental level may interfere with reflex integration. Detrusor contraction without urethral relaxation is called *reflex dyssynergia*.[14]

Reflex connections between the pelvic (parasympathetic) nerve afferents and the lumbar (sympathetic) motor neurons also have been demonstrated.[13] The effect seems to be similar to that observed in the pudendal (somatic) nerve—that is, as the pelvic motor neuron begins to fire to initiate a detrusor contraction, the hypogastric nerve becomes silent (see Fig. 3–2, records C and D). When the pelvic nerve stops firing as the bladder is emptied, the hypogastric nerve discharges once more. Presumably, the effect of the hypogastric nerve is on bladder relaxation and urethral contraction.

The Micturition Reflex

Urine is transported from the kidneys to the bladder through the ureters. Peristaltic waves move the urine into the bladder in spurts. Vesicoureteral reflux is prevented by the oblique course of the ureter through the bladder wall, resulting in the formation of a flap valve. The detrusor spirals around the ureter, assisting in the maintenance of the valve effect.

The bladder fills without a significant increase in pressure as the smooth muscle stretches (see Fig. 3–2, lines A and F). The sympathetic (adrenergic) pathways may assist by inhibiting parasympathetic (cholinergic) neurons or by direct relaxation of smooth muscle. If the bladder fills beyond the normal elasticity of the smooth muscle, pressure increases linearly with the increase in volume.

In the intact animal, as the limits of stretch of the smooth muscle are approached, stretch receptors in the bladder wall are excited and send sensory discharges through the pelvic nerves to the sacral spinal cord. These discharges are relayed up the spinal cord to the reticular formation in the pons. The activation of neuronal pools in the pons results in a motor discharge down the spinal cord to the sacral segments. Preganglionic parasympathetic motor neurons in the intermediate horn of the sacral gray matter are activated. The motor discharge passes down the pelvic nerves to activate postganglionic neurons in the pelvic ganglia and in the wall of the bladder, which in turn activate the bladder smooth muscle (detrusor). The sustained discharge of neurons through these pathways produces a coordinated, sustained contraction of the detrusor muscle (see Fig. 3–2, line A and record C).

The fibers of the detrusor muscle spiral into the neck of the bladder and help to maintain continence in the relaxed state. As the fibers contract, the bladder neck is pulled open into a funnel shape. Simultaneously, sensory discharges from the pelvic nerves are relayed to the lumbar segments, inhibiting the output of the sympathetic pathway, and to the pudendal motor neurons in the ventral horn of the sacral segments, inhibiting the tonic output in the nerves to the skeletal sphincter (see Fig. 3–2, records C–E).

The result is a coordinated contraction of the bladder and a relaxation of the sphincter, which is maintained until voiding is complete (see Fig. 3–2, line A and record B). Sustaining of the contraction also is enhanced by sensory fibers in the urethra, which respond to the flow of urine.

When the bladder is empty, the sensory discharge in the pelvic nerve stops, resulting in a cessation of motor discharge in the pelvic nerve and a return of activity in the sympathetic and pudendal nerves. The bladder relaxes, and the sphincter closes.

Disorders of Micturition

The neurogenic disorders of micturition are caused by abnormal detrusor or sphincter function, or both (Table 3–1). Detrusor or sphincter activity may be decreased, increased, or normal. Typical syndromes include inappropriate voiding; inadequate voiding with an overflow of urine; increased frequency, reduced capacity, or both; or incomplete voiding when normal voiding reactions are interrupted by abrupt contractions of the urethral sphincter.[8]

Clinical Signs

The clinical signs of abnormal micturition are summarized in Table 3–2.

Detrusor Areflexia with Sphincter Hypertonus. The most frequently recognized disorder of micturition is a loss of the detrusor reflex with increased tone in the urethral sphincter. Lesions from the pontine reticular formation to the L7 spinal cord segments may cause these complications. The most common cause is compression of the spinal cord, such as from a herniated disk, which disrupts the long pathways that are responsible for the detrusor reflex and the upper motor neuron (UMN) pathways to the skeletal muscle of the urethral sphincter. The animal is unable to void, the bladder becomes greatly distended, and it is difficult or impossible to express the bladder manually. The perineal reflex is intact.

Detrusor Areflexia with Normal Sphincter Tone. Lesions of the spinal cord or the brain stem may produce detrusor areflexia without producing increased tone in the urethral sphincter. Traumatic injuries of the pelvis may damage the pelvic plexus without damaging the pudendal nerve. The animal is unable to void, but manual expression can be accomplished. Females have a short skeletal sphincter so that even with UMN lesions, sphincter tone may not be excessive. Perineal reflexes are intact.

Detrusor Areflexia with Sphincter Areflexia. Lesions of the sacral spinal cord or the nerve roots, such as fractures of the L6 or L7 vertebrae, cause a loss of the detrusor and urethral sphincter reflexes. The bladder is easily expressed and may leak urine continuously. Perineal reflexes are diminished or absent.

Detrusor Areflexia from Overdistention. Loss of excitation–contraction coupling in the detrusor muscle may occur as a result of severe overdistention of the bladder. Manual expression of the bladder may be difficult, because the sphincter is normal. The animal may empty the bladder partially by abdominal contraction. Attempts to void indicate that sensory pathways are intact and suggests a primary detrusor muscle abnormality. The most frequent cause is obstruction of the outflow tract (e.g., by calculi or in the feline urologic syndrome).

Detrusor Hyperreflexia. Frequent voiding of small quantities of urine, often without warning, may be caused by partial lesions of the long pathways or of the cerebellum. Inflammation of the bladder (cystitis) may produce similar signs. There is little or no residual urine, the capacity of the bladder is reduced, and perineal reflexes are intact.

Reflex Dyssynergia. Normal initiation of voiding is followed by interruption of the stream through an involuntary contraction of the urethral sphincter. The stream of urine is normal at first. It is followed by short spurts, and then by a complete cessation of the flow. Frequently, the animal continues to strain with no success. Reflex dyssynergia is seen primarily in male dogs. The pathogenesis is not certain but is presumed to be the result of a partial UMN lesion, causing a loss of the normal inhibition of the pudendal nerves during the detrusor reflex. The detrusor reflex is present, and the perineal reflex is often hyperactive.

Normal Detrusor Reflex with Decreased Sphincter Tone. Loss of normal urethral resistance with a normal detrusor reflex causes leaking of urine when voiding is delayed. The animal can empty the bladder, but as soon as a small amount of urine accumulates, leakage occurs. The leakage may be related to an abdominal press (barking, coughing) or may occur during complete rest. The most frequent cause is the lack of sex hormones in a neutered animal. Hormone-responsive incontinence has been well documented in the ovariectomized bitch,[15] and less frequently

TABLE 3–1 Effect of Lesions of the Neuromuscular System on Micturition

		Bladder					**Sphincter**			
Location of Lesion	***Normal Function***	Voluntary Control	Sustained Detrusor Reflex	Tone	Volume	Residual Urine	Voluntary Control	Reflexes (Perineal)	Tone	Synergy with Detrusor
Cerebral cortex to brain stem	Voluntary control to detrusor and sphincter	Absent	Normal	Normal	May be greater or smaller than normal	None	Absent	Normal to hyperreflexic	Normal to increased	Normal
Cerebellum	Inhibition of detrusor reflex	Normal, but increased frequency	Possible hyperreflexia	Normal	Small	None	Normal	Normal	Normal	Normal
Brain stem to sacral spinal cord	Sustained detrusor reflex	Absent	Lost early; small unsynchronized contractions late	Atonic early; possibly increased late	Large	Large	Absent	Normal to hyperreflexic	Normal to increased	Absent
Partial lesions; brain stem to sacral spinal cord (reflex dyssynergia)	Coordination of detrusor and sphincter	May be present	May be present	Normal to atonic	Large	Small to large	May be normal	Normal	Normal to increased	Absent
Sacral spinal cord or roots	LMN to detrusor and sphincter	Absent	Absent	Atonic	Large	Large	Absent	Absent	Flaccid	Absent
Disruption of tight junctions of detrusor	Spread of excitation in detrusor	Absent	Absent	Atonic	Large	Large	Normal	Normal	Normal	Normal (cannot evaluate, however)

Modified from Oliver JE Jr, Osborne CA: Neurogenic urinary incontinence. In Kirk RW (ed): Current Veterinary Therapy, VI. Philadelphia, WB Saunders Co., 1977. Used by permission.

TABLE 3–2 Signs of Abnormal Micturition

Problem	*Voiding*	*Attempts to Void*	*Expression of Bladder*	*Residual Urine*	*Perineal Reflex*	*Probable Lesion*
Detrusor areflexia, sphincter hypertonus	Absent	No	Difficult	Large amount	Present	Brain stem to L7 spinal cord
Detrusor areflexia, normal sphincter tone	Absent	No	Possible, some resistance	Large amount	Present	Brain stem to L7 spinal cord
Detrusor areflexia, sphincter areflexia	Absent	No	Easy, often leaks	Large to moderate amount	Absent	Sacral spinal cord or nerve roots
Detrusor areflexia, (overdistention)	Absent	Yes	Possible, some resistance	Large amount	Present	Detrusor muscle
Detrusor hyperreflexia	Frequent, small quantity	Yes	Possible, some resistance	None	Present	Brain stem to L7, partial, or cerebellum; rule out inflammation of bladder
Reflex dyssynergia	Frequent, spurting, unsustained	Yes	Difficult	Small to large amount	Present	Brain stem to L7, partial
Normal detrusor reflex, incompetent sphincter	Normal, but with leakage of urine with stress, or full bladder	Yes	Easy	None	May or may not be present	Pudendal nerves, sympathetic nerves, hormone deficiency

in neutered male dogs. Both cases are responsive to hormone replacement therapy, with or without supplementation with adrenergic agents. A similar clinical picture may be seen in some animals that are not responsive to hormone therapy. The lesion may be a structural abnormality of the urethra, a loss of pudendal innervation, or a loss of sympathetic innervation to the urethra.[15]

Diagnosis

The minimum data base recommended for the evaluation of an animal with a problem associated with micturition is presented in Table 3–3. The minimum data base is designed to reveal any additional problems as well as to provide the information necessary to make a diagnosis and to formulate a prognosis. Figure 3–3 outlines the process of establishing a diagnosis. Specific steps in the process are discussed in the following sections.

History

In addition to the usual items in the history, the examiner should obtain some specific information pertinent to micturition.

Past History. The clinician should determine the animal's pattern of micturition habits from as early an age as possible. Age when house trained, frequency of micturition at various ages, and changes in habits may provide insights into the onset of a problem prior to the owner's recognition of its significance.

Signs of abnormality in the nervous system or the urinary tract or previous trauma are important. Previous operative procedures, especially

TABLE 3–3 Minimum Data Base for Diagnosis of Disorders of Micturition

History
Physical examination
  Includes: observation of voiding and measurement of residual urine
Neurologic examination
  Includes: sphincter reflexes
Clinical pathology
  Includes: CBC, urinalysis, BUN or creatinine determinations
Radiologic examination
  Includes: survey of abdomen and pelvis contrast cystography and urethrography intravenous pyelogram

Modified from Oliver JE Jr., Osborne CA: Neurogenic urinary incontinence. In Kirk RW (ed): Current Veterinary Therapy, VI. Philadelphia, WB Saunders Co., 1977.

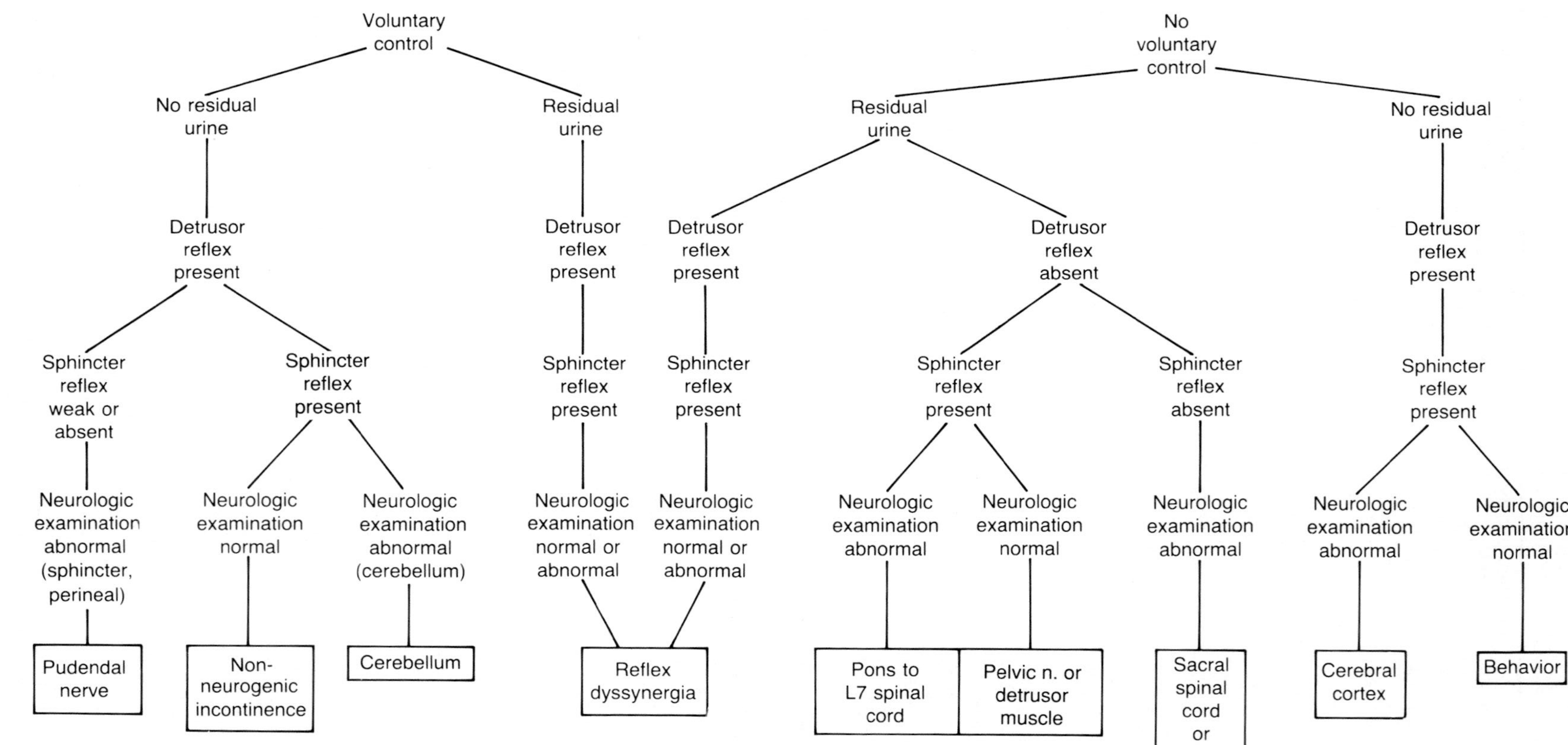

Figure 3–3 Algorithm for diagnosis of disorders of micturition. (From Oliver JE Jr, Osborne CA: Neurogenic urinary incontinence. In Kirk RW (ed): Current Veterinary Therapy, VII. Philadelphia, WB Saunders Co., 1980, pp 1122–1127. Used by permission.)

neurologic, abdominal, or pelvic surgery (e.g., ovariohysterectomy), should be analyzed in relation to the time of onset of the problem.

History of the Problem. Information regarding the onset and the chronological course of the problem will allow the examiner to construct a sign-time graph, which is useful for determining the etiology of the disease (see Chap. 1).

Voluntary control of micturition is often best established by the owner's perceptions, which are supplemented and confirmed by direct observation of the animal in natural surroundings (e.g., outside on the grass). If the animal can volitionally initiate voiding, the detrusor reflex probably is present. Voluntary control also implies that micturition can be withheld for a reasonable length of time (house training) and can be interrupted if necessary. Interruption of micturition is difficult to evaluate. A dog that is lead-trained can be interrupted by a pull on the lead and a command to "come." Individual interpretation of interruption is quite subjective.

Reflex dyssynergia begins with a normal initiation of voiding followed by a narrowing of the stream and a sudden interruption of the flow. The animal often strains and may continue voiding in brief spurts. Dyssynergia must be differentiated from *partial obstruction* (e.g., that caused by urethral calculi), which can be demonstrated by catheterization and urethral contrast-enhanced radiography.

Various types of incontinence may be described by the owner. Precipitate voiding (detrusor hyperreflexia), in which the animal voids suddenly in inappropriate places without apparent warning, is characteristic of cerebellar lesions and some partial spinal cord or brain stem lesions (see Table 3–2). Differentiation between precipitate voiding and loss of normal voluntary control, as in cortical lesions or behavioral changes, may be difficult on the basis of the history alone.

Dribbling of urine may result from loss of urethral resistance or overflow from an areflexic bladder (see Table 3–2).

Physical Examination

Observation of the animal may confirm the characteristics of micturition as described in the history. The differences in the various abnormalities of micturition may be subtle, so it is critical that the problem described by the owner be verified by the examiner.

The presence of a detrusor reflex can be assumed if voiding is sustained (see Fig. 3–3). However, bladder contractions with incomplete voiding are common in neurologic disorders. Such contractions are not the result of a true detrusor reflex. Therefore, the residual urine must be measured in every animal with a problem associated with micturition. After the animal has voided, preferably outside in natural surroundings, the bladder is catheterized and the residual urine is measured. Residual urine should be less than 10% of the normal volume. Most animals have less than 10 ml remaining (0.2–0.4 ml/kg).[9]

Except for urethral flaps, which are rare, obstructions in the urethra can be detected when a catheter is passed. A flap can be demonstrated only by excretory urethrography.[16]

Palpation of the bladder before and after the animal voids provides some information regarding bladder tone. The tone of the detrusor muscle is intrinsic and is not directly related to innervation; however, a normal bladder contracts to accommodate the volume of urine present. An overdistended bladder with rupture of the tight junctions does not contract. A chronically infected bladder is often small and has thickened, fibrotic walls. A small contracted bladder with infection may not be the primary problem, because bladder infection is a common sequela of urine retention from neurogenic disorders. Some of the nonneurogenic causes of incontinence, such as tumors or calculi, may be identified by palpation.

Manual expression of the bladder provides some information regarding urethral sphincter tone. Normally, expression of the bladder is more difficult in the male than in the female. Urethral sphincter tone is decreased in lesions of the sacral spinal cord, the sacral roots, or the pudendal nerve (lower motor neuron) and is increased in lesions between the L7 spinal cord segment and the brain stem (see Table 3–2). The sacral spinal cord segments lie within the body of the fifth lumbar vertebra in the dog, so that lesions of the vertebrae from L5–L6 caudad can affect the sacral roots. In large animals, lesions at the level of the midsacrum will affect the sacral segments and nerve roots.

Neurologic Examination

The complete neurologic examination was described in Chapter 1. Reflexes related to the sacral spinal cord segments are especially important in neurogenic bladder dysfunction.

The anal and urethral sphincters are innervated by the pudendal nerve, primarily from sacral segments 1 and 2, but occasionally with fibers from S3. Anal sphincter function is easy to observe or to palpate, whereas the urethral sphincter is evaluated best by electrodiagnostic procedures.

The tone of the anal sphincter can be observed, or the sphincter can be palpated with a gloved digit. Two sacral reflexes also can be evaluated. The *bulbocavernosus reflex* is a sharp contraction of the sphincter in response to a squeeze of the bulb of the penis or the clitoris. The *perineal reflex* is a contraction of the sphincter in response to a pinch or pinprick of the perineal region. The perineal reflex also is used to test sensory distribution in the perineal region. Unilateral lesions are detected in this manner.

Lesions of the sacral spinal cord, the sacral roots, or the pudendal nerves will abolish these reflexes, and the anal sphincter will be atonic.

The history, the physical examination, and the neurologic examination provide sufficient data to differentiate neurogenic from nonneurogenic bladder disorders and to localize the lesion in the nervous system if a neurogenic disorder is present (see Tables 3–1 and 3–2). Additional data are necessary for the formulation of an etiologic diagnosis and a prognosis.

Clinical Pathology

The minimum data base includes a complete blood cell (CBC) count, urinalysis, and a determination of blood urea nitrogen (BUN) or creatinine values. Each is essential for the formulation of a prognosis of urinary tract dysfunction and may assist in the diagnosis of nonneurogenic problems of micturition.

All animals with neurogenic bladder disorders are likely to have urinary tract infections. Constant surveillance and appropriate treatment, when indicated, are imperative if a favorable outcome is to be expected. Ureteral reflux is also a frequent complication of neurogenic bladder dysfunction. Reflux of infected urine may lead to pyelonephritis, uremia, and death.

Radiologic Examination

Radiography is important for the identification of nonneurogenic problems, for the evaluation of the extent of urinary tract disease, which may be a complication of neurogenic disorders, and for the assessment of the primary neurologic problem.

Contrast-enhanced cystourethrography, especially when performed in conjunction with cystometry, offers promise of more adequately evaluating the functional morphology of the lower urinary tract.[16]

Electrophysiologic Examination

Electrophysiologic tests were not included in the minimum data base described in Chapter 1 because they currently are not widely available. In some cases, however, electrophysiologic tests are necessary in order to make a definitive diagnosis.

The cystometrogram (CMG) measures intravesical pressure during a detrusor reflex (Fig. 3–4).[16–20] A sustained detrusor reflex is difficult to document clinically in most cases. Additionally, the CMG provides data on the threshold volume and pressure, the capacity, the ability of the bladder to fill at a normal pressure (a measure of elasticity of the bladder wall), and the presence of uninhibited bladder contractions (a sign of denervation). Normal data from the CMG of the dog and horse are presented in Table 3–4.

Simultaneous measurement of the CMG and urinary flow allows more complete assessment of the function of the bladder and urethra, especially in disorders of coordination of bladder contraction and urethral relaxation.[21,22] An electromagnetic flow transducer records the flow of urine collected in a funnel. The intravesical pressure is measured simultaneously. The major disadvantage of this technique is the necessity of placing two catheters through the abdominal wall into the bladder. Normal dogs have minimal problems, but we have had leakage from cystocentesis with 22-gauge needles in animals with neurogenic bladder. Therefore, this procedure must be used with caution.[23]

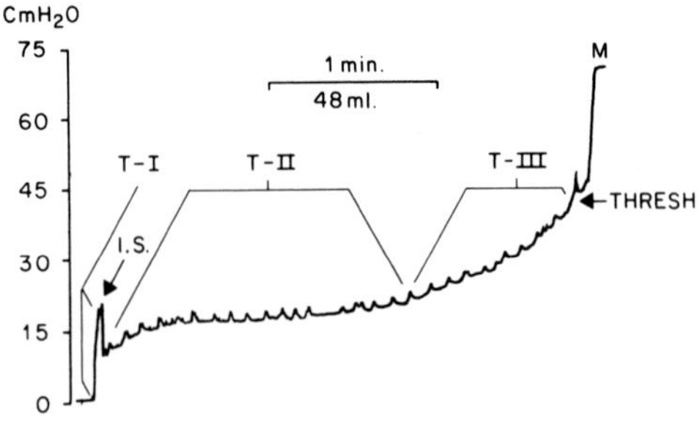

Figure 3–4 Cystometrogram of a dog showing segments of the tonus limb. *T-I*, resting pressure; *T-II*, bladder filling pressure change (smooth muscle elasticity); *T-III*, bladder filling pressure change after capacity is reached. Scale indicates time and volume. Thresh, threshold of detrusor reflex; *M*, maximal contraction; *I.S.*, initial spike, an artifact.

$$\text{T-II} = \frac{(\text{Pressure at inflection} - \text{Resting pressure}) \times 100}{\text{Volume}}$$

(From Oliver JE Jr, Young WO: Air cystometry in dogs under xylazine-induced restraint. Am J Vet Res 34:1433, 1973. Used by permission.)

TABLE 3–4 Normal Values for Cystometrograms (CMG) Using Xylazine for Restraint*

Measurement	Values of CMG	
	Dog	Horse
Tonus limb I	9.7 ± 4.3	1.9 ± 1.6
Tonus limb II	12.6 ± 12.2	1.0 ± 0.7
Threshold pressure	24.4 ± 10.0	22.0 ± 7.5
Threshold pressure Minus tonus limb I	14.4 ± 8.7	14.4 ± 10.6
Threshold volume	206.6 ± 184.4	2,554 ± 1,087
Maximal contraction Pressure	77.6 ± 33.8	100.1 ± 5.9

Data from Oliver JE Jr, and Young WO: Air cystometry in dogs under xylazine-induced restraint. Am J Vet Res 34:1433–1435, 1973; and Clark ES, Semrad SD, Bichsel P, Oliver JE: Cystometrography and urethral pressure profiles in healthy horse and pony mares. Am J Vet Res 48:552–555, 1987.

* All values are means ± SD and are given in cmH_2O except for threshold volume, which is given in ml air (see Fig. 3–4).

Electromyography (EMG) of the skeletal muscles of the anal and urethral sphincters and other muscles in the pelvic diaphragm provides direct evidence of the status of innervation. The perineal or bulbocavernosus reflex also can be tested while a recording is being taken directly from these muscles in cases in which clinical evaluation is equivocal.

An EMG recording that is taken from the anal sphincter while the urethra or the bladder is being stimulated with a catheter electrode is termed an *electromyelograph* (EMyG).[23] Urethral stimulation evokes a response similar to the bulbocavernosus reflex. Stimulation of the bladder wall evokes a comparable response, except that the sensory pathway is in the pelvic nerves. The evoked bladder response is difficult to record in most animals. An EMyG from bladder stimulation provides evidence of the integrity of the pelvic nerves. The main advantages of the electrical tests are the following: (1) the response is objective, (2) the response can be measured accurately, and (3) latencies are recorded that provide information about partial denervation.

The urethral pressure profile measures the pressure along the length of the urethra.[19,20,24–26] An EMG of the striated urethral sphincter can be recorded simultaneously. The maximum urethral closure pressure and the functional profile length are the most important parameters (Fig. 3–5). Normal values are listed in Table 3–5.

Averaged somatosensory-evoked responses can be recorded from the scalp (cortex) or the spinal cord during stimulation of the bladder or the urethra (see the section on the somatosensory-evoked response in Chap. 4). The cortical-evoked response is a method of evaluating the sensory pathways.

Results of these tests are useful for lesion localization. Table 3–6 summarizes the data provided by the physical examination findings and electrophysiologic tests.

The final diagnosis should include (1) the location of the lesion in the nervous system, (2) the etiology of the lesion, (3) the functional central nervous system (CNS) deficit, and (4) the functional deficit related to micturition.

Treatment

Management of a case depends on the final diagnosis. The treatment of primary CNS disease is described throughout this text. Functional deficits of micturition secondary to CNS disease may be temporary or permanent, depending on the reversibility of the CNS lesion and the maintenance of the integrity of the urinary system. If the bladder is severely infected and secondary fibrosis of the bladder wall occurs, normal function cannot be restored, even if the CNS lesion

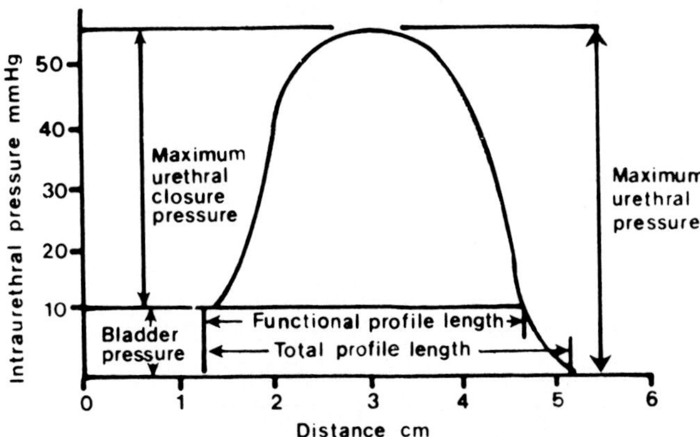

Figure 3–5 Schematic representation of the urethral closure pressure profile. (From Rosin A, Rosin E, Oliver JE Jr: Canine urethral pressure profile. Am J Vet Res 41:1113-1116, 1980. Used by permission.)

TABLE 3–5 Normal Values for Urethral Pressure Profiles*

Study Animal (Condition)	*Maximal Urethral Pressure (cm H_2O)*	*Maximal Urethral Closure Pressure (cm H_2O)*	*Functional Profile Length (cm)*
Female dogs (xylazine)	35.2 ± 16.2	31.0 ± 15.3	7.2 ± 1.9
Male dogs (xylazine)	42.5 ± 5.3	36.79 ± 5.2	28.3 ± 3.9
Female dogs (no sedation)	90.18 ± 4.48	79.72 ± 4.61	8.68 ± 0.57
Male dogs (no sedation)	109.77 ± 11.52	99.77 ± 11.71	24.00 ± 0.9
Female cats, intact (xylazine)	76.6 ± 26.7	71.4 ± 25	4.4 ± 1.5
Female cats, ovh. (xylazine)	81.3 ± 31.7	77.5 ± 31.3	5.78 ± 0.9
Male cats (xylazine)	163.2 ± 47.5	161.6 ± 47.1	10.53 ± 0.5
Female horse (xylazine)		43.4 ± 21.6	3.7 ± 1.4
Female horse (no sedation)		49.1 ± 19.4	5.0 ± 1.8

Data sources: Female and male dogs (xylazine): Rosin A, Rosin E, Oliver JE Jr: Canine urethral pressure profile. Am J Vet Res 41:1113–1116, 1980. (Values converted from mm Hg.) Female and male dogs, no sedation: Richter KP, Ling GV: Effects of xylazine on the urethral pressure profile of healthy dogs. Am J Vet Res 46:1881–1886, 1985. Female cats, intact vs. ovariohysterectomized (xylazine): Gregory CR, Willits NH: Electromyographic and urethral pressure evaluations: Assessment of urethral function in female and ovariohysterectomized female cats. Am J Vet Res 47:1472–1475, 1986. Male cats (xylazine): Gregory CR, Holliday TA, Vasseur PB, Bruhl-Day RAGA, Parker HR, and McNeal D: Electromyographic and urethral pressure profilometry: Assessment of urethral function before and after perineal urethrostomy in cats. Am J Vet Res 45:2062–2065, 1984. Female horse, xylazine or no sedation: Clark ES, Semrad SD, Bichsel P, Oliver JE: Cystometrography and urethral pressure profiles in healthy horse and pony mares. Am J Vet Res 48:552–555, 1987.

* Values are means ± SD. ovh. = ovariohysterectomized.

is corrected. Management of the urinary tract based on the functional disorder of micturition is presented in this section. Table 3–7 lists the most common drugs used in the pharmacologic management of disorders of micturition.

Medical therapy includes control of urinary tract infection and management of the functional abnormality of the bladder and urethra. Treatment of urinary tract infections is described in detail in most general medical books.

Detrusor Areflexia with Sphincter Hypertonus. Lesions from the pons to the L7 spinal cord segments may abolish the detrusor reflex and may produce a UMN-type sphincter characterized by hyperreflexia and increased tone (see Table 3–2). The animal is unable to void, and it is difficult if not impossible to express the bladder manually.

The primary consideration in all neurogenic bladder disorders is to evacuate the bladder completely at least three times daily. When tone in the urethra is exaggerated, manual expression is not only ineffective but also dangerous. Aseptic catheterization is required. In-

TABLE 3–6 Diagnostic Tests of Micturition

Test	*Detrusor Reflex*	*Detrusor Tone and Capacity*	*Complete Voiding*	*Sensation to Bladder*	*Urethral Resistance/ Obstruction*	*Synchrony of Bladder and Urethra*
Cystometrogram	+	+		+		
Urethral Pressure Profile					+	
Flow	+	+			+	+
Urethral EMG						
Evoked potentials				+		
Observation of voiding	+	+	+	+		+
Palpate bladder		+				
Measure residual urine			+			
Resistance to expression and catheterization					+	

Note: + = test evaluates this function or this anatomic component.

TABLE 3–7 Drugs Used in Treating Disorders of Micturition

Drug Action	*Drug*	*Dosage*	*Side Effects*
Increase detrusor contractility	Bethanochol (Urecholine)	2.5–15 mg PO q8h (dog) 1.25–5 mg PO q8h (cat)	Cholinergic: GI hypermotility, hypotension
Decrease detrusor contractility	Propantheline (Pro-Banthine)	7.5–15 mg PO q8h (dog) 5–7.5 mg PO q8h (cat)	Anticholinergic: decreased GI motility, decreased salivation, tachycardia
	Oxybutinin (Ditropan)	Not determined for small animals; human dosage = 5 mg PO	
Increase urethral resistance	Phenylpropanolamine	1.5 mg/kg PO q8–12h (dog and cat)	Sympathomimetic: Urine retention, hypertension
	Diethylstilbesterol (female)	0.1–1.0 mg/day PO for 3–5 days, then 1 mg/week (dog)	Estrogen: Estrus, bone marrow toxicity
	Testosterone, cypionate (male)	2 mg/kg IM at intervals of weeks to months	Androgen: Caution in animals with prostatic hyperplasia, perineal hernia, perianal adenoma
Decrease urethral resistance	Phenoxybenzamine (Dibenzyline)	0.25–0.5 mg/kg PO q12h	Sympatholytic: hypotension
	Diazepam (Valium)	0.2 mg/kg PO q8h	Tranquilizer and skeletal muscle relaxant: sedation
	Baclofen (Lioresal)	1–2 mg/kg PO q8h (dog)	Skeletal muscle relaxant: weakness

Modified with permission from Oliver JE, Hoerlein BF, Mayhew IG: Veterinary Neurology. Philadelphia, WB Saunders Co., 1987.

dwelling catheters are associated with a high risk of infection, and their use should be avoided. One exception is in cases of detrusor areflexia from overdistention (described later).

Urethral tone may be reduced pharmacologically, making management easier. Phenoxybenzamine, an alpha-adrenergic blocking agent, sometimes is effective in doses of 0.5 mg/kg/day divided into two doses (small animals). Hypotension is the most common side effect. Diazepam is used for relaxation of the striated sphincter. Bethanechol, a cholinergic agent, can be used to stimulate bladder contraction. We have not found it effective if the bladder is areflexic, however. If bladder contractions are present but are inadequate for good voiding, bethanechol in doses of 2.5 to 10 mg given subcutaneously t.i.d. may be beneficial. Side effects include increased motility of the gastrointestinal tract. Oral doses of up to 50 mg also may be effective. The combination of bethanechol and phenoxybenzamine may be necessary to reduce urethral resistance.[11,27,28]

Urinalysis is performed weekly or any time that the urine appears abnormal. At the first sign of infection, urine is obtained for quantitative culture and sensitivity tests.[16] Appropriate antibiotic therapy should be continued until urinalysis verifies correction of the problem. Animals receiving anti-inflammatory drugs such as corticosteroids are at increased risk for urinary tract infection. In addition, corticosteroids can suppress the inflammatory response to infection. Asymptomatic infection may go undetected unless urine is cultured repeatedly for microorganisms.

If catheterization is necessary for prolonged periods (over 1 week), prophylactic antibacterial agents such as methenamine may be indicated. These products do not replace an aseptic catheterization technique.

If the detrusor reflex returns with good voiding of urine, the bladder is catheterized periodically to ensure that there is no residual urine. Voiding is often incomplete in the early stages, and residual urine in quantities of 10 to 20 ml or more can result in a urinary tract infection.

Detrusor Areflexia with Normal Sphincter Tone. Some lesions of the spinal cord and the brain stem may abolish the detrusor reflex without producing hypertonus of the urethral sphincter. The bladder can be expressed manually in many of these cases. The urethra of the female dog is short, and the examiner will encounter less resistance with bitches than with male dogs. Manual expression may be effective even in the context of sphincter hypertonus. Manual expression, if adequate, is less likely to produce infection than is repeated catheterization.

Other aspects of management are the same as when sphincter tone is increased.

Detrusor Areflexia with Sphincter Areflexia. Lesions of the sacral spinal cord or the nerve roots will produce a lower motor neuron deficit of both the bladder and the sphincter. The management of the bladder is the same as that described previously.

An additional management problem is created by the constant leakage of urine through the incompetent sphincter. Frequent evacuation of the bladder reduces the problem but does not eliminate it. Continual soiling of the skin with urine quickly leads to irritation and formation of decubital ulcers. Frequent hydrotherapy and protective emollients are useful adjuncts.

The problem of long-term management of the patient with paralysis of the sphincter has not been solved. Surgical reconstruction of the bladder neck and the urethra is sometimes successful in humans but has had no significant trials in animals. Prosthetic devices have been developed that offer promise of a solution. The cost of these devices limits their applicability in veterinary medicine.

Detrusor Areflexia from Overdistention. Severe overdistention of the bladder can produce a separation of the tight junctions between the detrusor muscle fibers, which prevents excitation–contraction coupling. The neural elements may be normal.

The bladder must be treated early if an irreversible deficit is to be avoided. Complete evacuation of the bladder must be accomplished and maintained for 1 to 2 weeks. Manual expression is not recommended because of the increased stress on the detrusor muscle. Intermittent aseptic catheterization can be performed at least t.i.d. but preferably q.i.d. An indwelling catheter for the first 5 to 7 days followed by intermittent catheterization, if needed, is the procedure of choice. This is one of the few instances in which an indwelling catheter is recommended. Function should return in 1 to 2 weeks if the treatment is successful. Bethanechol may be of benefit, especially if partial contractions are present.

Antibiotics or urinary antiseptics are administered throughout the treatment period. Frequent urinalysis, with cultures when indicated, is mandatory. Infection in the overdistended bladder leads to fibrosis, and adequate function will not be restored in this case.

Detrusor Hyperreflexia. Frequent voiding of small volumes of urine, often without much warning and with little or no residual urine, is characteristic of detrusor hyperreflexia.[29] Partial long tract lesions or abnormalities of the cerebellum may produce these signs. The condition is not usually detrimental to the patient, but it may be an early sign of a progressive disease of the nervous system. Additionally, it is socially unacceptable in the house pet. The condition must be differentiated from the small, contracted, irritable bladder associated with chronic cystitis.

Anticholinergic medication may be of benefit. Propantheline (Pro-Banthine) is used in dosages of 15 to 30 mg t.i.d or q.i.d. The lowest dose should be tried first and the dose should be increased in small increments until a response is obtained. Oxybutinin may be more effective than propantheline in some cases. Overdosage may result in urine retention in addition to the other side effects characteristic of this group of drugs.[29]

Reflex Dyssynergia. Initiation of a detrusor reflex with voiding followed by an uncontrolled reflex contraction of the urethral sphincter is termed *reflex dyssynergia*. Partial lesions of the long tracts are presumed to be responsible, although the condition has been seen in a dog with a cauda equina lesion.[14]

The problem may be related to uninhibited reflexes of the external urethral sphincter (skeletal muscle) or to increased tonus in the smooth muscle related to adrenergic innervation. Limited reports in human beings and in dogs have not yet provided a definitive therapeutic regimen. Skeletal muscle reflexes may be reduced with diazepam or dantrolene. Sympathetic (adrenergic) activity can be reduced with an alpha-blocking agent such as phenoxybenzamine.

Normal Detrusor Reflex with Decreased Sphincter Tone. If hormone therapy is ineffective in an animal with normal voiding but leakage, an alpha-adrenergic-stimulating drug, such as phenylpropanolamine, may be effective. The dosage is 12.5 to 50 mg t.i.d given orally. Side effects include restlessness and irritability. Surgical management may be of benefit.[15]

Management of neurogenic bladder disorders is critical for the ultimate prognosis of both reversible and irreversible CNS disorders.

CASE HISTORIES

In the cases in this section, the reader should concentrate on the problem related to micturition, even though it may be only a part of the total deficit. Using Table 3–2, decide the location of the lesion that causes the problem.

Case History 3A

Signalment

Canine, Dachshund, male, 5 years old.

History

The dog became paralyzed in the pelvic limbs last night. The dog was alone in a fenced-in backyard when the owners found him.

Physical Examination

The bladder is large and easily palpated. It cannot be expressed, even with considerable pressure.

Neurologic Examination

The dog is alert and drags himself around the examination room. The thoracic limbs are normal. There are no voluntary movements of the pelvic limbs. The postural reactions are normal in the thoracic limbs and absent in the pelvic limbs. The spinal reflexes are normal in the thoracic limbs. The quadriceps reflex is exaggerated (+3) bilaterally, and the flexion reflexes are strong in the pelvic limbs. The perineal and bulbocavernosus reflexes are present. The anal sphincter has good tone. Hyperesthesia is evident on palpation of the T13–L2 area. The panniculus reflex is absent caudal to L1. Deep pain sensation is present in the pelvic limbs.

Case History 3B

Signalment

Canine, Pekingese, female, 6 years old.

History

The dog suddenly became paralyzed in the pelvic limbs while playing with the children of the owners. When first seen by the referring veterinarian 4 hours later, the dog had complete pelvic limb paralysis, increased tone in the pelvic limbs, exaggerated quadriceps reflexes, and no sensation caudal to L4. The dog was referred to you.

Physical Examination

The dog is seen 12 hours after the onset of paralysis. Urine has leaked during the trip to the clinic, and the dog is obviously in pain. The bladder is large and easily expressed on palpation.

Neurologic Examination

The dog is alert and anxious. The thoracic limbs are normal. The postural reactions and the spinal reflexes are absent in the pelvic limbs. The perineal reflex is absent, and the anal sphincter is dilated. There is no sensation caudal to T13.

Case History 3C

Signalment

Canine, Chihuahua, male, 3 years old.

History

The dog has had generalized seizures at least three times in the past 2 weeks. The previous medical history is noncontributory. Questioning about other changes reveals that the dog has started urinating in the house within the past 3 months, although before this problem he had not urinated in the house since he was a puppy. The dog has not been taking medication.

Physical Examination

The skull is dome-shaped, and the fontanelle is 1.5 cm in diameter. The bladder is empty.

Neurologic Examination

The postural reactions are judged to be a bit slow, but the rest of the examination is normal.

Assessment 3A

The neurologic examination indicates a UMN paralysis of the pelvic limbs. The sensory examination localizes the lesion to T13–L2. The bladder problem can be characterized as detrusor areflexia with sphincter hypertonia, which is typical of a lesion rostral to L7. Cystometry confirms detrusor areflexia. Management of the bladder should include intermittent aseptic catheterization (at least t.i.d). The dog has a herniated intervertebral disk, which is decompressed by hemilaminectomy. Seven days after surgery, voluntary movements of the pelvic limbs are seen, and voiding begins with minimal pressure of the abdomen. Voiding returns to normal in 10 days.

Assessment 3B

The dog has lower motor neuron paralysis of the pelvic limbs and the sphincters. This finding indicates a lesion from L4 through S3. The loss of sensation has progressed from L4 to T13 in 8 hours, indicating a progressive lesion. There is detrusor areflexia and sphincter areflexia, which is consistent with a lesion of the sacral segments of the spinal cord. The dog has a herniated disk with hemorrhagic myelomalacia (see Chap. 7). The prognosis is so poor that no other tests are performed. Cystometry would confirm the detrusor areflexia. The urethral pressure profile would be expected to show pressures below normal. EMG would demonstrate no voluntary or reflex activity, but fibrillation potentials would not be present this early. If management were attempted, manual evacuation of the bladder probably would be effective.

Assessment 3C

The seizures indicate abnormality of the cerebrum or diencephalon or a metabolic problem. The change in urinary habits also could be either cerebral or metabolic (polyuria). A laboratory evaluation is indicated to rule out metabolic diseases.

The evaluation was performed, and all tests were normal.

Rule-outs:

1. hydrocephalus,
2. encephalitis,
3. tumor (unlikely), and
4. idiopathic epilepsy.

The cystometrogram was normal and showed adequate capacity and a good detrusor reflex. An electroencephalogram showed high-voltage slow waves in all leads. This finding is typical of hydrocephalus. Computed tomography confirmed the diagnosis. The dog was treated with corticosteroids, and complete remission of the signs resulted. (See Chap. 13 for a discussion of hydrocephalus.) The voiding behavior was related to cerebral dysfunction.

REFERENCES

1. Oliver JE, Selcer RR: Neurogenic causes of abnormal micturition in the dog and cat. Vet Clin North Am 4:517–524, 1974.
2. Purinton PT, Oliver JE: Spinal cord origin of innervation to the bladder and urethra of the dog. Exp Neurol 65:422–434, 1979.
3. Oliver JE Jr, Bradley WE, Fletcher TF: Spinal cord representation of the micturition reflex. J Comp Neurol 137:329–346, 1969.
4. Gjone R, Setekleiv J: Excitatory and inhibitory bladder responses to stimulation of the cerebral cortex in the cat. Acta Physiol Scand 59:337–348, 1963.
5. Langworthy OR, Hesser FH: An experimental study of micturition released from cerebral control. Am J Physiol 115:694–700, 1936.
6. Bradley WE, Teague CT: Cerebellar influence on the micturition reflex. Exp Neurol 23:399–411, 1969.
7. Oliver JE, Bradley WE, Fletcher TF: Spinal cord distribution of the somatic innervation of the external urethral sphincter in the cat. J Neurol Sci 10:11–23, 1970.
8. Oliver JE: Disorders of micturition. In Hoerlein BF (ed): Canine Neurology, 3rd ed. Philadelphia, WB Saunders, 1978, pp 461–469.
9. Moreau PM: Neurogenic disorders of micturition in the dog and cat. Comp Cont Educ Pract Vet 4:12–22, 1982.
10. O'Brien D: Neurogenic disorders of micturition. Vet Clin North Am 18:529–544, 1988.
11. O'Brien D: Disorders of the urogenital system. Semin Vet Med Surg 5:57–66, 1990.
12. Purinton PT, Oliver JE, Bradley WE: Differences in routing of pelvic visceral afferent fibers in the dog and cat. Exp Neurol 73:725–731, 1981.
13. DeGroat WC: Nervous control of the urinary bladder of the cat. Brain Res 87:201–211, 1975.
14. Oliver JE: Dysuria caused by reflex dyssynergia. In Kirk RW (ed): Current Veterinary Therapy, VIII. Philadelphia, WB Saunders, 1983, p 1088.
15. Holt PE: Urinary incontinence in the bitch due to sphincter mechanism incompetence: Prevalence in referred dogs and retrospective analysis of sixty cases. J Small Anim Pract 26:181–190, 1985.
16. Barsanti JA: Diagnostic procedures in urology. Vet Clin North Am 14:3–14, 1984.
17. Oliver JE, Young WO: Air cystometry in dogs under xylazine-induced restraint. Am J Vet Res 34:1433–1435, 1973.
18. Johnson CA, Beemsterboer JM, Gray PR, et al: Effects of various sedatives on air cystometry in dogs. Am J Vet Res 49:1525–1528, 1988.
19. Barsanti J, Finco D, Brown J: Effect of atropine on cystometry and urethral pressure profilometry in the dog. Am J Vet Res 49:112–114, 1988.
20. Clark E, Semrad S, Bichsel P, et al: Cystometrography and urethral pressure profiles in healthy horse and pony mares. Am J Vet Res 48:552–555, 1987.
21. Moreau PM, Lees GE, Gross DR: Simultaneous cystometry and uroflowmetry (micturition study) for evaluation of the caudal part of the urinary tract in dogs: Studies of the technique. Am J Vet Res 44:1769–1773, 1983.
22. Moreau PM, Lees GE, Gross DR: Simultaneous cystometry and uroflowmetry (micturition study) for evaluation of the caudal part of the urinary tract in dogs: Reference values for healthy animals sedated with xylazine. Am J Vet Res 44:1774–1781, 1983.
23. Oliver JE: Urodynamic assessment. In Oliver JE, Hoerlein BF, Mayhew IG (eds): Veterinary Neurology. Philadelphia, WB Saunders, 1987, pp 180–184.
24. Kay AD, Lavoie J-P: Urethral pressure profilometry in mares. J Am Vet Med Assoc 191:212–216, 1987.
25. Gregory C, Willits N: Electromyographic and urethral pressure evaluations: Assessment of urethral function in female and ovariohysterectomized female cats. Am J Vet Res 47:1472–1475, 1986.
26. Richter KP, Ling GV: Effects of xylazine on the urethral pressure profile of healthy dogs. Am J Vet Res 46:1881–1886, 1985.
27. Moreau PM, Lappin MR: Pharmacologic management of urinary incontinence. In Kirk RW (ed): Current Veterinary Therapy. X. Small Animal Practice. Philadelphia, WB Saunders, 1989, pp 1214–1222.
28. Moreau PM: Management of micturition disorders in the dog and cat. In Proceedings of the Eighth Annual Veterinary Medical Forum, Washington, DC, 1990, pp 369–374.
29. Lappin MR, Barsanti JA: Urinary incontinence secondary to idiopathic detrusor instability: Cystometrographic diagnosis and pharmacologic management in two dogs and a cat. J Am Vet Med Assoc 191:1439–1442, 1987.

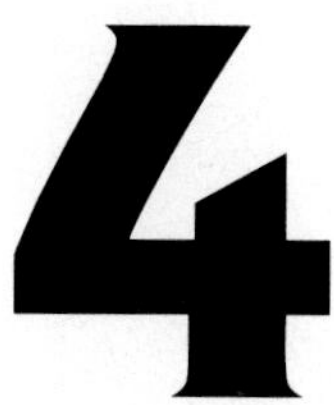

Confirming a Diagnosis

After the history has been taken and the physical and neurologic examinations have been completed, a list of problems is made. For each problem, the examiner makes a list of most likely diseases to be ruled out by appropriate diagnostic tests. Chapters 1 through 3 provided the information necessary for identifying the problem and making an anatomic diagnosis. Chapters 6 through 16 will elaborate on each problem in terms of arriving at a differential diagnosis through appropriate diagnostic tests. This chapter discusses the tests that are available, indicates the feasibility of performing them, suggests references for further reading on techniques and interpretation, and outlines the indications, contraindications, and limitations of the tests. The most useful tests for each major category of disease are listed in Table 4–1.

Clinical Laboratory Studies

Hematology, Blood Chemistry Analysis, and Urinalysis

Availability

All clinical practices should have the facilities to perform routine hematology studies, chemistry analysis, and urinalysis.

Indications

A minimum data base is required for all sick animals so that common diseases are not overlooked and the general status of the animal is assessed. In addition to the history, the physical examination, and the neurologic examination, a laboratory profile should be obtained (Table 4–2). The studies that are performed may vary, depending on the availability of automated chemistry profiles, the experience of the examiner in the practice, or the influence of economic considerations. The function of the major organ systems should be evaluated. Glucose and calcium levels always are included in the assessment of patients with seizures.

Cerebrospinal Fluid Analysis

Availability

Cerebrospinal fluid (CSF) analysis can be performed in any practice. CSF is collected routinely by cisternal puncture. The examiner should perform the procedure often enough to maintain confidence and accuracy. Lumbar puncture is less satisfactory in dogs because fluid is more difficult to obtain. It can be performed at the lumbosacral interspace in cats and in large animals.[1] Lumbar CSF is more likely to provide positive information in animals with spinal cord disease.

To avoid movement of the animal during needle placement, CSF is collected with the animal under general anesthesia. The skin is clipped and prepared for an aseptic procedure. The needle (a 22-gauge, 1.5-inch disposable spinal needle with a stylet for most small animals; a 20-gauge, 3.5-inch needle for most large animals) should be handled with sterile gloves. The landmarks for the midline are the occipital protuberance and the spinous process of the axis (C2) (Fig. 4–1). The needle is inserted on the midline near the cranial border of the wings of the atlas (C1). A slight loss of resistance is felt as the

TABLE 4–1 Selection of Diagnostic Tests

Site	Disease Category	Diagnostic Tests: Useful	Diagnostic Tests: Usually Diagnostic
Brain	Degenerative	EEG, CSF	Biopsy
	Anomalous	Examination	Radiography
	Neoplastic	EEG, radiography	CT or MR imaging
Spinal cord	Degenerative	Myelography, CSF	None
	Anomalous	Radiography	Myelography
	Neoplastic	CSF, radiography	Myelography
Vertebrae	Degenerative	CSF	Radiography, myelography
	Anomalous	Examination	Radiography
	Neoplastic	CSF	Radiography, myelography
	Inflammation	CSF	Radiography, myelography
Peripheral nerve, muscle	Demyelinating	EMG, EDT	Biopsy
	Inflammation	EMG, EDT, CPK	Biopsy
	Neoplastic	EMG, EDT	Biopsy
	Traumatic	EMG, EDT	Biopsy
	Toxic	EMG, EDT	Biopsy
Systemic or any site	Metabolic	History	Clinical laboratory profile
	Nutritional	History	Radiography
	Inflammation	History, examination	CSF, serology
	Traumatic	History, examination	Radiography
	Toxic	History	Clinical laboratory profile

needle penetrates the subarachnoid space. The stylet is withdrawn, and fluid is carefully removed as it flows from the hub of the needle. The syringe is not attached to the needle, because aspiration is likely to cause hemorrhage. If spinal fluid pressure is to be measured, a three-way valve is attached before any fluid is collected.[2] A spinal manometer is attached to the valve and fluid is allowed to rise in the manometer. The reading is taken at the bottom of the meniscus. Pulsations of the fluid indicate that the needle is patent. This additional manipulation of the needle increases the frequency of blood contamination of the fluid. Although spinal fluid pressure has some diagnostic value, we rarely measure it because the risk of contaminating the sample with blood outweighs the benefit.

TABLE 4–2 Minimum Data Base: Neurologic Problem

- History (see Chap. 1)
- Physical examination
- Neurologic examination (see Chap. 1)
- Clinical laboratory profile
  - Complete blood cell count, at least:
    - Packed cell volume
    - Hemoglobin level
    - WBC count and differential
  - Urinalysis
  - Chemistry profile
    - Recommended: Serum urea nitrogen level
    - Serum alanine transaminase level
    - Alkaline phosphatase level
    - Calcium level
    - Blood glucose level (with animal fasting at least 24 hours)
    - Total serum protein level
    - Albumin level

Total and differential white blood cell (WBC) counts are the most important parts of a CSF analysis. Unless a preservative is added, cell counts must be determined within 30 minutes of collection, as WBCs deteriorate rapidly. Total cell counts can be done with a hemacytometer. There are several methods for determining the differential count, including sedimentation and centrifugation techniques that can be done in practice. Techniques for RBC and WBC counts and differentials are described in the references.[3–5] Techniques for using a preservative and a filtration method of obtaining cell counts have been described by Roszel.[6] Not all laboratories are prepared to use this method. Referral institutions may also perform electron microscopy on the sample to identify microorganisms.

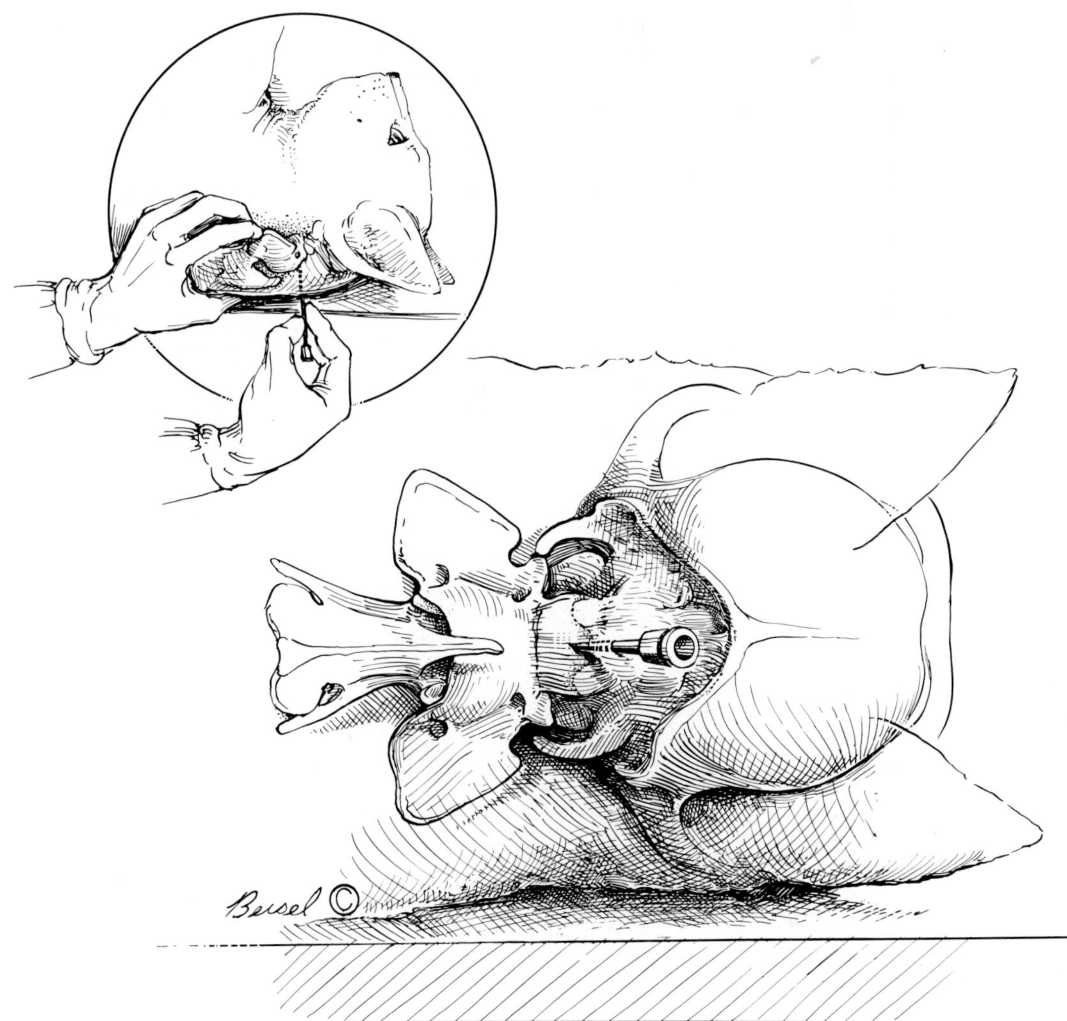

Figure 4—1 Landmarks for cerebrospinal fluid collection. (From Greene CE, Oliver JE Jr: Neurologic examination. In Ettinger SJ: Textbook of Veterinary Internal Medicine, 2nd ed. Philadelphia, WB Saunders, 1982. Used by permission.)

The examiner should observe the appearance of the CSF. Hemorrhage caused by the puncture produces a red tinge to the fluid that decreases as the fluid continues to flow. Centrifugation should leave a clear, colorless fluid. A yellowish tinge to the CSF is called xanthochromia and is caused by free bilirubin. Previous subarachnoid hemorrhage is the usual cause, although prolonged icterus can produce xanthochromia. Turbidity is caused by an increase in the cell content of the fluid. Usually, more than 500 cells/cu mm are required to produce turbidity. Shaking the sample will produce foam if the protein content is markedly elevated. Fibrin clots may be seen if the elevated protein includes fibrinogen.

Measurement of CSF protein levels is necessary for a complete examination. Simple qualitative studies such as the Pandy test are adequate, although quantitative methods are preferred. The Pandy test can be performed in the practice. Quantitative analysis also can be done in the practice, or the sample can be sent to a reference laboratory. Electrophoresis is used to quantitatively determine the levels of protein fractions or immunoglobulins in CSF. Increased albumin indicates a disturbance of the blood-brain barrier, while significant increases in immunoglobulins indicate synthesis intrathecally.[7–12]

Other chemical values, including glucose levels, creatine phosphokinase (CPK) levels, and lactic dehydrogenase (LDH) levels, may be determined. Quantities necessary for these tests are difficult to obtain from small animals, and the usefulness of the studies has not been demonstrated clearly. CSF glucose levels may be decreased in bacterial infections, but the increase in cells and protein is more significant. Increased CPK concentrations occur when nervous tissue is destroyed, but the increase usually parallels the increase in protein values. LDH concentrations have been reported to increase in central nervous system (CNS) lymphosarcoma.

A strong clinical suspicion of bacterial infection, an increase in WBCs, or the presence of neutrophils is an indication for CSF culture and sensitivity testing. Fluid should be obtained in two sterile syringes, one for laboratory analysis and one for culture.

Indications

CSF analysis is the best test for the diagnosis of CNS inflammatory disease. Increased WBC counts and increased protein levels are ex-

TABLE 4–3 Cerebrospinal Fluid

Disease	*Appearance*	*Pressure (mm H_2O)*	*White Blood Cells/cu mm*	*Cell Type*	*Protein (mg/dl)*	***same as dog*** *Other*
Normal dog	Clear	<140	<5	Mononuclear	<25	Glucose: 60%–70% of blood glucose
Normal cat	Clear	<100	<5	Mononuclear	<25	Same as dog
Normal horse	Clear	<500	<6	Mononuclear	<100	Same as dog
Normal cow	Clear	<200	<10	Mononuclear	<40	Same as dog
Normal pig	Clear		<30	Mononuclear	<40	Same as dog
Normal sheep	Clear		<10	Mononuclear	<40	Same as dog
Inflammatory						
Bacterial	Clear to turbid	Slight increase	Increased, usually >100	Mostly neutrophils	Increased, usually >100	Glucose decreased
Viral	Clear	Slight increase	Increased, usually <100	Mostly mononuclear	Increased, usually <100	EM: viral particles
Fungal	Turbid	Increased	Increased, usually >100	Mixed	Increased, usually >100	Organisms may be seen, especially *Cryptococcus*
Protozoal	Clear	Increased	Increased, may be >100	Mononuclear, sometimes neutrophils	Increased, usually >100	
Parasitic	Clear to xanthochromic	Increased	Increased, variable	Mixed, sometimes eosinophils	Increased, usually >100	
Degenerative, including compression	Clear	Normal	Normal to slight increase	Mononuclear	Increased, usually <100	
Neoplastic	Clear	Increased	Normal to increased	Mononuclear	Increased, usually <100	Tumor cells may be seen if tumor adjacent to subarachnoid space; usually contraindicated in suspected brain tumors
Traumatic	Xanthochromic	Increased	Normal to increased	RBCs, WBCs	Increased, variable	Usually contraindicated

Data from Hoerlein, BF: Canine Neurology: Diagnosis and Treatment, 3rd ed. Philadelphia, WB Saunders, 1978; Kornegay JN: Cerebrospinal fluid collection, examination, and interpretation in dogs and cats. Comp Cont Educ Pract Vet 3:85–92, 1981; deLahunta A: Veterinary Neuroanatomy and Clinical Neurology, 2nd ed. Philadelphia, WB Saunders, 1983; Mayhew IG, Whitlock RH, Tasker JB: Equine cerebrospinal fluid: Reference values of normal horses. Am J Vet Res 38:1271–1274, 1977; Simpson ST, Reed RB: Manometric values for normal cerebrospinal fluid pressure in dogs. J Am Anim Hosp Assoc 23:629–632, 1987.

pected with active inflammatory diseases. The WBCs are predominantly polymorphonuclear leukocytes in bacterial diseases and predominantly lymphocytes in viral diseases. Fungal and protozoal diseases may cause mixed populations of leukocytes (Table 4–3).

Any disease that causes degeneration of nervous tissue without inflammation will cause an increase in CSF protein with little or no increase in cells. Primary degenerative or demyelinating diseases, neoplasia, or any compression of the CNS may produce this change (see Table 4–3).

Free blood or xanthochromia may be seen following subarachnoid hemorrhage. Hemorrhage may be caused by trauma, primary vascular disease, or secondary vascular lesions from inflammation or neoplasia.

Contraindications

The animal should be anesthetized when CSF is collected; therefore, if anesthesia is contraindicated, CSF should not be obtained. When the animal is positioned for cisternal puncture, the anesthetist should be certain that the airway is patent and pulmonary ventilation is adequate.

CSF should not be collected if increased intracranial pressure is suspected. Removal of CSF from a cisternal or a lumbar puncture causes a pressure shift that pushes the cerebrum or the cerebellum in a caudal direction. Herniation of the cerebellum causes death of the animal from compression of the medullary respiratory centers or pathways. The slight increase in pressure associated with inflammatory disease is usually not sufficient to cause a problem. Increased pressure from brain tumors, large abscesses, or intracranial trauma can cause herniation. The information obtained from the CSF analysis may not be worth the risk to the animal in these cases.

Radiography

Radiography is the most frequently used and the most useful diagnostic tool in neurology (Table 4–4).

Availability

Most veterinary practices have radiographic capabilities adequate for the formulation of a neurologic diagnosis in small animals. Meticulous technique is essential for the detection of the subtle changes that are often the key to a diagnosis.[13] Positioning of the animal, correct exposure, and proper development are all imperative. Beyond these parameters, the only limitation is the interpretive skill of the veterinarian. Interpretive skill is developed through practice.

An approach to the interpretation of radiographs is as follows:

1. Scan the entire radiograph for quality of exposure, positioning, and presence of artifacts or motion. Recognize the limitations imposed by these factors.
2. Scan the structures on the radiograph that are not of primary interest, such as soft tissue, abdomen, chest, and so forth.
3. Systematically evaluate the area of primary interest.

Vertebral Column and Spinal Cord

a. Scan the entire vertebral column for contour: ventral surface of vertebral bodies, floor of vertebral canal, lamina, articulations, spinous processes. (See Table 4–5: "Displacement" and "Proliferation.")

b. Scan the entire vertebral column for changes in bone density, such as lytic or proliferative changes. (See Table 4–5: "Lysis" and "Proliferation.")

c. Scan the vertebral canal for changes in density, especially at the intervertebral foramina and the disk space.

d. Compare the size of adjacent intervertebral disk spaces, intervertebral foramina, and the joint space of facets. Narrowing of one or more of these spaces is suggestive of disk herniation.

e. Stand back and scan the vertebral column again. Changes in contour or spacing are sometimes more apparent from a distance.

Skull

a. Ventrodorsal and frontal (cranial-caudal) views are especially useful because the two sides can be compared.

b. Scan the periphery of the calvarium for asymmetry, cracks, deviations, or abnormal shape. (See Table 4–5: "Proliferation," "Lysis," and "Abnormal Shape.")

c. Compare the nasal passages, the frontal sinuses, and the bulla of the middle ear for similarity in density.

d. Survey the calvarium for changes in density (proliferative or lytic), normal digital impressions, presence of open suture lines or fontanelles, or linear fractures.

e. Evaluate the structures inside the calvarium—osseous tentorium cerebelli, foramina, petrous temporal bone.

Contrast-enhanced procedures, especially myelography, are within the capabilities of most

TABLE 4–4 Radiography

Test	*Indications*	*Possible Usefulness*	*Contraindications*	*Availability*
Spinal radiography	Degenerative disease (vertebral) Anomaly Neoplasia Inflammatory disease (vertebral) Trauma	High High Moderate High High	Anesthesia usually required	Practice
Myelography	Degenerative disease Anomaly Neoplasia Inflammatory disease Trauma	High High High Low High	Anesthesia required, not done if active inflammation is present or if intracranial pressure is increased	Specialty practice
Epidurography (primarily for evaluation of caudal lumbar and sacral area)	Degenerative disease Anomaly Neoplasia Inflammatory disease (vertebral) Trauma	High Variable High Variable Low	Anesthesia required	Specialty practice
Vertebral sinus venography	Same as those for epidurography	Low		
Skull radiography	Anomaly Neoplasia Inflammatory disease (especially otitis media) Trauma	High Low Low (except otitis media) High	Anesthesia required	Practice
Ventriculography	Anomaly (hydrocephalus) Neoplasia	High Low	Anesthesia required	Specialty practice
Ultrasonography	Hydrocephalus, with open fontanelles	High	None	Specialty practice
Cavernous sinus venography	Neoplasia (floor of skull)	Moderate	Anesthesia required	Specialty practice
Cranial thecography	Neoplasia (floor of skull)	Moderate	Anesthesia required	Specialty practice
Cerebral arteriography	Neoplasia	High	Anesthesia required	Specialty practice
Radioisotope scans	Neoplasia	Moderate	Anesthesia required	Institutions
Computed tomography and magnetic resonance imaging	Degenerative disease Anomaly Neoplasia Trauma	Moderate High High High	Anesthesia required; expensive	Institutions; local imaging centers

practices. As is the case with most procedures, however, they must be performed often enough that the veterinarian maintains confidence in both technique and interpretation. Table 4–4 indicates all special imaging techniques available in specialty practice. Arteriography and ventriculography are rarely performed with the advent of radioisotope brain scans, computed tomography (CT), and magnetic resonance (MR) imaging. Most institutions have one or more of these techniques available.[14–16] Practicing veterinarians often can have CT or MR imaging done at a local hospital or imaging center. In animals likely to have a brain tumor, one of these imaging methods should be the first diagnostic test performed after the minimum data base has been obtained.[16–19]

Indications

Nervous tissue has essentially the same radiographic density as other soft tissues. Radiographs of the head and the vertebral column demonstrate changes in the skull and the vertebrae. Lesions of nervous tissue, such as hemorrhage, tumor, or degeneration, are not detected, except in rare cases with calcification of the lesion or lytic change in adjacent bone. The most

TABLE 4–5 Radiographic Findings and Interpretation

Radiographic Change	Possible Causes
Vertebrae	
Proliferation	*Degenerative:* Spondylosis, dural ossification (linear density in vertebral canal) *Neoplastic:* Primary or metastatic vertebral tumor *Nutritional:* Ankylosing spondylosis, hypervitaminosis A *Inflammatory:* Osteomyelitis involving disk space, diskospondylitis (osteomyelitis usually is proliferative and lytic) *Traumatic:* Healing fracture
Lysis	*Neoplastic:* Primary or metastatic vertebral tumor, widening of vertebral canal (spinal cord tumor) widening of intervertebral foramen (nerve root tumor) *Nutritional:* Generalized loss of density, hypocalcemia, hyperparathyroidism *Inflammatory:* Osteomyelitis involving disk space, diskospondylitis (osteomyelitis usually is proliferative and lytic)
Abnormal shape of vertebrae	*Degenerative:* Cervical instability *Anomalous:* Hemivertebrae, spina bifida, fused vertebrae *Traumatic:* Compression fractures
Displacement	*Degenerative:* Cervical spondylopathy (Wobbler syndrome), lumbosacral spondylopathy, intervertebral disk herniation (narrowing of interspace, foramen, and facet space) *Anomalous:* Hemivertebrae, agenesis of dens (atlantoaxial luxation) *Neoplastic:* Pathologic fractures *Nutritional:* Pathologic fractures *Inflammatory:* Pathologic fractures *Traumatic:* Fractures, luxations
Skull	
Proliferation	*Degenerative:* Hypertrophic osteopathy of the mandible and skull (possibly inflammatory) *Neoplastic:* Primary or metastatic tumor *Inflammatory:* Osteomyelitis, otitis media, otitis interna
Lysis	*Anomalous:* Loss of digital markings, open fontanelles or suture lines, loss of osseous tentorium (may be caused by chronic hydrocephalus) *Neoplastic:* Primary or metastatic tumor *Nutritional:* Generalized loss of density, hypocalcemia, hyperparathyroidism *Inflammatory:* Osteomyelitis, otitis media, otitis interna
Abnormal shape	*Anomalous:* Hydrocephalus, rarely otocephaly, hydranencephaly, other cranial malformations *Traumatic:* Fractures
Alterations in shape of foramina	*Anomalous:* Occipital dysplasia, hydrocephalus *Neoplastic:* Tumor of a cranial nerve

common radiographic changes and their causes are listed in Table 4–5. Examples of radiographic changes associated with specific disease processes are included in the discussion of each disease (see Chaps. 6–16).

CT or MR imaging is used to confirm a suspected lesion that cannot be identified definitively on survey radiographs, or to identify the extent or the location of the lesion more precisely.

Myelography (radiographs made following the injection of contrast material into the subarachnoid space) is the most frequently used contrast-enhanced imaging procedure.[20–23] Masses that occupy space in the vertebral canal (e.g., tumors, abscesses, disks) cause alterations in the contrast column. The epidural, intradural-extramedullary, or intramedullary location can be determined by the type of distortion occurring in the contrast column (Fig. 4–2).[24] Focal degenerative changes in the spinal cord are recognized as a narrowing of the cord with a widening of the contrast column. Severe malacia may allow the contrast media to pool in the cord substance (Fig. 4–3).

Epidurography (radiographs made following the injection of contrast material into the epidural space of the vertebral canal) with the use of water-soluble contrast agents is indicated primarily for the evaluation of the lumbosacral region, where the subarachnoid space is very small or is not present.[25–27] The toxic effects of the procedure are minimized with the use of water-soluble contrast agents, and the technique is simple. Considerable experience with normal variations is required for proper interpretation of the radiographs.

Vertebral sinus venography requires filling the venous sinuses on the floor of the spinal canal with contrast material. This procedure has

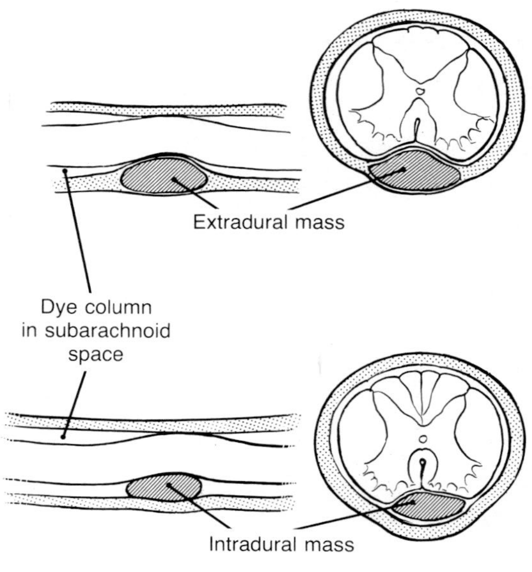

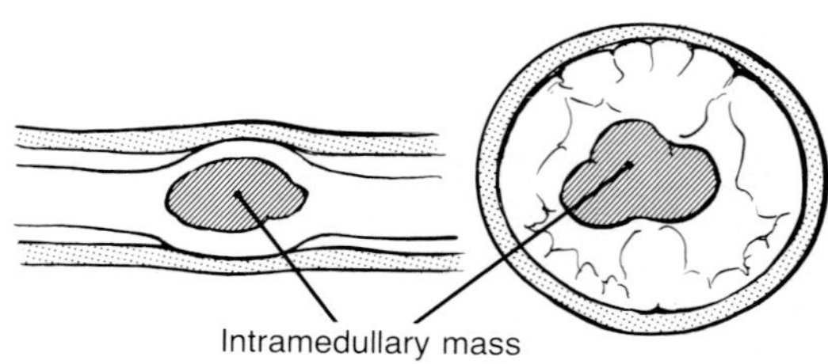

Figure 4–2 Effect of a mass lesion of a myelogram. *Top.* An extradural mass causes thinning or complete obliteration of the dye column. *Middle.* An intradural-extramedullary mass deviates the spinal cord and obstructs the dye column. The cranial and caudal borders of the mass may have a cup-shaped outline of contrast material. *Bottom.* An intramedullary mass expands the spinal cord, causing thinning or obliteration of the dye column on all sides.

limited value, since false positive results are common.

Ventriculography is the delineation of the cerebral ventricular system following the injection of air or a positive contrast agent (Fig. 4–4).[13] Ventriculography is the procedure of choice for the diagnosis of hydrocephalus unless CT or MR imaging is available. Ultrasonography is noninvasive and can be used if the fontanelle is open.[28] Masses in the cranial vault can be detected by shifts in the ventricular system. Precise localization is better accomplished with CT or MR imaging, which have essentially replaced ventriculography and arteriography for assessment of mass lesions.

Cavernous sinus venography is relatively easy to perform. Contrast material is injected into the angularis oculi vein.[29] The medium flows through the orbit into the cavernous sinuses on the floor of the cranial vault (Fig. 4–5). Compression or occlusion of the sinus from masses in the area of the pituitary gland can be demonstrated.

Intracranial thecography entails the injection of a water-soluble contrast agent into the subarachnoid space of the brain. The head is tilted down, and radiographs are taken in the dorsoventral projection. The floor of the cranial vault is outlined. The pituitary gland, optic nerves, and any mass lesion of this area may be seen. The procedure is safe and within the capability of most practices.[30,31]

Cerebral arteriography is performed by injecting contrast material into the internal carotid or vertebral arteries.[13] Arteriography is rarely used insofar as CT and MR imaging are noninvasive and provide more information on mass lesions. Primary arterial disease, a possible indication, is rare in animals.

CT or MR imaging is the procedure of choice for assessment of mass lesions (Fig. 4–6). Most animals with probable brain tumor should be referred to a facility with these imaging capabilities.[16]

Contraindications

Anesthesia is required for good-quality radiographs of the nervous system. Many patients with CNS disease are poor risks for anesthesia. The veterinarian must make a decision by weighing the risks of the procedure against the risk of doing nothing. For example, vertebral fractures usually require early decompression if spinal cord function is to be preserved. These patients may be in shock and may have several other injuries. The question of risk versus benefit must be resolved on an individual basis.

Increased intracranial pressure is a contraindication to spinal puncture; hence, myelography should not be performed in such cases. Because contrast media are irritating, myelography is usually not done in the presence of subarachnoid inflammation. When the puncture is made for myelography, a cell count of the CSF is determined. If the count indicates active inflammation, myelography is not performed unless it is considered essential for diagnosis and treatment (e.g., when there is strong suspicion of an abscess). CSF analysis before myelography is also important because the inflammation produced by the contrast agent precludes subsequent interpretation of CSF values.

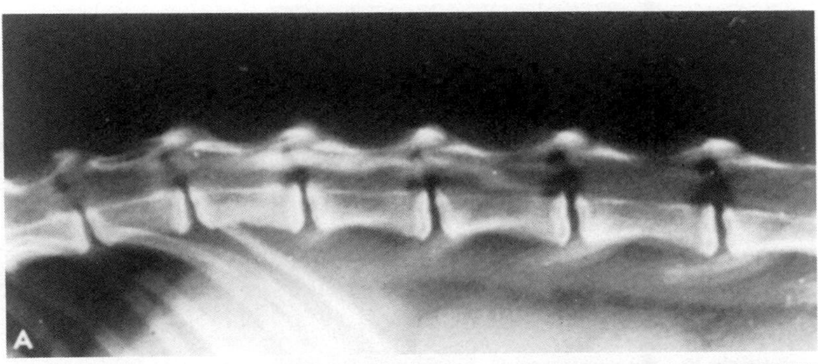

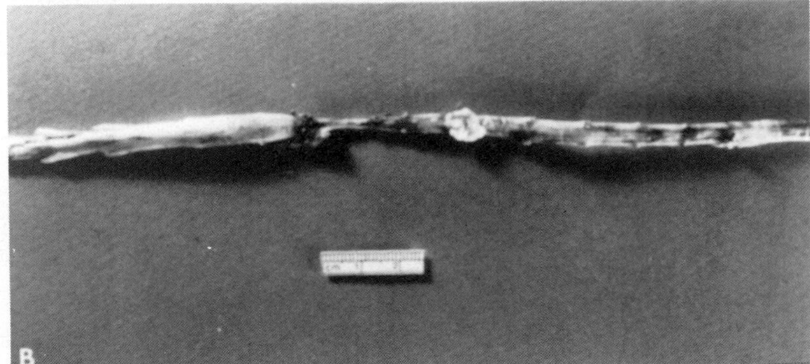

Figure 4–3 *A.* Myelogram of a cat with malacia in the spinal cord caused by an infarction. Note the contrast media pooled in the area of the malacia. *B.* Spinal cord showing the area of malacia.

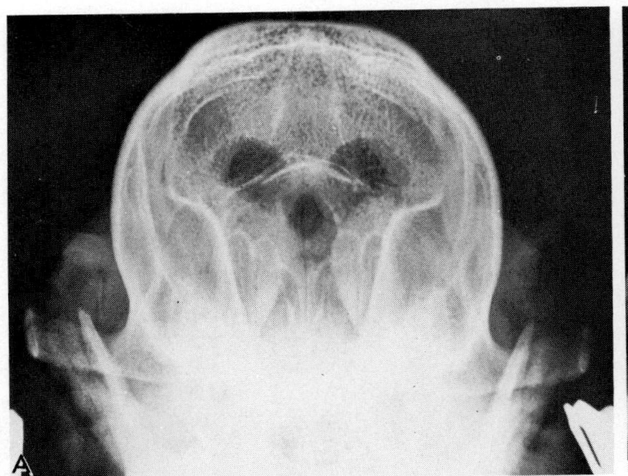

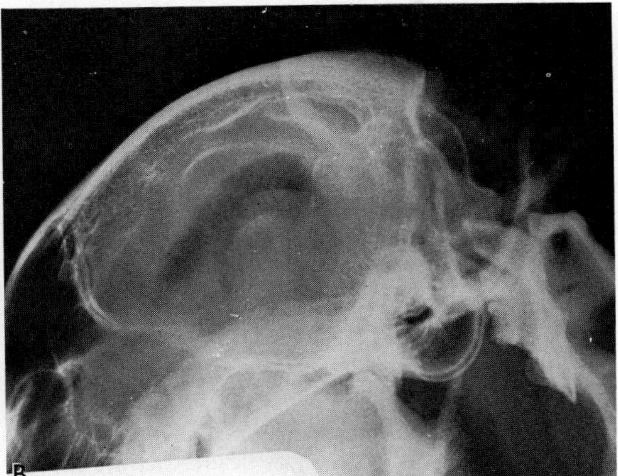

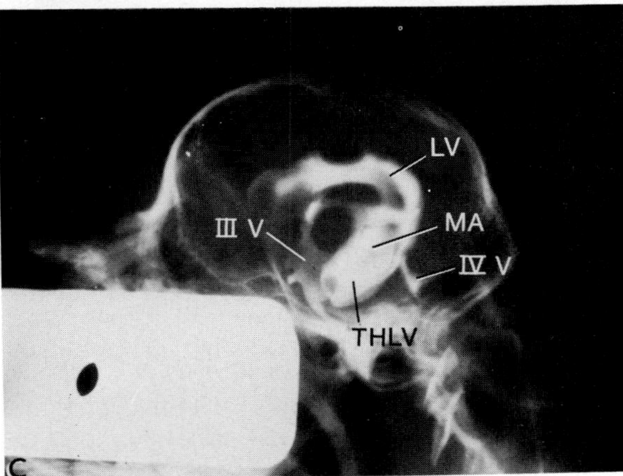

Figure 4–4 Frontal (*A*) and lateral (*B*) views of a pneumoventriculogram of a normal dog. The lateral ventricles are fillled with air. A portion of the third ventricle can be seen in the lateral view. *C.* Positive contrast ventriculogram. *LV*, lateral ventricle; *III V*, third ventricle; *MA*, mesencephalic aqueduct; *IV V*, fourth ventricle; *THLV*, temporal horn of lateral ventricle.

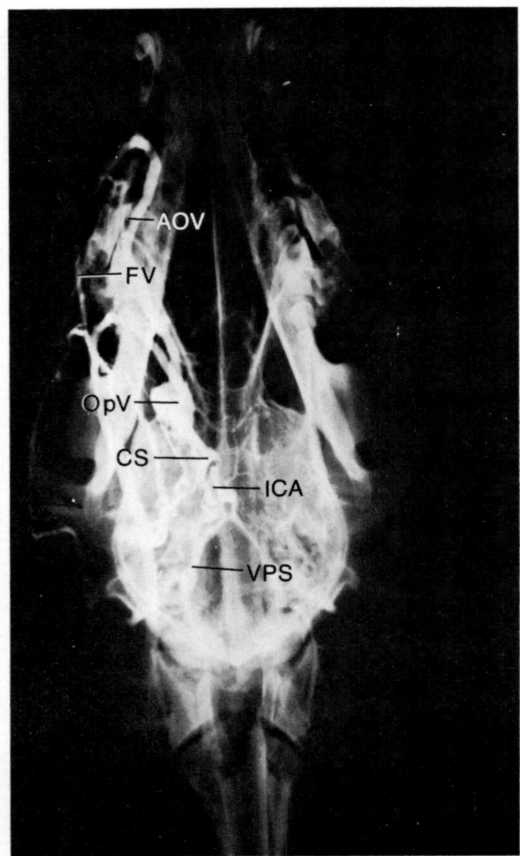

Figure 4–5 Cavernous sinus venogram of a normal dog. *AOV*, angularis oculi vein; *FV*, facial vein; *OpV*, ophthalmic vein; *CS*, cavernous sinus; *ICA*, internal carotid artery (negative image inside CS); *VPS*, ventral petrosal sinus.

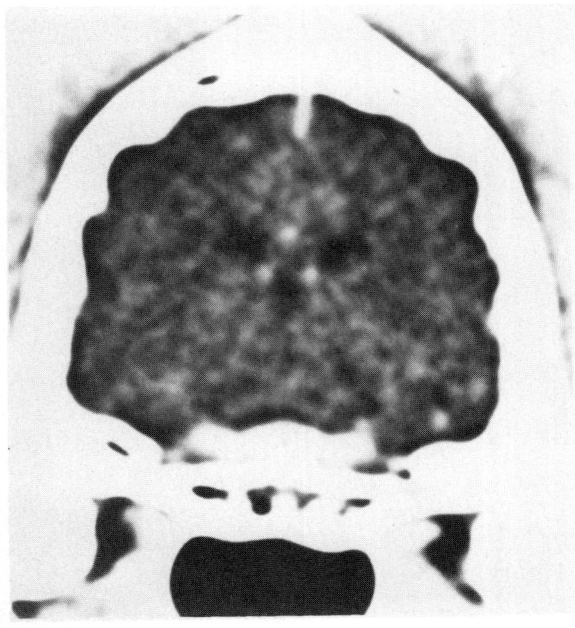

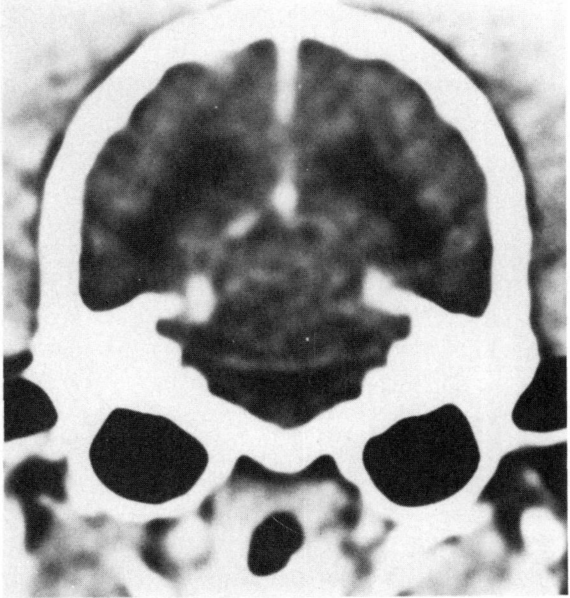

Figure 4–6 Computed tomographic scans of normal dogs. *A*. German shepherd dog, male, 1.5 years old, scan at the level of the thalamus. The two lateral ventricles and the midline third ventricle can be seen. *B*. Mixed breed dog, female, 15 years old, scan at the level of the brain stem and caudal cerebrum. The lateral ventricles and portions of the osseous tentorium can be seen. The lateral ventricles are significantly larger in the older dog, a normal finding with aging.

Electrophysiology

Availability

Equipment for electrophysiologic techniques is expensive and requires extensive training and experience for valid interpretation of results. These factors generally limit the availability of electrophysiologic studies to specialty practices and institutional settings. Electroencephalography (EEG) and electromyography (EMG) are the most widely used techniques and are available in a number of specialty practices. The other techniques are in varying stages of development for clinical application and are available primarily at research institutions (Table 4–6).

Indications

Electroencephalography, the graphic recording of the electrical activity of the brain, is useful for the evaluation of cerebral disease.[32,33] As with most diagnostic tools, the EEG often does not provide a specific diagnosis, but it supports the determination of a category of disease. The EEG varies with the level of consciousness: Low volt-

TABLE 4–6 Electrophysiology

Test	*Indications*	*Probable Usefulness*	*Contraindications*	*Availability*
Electroencephalography	Degenerative disease	Moderate	None	Specialty practice
	Anomaly	High		
	Metabolic disease	Moderate		
	Neoplasia	Moderate		
	Inflammatory disease	High		
	Trauma	Low		
	Toxic disease	Moderate		
Electromyography, nerve conduction, and nerve stimulation	Lower motor neuron diseases	High	None	Specialty practice
	Peripheral neuropathies	High		
	Myopathies	High		
Electroretinography	Retinal disease	High	None	Specialty practice
Evoked response (cortical, brain stem, and spinal)	Localization of lesions in pathways	Insufficient data in most areas	None	Specialty practice
Visual-evoked response	Cortical function	Moderate		
Auditory-evoked response	Test of hearing, location of brain stem lesions	High		
Somatosensory-evoked response	Spinal cord, plexus lesions	Moderate		
Echoencephalography	Midline shifts of cerebrum	Low	None	Institutions (few)
Urodynamics (cystometrogram, urethral pressure, sphincter reflexes)	Neurogenic bladder disorders	(See Chap. 3)		
Tympanometry	Otitis media, otitis interna, hearing disorders	Moderate	None	Institutions (few)

age and fast activity are seen in the alert animal, and higher voltage and slower activity occur during drowsiness and sleep. Drugs such as sedatives, tranquilizers, and anesthetics produce higher voltage and slower activity (similar to sleep patterns). The EEG usually can indicate that cerebral disease is present and whether it is focal or diffuse, acute or chronic, and inflammatory or degenerative.

The following general principles of EEG changes have been listed by Klemm and Hall:[34] (1) Low voltage, fast activity (LVFA) and spikes (very fast activity) indicate irritation from any cause (usually inflammatory disease). (2) High voltage, slow activity (HVSA) suggests neuronal death or compression. (3) Neither change is diagnostic of a disease; rather, it reflects the kind of process occurring (e.g., inflammation or degeneration). (4) A focal EEG abnormality indicates a focal cortical lesion. (5) A generalized EEG abnormality indicates diffuse cortical disease or a subcortical abnormality that alters the activity of the majority of the cerebral cortex. (6) The EEG can change with time, suggesting the progression or resolution of the disease process.

Electromyography, the measurement of the electrical activity of muscle, and measurement of nerve conduction velocity (NCV) are performed on the same equipment, usually during the same examination. EMG and NCV are the best diagnostic tools for the evaluation of neuropathies and myopathies.[35] The information provided by these procedures regarding the location and the extent of the abnormality may support an etiologic diagnosis.

The EMG examination includes evaluation of the electrical activity of the muscle at the following times: (1) during insertion or movement of the electrode (insertion activity), (2) when the muscle is resting (resting activity), (3) during muscle contraction (voluntary or reflex), and (4) in response to electrical stimulation of the motor nerve (also called electrodiagnostic testing [EDT]). Mechanical distortion of the muscle membrane by the needle electrode causes the membrane to depolarize, producing a brief burst of electrical activity (i.e., insertion activity). Resting muscle is electrically silent.

Loss of nerve supply to a muscle causes an increase in the excitability of the muscle membrane. Insertion activity is greatly prolonged. Small, abnormal potentials (called *fibrillation potentials* and *positive sharp waves*) are produced spontaneously while the muscle is at rest. Contraction of the muscle voluntarily, by activation of a reflex or by direct stimulation of a nerve, usually is reduced because of denervation.

Myopathies may be associated with EMG changes similar to those of neuropathies, except that muscle activation is possible and may even be hyperactive. In addition, many myopathies are characterized by prolonged complex repetitive discharges that sound like divebombers or motorcycles on the speaker of the EMG unit.

Localization to a spinal cord segment, a spinal nerve root, or a peripheral nerve is determined on the basis of the distribution of abnormal findings. Lesions of spinal cord segments and roots typically cause partial denervation of several muscle groups, whereas peripheral nerve lesions are more likely to cause complete denervation of the distribution of that nerve. Spinal cord segment lesions are more likely to be bilateral.

Electroretinography (ERG) is the electrical recording of the retinal response to light. Simple strip chart recorders can be used, but a cathode ray oscilloscope is necessary in order to obtain better results. Signal-averaging computers provide even better resolution,[36] and allow the recording in nonsedated animals. The ERG is helpful for differentiating retinal blindness from central blindness.

The *visual-evoked response* (VER) is the cortical electrical activity that occurs in response to a light stimulus administered to the eye. A signal-averaging computer is needed to record this response. The response provides an objective evaluation of central visual pathways.[37,38] Use of pattern stimuli, light-emitting diode goggles, or a red filter has made this technique more useful.[39,40]

The *brain stem auditory-evoked response* (BAER) entails the recording of brain stem potentials in response to a click stimulus in the ear canal. A signal-averaging computer is necessary to record this response.[41–44] The peripheral auditory system can be evaluated rapidly and accurately with this system. Partial hearing losses require pure tone stimuli, which present more difficult technical problems. Brain stem function also can be evaluated. The recording consists of a series of waves that represent electrical activity at successive levels of the brain stem. A lesion at one level of the brain stem will block the responses at that level and at all succeeding levels. The BAER is used to evaluate cochlear lesions and the level of brain stem lesions and to confirm a diagnosis of complete loss of brain stem function when brain death has occurred.

Impedance audiometry (IA) is a method of assessing the integrity of the middle ear system. IA measures the compliance of the tympanic membrane at rest, with changes in pressure, and in response to auditory stimuli. Middle ear effusion, occlusion of the auditory (eustachian) tube, conduction alterations in the ossicles, retrocochlear hearing loss, and facial motor nerve function (through the stapedial reflex) can be identified through IA.[45,46]

Somatosensory-evoked potentials (SEPs) are the potentials recorded from spinal cord, brain stem, or brain in response to a stimulus administered to a peripheral nerve.[47,48] A signal-averaging computer is required. The SEP is used to determine the functional capacity of sensory pathways, for example, in a paraplegic animal with questionable sensory function on neurologic examination. Adequate information is not yet available to determine the clinical value of this test. The fastest potentials recorded are those of the faster pathways (e.g., the dorsal columns). More trials are needed before it can be determined whether the slower-conducting pain pathways can be evaluated in clinical patients.[49]

Echoencephalography uses pulsed ultrasound (1 to 2 MHz) to record the location of tissue interfaces. Midline structures of the brain can be determined in relation to the bony calvarium. Shifts of the midline structures caused by masses in the cranial vault (tumor, hemorrhage) can be detected. The technique is noninvasive and requires minimal patient cooperation. It appears to be reliable, although there have been limited trials in veterinary medicine. CT and MR imaging have replaced this technique in many institutions. Ultrasonography can be used if there is a bony defect in the skull. It has been used to assess hydrocephalics with open fontanelles.[50,51]

Urodynamics includes cystometrography (CMG), urethral pressure profiles (UPP), and electrophysiologic testing of bladder and sphincter reflexes (see Chap. 3 for details).

Contraindications

There are no significant contraindications to any of the electrophysiologic tests. Anesthesia or tranquilization may be necessary for some procedures, and may be contraindicated in some animals.

Biopsy

Availability

A biopsy of neural or muscular tissue can be performed by any veterinary surgeon; however, the difficulties in obtaining good diagnostic samples generally limit the use of this procedure to specialty practices and institutions. Histopathologic evaluation requires a trained pathologist.

Indications

Brain biopsy is used to confirm a diagnosis of a diffuse encephalopathy, such as viral inflammation or storage disease.[52] Samples of the cerebral cortex or the cerebellum can be obtained. Many of these diseases cannot be diagnosed ante mortem with other procedures. Because of the invasive nature of the procedure, it is not generally recommended; however, it is very useful for establishing the diagnosis in a potential animal model of neurologic disease or when the owner of the animal wants a definitive diagnosis of a potentially untreatable disease. Minimal deficits in neurologic function are produced by removal of small samples of the cerebral or cerebellar cortex.

Fine-needle aspiration of spinal cord masses can be accomplished using fluoroscopy.[53] Lymphosarcoma is readily identified, and we have obtained a histologic diagnosis on parenchymal tumors as well.

A biopsy of a peripheral nerve is indicated in peripheral neuropathies. Excision of a few fascicles of a mixed nerve is preferred if a motor neuropathy is suspected, but small sensory nerves may be used in many disorders.[54,55]

A muscle biopsy usually is performed simultaneously with a peripheral nerve biopsy in order to differentiate neuropathies from myopathies. Tissues must be handled properly for satisfactory histopathologic evaluation. The nerve or muscle specimen must be maintained straight, without excess tension, during fixation. This positioning usually is attained by suspending the nerve with a weight on the end, tying or pinning the ends of the nerve to a tongue depressor, or using double clamps on the muscle.[54] The pathologist should be consulted regarding the proper handling of the tissues.

Ventricular puncture is indicated primarily for confirmation of hydrocephalus[56] rather than for procurement of CSF. The thickness of the cerebral cortex can be estimated from the depth of the needle in the site where CSF is first obtained. Questionable cases can be confirmed with pneumoventriculography. Animals with open fontanelles or suture lines can be tapped easily. If the skull is closed, the procedure is more difficult.

Contraindications

The invasive nature of these procedures must be weighed against the benefits of the information to be derived. A brain biopsy usually is reserved for animals with serious, usually untreatable, encephalopathies. The brain biopsy has gained favor as a procedure for the diagnosis of certain human viral encephalitides, such as herpes encephalitis. The deficits produced by the biopsy are minimal. A spinal cord biopsy is contraindicated, because the procedure seriously compromises spinal cord function. However, fine-needle aspiration of mass lesions in the vertebral canal are useful and produce little damage. Peripheral nerve and muscle biopsies are performed more commonly and do not produce serious deficits if care is exercised in the selection of the peripheral nerve. A ventricular tap not only is diagnostic but also may be therapeutic in an animal with increased intracranial pressure. Excessive removal of fluid can cause collapse of the cerebral cortex and subdural hematoma.

CASE HISTORIES

The case studies presented in Chapters 1 and 2 involved the history (Chap. 1), which was used to develop a sign-time graph and a list of probable categories of disease (rule-outs); the neurologic examination (Chap. 1); and, from it, localization of the lesion (Chap. 2). At this point in each case, an anatomic diagnosis and a list of rule-outs have been established. The next step is to perform appropriate diagnostic tests to confirm or exclude the possible causes of the problem and, in some cases, to pinpoint the location of the lesion. The signalment, the localization, and the list of rule-outs will be repeated. The reader should decide which diagnostic tests are appropriate in each case before reading the diagnostic plan.

Case History 4A

Signalment

Canine, West Highland white terrier, female, 6 years old.

Problems

Right hemiparesis, slight paresis in left pelvic limb.

Localization

(See Chap. 2.) Spinal cord, C6–T2, primarily the right side.

Rule-outs

(See Chap. 1.)
1. vascular lesion,
2. trauma, and
3. inflammation.

Case History 4B

Signalment

Canine, German shepherd, female, 7 years old.

Problems

Pelvic limb ataxia and paresis.

Localization

(See Chap. 2.) Spinal cord, T3–L3, symmetric.

Rule-outs

(See Chap. 1.)
1. degenerative disease,
2. neoplasia, and
3. inflammation.

Case History 4C

Signalment

Feline, domestic short hair, female, 3 months old.

Problems

Ataxia and dysmetria, nystagmus, and menace deficit.

Localization

(See Chap. 2.) Cerebellum.

Rule-outs

(See Chap. 1.)
1. anomaly and
2. trauma.

Case History 4D

Signalment

Feline, Siamese, male, 2 years old.

Problems

1. depression,
2. head tremor,
3. left hemiparesis, and
4. uveitis in left eye.

Localization

(See Chap. 2.)
1. left C6–T2 spinal cord,
2. cerebellum, and
3. possibly cerebrum or brain stem.

Rule-outs

(See Chap. 1.)
1. inflammation,
2. neoplasia, and
3. degenerative disease.

Case History 4E

Signalment

Canine, Yorkshire terrier, male, 8 months old.

Problems

1. mental status: episodic depression and agitation; and
2. compulsive walking with slight dysmetria and mild postural reaction deficits.

Localization

(See Chap. 2.) Cerebrum, diffuse.

Rule-outs

(See Chap. 1.)
1. metabolic disease and
2. toxic disease.

Assessments

Diagnostic Plan 4A

Radiography: Rule out trauma (vertebral fracture or luxation). Survey radiographs were normal.

Cerebrospinal fluid (CSF) analysis: Rule out inflammation. Possible evidence of hemorrhage. The protein level was 50 mg/dl, with 1 WBC per cu mm in the CSF.

Myelography: Rule out compression from trauma. Check for possible swelling of the spinal cord, which may be seen with a vascular lesion. The myelogram was normal, ruling out trauma.

The probable diagnosis is spinal cord infarction. Infarctions usually are diagnosed by exclusion, as in this case. The CSF may have a slight increase in protein and, more rarely, may be xanthochromic. See Chapter 7 for a discussion of spinal cord infarction.

Diagnostic Plan 4B

Radiography: Rule out vertebral inflammation (diskospondylitis) or vertebral neoplasia.

CSF analysis: Rule out inflammation.

Myelography: Rule out degenerative disk disease and spinal cord tumor. Primary degenerative diseases of the spinal cord or the brain are diagnosed by exclusion, because the lesion is microscopic. Tumors and herniated intervertebral disks also may cause these signs, so they must be ruled out. This dog had a protruding disk that was demonstrated on the myelogram and was corrected surgically. For a discussion of these diseases, see Chapter 7.

Diagnostic Plan 4C

This kitten has been abnormal since birth—a congenital lesion. Trauma is a possible diagnosis if we consider the possibility of a birth injury. The problem has been present for at least 6 to 8 weeks (from the time of significant motor activity) and probably since birth (poor nursing). The lack of progression and the severity of the signs suggest a static lesion, which is not likely to be treatable. This syndrome is typical of cerebellar malformations associated with in utero infections of panleukopenia virus. Diagnostic tests other than a cerebellar biopsy or CT scan are not likely to be rewarding. Sometimes the client should be advised not to waste any more money on diagnostic procedures. The cat can live a reasonably normal life if she stays in the house. See Chapter 9 for a discussion of this syndrome.

Diagnostic Plan 4D

Funduscopic examination: Characterize the eye lesion. Hematology and chemistry analysis: Rule out systemic disease.

CSF analysis: Rule out inflammation and neoplasia.

Serum titers: Rule out feline infectious peritonitis and feline leukemia virus. Radiography and myelography are performed if these tests are negative. Rule out neoplasia. The funduscopic examination is an integral part of the neurologic examination. Inflammatory and neoplastic diseases of the nervous system often produce retinal lesions as well. Hematology and chemistry analyses should be performed for any animal with neurologic disease (see the section on the minimum data base in Chapter 1), but they are likely to provide positive evidence in this case. The chronic progressive history and the multifocal signs are most likely caused by an infectious agent or a metastatic neoplasia. Feline infectious peritonitis (FIP) and feline leukemia virus (FeLV) are the most likely causes of this syndrome. Specific immunologic tests for these diseases are available and should be used if the results are questionable. It is unlikely that radiographs are needed. This cat had an increased plasma protein (9.2 mg/dl), primarily in the globulin fraction (6.2). A granulomatous uveitis and retinitis were seen on ophthalmoscopic examination. The CSF protein level was 400 mg/dl, with 300 WBCs cu mm, which were 80% neutrophils and 20% lymphocytes. These findings are typical of FIP. The FeLV test was positive, and the FIP titer was high. For a discussion of these diseases, see Chapter 16.

Diagnostic Plan 4E

Consider the results of the minimum data base (see Chap. 1) before proceeding. The history and clinical findings are typical of hepatic encephalopathy. Any suggestion of liver disease in the minimum data base will indicate the need for specific tests. Levels of serum enzymes that indicate acute liver disease (alkaline phosphatase) may be normal. Decreased values of serum urea nitrogen (BUN) and serum albumin are significant. Specific tests include sulfobromophthalein sodium excretion (BSP), serum bile acids, blood ammonia levels, and the ammonia tolerance test. For a discussion of hepatic encephalopathy, see Chapter 16.

REFERENCES

1. Mayhew I: Collection of cerebrospinal fluid from the horse. Cornell Vet 65:500–511, 1975.
2. Simpson ST, Reed RB: Manometric values for normal cerebrospinal fluid pressure in dogs. J Am Anim Hosp Assoc 23:629–632, 1987.
3. Duncan JR, Oliver JE, Mayhew IG: Laboratory examinations. In Oliver JE, Hoerlein BF, Mayhew IG: Veterinary Neurology. Philadelphia, WB Saunders, 1987, pp 57–64.
4. Kornegay JN: Cerebrospinal fluid collection, examination, and interpretation in dogs and cats. Comp Cont Educ Pract Vet 3:85–94, 1981.
5. Jamison EM, Lumsden JH: Cerebrospinal fluid analysis in the dog: Methodology and interpretation. Semin Vet Med Surg 3:122–132, 1988.
6. Roszel J: Membrane filtration of canine and feline cerebrospinal fluid for cytologic evaluation. J Am Vet Med Assoc 160:720–725, 1972.
7. Bichsel P, Vandevelde M, Vandevelde E, et al: Immunoelectrophoretic determination of albumin and IgG in serum and cerebrospinal fluid in dogs with neurological diseases. Res Vet Sci 37:101–107, 1984.
8. Krakowka S, Fenner W, Miele JA: Quantitative determination of serum origin cerebrospinal fluid proteins in the dog. Am J Vet Res 42:1975–1977, 1981.
9. Sorjonen DC, Warren JN, Schultz RD: Qualitative and quantitative determination of albumin, IgG, IgM and IgA in normal cerebrospinal fluid in dogs. J Am Anim Hosp Assoc 17:833–839, 1981.
10. Sorjonen D: Total protein, albumin quota, and electrophoretic patterns in cerebrospinal fluid of dogs with central nervous system disorders. Am J Vet Res 48:301–305, 1987.
11. Kristensen F, Firth EC: Analysis of serum proteins and cerebrospinal fluid in clinically normal horses, using agarose electrophoresis. Am J Vet Res 38:1089–1092, 1977.
12. Rand JS, Parent J, Jacobs R, et al: Reference intervals for feline cerebrospinal fluid: Biochemical and serologic variables, IgG concentration, and electrophoretic fractionation. Am J Vet Res 51:1049–1054, 1990.
13. Barber DL, Oliver JE, Mayhew IG: Neuroradiography. In Oliver JE, Hoerlein BF, Mayhew IG (eds): Veterinary Neurology. Philadelphia, WB Saunders, 1987, pp 65–110.
14. Fike JR, LeCouteur RA, Cann CE: Anatomy of the canine brain using high resolution computed tomography. Vet Radiol 22:236–243, 1981.
15. LeCouteur RA, Fike JR, Cann CE, et al: X-ray computed tomography of brain tumors in cats. J Am Vet Med Assoc 183:301–305, 1983.
16. Kornegay JN: Imaging brain neoplasms: Computed tomography and magnetic resonance imaging. Vet Med Rep 2:372–390, 1990.
17. Turrel J, Fike J, LeCouteur R, et al. Computed tomographic characteristics of primary brain tumors in 50 dogs. J Am Vet Med Assoc 188:851–856, 1986.
18. LeCouteur RA, Fike JR, Cann CE, et al: Computed tomography of brain tumors in the caudal fossa of the dog. Vet Radiol 22:244–251, 1981.

19. Fike JR, LeCouteur RA, Cann CE, et al: Computerized tomography of brain tumors of the rostral and middle fossas in the dog. Am J Vet Res 42:275–281, 1981.
20. Cox F, Jakovljevic S: The use of iopamidol for myelography in dogs: A study of twenty-seven cases. J Small Anim Pract 27:159–165, 1986.
21. May S, Wyn-Jones G, Church S: Iopamidol myelography in the horse. Equine Vet J 18:199–202, 1986.
22. Wheeler SJ, Davies JV: Iohexol myelography in the dog and cat: A series of one hundred cases, and a comparison with metrizamide and iopamidol. J Small Anim Pract 26:247–256, 1985.
23. Wood AK: Iohexol and iopamidol: New nonionic contrast media for myelography in dogs. Comp Cont Educ Pract Vet 10:31–36, 1988.
24. Suter PF, Morgan JP, Holliday TA, et al: Myelography in the dog: Diagnosis of tumors of the spinal cord and vertebrae. J Vet Radiol Soc 12:29–44, 1971.
25. Selcer BA, Chambers JN, Schwensen K, et al: Epidurography as a diagnostic aid in canine lumbosacral compressive disease: 47 cases (1981–1986). Vet Comp Orthop Trauma 2:97–103, 1988.
26. Feeney DA, Wise M: Epidurography in the normal dog: Technic and radiographic findings. Vet Radiol 22:35–39, 1981.
27. Klide AM, Steinberg SA, Pond MJ: Epiduralograms in the dog: The uses and advantages of the diagnostic procedure. J Vet Radiol Soc 8:39–44, 1967.
28. Hudson JA, Cartee RE, Simpson ST, et al: Ultrasonographic anatomy of the canine brain. Radiology 30:13–21, 1989.
29. Oliver JE: Cranial sinus venography in the dog. J Am Vet Radiol Soc 10:66–71, 1969.
30. LeCouteur RA, Scagliotti RH, Beck KA, et al: Indirect imaging of the optic nerve, using metrizamide (optic thecography). Am J Vet Res 43:1424–1428, 1982.
31. Voorhout G, Rijnberk A: Cisternography combined with linear tomography for visualization of pituitary lesions in dogs with pituitary dependent hyperadrenocorticism. J Vet Radiol 31:74–78, 1990.
32. Redding RW, Knecht CE: Atlas of Electroencephalography in the Dog and Cat. New York, Praeger, 1984.
33. Redding RW: Electroencephalography. Prog Vet Neurol 1:181–188, 1990.
34. Klemm WR, Hall CL: Current status and trends in veterinary electroencephalography. J Am Vet Med Assoc 164:529–532, 1974.
35. Bowen JM: Electromyography. In Oliver JE, Hoerlein BF, Mayhew IG (eds): Veterinary Neurology. Philadelphia, WB Saunders, 1987, pp 145–168.
36. Acland GM: Diagnosis and differention of retinal diseases in small animals by electroretinography. Semin Vet Med Surg 3:15–27, 1988.
37. Sims MH, Laratta LJ, Bubb WJ, et al: Waveform analysis and reproducibility of visual-evoked potentials in dogs. Am J Vet Res 50:1823–1828, 1989.
38. Strain GM, Claxton MS, Olcott BM, et al: Visual-evoked potentials and electroretinograms in ruminants with thiamine-responsive polioencephalomalacia or suspected listeriosis. J Am Vet Med Assoc 51:1513–1517, 1990.
39. Sims MH, Laratta LJ: Visual-evoked potentials in cats, using a light-emitting diode stimulator. Am J Vet Res 49:1876–1881, 1988.
40. Bichsel P, Oliver JE, Coulter DB, et al: Recording of visual-evoked potentials in dogs with scalp electrodes. J Vet Intern Med 2:145–149, 1988.
41. Rolf SL, Reed SM, Melnick W, et al: Auditory brain stem response testing in anesthetized horses. Am J Vet Res 48:910–914, 1987.
42. Sims MH, Moore RE: Auditory-evoked response in the clinically normal dog: Early latency components. Am J Vet Res 45:2019–2027, 1984.
43. Holliday TA, Te Selle ME: Brain stem auditory-evoked potentials of dogs: Wave forms and effects of recording electrode positions. Am J Vet Res 46:845–851, 1985.
44. Strain GM, Olcott BM, Thompson DR, et al: Brainstem auditory-evoked potentials in Holstein cows. J Vet Intern Med 3:144–148, 1989.
45. Penrod JP, Coulter DB: The diagnostic uses of impedance audiometry in the dog. J Am Anim Hosp Assoc 16: 941–948, 1980.
46. Sims M, Weigel J, Moore R: Effects of tenotomy of the tensor tympani muscle on the acoustic reflex in dogs. Am J Vet Res 47:1022–1032, 1986.
47. Oliver JE, Purinton PT, Brown J: Somatosensory evoked potentials from stimulation of thoracic limb nerves of the dog. Prog Vet Neurol 1:433–443, 1990.
48. Strain GM, Taylor DS, Graham MC, et al: Cortical somatosensory-evoked potentials in the horse. Am J Vet Res 49:1869–1872, 1988.
49. Holliday T, Ealand B, Weldon N: Ascending pathways of average evoked spinal cord potentials of dogs. In: Proceedings of the ACVIM, Seattle, 1979, p 104.
50. Spaulding KA: Ultrasonographic imaging of the lateral cerebral ventricles in the dog. J Vet Radiol 31:59–64, 1990.
51. Hudson JA, Simpson ST, Buxton DF, et al. Ultrasonographic diagnosis of canine hydrocephalus. J Vet Radiol 31:50–58, 1990.
52. Swaim SF, Vandevelde M, Faircloth JC: Evaluation of brain biopsy techniques in the dog. J Am Anim Hosp Assoc 15:627–633, 1979.
53. Irving G, McMillan MC: Fluoroscopically guided percutaneous fine-needle aspiration biopsy of thoracolumbar spinal lesions in cats. Prog Vet Neurol 1:473–475, 1990.
54. Braund KG: Nerve and muscle biopsy techniques. Prog Vet Neurol 2:35–56, 1991.
55. Braund K, Walker T, Vandevelde M: Fascicular nerve biopsy in the dog. Am J Vet Res 40:1025–1030, 1979.
56. Savell CM: Cerebral ventricular tap: An aid to diagnosis and treatment of hydrocephalus in the dog. J Am Anim Hosp Assoc 10:500–501, 1974.

5

Principles of Medical Treatment

Primary neurologic disorders that require medical treatment include infections, and physical therapy for rehabilitation. Seizures (see Chap. 14), neoplasia (see Chap. 16), and other diseases requiring specific treatment are covered in the descriptions of the diseases. The management of central nervous system (CNS) edema is discussed in Chapter 13 in the section on brain trauma. Management of pain is reviewed in Chapter 15.

Management of Central Nervous System Infections

Effective therapy for CNS infections depends on identification of the cause and selection of the appropriate antimicrobial agent. Identification is based on cerebrospinal fluid (CSF) analysis and culture. Selection of the appropriate antimicrobial agent depends on two principles: (1) The agent must be effective against the microbial target without severely injuring the patient, and (2) it must be delivered to and must penetrate the CNS. Unfortunately, anatomic and physiologic barriers to successful therapy for CNS infections exist, especially when certain drugs are used. The combined effects of these obstacles create a functional blood-brain barrier.

The Blood-Brain Barrier

The combined functions of the CNS capillaries and the choroid plexus create a barrier to the movement of drugs from the capillary or pericapillary fluid into nervous tissue or CSF. Discrepancies between serum and CNS drug concentrations occur because of two factors: the special anatomy of CNS capillaries and the secretory selectivity of the choroid plexus. In capillaries outside the CNS, drugs and other agents pass from the blood through clefts between endothelial cells and through fenestrations in the capillary basement membrane. In the CNS, capillary endothelial cells are joined by tight junctions that seal the intercellular clefts. The capillary basement membrane has no fenestrations. In addition, glial cell foot processes surround the capillaries. In the CNS, a drug must penetrate an inner bimolecular lipid membrane, the endothelial cell cytoplasm, an outer lipid membrane, and a basement membrane; finally, it must traverse the glial foot processes.[1] Penetration of a drug is largely a function of its endothelial membrane solubility. Membrane solubility is favored by (1) a low degree of ionization at physiologic pH, (2) a low degree of plasma protein binding, and (3) a high degree of lipid solubility of the un-ionized drug.[2] Certain highly lipid-soluble drugs bind strongly to tissue sites in the brain, permitting high concentrations to be achieved within nervous tissue.

Regulation of CSF solutes occurs at the choroid plexus. Plasma dialysate that filters through fenestrated capillaries is selectively secreted by choroid epithelial cells. Certain CSF constituents also are actively reabsorbed by the choroidal epithelial cell, which tends to clear these substances from the CSF and from nervous tissue. This active transport system for weak organic acids removes such drugs as penicillin and gentamicin. Inflammation may block this active transport system, allowing drug concentrations to increase. In addition, inflammation may increase the permeability of endothelial membranes to certain antibiotics, allowing these drugs to penetrate nervous tissue in cases of disease. In the normal animal, these antibiotics penetrate poorly. Therefore, as the inflammation decreases, penetration of the antibiotic also decreases.

Use of Antimicrobial Agents in Treating Infections

Antimicrobial agents are grouped by their capacity to achieve concentrations in CSF sufficient to inhibit microorganisms throughout the period of therapy.[2] Table 5–1 lists these drugs relative to achievable concentrations in CSF. Microbicidal drugs are preferred to microbistatic drugs whenever possible. Antibiotics such as the aminoglycosides diffuse poorly, even in the presence of inflammation. Intrathecal administration may be required in order for adequate CSF concentrations to be achieved, but this route is rarely used in animals because of the necessity for anesthesia for each injection.

TABLE 5–1 Antimicrobial Drugs: Ability to Penetrate the Blood-Brain Barrier

Good	*Intermediate*	*Poor*
Microbicidal		
Trimethoprim	Penicillin G*	Penicillin G benzathine
Moxalactam	Ampicillin*	Cephalosporins‡
Cefotaxime	Methicillin*	Aminoglycosides
Cefatazidime	Nafcillin*	
Metronidazole	Carbenicillin*	
Enroflaxcin	Oxacillin	
	Vancomycin	
Microbistatic		
Chloramphenicol	Tetracycline	Amphotericin B§
Sulfonamides	Flucytosine	Erythromycin‖
Isoniazid		
Minocycline†		
Doxycycline†		
Rifampin		

* High intravenous doses are needed to achieve the maximal effect.

† Lipid-soluble tetracyclines that achieve higher concentrations in CSF than do other tetracyclines.

‡ First and second generation, may be effective early in bacterial meningitis; concentrations dramatically decrease with repair of the blood-brain barrier.

§ May be effective in cryptococcal meningitis.

‖ Penetration in the face of inflammation is unpredictable.

Placement of intraventricular catheters can be used to facilitate injection of drugs into the CSF.

Bacterial Infections

Bacterial Meningitis

Primary bacterial meningitis is more common in dogs and cats than was once believed. It occurs primarily in association with bacteremia or endocarditis or as an extension of an infection in structures surrounding the nervous system such as the nose, sinuses, and ear. In the dog, organisms associated with canine bacterial meningitis include the *Pasteurella* spp., especially *Pasteurella multocida*, and the *Staphylococcus* spp. *S. aureus*, *S. epidermidis*, and *S. albus*.[3] *Staphylococcus aureus* is the most frequent isolate in our clinic. Gram-negative septicemia with *Salmonella*, *Escherichia coli*, *Proteus*, and *Pseudomonas* is occasionally associated with purulent meningoencephalomyelitis. Bacterial meningitis is common in neonatal foals, calves, and lambs.[4] Septicemia may lead to showering of emboli in these species. Organisms include *Pasteurella* spp., *Corynebacterium*, *Hemophilus*, *Actinobacillus*, and *Streptococcus* spp. Coliforms are also frequent causes of meningitis.

Definitive treatment of bacterial meningitis is based on isolation of the organism from the CSF and determination of its antibiotic sensitivity. In addition, the source of infection (i.e., endocarditis, bacteremia) should be identified and should be managed therapeutically. The initial therapy for bacterial meningitis in small animals is based on the assumption that staphylococcal organisms are the cause. The antibiotics of choice for both large and small animals are penicillin, ampicillin, or a penicillinase-resistant antibiotic such as methicillin. We prefer to use penicillin G, 10,000–20,000 units/kg every 4 to 6 hours, or ampicillin, 10–15 mg/kg every 6 hours. The antibiotics are given intravenously (IV) for at least 7 days. Chloramphenicol, 50 mg/kg every 4 to 6 hours IV, can also be used as a substitute for penicillin; however, many strains of staphylococcal organisms are resistant to this antibiotic.[3,5] Chloramphenicol should be used only when the organism has been determined to be sensitive to its action. Although the aminoglycoside antibiotics penetrate very poorly into nervous tissue, gentamicin commonly is combined with penicillin or ampicillin. The basis for this combination is the assumption that the source of infection is not the CNS. The drug is given IV or intramuscularly (IM) at a dosage of 2 mg/kg every 8 hours. Renal function must be monitored carefully, and treatment should not exceed 14 days. *Under no circumstances should gentamicin or any other aminoglycoside antibiotic be given as the sole antimicrobial agent in bacterial meningitis.* Antibiotic therapy should be modified if results of culture and sensitivity testing suggest that the initial therapy will not be effective. Third-generation cephalosporins have a broad spectrum of activity and penetrate the CNS well. However, they must be given by injection and are expensive. Other alternatives we have found effective in difficult cases include enrofloxacin (dogs, 2.5 mg/kg per os twice daily),[6] metronidazole (10–15 mg/kg per os three times daily), and combining rifampin with other agents. Metronidazole and enrofloxacin have potential for CNS toxicity, so prolonged administration is not recommended.

After 7 to 14 days, IV therapy can be stopped and oral antibiotics begun. Antibiotics should be given for 4 to 6 weeks in order to prevent relapse. The prognosis for recovery is fair to good.

Gram-negative meningoencephalomyelitis presents some unusual problems in therapy, inasmuch as the effective antibiotics may not penetrate the CNS, even in the presence of inflammation. The third-generation cephalosporins are the treatment of choice. An alternative is the concomitant administration of chloramphenicol and gentamicin parenterally. Intrathecal gentamicin, 5–10 mg/day, can be considered. Because the intrathecal use of antibiotics in dogs or cats requires multiple anesthetic episodes, it is rarely used. If *Pseudomonas aeruginosa* is isolated, the optimal therapy is a combination of sodium carbenicillin and gentamicin. In systemic salmonellosis with CNS involvement, chloramphenicol is the initial drug of choice, unless it is contraindicated by sensitivity testing. Alternative regimens include trimethoprimsulfa or ampicillin-gentamicin combinations. Other gram-negative infections should be treated according to culture and sensitivity results.

Occasionally, systemic infection extending to the nervous system occurs from *Brucella canis*. The best therapy for brucellosis includes a combination of streptomycin and minocycline. Streptomycin should be administered for 2 weeks by parenteral injection. Minocycline should be given orally for 4 weeks, in combination with the 2-week schedule for streptomycin.[7,8]

Cats may have meningitis secondary to abscesses that are frequently caused by anaerobic bacteria. Penicillin or amoxicillin are effective and reasonable in cost. Clindamycin or metronidazole are good alternatives in resistant infections.[9]

Bacterial Brain Abscess

An abscess of the brain usually results from extension of purulent otitis media and otitis interna or from rhinitis or sinusitis. Brain abscesses are more common in large animals than in cats and dogs. An abscess can occur in association with foreign body penetration or migration through the CNS. The causative agents are usually *Staphylococcus*, *Streptococcus*, or *Pasteurella* organisms. Successful treatment includes appropriate antibiotics and surgical drainage or removal of the abscess. Because of the organisms involved, penicillin, ampicillin, methicillin, and chloramphenicol are the antibiotics of choice. The treatment of bacterial brain abscess is difficult, the relapse rate is high, and the prognosis is very poor. Surgical drainage may be efficacious if the lesion can be localized by computed tomography (CT).

Diskospondylitis

The most common cause of diskospondylitis in dogs is *Staphylococcus aureus*; occasionally *Brucella canis* organisms are the source.[10] The disease is associated with a high incidence of urinary tract infection and bacteremia. In staphylococcal diskospondylitis, penicillinase-resistant antibiotics should be chosen. Cephalosporins or semisynthetic penicillins are usually effective. Medical treatment should be tried before surgical treatment is considered. Severe paresis may require decompression. Vertebral curettage in addition to antibiotic therapy for 4 to 6 weeks may achieve resolution if medical treatment is unsuccessful.

In *Brucella canis* diskospondylitis, therapy is expensive and may not eradicate the infection effectively. Streptomycin-minocycline combinations are used as described for meningitis.[8] The dog should be neutered and should be isolated from other dogs. Human infection has occurred with this organism.

Mycotic Infections

The more common mycotic infections of the CNS are caused by *Cryptococcus neoformans*, *Blastomyces dermatitidis*, *Histoplasma capsulatum*, and *Coccidioides immitis*. A definitive diagnosis is made by isolation or identification of the organism in the CSF or other body secretions. Except for cryptococcal meningitis, each of these diseases is treated in nearly the same way as the others.

Cryptococcal Meningitis

The mainstay of therapy for the deep mycotic agents is amphotericin B. This drug is poorly absorbed from the gastrointestinal tract and must be given IV for a full therapeutic effect. Amphotericin B diffuses very poorly into the CSF; however, it remains the drug of choice for many CNS mycotic infections. Several therapeutic regimens have been described. Commonly, 50 mg of amphotericin B is dissolved in 10 ml of sterile water, divided into small portions, and frozen. Each week a vial is thawed and diluted in a small volume of 5% dextrose for treatment. The dose for each treatment is 0.1–0.5 mg/kg IV, given slowly over 3 to 5 minutes. The treatment is repeated three times a week until a total cumulative dose of 4–10 mg/kg has been given. Renal function must be monitored during treatment. The dose must be lowered or a dose skipped if the blood urea nitrogen (BUN) increases.[11]

Amphotericin B is a very toxic antibiotic. Untoward effects include fever, vomiting, and phlebitis at the site of the injection. The drug is very irritating to tissues, and care must be exercised to avoid extravascular spillage. Serious side effects include acute hepatic failure and irreversible renal failure. Decreased renal function is expected in most patients given amphotericin B; however, critical monitoring of the animal allows the clinician to suspend therapy before renal failure becomes irreversible. Renal effects include a reversible decrease in glomerular filtration and concentrating ability of relatively short duration. A more prolonged decrease in renal blood flow occurs. These effects usually disappear when therapy is stopped and do not contraindicate retreatment.

Intrathecal amphotericin B may be helpful. Five ml of spinal fluid is removed and mixed with 10 to 20 mg of soluble hydrocortisone or methylprednisolone. The solution is instilled slowly intrathecally. After 5 to 10 minutes, 5 ml of spinal fluid is removed again, and a solution containing 0.1 to 0.5 mg of amphotericin B is added. The mixture is injected slowly intrathecally. The procedure is repeated two to three times per week until a total dose of 10 to 15 mg has been given. Spinal arachnoiditis and cranial toxic neuropathy are major hazards, even if the clinician takes precautions.

Flucytosine, when combined with amphotericin B, acts synergestically in vitro against *Cryptococcus neoformans*. It achieves satisfactory concentrations in CSF. The oral dose of flucytosine is 50–75 mg/kg every 8 hours.[11,12] The rate of relapse is considerably lower with the combined therapy. Side effects include leukopenia, thrombocytopenia, vomiting, and diarrhea.

Ketoconazole and itraconazole (investigational drug) may also be used as an adjunct to amphotericin B and continued after amphotericin B is discontinued. The dose of ketoconazole is 5–10 mg/kg twice daily for 4 to 5 months. Absorption is enhanced if the drug is given with food. The dosage of itraconazole is similar, but the drug appears to have fewer side effects.[13] Ketoconazole may cause hepatotoxicity at the dosages recommended.

Coccidioidal Meningitis

Coccidioides immitis is not susceptible to the synergistic activity of combined amphotericin B and flucytosine therapy. The levels of amphotericin B achieved in CSF following IV administration are usually below the levels needed to inhibit most coccidioidal strains. Intrathecal administration of amphotericin B may be needed for the management of coccidioidal meningitis. Combination therapy may be advantageous, as in cryptococcal infections. Ketaconazole is effective if the CNS is not involved.

Other Systemic Fungal Infections of the Meninges

Histoplasma capsulatum, *Blastomyces dermatidis*, *Aspergillus* spp., *Candida* spp., and *Sporothorix schenckii* are occasionally involved in meningitis. Treatment is the same as for cryptococcosis.

Actinomycetes Infections

Tuberculous Meningitis

Although it is nearly nonexistent in dogs and cats, this disease occurs occasionally in primates. Most of the antituberculous drugs readily penetrate the CNS. A combination of isoniazid and ethambutol is suggested. Other effective drugs include rifampin, ethionamide, pyrazinamide, and cycloserine.

Nocardiosis

The drugs of choice have been triple sulfonamides or trimethoprim-sulfa combinations. However, their in vitro effect has not been duplicated in vivo. The drugs should be given in high doses, and precautions should be taken to prevent nephrotoxicity. Alternative drugs include minocycline, amikacin, and erythromycin combined with ampicillin.[14]

Actinomycosis

The drug of choice is penicillin G, given IM or subcutaneously at 100,000 units/kg/day.[14] Therapy is continued with clindamycin, erythromycin, or chloramphenicol.

Viral Infections

Viral infection of the CNS may fit into one of four categories: (1) viral invasions resulting in inflammation (viral meningitis, encephalitis, or poliomyelitis), (2) postinfectious, noninflammatory encephalopathic states, (3) postinfectious and postvaccinal inflammatory states ("old dog" encephalitis, perhaps polyradiculoneuritis, brachial plexus neuropathy), and (4) slow virus infections (scrapie, bovine spongiform encephalopathy, Aleutian mink disease). There are no specific treatments for any viral disease. Supportive care is necessary.

Viral diseases of all species are described in Chapter 16.

Rickettsial Infections

In addition to vasculitis and hematologic disorders, the agents of Rocky Mountain spotted fever and canine ehrlichiosis may also cause meningitis. Both diseases are transmitted by ticks and are limited to areas harboring the appropriate vector. Treatment is with tetracycline, minocycline, or doxycycline. Chloramphenicol is usually effective, but our experience suggests that better results are achieved with the tetracyclines.

Physical Therapy

Physical rehabilitation is often as important as specific medical or surgical treatment in the outcome of a patient with neurologic disease. However, physical therapy is often neglected in veterinary practice. It is time-consuming and labor-intensive and is often boring. Pet owners can be taught to help, and many do a better job than veterinarians.

Hydrotherapy

Exercises performed in water or whirlpools are very effective for relaxing contracted muscles, maintaining joint mobility, and stimulating circulation in atrophied muscles. Most important, they also help to keep the patient clean.

Paralyzed dogs should undergo hydrotherapy sessions twice a day. Muscles and legs should be exercised passively. Sodium hypochlorite is used as a disinfectant in bathtubs and whirlpools to help suppress wound infections.

Exercise

Exercise can be passive or active, depending on the degree of neurologic dysfunction. If possible, dogs should be exercised outdoors, with a towel used as a sling. Walkers, dog carts, or slings may be useful for long-term rehabilitation. Limbs should be massaged vigorously to stimulate muscle tone and delay muscle contracture. Muscle massage with warm mineral oil is also helpful. Proper exercise seems to encourage dogs to walk and improves their mental status.

Bladder Care

Many neurologic lesions disrupt voluntary micturition, resulting in urinary incontinence, retention cystitis, and bladder atony. Urinary bladders should be expressed or emptied by intermittent catheterization at least three times a day. Urinary tract infections should be treated with appropriate antibiotics. See Chapter 3 for details and for the use of pharmacologic agents to assist micturition.

Cage Care

Paralyzed dogs must be turned frequently and must be kept on soft beds to prevent decubital ulcers and wound infections. Waterbeds, sealed foam mattresses, and air mattresses are helpful. The primary concern is to keep the cage clean and free of bacterial contamination. Paralyzed dogs, especially large breed dogs, are predisposed to wound infections, respiratory infections, and urine soiling. They must be cleaned frequently and nursed compassionately in order to be rehabilitated.

REFERENCES

1. Milhorat TH: Cerebrospinal Fluid and the Brain Edemas. New York, Neuroscience Society of New York, 1987.
2. Fenner WR: Bacterial infections of the central nervous system. In Greene CE (ed): Infectious Diseases of the Dog and Cat. Philadelphia, WB Saunders, 1990, pp 184–196.
3. Kornegay JN, Lorenz MD, Zenoble RD: Bacterial meningoencephalitis in two dogs. J Am Vet Med Assoc 173:1334–1336, 1978.

4. Mayhew IG: Large Animal Neurology: A Handbook for Veterinary Clinicians. Philadelphia, Lea & Febiger, 1989.
5. Watson ADJ: Chloramphenicol. 2. Clinical pharmacology in dogs and cats. Aust Vet J 68:2–5, 1991.
6. Bahri LE, Blouin A: Fluoroquinolones: A new family of antimicrobials. Comp Cont Educ Pract Vet 13:1429–1434, 1991.
7. Greene CE: Infectious diseases affecting the nervous system. In Kornegay JN (ed): Neurologic Disorders. New York, Churchill Livingstone, 1986, pp 57–77.
8. Carmichael LE, Greene CE: Canine brucellosis. In Greene CE (ed): Infectious Diseases of the Dog and Cat. Philadelphia, WB Saunders, 1990, pp 573–584.
9. Greene CE (ed): Infectious Diseases of the Dog and Cat. Philadelphia, WB Saunders, 1990.
10. Kornegay JN: Vertebral diseases of large breed dogs. In Kornegay JN (ed): Neurologic Disorders. New York, Churchill Livingstone, 1986, pp 197–215.
11. Medleau L, Barsanti JA: Cryptococcosis. In Greene CE (ed): Infectious Diseases of the Dog and Cat. Philadelphia, WB Saunders, 1990, pp 687–695.
12. Cook JR, Evinger JV, Wagner LA: Successful combination chemotherapy for cryptococcal meningoencephalitis. J Am Anim Hosp Assoc 27:61–64, 1991.
13. Medleau L, Greene CE, Rakich PM: Evaluation of ketoconazole and itraconazole for treatment of disseminated cryptococcosis in cats. Am J Vet Res 51:1454–1458, 1990.
14. Hardie EM: Actinomycosis and nocardiosis. In Greene CE (ed): Infectious Diseases of the Dog and Cat. Philadelphia, WB Saunders, 1990, pp 585–591.

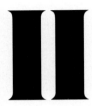

Clinical Problems: Signs and Symptoms

6

Paresis of One Limb

The term *monoparesis*, or *monoparalysis*, denotes partial or complete loss of motor function in one limb resulting from neurologic dysfunction. With mild neurologic dysfunction, the clinical signs may suggest lameness or pain from musculoskeletal disease. With more severe neurologic disease, paresis or paralysis is usually obvious, and the clinician's attention is immediately directed to the nervous system. Thus, when movement disorders occur in only one limb, the initial step in diagnosis is to localize the problem to either the musculoskeletal system or the nervous system (see Chaps. 1 and 2). In a few cases, electrodiagnostic techniques are necessary in order to differentiate musculoskeletal disorders from primary neurologic disorders.

Physical injury to the peripheral or spinal nerves is a significant cause of movement disorders involving one limb and often results from skeletal fractures or luxations. Thus, careful evaluation of both systems is extremely important, because injury to the musculoskeletal system may produce injury or dysfunction of nerves. In general, the prognosis for recovery is better with skeletal injuries than with neurologic injuries.

Lesion Localization

The basic anatomic and physiologic principles that enable a clinician to localize lesions based on motor or sensory deficits were presented in Chapter 2. A brief review of these concepts as they relate to the localization of lesions producing monoparesis or monoparalysis will be presented here (Fig. 6–1).

Monoparesis usually is caused by disease or injury to the lower motor neurons (LMNs) innervating the affected limb. Thus, dysfunction of the neuron (motor nerve cell body), the axon (ventral root, spinal nerves, peripheral nerves), or the neuromuscular end-plate results in motor dysfunction and denervation atrophy. Disruption of the axon (especially the spinal and peripheral nerves) is the most common cause of monoparesis, although in rare circumstances, selective disease of motor neurons in the ventral gray matter of the spinal cord also may produce this problem. In most cases, unilateral spinal cord lesions rostral to T3 produce signs of hemiparesis and bilateral lesions produce tetraparesis. Unilateral spinal cord lesions caudal to T2 may produce paresis or paralysis of the ipsilateral pelvic limb. Obviously, bilateral lesions caudal to T2 produce bilateral pelvic limb paresis. Thus, when lesions are localized in cases of neurologic dysfunction of one thoracic limb (with the rest of the limbs normal), primary consideration is given to the brachial plexus or the peripheral nerves (Table 6–1). Spinal cord disease is not likely to be present, because disease in spinal cord segments C1–T2 affects the upper motor neurons (UMNs) to the ipsilateral pelvic limb. Rarely, lesions confined solely to ventral gray matter (C6–T2) result in thoracic limb monoparesis. Lesion locations for neurologic dysfunction of one pelvic limb may be in the ipsilateral spinal cord from T3–S1. More com-

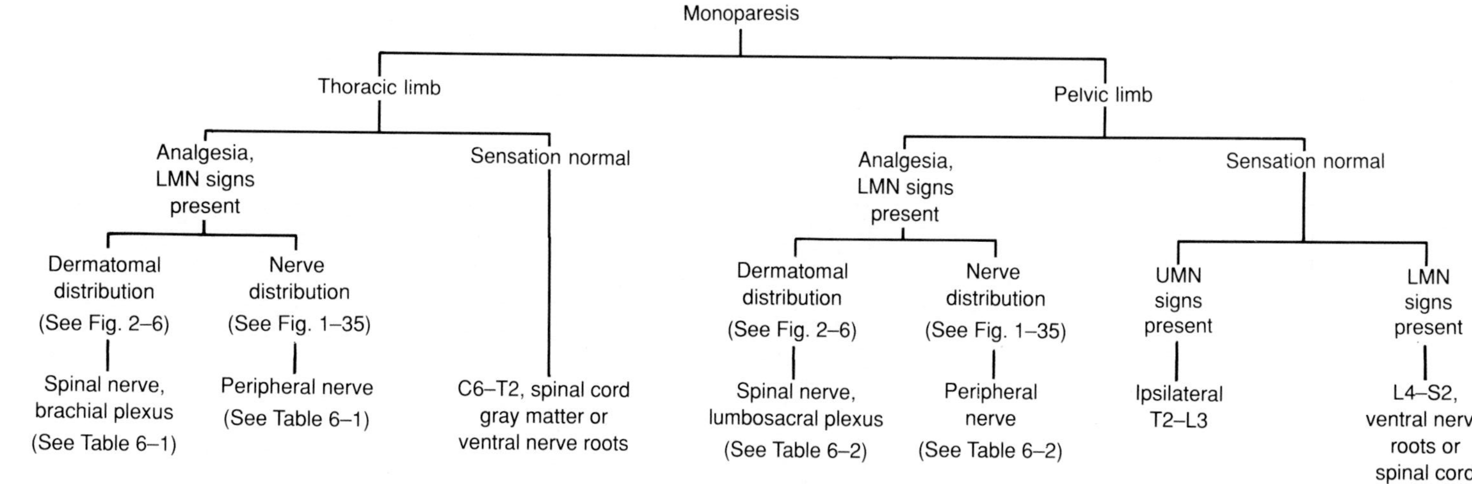

Figure 6–1 An algorithm for the localization of lesions that produce monoparesis.

TABLE 6–1 Nerves of the Brachial Plexus

Nerve	*Spinal Cord Segments**	*Motor Function*	*Cutaneous Sensory Distribution*	*Signs of Dysfunction*
Suprascapular	*C6*, C7	Extension and lateral support of the shoulder	None	Little gait abnormality, pronounced atrophy of supraspinatus and infraspinatus muscles (sweeney)
Brachiocephalicus	*C6*, C7	Advance limb	Cranial surface of brachium	Little gait abnormality, analgesia of cranial brachium
Musculocutaneous	C6, *C7*, C8	Flexion of the elbow	Medial antebrachium	Little gait abnormality, weakened flexion of the elbow; analgesia of medial antebrachium
Axillary	C6, *C7*, C8	Flexion of the shoulder	Dorsolateral brachium	Little gait abnormality, decreased shoulder flexor reflex; analgesia of lateral side of brachium
Radial	*C7*, *C8*, *T1*, T2	Extension of the elbow, the carpus, and the digits	Dorsal surface of the foot and dorsal and lateral parts of the antebrachium	Loss of weight bearing, knuckling of pes, decreased extensor and triceps reflex, analgesia of dorsal surface below elbow
Median and ulnar	*C8*, *T1*, T2	Flexion of the carpus and the digits	Palmar surface of the foot; caudal antebrachium	Little gait abnormality, slight sinking of the carpus; loss of carpal flexion on withdrawal reflex; partial loss of sensation of the palmar surface of the foot and caudal antebrachium
Lateral thoracic	*C8*, *T1*	Cutaneous muscle of trunk	None	Absent cutaneous reflex, normal sensation
Sympathetic†	T1, T2, T3	Dilation of the pupil	None	Miosis, ptosis, enophthalmos and protrusion of third eyelid

* Italics indicate the major spinal cord segment that forms the peripheral nerve.
† The sympathetic nerve is not considered a part of the brachial plexus; however, its nerve fibers travel along the roots of the brachial plexus as they exit from the vertebral column.

monly, however, pelvic limb monoparesis results from damage to spinal or peripheral nerves. Unilateral spinal cord lesions (T3–L3) produce UMN signs in the ipsilateral limb, whereas lesions in the region of L4–S2 or in the spinal or peripheral nerves result in LMN signs.

Disease of the spinal or peripheral nerves produces both sensory and motor dysfunction distal to the lesion, because these nerves contain both motor and sensory fibers. In contrast, lesions that originate in the spinal cord and are confined to the ventral gray matter (motor neurons only) do not produce sensory loss in the affected limbs. Also, unilateral spinal cord lesions (T3–L3) do not produce analgesia of the affected limb because of the bilateral, multisynaptic anatomy of the deep pain pathways (see Chap. 1). The presence of analgesia in the affected limb is very suggestive of peripheral or spinal nerve lesions. If sensory loss cannot be detected in the affected limb, lesions in the spinal cord gray matter or the ventral spinal roots are suspected. It should be remembered that unilateral spinal cord lesions involving segments T3–L3 produce paresis of the ipsilateral pelvic limb, but sensory loss usually is not detectable. However, lesions in this region of the spinal cord produce UMN signs in the affected limb, in contrast to the LMN signs produced by lesions in the L4–S2 segments. Figure 6–1 outlines the localization of lesions that produce monoparesis of the thoracic and pelvic limbs.

The distribution of sensory loss in an affected limb has great localizing value, because lesions can be pinpointed to a particular nerve or to within two to three spinal cord segments (see Fig. 1–35). In addition, the degree of sensory loss influences the prognosis for functional recovery. The pattern of denervation atrophy also is helpful for the localization of lesions to a particular nerve or nerve group. Tables 6–1 and 6–2 outline the motor and sensory distribution of the brachial and lumbosacral plexus. The neurologic signs associated with lesions in each major nerve also are summarized in these tables.

Lesions in the gray matter of the spinal cord (T1–T3) or in the roots of the brachial plexus may injure the LMNs of the sympathetic nerve fibers that form the cranial sympathetic trunk. Loss of sympathetic stimulation to the ipsilateral eye produces signs of miosis, enophthalmos with extrusion of the third eyelid, and ptosis (Horner's sign). In the horse, the miosis is not as obvious and sweating is seen on the

TABLE 6–2 Nerves of the Lumbosacral Plexus

Nerve	Spinal Cord Segments*	Motor Function	Cutaneous Sensory Distribution	Signs of Dysfunction
Obturator	L4, *L5, L6*	Adduction of pelvic limb	None	Little gait abnormality, abduction on slick surface
Femoral	L3, *L4, L5,* L6	Extension of stifle, flexion of hip	Saphenous branch supplies medial surface of limb and medial digit	Severe gait dysfunction, no weight bearing, decreased or absent knee jerk reflex, loss of sensation in medial limb and medial digit
Sciatic	*L6, L7, S1,* S2	Extension of hip, extension and flexion of stifle (see *tibial and peroneal branches*)	Caudal and lateral surfaces of limb distal to stifle (see *tibial and peroneal branches*)	Severe gait dysfunction; paw is knuckled, but weight bearing occurs; hip cannot be extended, hock cannot be flexed or extended (in more central lesions, hip is flexed and drawn toward the midline); loss of cutaneous sensation distal to stifle (except for areas supplied by saphenous nerve); absent withdrawal reflex
Peroneal	*L6, L7,* S1, S2	Flexion of hock, extension of digits	Cranial surface of limb distal to stifle	Hock is straightened and foot tends to knuckle; loss of sensation on cranial surface of limb below stifle, poor hock flexion on withdrawal reflex†
Tibial	L6, *L7, S1,* S2	Extension of hock, flexion of digits	Caudal surface of limb distal to stifle	Hock is dropped, loss of sensation on caudal surface of limb distal to stifle†

* Italics indicate the major spinal cord segments that form the peripheral nerve.
† Peroneal and tibial nerve paralysis commonly occur in association with each other. The signs of peroneal nerve damage tend to predominate.

face and neck to the level of C2 on the side of the lesion.[1] Horner's sign commonly is associated with traumatic injuries of the brachial plexus. Similarly, lesions of the C8–T1 gray matter or spinal nerves affect the lateral thoracic nerve that is the motor component of the cutaneous (panniculus) reflex. Therefore, lesions of the brachial plexus may cause an LMN paresis of the limb, Horner's sign, and loss of the cutaneous reflex on the same side.

Mononeuropathy refers to a disease or an injury of a specific peripheral nerve or its nerve roots. If a large nerve, such as the sciatic or radial nerve, is injured, a severe monoparesis may occur. In most cases, mononeuropathies result from physical injury secondary to compression, laceration, or contusion or from the intramuscular injection of drugs. In addition to motor dysfunction and atrophy, variable degrees of sensory loss are encountered, because peripheral nerves innervating the limbs contain both motor and sensory fibers. *Polyneuropathy* refers to a disease or an injury of several peripheral nerves or their nerve roots. As the term is generally used, a polyneuropathy is the systemic involvement of many nerves. In regard to monoparesis, the term polyneuropathy suggests an injury or a disease of the brachial plexus, the lumbosacral plexus, or the cauda equina. As is true for mononeuropathies, the most important category of disease resulting in monoparesis from polyneuropathies is physical injury. Occasionally, neoplasia of a specific peripheral nerve, nerve root, or nerve plexus is encountered. The incidence of this problem is low, however, and the clinical course is slowly progressive, in contrast to the acute nonprogressive course that tends to characterize physical injuries.

Neurapraxia is a transient loss of function of a nerve. It is usually caused by a loss of blood supply, such as that produced by application of a tourniquet or by pressure from the weight of the animal during anesthesia. Neurapraxia may last for days to months. It should be assumed that demyelination has occurred if the dysfunction lasts more than a few days. Remyelination takes 3 to 4 weeks to effect any clinical improvement. Axonotmesis denotes disruption of the continuity of the axon within the nerve, but with the supporting structures intact. The axon distal to the injury degenerates and stops conducting in 3 to 5 days. Regeneration of the axon may occur beginning in about a week and progressing at a rate of approximately 1 mm a day (1 inch a month). Neurotmesis denotes complete severance of the nerve. Regeneration may occur, but neuroma formation is likely.

Electromyography (EMG) and nerve conduction studies are useful for confirming a diagnosis and may be helpful in estimating the prognosis. EMG changes appear about a week after injury (see Chap. 4 for details). The presence of motor unit action potentials indicates an incomplete injury. The EMG can also be used to monitor the progress of recovery.

Monoparesis of the Pelvic Limbs

Peripheral Nerve Injuries

Sciatic Nerve Injury

The sciatic nerve is a mixed nerve that arises from spinal cord segments L6–S2 (see Table 6–2). Because the spinal cord ends at the middle of the sixth lumbar vertebra in the dog, the sciatic nerve fibers travel caudally within the vertebral canal before exiting from the vertebrae. The course of these nerve fibers makes them particularly subject to injury from lumbosacral fractures and subluxations, lumbosacral stenosis, and pelvic fractures. Sciatic nerve paralysis is a common calving injury in cattle. Damage to the fibers within the vertebral canal usually results in bilateral injury, producing pelvic limb paresis. Occasionally the injury is asymmetric, involving only the fibers of one sciatic nerve. Traumatic injuries of the lumbosacral area rarely result in a true mononeuropathy, because fibers forming the pudendal, pelvic, and caudal nerves are also injured. However, in degenerative lumbosacral stenosis the L7 root may be entrapped in the L7–S1 foramen, causing a lameness or monoparesis.

After giving off branches within the pelvis, the major portion of the sciatic nerve exits at the greater ischiatic foramen and courses caudal to the coxofemoral joint, between and deep to the tuber ischii and the greater trochanter of the femur. It continues distally between the semimembranosus and biceps femoris muscles. Branches of the sciatic nerve supply muscles that help extend the hip and flex the stifle. Between the hip and the stifle, the sciatic nerve branches into the peroneal and tibial nerves. These latter nerves supply all muscles below the stifle and provide sensation to all areas of the foot except the medial digit, which is innervated by the saphenous branch of the femoral nerve.

Injuries below the distal third of the femur produce signs from loss of function of the peroneal and tibial nerves. These injuries will be described later. Damage to the proximal sciatic nerve results in severe monoparesis, because the extensor muscles of the stifle are the only group that remains functional. Although the animal may bear weight, the stifle does not flex. The hock and the digits will not flex or extend because of tibial and peroneal nerve involvement. The animal stands "knuckled over," and the hock usually is dropped. Sensation below the stifle is severely compromised, but normal sensation is perceived from the medial surface of the limb or the medial digit (innervated by the femoral nerve). The dorsal surface of the foot frequently is ulcerated from the animal's dragging or walking on the knuckled-over foot (Fig. 6–2). The sciatic nerve is the major nerve evaluated by the pelvic limb flexor reflex. In proximal sciatic nerve injuries, the digits, the hock, and the stifle do not flex when the toes are stimulated. Stimulation of the medial digit or the medial distal leg elicits a pain response and flexion of the hip, but the remainder of the joints of the affected limb do not flex. Atrophy of the caudal thigh muscles and the muscles below the stifle may be severe.

The proximal portion of the sciatic nerve is most frequently damaged by fractures of the shaft of the ilium, acetabular fractures, fractures of the proximal femur, following retrograde placement of intramedullary pins in the femur, and during calving injuries in cattle.[2–6] Less common causes include severe hip dysplasia and surgical procedures involving the coxofemoral joint.[7,8] The prognosis is poor if these injuries are complete. Partial deficits may be temporary. Surgical relief of compression injuries may be rewarding.

Damage to the sciatic nerve, or to the peroneal or tibial nerves along the caudal aspect of the femur, may occur in association with injection injuries or femoral fractures. Injections intended for the biceps femoris or semimembranosus muscles may go into the fascial plane between these muscles.[9] Injury may be from direct laceration of the nerve by the needle, from the agent being injected directly into the nerve, or from secondary scarring around the nerve. Injection injuries may be prevented by using

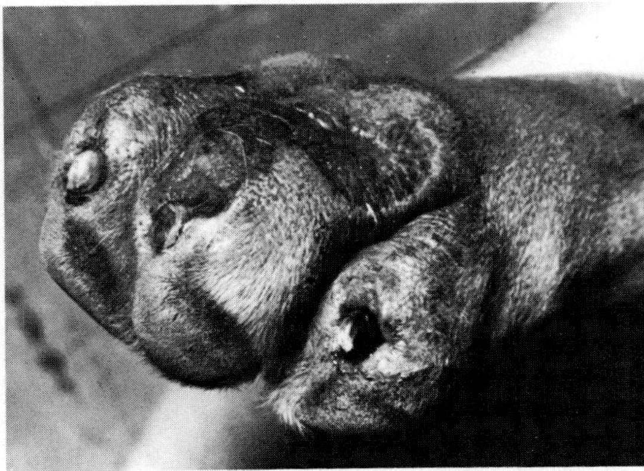

Figure 6–2 Ulcerated digits of the pelvic limb in a dog with peroneal nerve paralysis.

another site for intramuscular injections, such as the quadriceps or lumbar muscles. The diagnosis is based on the history and the lack of another explanation. Absolute proof of the cause is unlikely to be obtained, which may be important from a medicolegal standpoint. The prognosis and the management plan depend on the severity of the injury. Careful assessment of the motor and sensory function determines if both peroneal and tibial components are affected. Tibial paralysis is more easily accommodated than peroneal paralysis. If both components are affected, the sensory evaluation is important to determine if the lesion is complete. If there is some remaining function, especially in the peroneal distribution, conservative treatment is recommended and a fairly good prognosis is given. Many of these injuries are apraxias, and function will recover. If the lesion is complete, more aggressive treatment is indicated. Conservative treatment includes protecting the foot from injury with a boot or splint, and physical therapy to maintain muscle mass and range of motion. Boots for dogs are available from several sources, usually advertised in hunting magazines. Surgical exploration of the nerve, with debridement of surrounding tissues, and neurolysis are the alternative. If the injury is severe, resection of the damaged area and anastomosis are required.

Peroneal Nerve Injury

The peroneal nerve supplies the muscles that flex the hock and extend the digits or the feet. It provides cutaneous sensory innervation to the dorsal aspect of the foot and the cranial surface of the hock and the tibia. This nerve is subject to injury where it crosses the lateral aspect of the stifle joint. In large animals, prolonged recumbency may injure the nerves at this site. In small animals and calves, injuries usually result from the intramuscular injection of drugs into or near the nerve. The foot tends to "knuckle over," and the hock may be overextended. The cranial tibial muscle and the digital extensor muscles are atrophied in small animals. Loss of sensation occurs from the dorsal areas of the foot and the cranial surface of the hock and the tibia. The flexor reflex is severely depressed when the dorsal aspects of the foot or the digits are stimulated. Pinching the plantar surface of the digits or the foot elicits a definite pain response, and the flexor reflex is present, but the animal may not actively flex the hock joint. The examiner must exercise care in evaluating the flexor reflex, because some passive flexion of the hock may occur as the stifle actively flexes. Although the foot tends to knuckle over, the dorsal surface usually does not become abraded or ulcerated as severely as it does in higher sciatic nerve lesions (see Fig. 6–2). Dogs soon learn to place the foot by greater flexion of the hip and extension of the stifle. Horses reportedly have minimal gait deficits 3 months after injury.[1]

Tibial Nerve Injury

The tibial nerve supplies the muscles that extend the hock and flex the digits. It provides cutaneous sensory innervation to the plantar surface of the foot and the caudal surface of the leg. In a pure tibial nerve injury, the hock joint is dropped when the animal walks or supports weight (Fig. 6–3). The gastrocnemius muscle is

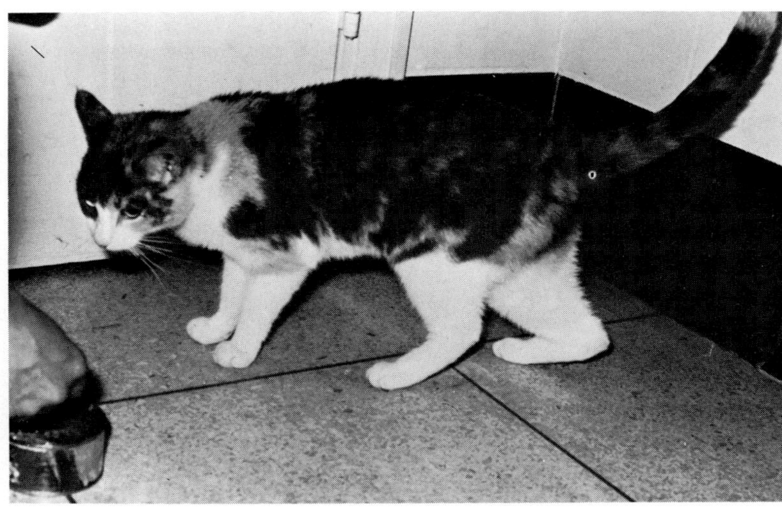

Figure 6–3 Tibial nerve paralysis in a cat, resulting from an injection injury. Note the dropped hock of the right pelvic limb, a result of paralysis of the gastrocnemius muscle.

atrophied. Loss of sensation occurs from the plantar aspect of the foot. This problem may cause the formation of large ulcers in the digital pads of small animals. Apparently, the lack of sensation allows the pads to be ground into hard surfaces during weight bearing. The flexor reflex is severely depressed when the plantar surface of the foot is stimulated. Pinching the dorsal surface of the foot elicits a definite pain response, and the flexor reflex is present even though the toes are not flexed. Isolated tibial nerve injury may follow injections into the thigh muscles. In most animals, tibial nerve lesions usually occur in association with peroneal nerve injuries, and a mixture of neurologic signs is encountered.

Femoral Nerve Injury

The femoral nerve arises from lumbar segments 4, 5, and 6 and supplies the extensor muscles of the stifle, which are the major weight-bearing muscles of the pelvic limb. The major motor component is from L5.[10] The saphenous branch of the femoral nerve is the sensory pathway from the skin on the medial surface of the foot, the leg, the stifle, and the thigh. Peripheral injuries to this nerve are not common, because it is well protected. Rarely, unilateral damage restricted to the ventral gray matter of lumbar segments 4, 5, and 6 results in a neuronopathy involving the femoral nerve. Bilateral femoral nerve injury has been seen in dogs following extreme extension of the hips. With femoral nerve lesions, the stifle cannot be fixed (extended) for weight bearing. The leg usually is carried, and the dog hops on the opposite limb. Lesions involving the peripheral femoral nerve produce analgesia in areas innervated by the saphenous nerve. Selective lesions involving the gray matter of the spinal cord produce motor dysfunction only. Sensation through the saphenous nerve is preserved. The knee jerk (patellar) reflex is absent or diminished; however, the flexor reflex is normal, except for decreased flexion of the hip. The hopping reaction is greatly decreased in the affected leg, because weight bearing is inhibited.

In large animals, femoral nerve paralysis results in a severe monoparesis. The affected limb is poorly advanced and collapses during weight bearing. In calves and foals, femoral nerve paralysis results from trauma during parturition. Forced extraction from the "hip-lock" position may hyperextend the hip and overstretch the nerve where it enters the quadriceps muscle. Apparently, there is an increased incidence in the heavy-muscled breeds of cattle.

Obturator Nerve Injury

Injuries to the obturator nerve in the dog or the cat do not result in monoparesis, although the affected leg may slide laterally when the animal stands on a smooth surface. Injuries to this nerve are not clinically important in small animals.

Obturator paralysis is a common injury during partiturition in cows. The obturator nerve innervates the adductor muscles of the limb, and injuries to this nerve produce marked pelvic limb ataxia, especially on slippery surfaces. The limbs may be placed in a wide-based stance, and this posture is exaggerated as the animal runs. Unilateral paralysis produces less of a gait abnormality, since the signs are associated with only one limb. Most calving injuries damage the branches to the sciatic nerve as well as the obturator nerve.[3]

Spinal Cord Diseases

Unilateral spinal cord lesions involving segments L4–S2 result in monoparesis. Because these lesions may damage the motor neurons that form the nerves of the lumbosacral plexus, LMN dysfunction occurs. Infarctions are the most common cause of unilateral lesions. Occasionally, spinal cord trauma or neoplasia has a unilateral distribution and will produce monoparesis. Rarely, inflammatory disease of the spinal cord is restricted to one side, and monoparesis may be the presenting complaint. Some degree of sensory loss usually accompanies the motor dysfunction. In rare cases in which the spinal cord lesions are restricted to ventral gray matter, sensation will be normal. In most cases, several spinal cord segments are involved, and dysfunction of several nerves (polyneuropathy) occurs.

Unilateral spinal cord lesions involving segments T2–L3 also result in monoparesis, but it is of the UMN type. The usual cause is infarction, but occasionally trauma, inflammation, or neoplasia may produce unilateral or pronounced asymmetric signs. Pertinent disorders that produce unilateral spinal cord lesions will be discussed in the chapters on pelvic limb paresis (Chap. 7) and tetraparesis (Chap. 8).

Monoparesis of the Thoracic Limbs

Peripheral Nerve Injuries

The nerves that innervate the muscles of the thoracic limbs and the clinical signs associated with injuries of these nerves are presented in

Table 6–1. Triceps paralysis (radial nerve) causes a dropped elbow and a loss of weight bearing. Biceps and brachialis muscle paralysis (musculocutaneous nerve) prevents flexing the elbow. Carpal extension (radial nerve) is essential for placing the foot in a normal position. Paralysis of carpal flexors is more subtle, causing overextension of the carpus during weight bearing. Reflexes help identify which muscle groups are functional. The flexor reflex is useful to assess muscle strength, identifying partial lesions. The sensory evaluation is essential to map the area of decreased sensation (see Chap. 1). In this section, injuries to the brachial plexus, the radial nerve, and the suprascapular nerve are discussed, because they are of greatest clinical importance.

Avulsion of the Brachial Plexus

The nerves of the brachial plexus have their origin from spinal cord segments C6–T2 (see Table 6–1). In addition, the sympathetic nerves that innervate the eye originate from neurons in the first three thoracic segments and travel along the roots of the brachial plexus as they exit from the vertebral column. Injuries to the brachial plexus result in monoparesis of the affected limb and, in some cases, an ipsilateral partial Horner's syndrome. Avulsion of the brachial plexus is a common traumatic injury in the dog and results from severe abduction of the limb. The nerve roots of the brachial plexus are torn or stretched from their spinal cord attachments.[11–15] The avulsion of the roots may damage the spinal cord, causing some UMN paresis of the ipsilateral pelvic limb. Rarely, the plexus is damaged by a direct blow to the shoulder, causing contusion or hemorrhage. This lesion is usually not complete.

The avulsion may be of the cranial or caudal portions of the plexus, or of the total plexus. The sensory and motor examination can differentiate these syndromes.[12,13] The major signs of motor dysfunction are related to damage to the roots of the radial nerve and, to a lesser extent, to the other nerves of the plexus. The proximal radial nerve innervates the triceps muscle, which is the major weight-bearing muscle in the thoracic limb. The distal branches of the radial nerve innervate the extensors of the carpus and the digits. An injured animal bears little or no weight on the limb, and the paw is knuckled over and usually drags on the ground (Fig. 6–4). The dorsal aspect of the paw may become severely abraded and ulcerated. The hopping and proprioceptive positioning reactions are decreased or absent. The flexor, extensor carpi radialis, and triceps reflexes are weak or absent. Injury of the musculocutaneous, ulnar, and median nerves causes a loss of the flexor reflex. Muscle atrophy of the thoracic limb may begin in about 1 week and become severe, depending on the number of nerve roots injured. Because sympathetic nerve roots may be injured, an ipsilateral partial or complete Horner's syndrome is present in over 50% of cases. Mapping the area of sensory loss is the best test for estimating the extent of damage to the plexus. Cranial avulsions will cause loss of sensation to the cranial surface of the limb distal to the elbow (radial nerve), but the caudal surface will have intact sensation. The autonomous zone (AZ) of the brachiocephalicus and axillary nerves on the cranial and lateral surface of the brachium will be affected. Caudal avulsions will cause

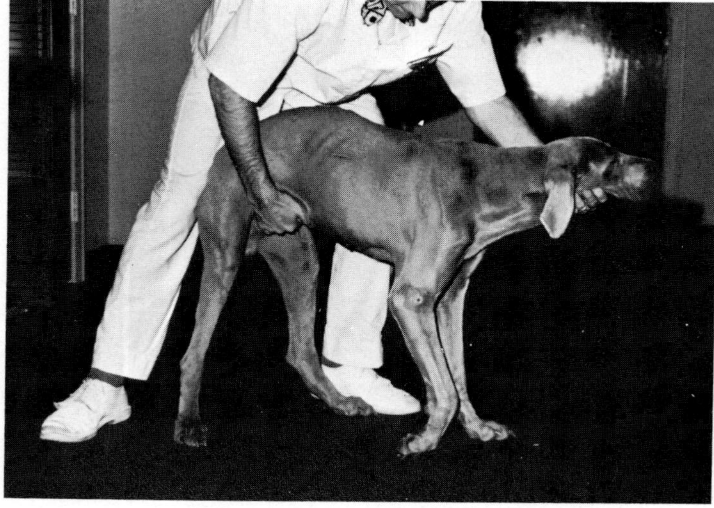

Figure 6–4 Brachial plexus injury in a dog, a result of a car accident. Note the knuckled paw, and the inability to support weight on the limb. Atrophy is present in the scapular and triceps muscles.

loss of sensation on the caudal surface of the limb below the elbow, and a variable loss on the cranial surface. The brachiocephalicus and axillary AZ will be normal. Total avulsion will cause loss of sensation of the entire limb below the elbow, as well as the AZ of the brachiocephalicus and axillary nerves (Fig. 6–5).

The prognosis for use of the affected limb is poor if a proximal radial nerve injury is present. The more proximal branches of the radial nerve innervate the triceps muscle, which must be functional for weight bearing. Corrective orthopedic procedures such as carpal arthrodesis or tendon transplantation are not indicated when the nerves to the triceps muscle are injured. These procedures may be helpful in selected cases in which the injury has spared the proximal branches of the radial and the musculocutaneous nerve. An EMG is useful for evaluating these muscles for evidence of denervation when corrective surgery is contemplated.

Occasionally, bilateral brachial plexus injuries are encountered. These injuries have been observed in animals that have fallen from great heights and have landed in a sternal position, severely abducting both thoracic limbs. In addition to the signs of bilateral plexus injury, the diaphragm may be paralyzed if the roots of the phrenic nerve are damaged. The phrenic nerve arises from cervical segments 5, 6, and 7 but is not considered part of the brachial plexus. Rarely, the injury may involve these nerve roots; however, dyspnea resulting from diaphragmatic paralysis is uncommon.

Suprascapular Nerve Injury

Suprascapular paralysis occurs most frequently in large animals secondary to trauma or fracture of the scapula. The nerve innervates the supraspinatus and infraspinatus muscles. These muscles may atrophy severely, resulting in sweeney. Weight bearing is usually unaffected; however, the stride may be shortened and the shoulder may luxate laterally when weight is borne on the leg. Cattle may be injured in malfunctioning chutes or from striking the head gate with the shoulders. Work horses may be injured from poorly fitting collars. EMG is useful to be certain that other nerves are not affected. Surgical decompression of the nerve as it passes around the cranial surface of the scapula is recommended if there is no improvement. Recommendations vary on early versus delayed surgery.[1] The results are probably best with exploration after about 1 month. However, waiting for 3 months to be sure that spontaneous recovery is not occurring is an alternative.

Contracture of the infraspinatus muscle occurs in dogs and results in a thoracic leg lameness. The elbow and the foreleg are abducted as the dog runs. The forward stride of the limb may be slightly shortened. Characteristically, the foot is moved laterally as the limb is advanced. The cause is presumed to be trauma to the muscle and possibly to the vasculature or the suprascapular nerve supplying the muscle.[16] Cutting the insertion of the infraspinatus muscle is beneficial.

Radial Nerve Injury

The entire radial nerve may be injured by fractures of the first rib or in avulsion of the brachial plexus. Fractures of the humerus may injure the nerve distal to the branches that supply the triceps muscle. In large animals, radial nerve injuries occur most commonly during anesthetic procedures or when the animal is in lateral recumbency on a hard surface for extended periods. Distal radial injuries produce less severe gait abnormalities than do brachial

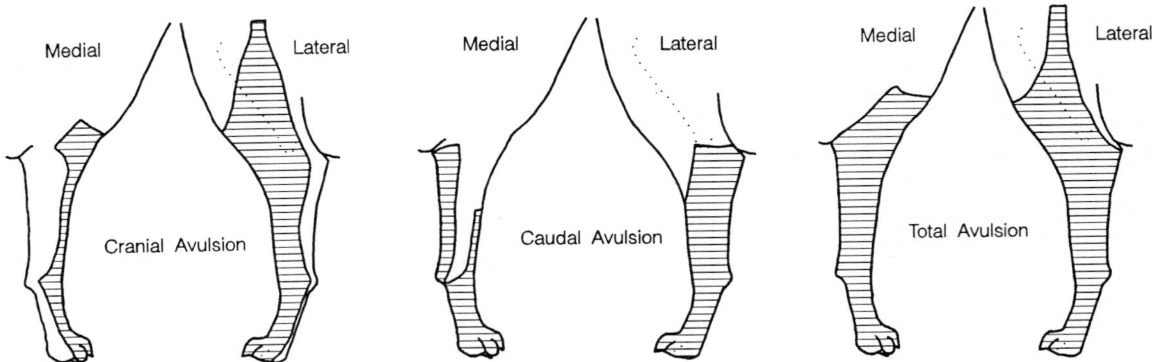

Figure 6–5 Maps of sensory loss in cranial, caudal, and total brachial plexus avulsions. (Data from Bailey CS: Patterns of cutaneous anesthesia associated with brachial plexus avulsions in the dog. J Am Vet Med Assoc 185:889, 1984.)

plexus injuries. The elbow can be extended; however, the foot tends to knuckle over when the animal walks, because the extensors of the carpus and the digits are paralyzed. Sensation is lost from the dorsal and cranial aspects of the limb below the elbow. Surgical exploration of the injured nerve with neurolysis or anastomosis is indicated, especially in distal radial nerve injuries. Carpal arthrodesis or transposition of a flexor tendon may be helpful. The loss of sensation frequently leads to self-mutilation, however.

Spinal Cord Diseases

Unilateral spinal cord lesions restricted to the gray matter (C6–T2) may destroy the motor neurons of the brachial plexus, resulting in LMN monoparesis. Unlike peripheral nerve injuries, which involve both motor and sensory nerve fibers, lesions in this area result in paresis or paralysis, but sensation to the leg may be preserved, depending on the degree of involvement of the dorsal horn sensory relay neurons. Vascular occlusions that infarct this area of the spinal cord and, rarely, neoplasia or inflammatory diseases produce this problem. Spinal cord lesions at this level usually involve the motor and proprioceptive pathways to the ipsilateral pelvic limb. Unilateral spinal cord lesions (C6–T2), therefore, usually result in hemiparesis with UMN signs in the ipsilateral rear limb and LMN signs in the thoracic limb. Avulsion of the brachial plexus may be associated with paresis or paralysis of the ipsilateral pelvic limb if the spinal cord is compressed, contused, or otherwise damaged at the time of trauma. Spinal cord diseases will be discussed in the chapters on pelvic limb paresis and tetraparesis.

Prognosis

The prognosis of peripheral nerve injuries depends on the type of damage and the severity of neurologic dysfunction. Nerve fibers that have been contused, compressed, or stretched may regain function slowly. Nerves that have been lacerated or avulsed from their spinal cord attachments, however, seldom regain function. Unfortunately, in routine practice it is sometimes difficult to establish which of these situations has occurred at the time of the initial examination. In order for nerve fibers to regenerate, the nerve sheath must remain intact. Compressive lesions may cause demyelination without disrupting the axon. The recovery begins in about 3 to 4 weeks and continues for 1 to 2 months. Axonal regeneration occurs slowly, at a rate of approximately 1 inch a month; however, an intact sheath must be present in order to guide the axon to the denervated muscle. Motor function in affected muscles may be regained by the sprouting and innervation of these muscle fibers by adjacent intact neurons. Regardless of the repair process involved, return to function may take several months and may never be complete. As a general rule, reinnervation must occur in 12 months or less to be effective. Therefore, regeneration for distances greater than 12 inches is unlikely.

In general, the prognosis for functional recovery for animals with severe motor dysfunction and complete analgesia is poor. These lesions are usually severe and may involve complete disruption of nerve fibers. Some animals regain function; however, the outcome is often unsatisfactory. The prognosis is better for animals with partial loss of motor or sensory function, because the damage to the axons may be transitory, and reinnervation from adjacent, intact nerve fibers is more predictable. In addition, animals with partial dysfunction may learn to compensate for their problem by using other, uninvolved muscle groups. In most cases, the distribution and the severity of sensory loss are considered when a prognosis is established.

If available, an EMG examination, including nerve conduction and evoked potentials, is useful for formulating a prognosis and assessing the recovery of peripheral nerve injuries. This technique helps the clinician establish the severity and the distribution of the nerve injury. A total lack of voluntary motor potentials, an absence of responses to nerve stimulation, and evidence of diffuse denervation are highly correlated with a poor prognosis. The presence of some motor unit activity and patchy denervation suggests that the lesion is not complete and that a better chance for nerve regeneration exists. EMG examinations can be repeated periodically over several months to determine if reinnervation is occurring. If tendon transplant surgery is contemplated, an EMG examination of the involved muscles is performed. The muscles should be free of fibrillation potentials and positive sharp waves.

Treatment

The initial therapy for a nerve injury consists of corticosteroid administration to relieve inflammation and immobilization of the limb to prevent further trauma. Nerve decompression or anastomosis is indicated if the site of injury is accessible for surgical manipulation. Long-term management consists of physical therapy to help prevent muscle atrophy and trauma to the foot. Tendon transplantation and joint arthrodesis are performed primarily for distal radial nerve and peroneal injuries in small animals. Probably the most important aspect of long-term management is prevention of trauma to the distal extremity. There are commercially available boots that help protect the foot, are easily applied by the owner, and are well tolerated by the dog. Owners frequently request amputation of the affected limb because of distal extremity trauma. Prevention of this problem spares the limb for a period that is sufficient for the veterinarian to see if nerve regeneration will occur. Generally, amputation of the limb should be delayed for 6 months, unless traumatic complications cannot be prevented. The owner should be warned that recovery is slow and that amputation is an irreversible solution to the problem. A "wait-and-see" approach should be recommended.

Many peripheral nerve injuries can be avoided by proper management of large animals placed in lateral recumbency. Adequate padding must be provided at all times, and recumbent animals should be turned frequently (at least three times a day). Excessive traction on limbs should be avoided during anesthesia, animal movement, or fetal extraction. Injured limbs should be protected by bandages, splints, or casts. Cattle with obturator paralysis must be kept on good footing. Hobbles on the pelvic limbs may be helpful. Recumbent animals should be supported with slings whenever possible.

Peripheral Nerve Tumors

Nerve sheath tumors arise from Schwann cells or connective tissue surrounding the nerves. The definitive terminology for these tumors in animals is still debated, so the term nerve sheath tumor will be used.[17] Nerve sheath tumors are relatively rare in all species and can occur on any peripheral nerve. They are probably most common in cattle, but do not usually cause clinical signs.[18] Most clinical cases in dogs involve the nerves of the brachial plexus. The tumor may start distally or in the nerve root. Spread of the tumor proximally may result in compression of the spinal cord. Typically, an affected animal starts with a lameness of obscure origin. With time, there is significant atrophy of selected muscle groups, and eventually the spinal cord compression causes paresis of other limbs.

The diagnosis is difficult to establish in the early stages. If the spinal cord is involved, there may be enlargement of the intervertebral foramen, and spinal cord compression demonstrated with myelography (see Fig. 7–12). The mass is frequently intradural-extramedullary in appearance on the myelogram (see Chap. 4). Brachial plexus tumors in small animals may be extremely painful on deep palpation in the axilla, and occasionally the mass can be palpated.

Treatment entails complete removal of the tumor. Unfortunately, this is difficult because of the extent of the tumor. Amputation of the limb, laminectomy, and resection of the nerve roots is often necessary. Even with radical resection, recurrence is common.[19]

CASE HISTORIES

Case History 6A

Signalment

Canine, weimaraner, male, 6 years old.

History

The dog was hit by a car 20 days ago. Since that day, he has been unable to use the right thoracic limb. He has been dragging the foot and is unable to advance the leg or bear weight. Open sores have developed on the dorsum of the foot.

Physical Examination

No abnormalities were uncovered other than the neurologic problems described in the next section.

*Neurologic Examination**

A. Observation
   1. Mental status: Alert.
   2. Posture: Normal; see Gait.
   3. Gait: Severe paresis of the right thoracic limb. Drags the leg and the foot. The paw knuckles over, and the dog can bear little weight on the limb.

B. Palpation: Atrophy of the triceps, supraspinatus, infraspinatus, biceps, and flexor carpi radialis muscles of the right thoracic limb.

C. Postural Reactions

Left	Reactions	Right
	Proprioceptive positioning	
+2	PL	+2
+2	TL	0
+2	Wheelbarrowing	0

* *Key*: 0 = absent, + 1 = decreased, +2 = normal, +3 = exaggerated, +4 = very exaggerated or clonus, PL = pelvic limb, TL = thoracic limb.

Left	Reactions	Right
+2	Hopping, PL	+2
+2	Hopping, TL	0
+2	Extensor postural thrust	+2
+2	Hemistand-hemiwalk	0
+2	Placing, tactile PL	+2
+2	TL	0
+2	Placing, visual TL	0

D. Spinal Reflexes

Left	Reflex Spinal Segment	Right
+2	Quadriceps L4–L6	+2
+2	Extensor carpi radialis C7–T1	0
+2	Triceps C7–T1	0
+2	Flexion, PL L5–S1	+2
+2	Flexion, TL C6–T1	0
0	Crossed extensor	0
+2	Perineal S1–S2	+2

E. Cranial Nerves

Left	Nerve + Function	Right
+2	CN II vision menace	+2
Nor.	CN II + III pupil size	Constricted
+2	Stim. left eye	+2
+2	Stim. right eye	+2
Nor.	CN II fundus	Nor.
	CN III, IV, VI	
0	Strabismus	0
0	Nystagmus	0
+2	CN V sensation	+2
Nor.	CN V mastication	Nor.
Nor.	CN VII facial muscles	Nor.
+2	Palpebral	+2
Nor.	CN IX, X swallowing	Nor.
Nor.	CN XII tongue	Nor.

F. Sensation: Location.
Hyperesthesia: None.
Superficial pain: 0 right TL.
Deep pain: 0 to +1 right TL.

Complete sections G and H before reviewing Case Summary.

G. Assessment (Anatomic diagnosis and estimation of prognosis)

H. Plan (Diagnostic)

Rule-outs *Procedure*

1.
2.
3.
4.

Case History 6B

Signalment

Canine, boxer, male, 1 year old.

History

The dog was hit by a car 10 months ago and was treated for shock and multiple pelvic fractures. He was referred 2 days after the initial injury because of severe dyspnea. Massive pleural effusion was treated with chest drains. The examination disclosed moderate paresis in the right pelvic limb and hypalgesia below the stifle. No treatment was given, and the dog was discharged 4 days later. He returned 10 months after the initial injury for follow-up examination, at which time no improvement in the right pelvic limb was noted.

Physical Examination

Negative except for the neurologic problems.

*Neurologic Examination**

A. Observation
1. Mental status: Alert.
2. Posture: Normal.
3. Gait: Moderate paresis of the right pelvic limb, with hyperflexion of the stifle. The paw knuckles over and the hock sinks during weight bearing. All other limbs are normal.

B. Palpation: Atrophy of the cranial tibial muscle and flexors and extensors of the hock and digits. Deep ulcers in the plantar surfaces of the middle two digital pads. These toes are swollen.

C. Postural Reactions

Left	Reactions	Right
+2	Proprioceptive positioning PL	0
+2	TL	+2
+2	Wheelbarrowing	+2
+2	Hopping, PL	0

*Key: 0 = absent, + 1 = decreased, +2 = normal, +3 = exaggerated, +4 = very exaggerated or clonus, PL = pelvic limb, TL = thoracic limb.

+2	Hopping, TL	+2
+2	Extensor postural thrust	0
+2	Hemistand-hemiwalk	0
+2	Placing, tactile PL	0 to +1
+2	TL	+2
+2	Placing, visual TL	+2

D. Spinal Reflexes

Left	Reflex	Right
	Spinal Segment	
+2	Quadriceps L4–L6	+2
+2	Extensor carpi radialis C7–T1	+2
+2	Triceps C7–T1	+2
+2	Flexion, PL L5–S1	Flexes hip and stifle—0 below stifle
+2	Flexion, TL C6–T1	+2
0	Crossed extensor	0
+2	Perineal S1–S2	+2

E. Cranial Nerves

Left	Nerve + Function	Right
+2	CN II vision menace	+2
Nor.	CN II + III pupil size	Nor.
+2	Stim. left eye	+2
+2	Stim. right eye	+2
Nor.	CN II fundus	Nor.
	CN III, CN IV, CN VI	
0	Strabismus	0
0	Nystagmus	0
Nor.	CN V sensation	Nor.
Nor.	CN V mastication	Nor.
Nor.	CN VII facial muscles	Nor.
+2	Palpebral	+2
Nor.	CN IX, X swallowing	Nor.
Nor.	CN XII tongue	Nor.

F. Sensation: Location.
 Hyperesthesia: None.
 Superficial pain: Blunted below stifle in right PL.
 Deep pain: 0 from middle two digits in right PL.

Complete sessions G and H before reviewing Case Summary.

G. Assessment (Anatomic diagnosis and estimation of prognosis)

H. Plan (Diagnostic)

Rule-outs	*Procedure*
1.	
2.	
3.	
4.	

Case History 6C

Signalment

Feline, domestic, female, 7 years old.

History

Mild lameness was noted in the right thoracic limb 6 to 8 weeks ago. The condition has slowly worsened, and the cat now cannot bear weight on the leg. She holds the leg extended with the paw flexed and is knuckling occasionally on the right pelvic limb.

Physical Examination

Negative except for the neurologic problems.

*Neurologic Examination**

A. Observation
 1. Mental status: Alert.
 2. Posture: Normal.
 3. Gait: Severe paresis of the right thoracic limb. The cat occasionally drags and knuckles the right pelvic paw.

B. Palpation: Mild atrophy in right scapular muscles.

C. Postural Reactions

Left	Reactions	Right
+2	Proprioceptive positioning PL	+1
+2	TL	0
+2	Wheelbarrowing	0
+2	Hopping, PL	+1
+2	Hopping, TL	0
+2	Extensor postural thrust	+1
+2	Hemistand-hemiwalk	0
+2	Placing, tactile PL	+1

**Key*: 0 = absent, + 1 = decreased, +2 = normal, +3 = exaggerated, +4 = very exaggerated or clonus, PL = pelvic limb, TL = thoracic limb.

+2	TL	0
+2	Placing, visual TL	0

D. Spinal Reflexes

Left	Reflex	Right
+2	Spinal Segment Quadriceps L4–L6	+3
2	Extensor carpi radialis C7–T1	0 to +1
+2	Triceps C7–T1	0 to +1
+2	Flexion, PL L5–S1	+2
+2	Flexion, TL C6–T1	0
0	Crossed extensor	0
S1–S2	Perineal +2	+2

E. Cranial Nerves

Left	Nerve + Function	Right
+2	CNII vision menace	+2
Nor.	CN II + III pupil size	Constricted
+2	Stim. left eye	+2
+2	Stim. right eye	+2
Nor.	CN II fundus	Nor.
 0 0	CN III, IV, VI Strabismus Nystagmus	 0 0
Nor.	CN V sensation	Nor.
Nor.	CN V mastication	Nor.
Nor. +2	CN VII facial muscles Palpebral	Nor. +2
Nor.	CN IX, X swallowing	Nor.
Nor.	CN XII tongue	Nor.

F. Sensation: Location.
Hyperesthesia: None.
Superficial pain: Normal.
Deep pain: Normal.

Complete sections G and H before reviewing Case Summary.

G. Assessment (Anatomic diagnosis and estimation of prognosis)

H. Plan (Diagnostic)

Rule-outs	*Procedure*
1.	
2.	
3.	
4.	

Assessment 6A

Anatomic diagnosis. The dog has a monoparesis affecting the right thoracic limb and a partial Horner's sign of the right eye. LMN signs with sensory deficits in several nerves suggest a lesion of the right brachial plexus. A C6–T2 spinal cord lesion is discounted because the right pelvic limb is normal.

1. A brachial plexus injury.
2. An injury to the roots of the right sympathetic nerve that causes Horner's sign.

Diagnostic plan (rule-outs).

1. Caudal cervical trauma – Radiography (negative).
2. Brachial plexus injury – EMG (fibrillation potentials and positive sharp waves in several muscle groups).

Therapeutic plan.

1. Protect the foot with a boot.
2. Perform physical therapy.

Client education. The prognosis is very poor for functional use of the leg, because the nerve roots have been severely injured. Amputation may be needed in the future.

Case summary.

1. Diagnosis: Brachial plexus injury.
2. Result: The dog regained partial use of the leg in 6 months; however, he must wear a boot continually to protect the foot. Persistent mild pupil constriction is present in the right eye.

Assessment 6B

Anatomic diagnosis. The dog has monoparesis of the right pelvic limb. LMN signs with sensory deficits below the stifle localize the lesion to the distal sciatic nerve. A distal sciatic nerve (peroneal and tibial nerves) injury was diagnosed.

Diagnostic plan (rule-outs):

1. Pelvic fracture – Pelvic radiography (multiple pelvic fractures that are now healed but are displaced).
2. Injection injury – EMG (diffuse denervation below the stifle; few fibrillation potentials and positive sharp waves in the gastrocnemius, the semitendinosus, and the semimembranosus muscles; evidence of reinnervation in some muscles).

Therapeutic plan.

1. Physical therapy should be performed.
2. The middle two digits are infected and require antibiotic therapy.
3. A boot should be fitted on the dog to prevent further trauma.

Client education. Because the sciatic nerve injury is partial and evidence of reinnervation is present, the dog may regain functional use of the limb.

Case summary. One must debate the cause of

the nerve injury, i.e., a pelvic fracture versus a needle (injection) injury. The neurologic examination is more consistent with the diagnosis of a needle (injection) injury, because nerve damage usually occurs at the origin of the peroneal and the tibial nerves in the area caudal to the femur. The EMG, however, provides evidence that the lesion is more central. Denervation of the semitendinosus and semimembranosus muscles probably is a result of the pelvic fractures, as these muscles are rarely affected by injections in the thigh muscles.

Final diagnosis. Sciatic nerve injury from a pelvic fracture.

Result. The dog regained good use of the leg, and the boot eventually was removed.

Assessment 6C

Anatomic diagnosis. LMN signs are present in the right thoracic limb, and UMN signs are present in the right rear leg. In addition, there is a mild Horner's sign in the right eye. A unilateral right C6–T3 spinal cord lesion would explain these signs. The history suggests that the lesion may have begun in the brachial plexus and moved centrally.

Diagnostic plan (rule-outs).

1. Neoplasia—Radiology (survey films negative), myelography (intradural-extramedullary mass at the right side of the cord at C7–T1 intervertebral space).
2. Inflammation—CSF tap (0 cells, 20 mg/dl protein).

Therapeutic plan. Administer dexamethasone to help relieve spinal cord edema. Surgical removal may be possible but probably will cause denervation of the limb, requiring amputation.

Case summary. A neurofibroma of the right brachial plexus is present with cord compression of C6, C7, C8, and T1. The history is typical for a nerve sheath tumor of the brachial plexus.

REFERENCES

1. Mayhew IG: Large Animal Neurology: A Handbook for Veterinary Clinicians. Philadelphia, Lea & Febiger, 1989.
2. Chambers J, Hardie E: Localization and management of sciatic nerve injury due to ischial or acetabular fracture. J Am Anim Hosp Assoc 22:539–544, 1986.
3. Cox V, Breazile J, Hoover T: Surgical and anatomic study of calving paralysis. Am J Vet Res 36:427–430, 1975.
4. Walker T: Ischiadic nerve entrapment. J Am Vet Med Assoc 178:1284–1288, 1981.
5. Palmer RH, Aron DN, Purinton PT: Relationship of femoral intramedullary pins to the sciatic nerve and gluteal muscles after retrograde and normograde insertion. Vet Surg 17:65–70, 1988.
6. Fanton J, Blass C, Withrow S: Sciatic nerve injury as a complication of intramedullary pin fixation of femoral fractures. J Am Anim Hosp Assoc 19:687–694, 1983.
7. Stanton ME, Weigel JP, Henry RE: Ischiatic nerve paralysis associated with the biceps femoris sling: Case report and anatomical study. J Am Anim Hosp Assoc 24:429–432, 1988.
8. Sorjonen DC, Milton JL, Steiss JE, et al: Hip dysplasia with bilateral ischiatic nerve entrapment in a dog. J Am Vet Med Assoc 197:495–497, 1990.
9. Autefage A, Fayolle P, Toutain P–L: Distribution of material injected intramuscularly in dogs. Am J Vet Res 51:901–904, 1990.
10. Wilson J: Relationship of the patellar tendon reflex to the ventral branch of the fifth lumbar spinal nerve in the dog. Am J Vet Res 39:1774–1777, 1978.
11. Griffiths I: Avulsion of the brachial plexus: 1. Neuropathology of the spinal cord and peripheral nerves. J Small Anim Pract 15:165–176, 1974.
12. Griffiths I, Duncan I, Lawson D: Avulsion of the brachial plexus: 2. Clinical aspects. J Small Anim Pract 15:177–182, 1974.
13. Bailey C: Patterns of cutaneous anesthesia associated with brachial plexus avulsions in the dog. J Am Vet Med Assoc 185:889–899, 1984.
14. Steinberg HS: Brachial plexus injuries and dysfunctions. Vet Clin North Am 18:565–580, 1988.
15. Wheeler S, Jones C, Wright J: The diagnosis of brachial plexus disorders in dogs: A review of twenty-two cases. J Small Anim Pract 27:147–157, 1986.
16. Bennett R: Contracture of the infraspinatus muscle in dogs: A review of 12 cases. J Am Anim Hosp Assoc 22:481–487, 1986.
17. Braund KG: Neoplasia. In Oliver JE, Hoerlein BF, and Mayhew IG (eds): Veterinary Neurology. Philadelphia, WB Saunders, 1987, pp 278–284.
18. de Lahunta A: Veterinary Neuroanatomy and Clinical Neurology, 2nd ed. Philadelphia, WB Saunders, 1983.
19. Bradley RL, Withrow SJ, Snyder SP: Nerve sheath tumors in the dog. J Am Anim Hosp Assoc 18:915–921, 1982.

7

Pelvic Limb Paresis, Paralysis, or Ataxia

Bilateral motor dysfunction of the pelvic limbs is termed *paraparesis* or *paraplegia*, depending on the severity of the motor loss. Loss of proprioception from the pelvic limbs results in sensory ataxia. In addition, loss of pain perception from the pelvic limbs may accompany the motor dysfunction. Lesion localization has been discussed in Chapter 2 and is summarized in Figure 7–1. A brief review follows.

Lesion Localization

Animals with pure pelvic limb paresis and ataxia have neurologic disease caudal to the second thoracic spinal cord segment. Lesions in the region of T3–L3 produce paraparesis of the upper motor neuron (UMN) type. The pelvic limb lower motor neurons (LMNs), located in the segments L4–S2, remain intact and are capable of reflex motor activity; however, voluntary motor control from the brain is lost, because the motor pathways in the spinal cord are damaged. The spinal reflexes are normal or exaggerated. Exaggerated reflexes result when UMN inhibitory influence on the LMNs is lost. Similarly, extensor hypertonus also may develop. Ataxia results from damage to the spinal cord proprioceptive pathways, which transmit position sense signals from receptors in the pelvic limbs to the brain. Hypalgesia or analgesia distal to the lesion results from disruption of pain pathways from the pelvic limbs to the brain. Deep pain sensation is lost only if the lesions are bilateral and severe. Voluntary visceral functions (see Chap. 3), such as micturition, may be lost when motor or sensory pathways in the spinal cord are damaged. Muscle atrophy due to disuse may develop with time.

In summary, spinal cord lesions in the region of T3–L3 result in paresis, ataxia, decreased or absent postural reactions, normal reflexes or hyperreflexia, impaired micturition, and variable degrees of sensory loss caudal to the lesion. Examination of the thoracolumbar dermatomes may be helpful in the localization of lesions to spinal segments within this spinal cord region (see Chap. 2).

Lesions in the area of L4–S2 or those that involve the cauda equina produce pelvic limb paresis of the LMN type. Lesions involving spinal cord segments L4–S2 injure the motor neurons that form the lumbosacral plexus. Abnormalities related to femoral, sciatic, pudendal, and pelvic nerves are encountered in these patients. Pelvic limb reflexes are depressed or absent, and the muscles may be hypotonic. Neurogenic muscle atrophy will develop. Sensory dysfunction (ataxia, hypalgesia, analgesia) results from an injury to the sensory neurons and the nerve fibers located in this region of the spinal cord. Abnormalities of visceral function result from an injury to the motor and sensory neurons that innervate the bladder and the anus. Lesions involving the caudal segments of the spinal cord and the cauda equina damage nerve fibers that form the sciatic, pudendal, pelvic, and caudal nerves. Because the femoral nerve is spared, the animal is able to support weight on the pelvic limbs. The knee jerk reflex

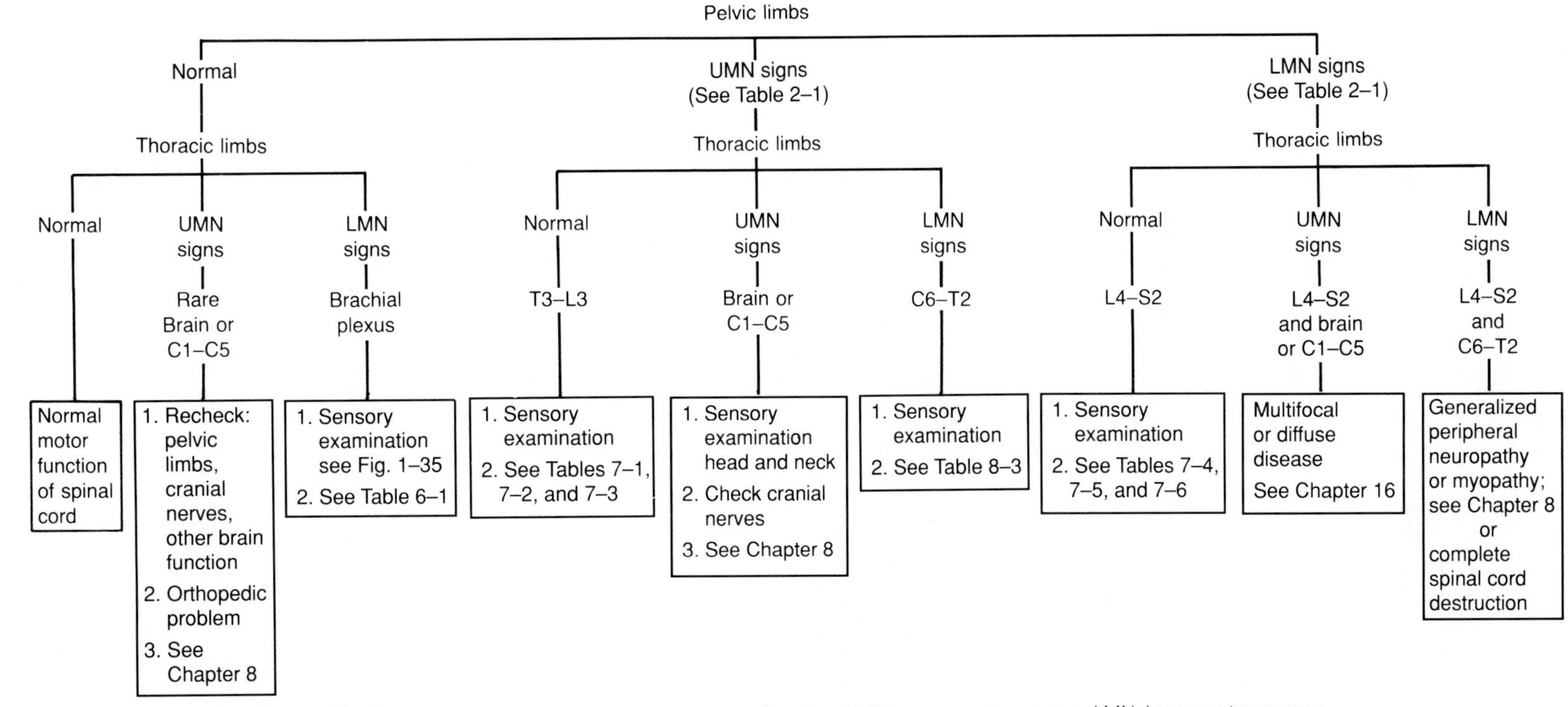

Figure 7–1 Localization of lesions based on motor function. *UMN*, upper motor neuron; *LMN*, lower motor neuron; *C*, cervical; *T*, thoracic; *L*, lumbar; *S*, sacral. (From Hoerlein BF: Canine Neurology: Diagnosis and Treatment, 3rd ed. Philadelphia, WB Saunders, 1978. Used by permission.)

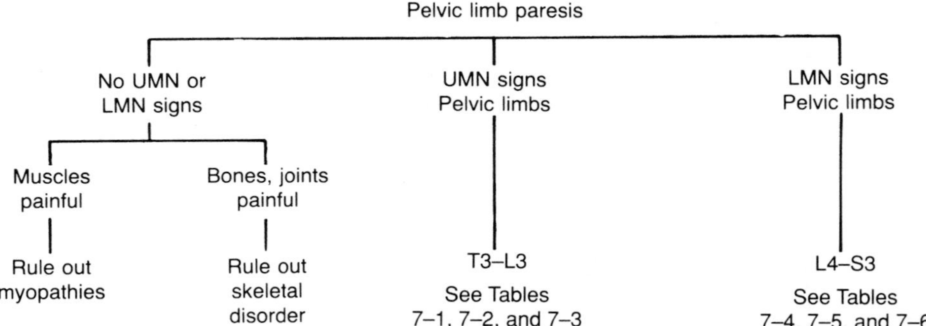

Figure 7–2 Algorithm for the localization of lesions causing pelvic limb paresis.

is normal, and pain is perceived from the medial digit and the thigh. The clinical signs relate to motor and sensory dysfunction of the involved nerves. Figure 7–2 summarizes lesion localization for the problem of pelvic limb paresis based on motor signs.

Diseases

The disorders or diseases that affect the spinal cord segments T3–L3 are classified in Tables 7–1, 7–2, and 7–3. Disorders that affect spinal cord segments L4–S2 and the cauda equina are

TABLE 7–1 Small Animal Thoracolumbar Spinal Cord Diseases: Differential Diagnosis of T3–L3 Spinal Cord Disease Based on Clinical Course and Etiologic Categories*

Etiologic Category	*Acute Nonprogressive*	*Acute Progressive*	*Chronic Progressive*
Degenerative	None	Type I disk disease (7) Hemorrhagic myelomalacia (7)	Type II disk disease (7) Degenerative myelopathy (7) Spondylosis deformans (7) Afghan hound myelopathy (7) Demyelinating diseases (8) Neuronopathies (8)
Anomalous	None	None	Spinal dysraphism (7) Vertebral anomalies (7)
Metabolic	None	None	Endocrine neuropathies (8)
Neoplastic (7)	None	Metastatic Primary Skeletal Lymphoreticular	Primary Lymphoreticular Skeletal Metastatic
Nutritional	None	None	Hypervitaminosis A (cats) (16)
Inflammatory	None	Distemper myelitis (16) Bacterial myelitis (15) Diskospondylitis (7) Protozoal myelitis (16) Mycotic myelitis (16)	Feline infectious peritonitis (16) Distemper myelitis (16) Granulomatous meningoencephalomyelitis (16) Immune meningoencephalomyelitis (16)
Toxic	None	None	Various neuropathies (8, 16)
Traumatic	Fractures (7) Luxations (7) Contusions (7) Intervertebral disk rupture (7)	Hemorrhagic myelomalacia (7) Intervertebral disk rupture (7)	None
Vascular	Fibrocartilaginous embolism (7) Aortic thromboembolism (7)	None	None

* Numbers in parentheses refer to chapters in which the entities are discussed.

TABLE 7–2 Equine Thoracolumbar Spinal Cord Diseases: Differential Diagnosis of T3–L3 Spinal Cord Disease Based on Clinical Course and Etiologic Categories*

Etiologic Category	*Acute Nonprogressive*	*Acute Progressive*	*Chronic Progressive*
Degenerative	None	Degenerative myeloencephalopathy (8)	Spondylosis deformans (7) Neuronopathies (8) Demyelinating diseases (8) Axonopathies (8)
Anomalous	None	None	Vertebral anomalies (7) Spinal dysraphism (7)
Neoplastic (7)	None	Metastatic Primary Skeletal Lymphoreticular	Primary Skeletal Lymphoreticular
Inflammatory	None	Herpesvirus 1 (7) Protozoal myelitis (7) Verminous migrations (7) Vertebral osteomyelitis (7) Mycotic myelitis (7)	See acute progressive
Toxic	None	None	Various neuropathies (8, 16)
Traumatic	Fractures (7) Luxations (7)		
Vascular	Embolic myelopathy (7) Fibrocartilaginous emboli (7) Postanesthetic myelopathy	None	None

* Numbers in parentheses refer to chapters in which the entities are discussed.

TABLE 7–3 Food Animal Thoracolumbar Spinal Cord Diseases: Differential Diagnosis of T3–L3 Spinal Cord Disease Based on Clinical Course and Etiologic Categories*

Etiologic Category	*Acute Nonprogressive*	*Acute Progressive*	*Chronic Progressive*
Degenerative	None		Progressive ataxia of Charolais cattle – B (8) Degenerative myeloencephalopathy – B (8) Spondylosis deformans – All (7) Arthrogryposis – All (8) Demyelinating diseases – B (8) Neuronopathies – O (8)
Anomalous	None	None	Spinal dysraphism – All (7) Vertebral anomalies – All (7)
Neoplastic (7)	None	Metastatic Primary Skeletal Lymphoreticular	Primary Lymphoreticular Skeletal Metastatic
Nutritional	None	None	Enzootic ataxia, copper deficiency – C, O (16)
Inflammatory	None	Caprine arthritis-encephalomyelitis – C (7) Bacterial myelitis – All (15) Vertebral osteomyelitis – All (7) Protozoal myelitis (16) Mycotic myelitis (16)	Visna-Maedi – O (16) Verminous migration – All (7)
Toxic	None	None	Various neuropathies (8, 16)
Traumatic	Fractures (7) Luxations (7) Contusions (7)		None
Vascular	Fibrocartilaginous embolism – B (7) Aortic thromboembolism – B (7)	None	None

* Numbers in parentheses refer to chapters in which the entities are discussed. B = bovine, C = caprine, O = ovine, P = porcine.

TABLE 7–4 Small Animal Lumbosacral and Cauda Equina Diseases: Differential Diagnosis of L4–S3 and Caudal Spinal Cord Disease Based on Clinical Courses and Etiologic Categories*

Etiologic Category	*Acute Nonprogressive*	*Acute Progressive*	*Chronic Progressive*
Degenerative	None	Type I disk disease (7) Hemorrhagic myelomalacia (7)	Type II disk disease (7) Degenerative myelopathy (7) Degenerative lumbosacral stenosis (7) Spondylosis deformans (7) Neuronopathies (8)
Anomalous	None	None	Spinal dysraphism (7) Vertebral anomalies (7)
Metabolic	None	None	Endocrine neuropathies (8)
Neoplastic (7)	None	Metastatic Primary Skeletal Lymphoreticular	Primary Lymphoreticular Skeletal Metastatic
Inflammatory	None	Distemper myelitis (16) Bacterial myelitis (15) Diskospondylitis (7) Protozoal myelitis (16) Mycotic myelitis (16)	Feline infectious peritonitis (16) Distemper myelitis (16) Granulomatous meningoencephalomyelitis (16) Immune meningoencephalomyelitis (16) Postvaccinal rabies
Toxic	None	None	Various neuropathies (8, 16)
Traumatic	Fractures (7) Luxations (7) Contusions (7) Intervertebral disk rupture (7)	Hemorrhagic myelomalacia (7) Intervertebral disk rupture (7)	None
Vascular	Fibrocartilaginous embolism (7) Aortic thromboembolism (7)	None	None

* Numbers in parentheses refer to chapters in which the entities are discussed.

TABLE 7–5 Equine Lumbosacral and Cauda Equina Diseases: Differential Diagnosis of L4–S2 and Caudal Disease Based on Clinical Course and Etiologic Categories*

Etiologic Category	*Acute Nonprogressive*	*Acute Progressive*	*Chronic Progressive*
Degenerative	None	None	Spondylosis deformans (7) Neuronopathies (8) Demyelinating diseases (8) Axonopathies (8)
Anomalous	None	None	Vertebral anomalies (7) Spinal dysraphism (7)
Neoplastic (7)	None	Metastatic Primary Skeletal Lymphoreticular	Primary Skeletal Lymphoreticular
Inflammatory	None	Herpesvirus 1 (7) Protozoal myelitis (7) Verminous migrations (7) Vertebral osteomyelitis (7) Mycotic myelitis (7)	Neuritis of the cauda equina (7) (see also acute progressive)
Toxic	None	None	Various neuropathies (8, 16) Sorghum cystitis (7)
Traumatic	Fractures (7) Luxations (7) Postfoaling paralyses (6)	None	None
Vascular	Embolic myelopathy (7) Fibrocartilaginous emboli (7) Postanesthetic myelopathy	None	None

* Numbers in parentheses refer to chapters in which the entities are discussed.

TABLE 7–6 Food Animal Lumbosacral and Cauda Equina Diseases: Differential Diagnosis of L4–S3 and Caudal Disease Based on Clinical Course and Etiologic Categories*

Etiologic Category	*Acute Nonprogressive*	*Acute Progressive*	*Chronic Progressive*
Degenerative	None	None	Spondylosis deformans—All (7) Arthrogryposis—All (8) Neuronopathies—O (8)
Anomalous	None	None	Spinal dysraphism—All (7) Vertebral anomalies—All (7)
Neoplastic (7)	None	Metastatic Primary Skeletal Lymphoreticular	Primary Lymphoreticular Skeletal Metastatic
Nutritional	None	None	Enzootic ataxia, cooper deficiency—C, O (16)
Inflammatory	None	Bacterial myelitis—All (15) Vertebral osteomyelitis—All (7) Protozoal myelitis—All (16) Mycotic myelitis—All (16)	Verminous migration—All (7)
Toxic	None	None	Various neuropathies (8, 16)
Traumatic	Fractures (7) Luxations (7) Contusions (7) Postcalving paralyses—B (6)	None	None
Vascular	Fibrocartilaginous embolism—B (7) Aortic thromboembolism—B (7)	None	None

* Numbers in parentheses refer to chapters in which the entities are discussed. B = bovine, C = caprine, O = ovine, P = porcine.

presented in Tables 7–4, 7–5, and 7–6. These tables are organized according to the logic used in the formulation of a neurologic diagnosis, which was discussed in Chapter 1. After the lesion has been localized to a region or segment of the spinal cord or nerve root, consideration is given to the possible etiologic categories that could produce the lesion. The etiologic categories are listed in the left-hand column of these tables and follow the DAMNIT scheme described in Chapter 1. The diseases are further divided into acute progressive, acute nonprogressive, and chronic progressive categories based on historical information or by following the clinical course of the illness. Most diseases have been included in the tables. The most important disorders will be described in subsequent sections of this chapter. They will be reviewed briefly, with an emphasis on diagnosis and treatment. Some diseases are discussed in other chapters, as noted in the tables.

Acute Progressive Diseases, T3–L3

Thoracolumbar Intervertebral Disk Disease

Intervertebral disk disease is one of the most common disorders producing pelvic limb paresis in the dog. Disk disease occurs in approximately 2% of canine patients seen at teaching hospitals.[1] It is rarely a problem in the cat, horse, or food animals. Degenerative changes within the disk tend to lead to protrusion or herniation of the disk substance into the vertebral canal. Basically, two types of disk degeneration that result in different clinical syndromes have been described (Fig. 7–3). Hansen type I disk degeneration occurs primarily in the chon-

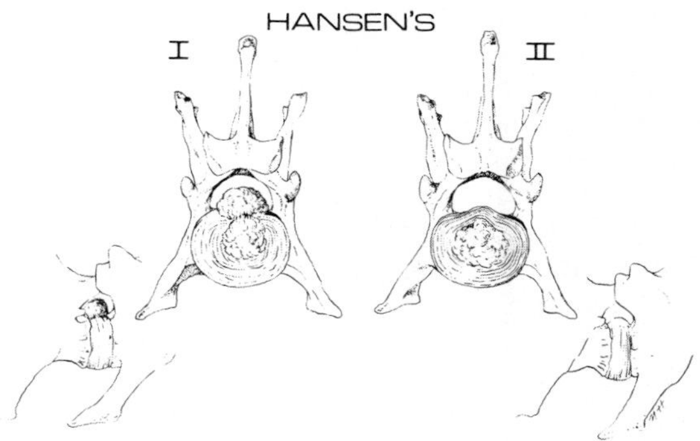

Figure 7–3 Drawings of Hansen type I and type II disk protrusions. (From Hoerlein BF: Canine Neurology: Diagnosis and Treatment, 3rd ed. Philadelphia, WB Saunders, 1978. Used by permission.)

drodystrophoid breeds (small poodle, dachshund, beagle, cocker spaniel, Pekingese, or mixed chondrodystrophoid breeds). It develops when the animal is young (2 to 9 months), and clinical signs are present by the time the animal is 3 to 6 years of age. The disk degeneration is basically a chondroid metaplasia of the nucleus pulposus with degeneration and weakening of the annulus fibrosus. The weakened annulus cannot restrain the degenerative nucleus, and normal movements of the vertebral column are sufficient to initiate acute disk prolapse. These extrusions of disk material result primarily in an acute focal compressive myelopathy. In some cases a severe progressive myelopathy, known as ascending–descending myelomalacia, follows acute "blowouts" of the nuclear material.[2]

Hansen type II disk degeneration occurs in nonchondrodystrophoid breeds, such as German shepherds and Labrador retrievers.[1] It develops at a slower rate, and clinical signs occur when the animal is 5 to 12 years of age. The disk degeneration is basically a fibroid metaplasia that may result in the gradual protrusion of disk material contained within an intact, but degenerate, annulus. True extrusion of free nuclear material into the epidural space does not occur. Compression from this protrusion results in a slowly progressive focal myelopathy. This syndrome will be discussed in the section on chronic progressive spinal cord disorders.

Compressive myelopathy has been attributed primarily to the mechanical derangement of nerve tissue and hypoxic changes resulting from pressure on the vascular system in the spinal cord. Vascular factors that result in ischemia and edema undoubtedly play a role in the development of more severe spinal cord degeneration and the syndrome of hemorrhagic myelomalacia. The severity of the spinal cord lesion is influenced by the magnitude of the protrusion and its rate of development. The inflammatory reaction induced by the extruded material and the diameter of the vertebral canal are also related to the severity of the clinical signs. Acute protrusions produce more severe spinal cord lesions than chronic progressive protrusions, and less severe lesions occur in areas in which the vertebral canal is large (such as the cervical area). Changes progress from edema, demyelination, and necrosis of myelin and axons to myelomalacia.

Progressive myelomalacia has an unknown pathogenesis, but vascular lesions leading to severe ischemia probably are important. This syndrome follows severe acute spinal cord trauma of any cause and results in nearly complete nervous tissue destruction. The clinical signs result from necrosis of the motor neurons and the sensory fibers. LMN signs develop in the muscles supplied by the affected spinal cord segments. Analgesia develops caudal to the cranial edge of the lesion. This syndrome should be suspected in all animals that develop ascending or descending signs of LMN dysfunction and ascending analgesia following spinal trauma and severe compression. Affected animals usually die of respiratory failure 2 to 4 days after the onset of clinical signs. The lesion is irreparable, and euthanasia should be performed on affected animals in order to prevent needless suffering.

Clinical Signs. In addition to the signs of paresis or paralysis that characterize lesions in this region of the spinal cord, disk disease is associated with considerable pain in the area of the protrusion. The extruded material irritates the nerve roots and the meninges, resulting in severe pain and hyperesthesia when the vertebral column is manipulated. An animal may arch its back and tense its abdominal muscles—motions that are suggestive of acute abdominal disorders, such as pancreatitis. Sensory examinations, such as pinching the skin and palpating the vertebra, are important, because they allow the clinician to localize the lesion to two or three spinal cord segments. Lesions that affect the superficial pain pathways will abolish the cutaneous reflex caudal to the lesion. This reflex is normally most apparent when the skin over the thoracolumbar junction is stimulated. Students incorrectly believe that this apparent exaggeration of the skin twitch represents hyperesthesia and thus correlates with lesion location. Hyperesthesia is an exaggerated cerebral response to painful stimuli. Cooperative animals that cry out or try to bite when an area is palpated or pinched may be experiencing hyperesthesia, and the lesion is usually one or two segments cranial to the point at which the response was induced. In animals that are analgesic in the pelvic limbs, the point of analgesia along the spine should be found. The lesion is usually one or two segments cranial to the point at which the animal first feels painful stimuli.

Thoracolumbar disk disease may develop at intervertebral disk spaces T9–T10 to L7–S1. The intercapital ligament usually prevents protrusion of the cranial and midthoracic disks. Over 65% of disk protrusions occur at sites T11–T12, T12–T13, T13–L1, and L1–L2. These areas should be evaluated carefully in animals with suspected thoracolumbar disk disease. Less frequently, disk protrusions occur in sites caudal to L3–L4. Protrusions at these sites produce

LMN signs in the pelvic limbs, because the compressive myelopathy affects the motor neurons that form the lumbosacral plexus. These cases may be differentiated from those of descending myelomalacia as the result of a more cranial lesion by the location of hyperesthesia or the cranial level of decreased sensation.

Animals that develop progressive myelomalacia have ascending or descending signs of progressive LMN dysfunction and ascending levels of analgesia. Typically, affected dogs develop hypotonic abdominal muscles and hypotonic, areflexic pelvic limbs. The anus may be dilated, and the perineal reflex is weak or absent. The bladder is usually distended and easily expressed because of poor tone in the urethral sphincter.

Ascending signs of LMN paralysis include a loss of intercostal respirations and an inability to remain sternal because of paralysis of the paraspinal muscles. The thoracic limbs may be rigidly extended, and hyperesthesia may develop in the feet a few hours before the necrosis affects the lower cervical cord. Animals die of respiratory failure when the necrosis ascends to the level of the fifth and sixth cervical cord segments and thus destroys the neurons of the phrenic nerves. This syndrome apparently occurs with greatest frequency in dogs that develop acute paralysis and sensory loss. Owners should be warned of this possibility, particularly in cases in which surgical therapy is contemplated.

Diagnosis. A tentative diagnosis of thoracolumbar disk disease is based on an assessment of the clinical signs, a knowledge of the typical breed involvement, and the results of the neurologic evaluation. For example, an animal with asymmetric paresis and little hyperesthesia is more likely to have an infarct than a compressive lesion from a disk. The diagnosis can be confirmed by a conventional radiographic examination of the spine with the x-ray beam centered over the probable lesion site, which is established by the neurologic examination (Figs. 7–4, 7–5, and 7–6). General anesthesia is required for making diagnostic spinal radiographs. In our hospital, radiographs are taken when the animal is treated surgically. For cases treated by conservative medical procedures, radiographs are not routinely made unless another disease, such as diskospondylitis, is to be excluded. It is difficult to justify the expense and risk of anesthesia in a dog that probably has this disease, if medical therapy is contemplated. Survey radiographic changes include narrowing of the intervertebral disk space, narrowing of the articular space, and a smaller intervertebral foramen with some increase in density in the foramen as compared to adjacent spaces. In some cases, myelography is needed to determine the site of the compression, particularly if the survey radiographs suggest several potential sites. Myelographic changes are consistent with an extradural compression, although if there is significant spinal cord swelling, the column of contrast agent may be absent for some distance. Some surgeons require myelography for all disk problems to be certain of the lesion site, to increase the probability of identifying the side of the protrusion, and to rule out other diseases. In some hospitals, magnetic resonance (MR) imaging and computed tomography (CT) may be useful to document more obscure disk herniations.

Treatment. Many dogs with intervertebral disk disease respond at least temporarily to attentive nursing care that promotes the sponta-

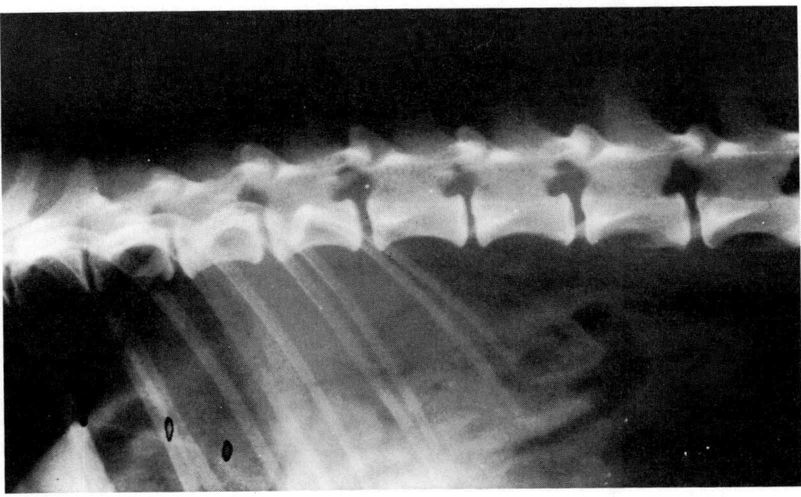

Figure 7–4 Lateral thoracolumbar radiograph showing narrowing of the intervertebral space, intervertebral foramen, and articular space between the facets at L1–L2, a common radiographic lesion in type I intervertebral disk disease.

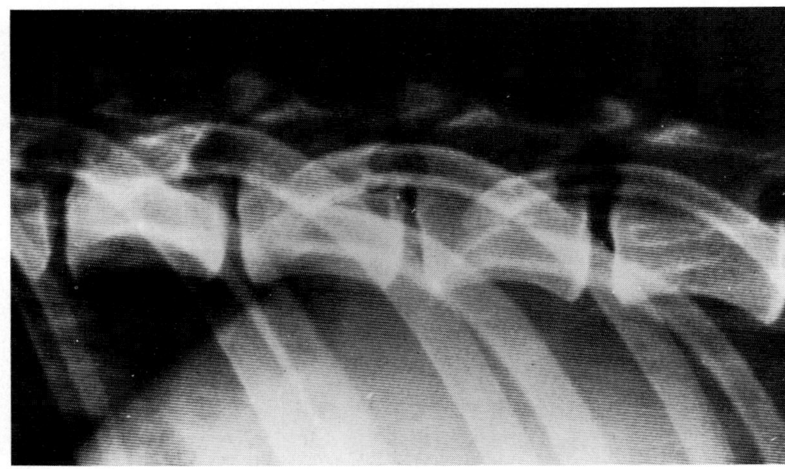

Figure 7–5 Lateral thoracolumbar radiograph showing wedging of the intervertebral space at T12–T13. This is another radiographic lesion indicative of disk protrusion.

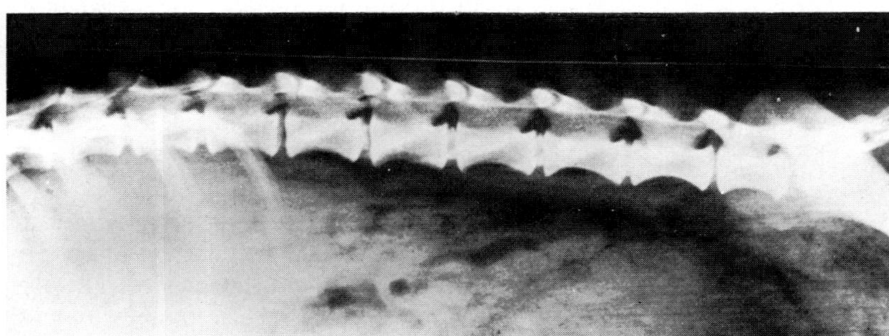

Figure 7–6 Lateral thoracolumbar radiograph showing numerous calcified disks. The active site of disease is L1–L2, where the disk space is narrowed. Calcified disks in situ seldom cause active disease but are likely to herniate later.

neous healing processes. Because of this finding it is extremely difficult to cite clear-cut evidence of the superiority of one therapy over another. The major treatment controversy centers on the benefit of surgery versus conservative medical management. In addition, the relative benefits of the various surgical procedures are still being debated. In comparing any treatment protocols it must be recognized that the severity and duration of the problem are critical factors in recovery, regardless of treatment.[1] When those factors are constant, the literature is reasonably clear on appropriate treatment. Table 7–7 summarizes the indications for treatment and the forms of management currently recommended.

MEDICAL THERAPY Medical therapy is indicated for animals that experience an initial episode of mild neurologic dysfunction or pain, or those that have other medical problems pre-

TABLE 7–7 Treatment of Thoracolumbar Intervertebral Disk Herniation

Therapy	*Indications Based on History and Clinical Signs*
Medical	Pain only – first episode
	Mild ataxia and paresis – first episode
	Medical condition precludes surgery
	Paralyzed – deep pain response absent ≥ 48 hr
	Progressive myelomalacia
Surgical	
Fenestration only	Multiple episodes of pain only
Decompression (hemilaminectomy) with fenestration	Paresis and ataxia – second episode
	No improvement or deterioration of signs with medical therapy
	Moderate paresis or paralysis, deep pain response present – first episode
	Paralysis, deep pain response absent < 48 hr (very guarded prognosis)

cluding surgery. Therapy should support the normal healing processes but should not totally relieve pain or totally inhibit the beneficial inflammatory process induced by the extruded disk material. Analgesics and anti-inflammatory drugs (aspirin, meperidine, phenylbutazone, corticosteroids) should be used with caution so that complete relief of pain is not produced. Total relief of pain may allow overactivity of the animal, which may result in further disk extrusion and rapidly worsening clinical signs. The most important aspect of therapy is enforced cage rest, preferably under direct veterinary supervision.

Owners often are told to place the animals in a baby crib or playpen. In our opinion, this is poor advice, because this form of confinement encourages the animal to jump in an attempt to get out. Confinement at home should be in a small airline crate placed in a quiet room where the animal will not be disturbed. The animal should be exercised twice a day on a leash, away from other dogs or cats. Analgesics or other anti-inflammatory drugs should not be used at home unless the client agrees to cooperate fully with the instructions for strict cage rest. The most common mistake made by veterinarians is to administer corticosteroids and send the animal home. Predictably, these animals return in 36 to 48 hours with severe neurologic signs. Generally, dogs should be hospitalized for 1 week. Prednisolone, 0.25 mg/lb, is given every 12 hours for 72 hours and then discontinued. The animal is sent home with instructions for cage confinement of 3 weeks' duration. If satisfactory progress is made, exercise is restricted to a leash for an additional 3 weeks. If followed closely, these procedures result in considerable improvement; however, the owner must be aware that further attacks will occur in over 50% of cases, and that the recurrence may be severe. If the animal's signs deteriorate at any time, surgery should be performed immediately.

Paralyzed animals that have lost deep pain sensation for 48 hours or more have a grave prognosis (less than 5% chance for recovery) with or without surgery. The absence of deep pain perception represents a severe, usually irreparable spinal cord injury. Unless the owner definitely wants to try surgery in the face of these odds, the animal should be treated medically. Methylprednisolone sodium succinate, 30 mg/kg, is given intravenously (IV) upon presentation, followed by a continuous infusion of 5 mg/kg/hr for 24 hours. Other corticosteroids have not been shown to have the same effect (see Chap. 13 for a complete discussion of the use of corticosteroids in CNS trauma). Mannitol, 0.5 g/kg, may also be given. The steroids are not given after 24 hours. They are not likely to be of benefit unless administration is started within a few hours of the onset of the injury to the spinal cord. Physical therapy then is initiated. No improvement in clinical signs in 3 weeks is an indication for euthanasia. Corticosteroid therapy, if continued longer than 5 to 7 days, may result in gastrointestinal ulceration and may aggravate urinary tract infection in those dogs with urine retention from a paralyzed detrusor muscle.

SURGICAL THERAPY The various forms of surgical therapy have been reviewed extensively by Hoerlein.[1] There appears to be general agreement that disk fenestration is indicated for animals with recurrent pain or minimal paresis and ataxia. Although there is no decompression, fenestration helps prevent further protrusion. This surgical procedure may also produce an acute inflammatory process that stimulates phagocytosis, the resorption of necrotic disk material, and the formation of fibrosis, which helps to stabilize the disk.

In dogs with moderate to severe paresis and ataxia, decompressive surgery should be performed immediately. This recommendation is supported by several clinical and experimental studies that compared the speed and duration of spinal cord compression with the rate of recovery. Tarlov and co-workers have demonstrated that acute spinal cord compression with a force sufficient to produce complete sensorimotor paralysis results in complete recovery if the compression is less than 2 hours in duration.[3,4] Furthermore, the rate of recovery in Tarlov's study correlated directly with the duration of compression. After 10 minutes of acute compression, 2 to 3 days were required for initial improvement in neurologic function. With 50 to 120 minutes of acute compression, 20 to 30 days were required for initial improvement. Gradual compression of the spinal cord was better tolerated, and irreversible changes developed at a slower rate in these animals. Gradual compression to paralysis in 75 minutes resulted in full recovery if the compressive force was removed within 9 hours. One to three days were required for initial improvement. Thus, early decompressive surgery may have a positive influence on both the quality of restored function and the rate of recovery. *When indicated, spinal cord decompression should be performed without delay.* The common practice of medically treating dogs with moderate to severe paresis or paraplegia for 24 to 48 hours and then performing surgery if no improvement occurs should be condemned. This procedure discounts the experimental data regarding the effects of spinal compression over variable periods and the clinical experience of many veterinary surgeons.[1]

Dogs with acute paralysis and no deep pain responses should undergo decompression within 2 hours for possible functional recovery. Surgery is recommended for dogs with absence of deep pain sensation for up to 48 hours; however, the rate and quality of recovery are much less predictable. After 48 hours, the chance for recovery is probably less than 5%. These dogs are surgically treated only at the owner's insistence.

If a paralyzed dog is to be referred to a surgeon for decompression, the administration of steroids as outlined in the medical treatment is indicated.

SUPPORTIVE CARE OF THE PARAPLEGIC Supportive care of the "downer dog" is directed at preventing the development of decubital ulcers, urinary tract infection, and muscle atrophy. Physical therapy is described in Chapter 5. Bladder care is described in Chapter 3.

The rate of return to acceptable pelvic limb function and micturition is highly correlated with the duration and rate of the spinal cord compression. Generally, if paraplegia has lasted longer than 48 hours, voluntary motor function, micturition, and normal pain responses return within 2 to 3 weeks. Good voluntary motor activity should return within 4 to 5 weeks, and the unassisted ability to support weight usually is restored within 6 to 8 weeks. Proprioception is the last function to return. Once again, it must be stressed that *early* decompression hastens the return of neurologic function. Animals decompressed in the first 24 hours may be walking in the next 24 hours.

Equine Herpesvirus 1 (Rhinopneumonitis) Myeloencephalitis

Equine herpesvirus 1 (EHV-1) myeloencephalitis is an acute progressive neurologic disease that usually affects adult horses, but disease in foals also has been reported.[5] Multifocal neurologic lesions, primarily a severe vasculitis and necrosis, occur in the brain and the spinal cord;[6] however, the spinal cord lesions usually produce the majority of clinical signs. The pathogenesis of this disease is not related to direct viral infection of the central nervous system (CNS). An immune-mediated, Arthus-type reaction involving a viral antigen and an antibody may induce the severe neurologic vasculitis characteristic of this disease.

Clinical Signs. EHV-1 myeloencephalitis usually occurs within 1 to 2 weeks after outbreaks of upper respiratory tract infections or abortions. Pregnant mares may be more susceptible to the development of severe spinal cord lesions and may abort if infected in the last trimester of pregnancy. Neurologic signs develop acutely; however, progression of the signs is variable, depending on the severity of the initial spinal cord lesions. Affected horses may recover in 24 to 48 hours, or they may progress rapidly to severe tetra- or paraplegia. Neurologic signs vary according to the area of the spinal cord involved. Usual neurologic signs include dysuria, ataxia of the pelvic limbs, and a flaccid anus and tail. Signs may progress to severe pelvic limb paresis or paralysis. Tetraparesis may be severe if cervical spinal cord lesions are extensive. In a few cases, involvement of the cerebral cortex or the brain stem may produce seizures, cranial nerve dysfunction, or vestibular signs. In most cases the clinical signs are those of thoracolumbar cord dysfunction. One must remember that both UMN and LMN signs may develop relative to the site of development of vascular lesions in the spinal cord. In addition, neurologic signs may be symmetric or lateralizing, depending on the site of involvement.

Diagnosis. EHV-1 myeloencephalitis is a sporadic disease of horses and must be suspected when neurologic disease appears to follow outbreaks of respiratory tract infection or abortion. Analysis of the cerebrospinal fluid (CSF) reveals significant elevations in protein levels (150 mg/dl or greater) with normal or slightly elevated cell counts. The CSF may be xanthochromic. The definitive diagnosis is made by isolation of the virus from nervous tissue or by serologic methods. Because viral isolation is difficult, comparison of antibody titers at the onset of clinical signs and during convalescence is the preferred method for confirming a clinical diagnosis. In experimental studies, a sharp rise in serum antibody neutralization titers occurs within 5 to 7 days after inoculation.

Treatment. There is no definitive treatment for this disease. Because an immune mechanism may be responsible, some authors have suggested the use of corticosteroids (dexamethasone, 0.1–0.25 mg/kg).[5,7] The benefits of this therapy are hard to document, insofar as many animals recover if given supportive nursing care, including catheterization of the urinary bladder. A killed intramuscular (IM) vaccine is available that probably provides immunity to the respiratory disease, but not to infection of the placenta or CNS. Therefore, vaccinated animals may still have abortions or neurologic disease.

Equine Protozoal Myeloencephalomyelitis

Equine protozoal myelitis-encephalitis is a neurologic syndrome of horses that is characterized by *sudden* or *gradual* onset of pelvic limb paresis and ataxia. Because lesions may be multifocal in the spinal cord or brain, neurologic signs may indicate involvement of any part of the CNS. Equine protozoal myelitis-encephalitis is caused by an unidentified sporozoan parasite resembling *Sarcocystis cruzi*.[5,8] It occurs most frequently in the eastern United States and has been reported from many other locations.[5,9–11]

Lesions within the CNS are focal or multifocal and usually are asymmetric. The histopathologic lesion is a nonsuppurative myelitis affecting both gray and white matter. The disease is most common in young to middle-aged horses of the light breeds.

Clinical Signs. Clinical signs usually develop suddenly and progress slowly over days to weeks, but rapid progression is sometimes the case. Asymmetric ataxia and paresis of the pelvic limbs are the usual predominant manifestations. Because lesions may be multifocal, however, a mixture of UMN and LMN signs may be present in the pelvic and thoracic limbs, and brain stem signs may be present. If the lesion occurs in the brachial intumescence, the thoracic limb signs may be worse than the pelvic limb signs. These animals move with the thoracic limbs extended forward and the head held low. The clinical signs may resemble those observed in the equine wobbler syndrome and EHV-1 myeloencephalitis; however, the asymmetry that is seen helps in the clinical differentiation of protozoal myelitis-encephalitis from the other two diseases.

Diagnosis. In protozoal myelitis-encephalitis, unlike EHV-1 encephalomyelitis, there are few CSF abnormalities. Mildly increased concentrations of mononuclear cells and protein occasionally are found. Cervical radiographs are normal (differentiating this disease from equine wobbler syndrome). Electromyography (EMG) can help identify multifocal LMN damage, which is more common in this disease than in the others that resemble it.

Treatment. Therapy may be effective, especially if it is started before profound signs are present. Although no definitive therapy is known, pyrimethamine (not licensed for the horse) is given in a loading dose of 0.5 mg/kg orally, followed by 0.1–2.5 mg/kg once daily and trimethoprim and sulfadiazine at a dosage of 15–20 mg/kg orally, twice daily. This regimen should be continued for 1 to 3 months.[5] The hemogram should be monitored for depression of blood cell production. Vitamin B complex can be given to help counteract the folic acid inhibition.

Verminous Migration

Equine. The migration of several parasites through the spinal cord of horses has been described. The most important of these organisms include *Micronema deletrix*, *Strongylus vulgaris*, *Draschia megastoma*, and *Hypoderma lineatum*. The clinical signs depend on the location of the parasite and may be asymmetric, focal, or multifocal. Embolization of *Strongylus vulgaris* larvae into spinal or cerebral arteries may produce severe acute progressive or nonprogressive clinical signs.

A confirmed clinical diagnosis is difficult to make. The CSF may contain increased concentrations of eosinophils, neutrophils, macrophages, and red blood cells. It is not xanthochromic, in contrast to the CSF of animals with EHV-1 myelitis.

No definitive therapy is known. In suspected cases, thiabendazole (440 mg/kg), oxfendazole (10 mg/kg), diethylcarbamazine (50 mg/kg), or ivermectin (200 μg/kg) have been recommended.[5] Glucocorticosteroids can be used to decrease the inflammatory response to the dying worms. Many animals will have permanent disability, but the response can be very good if treatment is started early.

Bovine. The larvae of *Hypoderma bovis* migrate through the epidural space of cattle. Infestation usually occurs during the months of July through October. If the larvae die or are killed while in the epidural space, a severe immunologic reaction occurs, resulting in spinal cord injury. The clinical signs usually appear in cattle treated with organophosphate insecticides during the period of epidural larvae migration. Clinical signs develop acutely hours to days after treatment and usually are caused by thoracolumbar spinal cord injury. Prominent signs include pelvic limb ataxia and paresis. If the lumbosacral cord is involved, LMN signs may be detected in the pelvic limbs. The signs are usually asymmetric. The diagnosis is based on the history and the clinical signs. The CSF changes reflect signs of degeneration (moderate increases in protein and cell concentrations). Eosinophils may not be present in the

CSF. Affected animals should be treated with corticosteroids or phenylbutazone to reduce the inflammatory reaction. If signs develop several days to weeks after organophosphate application, the possibility of organophosphate intoxication should be considered.

Ovine, Caprine. Sheep and goats may serve as aberrant hosts for the meningeal worm of white-tailed deer, *Parelaphostrongylus tenuis*. Migration of this parasite through the CNS produces a variety of clinical signs, including pelvic limb paresis and ataxia. The clinical course is variable and may include progression, stasis, or improvement in clinical signs. Affected animals have a history of grazing in pastures that have been exposed to white-tailed deer. The CSF of these animals usually contains increased concentrations of protein and cells. A mononuclear and eosinophilic pleocytosis is usually encountered. Treatment with diethylcarbamazine, levamisole, or thiabendazole is recommended. The prognosis is guarded.

Porcine. The kidney worm of swine, *Stephanurus dentatus*, may migrate through the spinal cord, producing pelvic limb paresis and ataxia. This organism must be considered in individual swine that develop acute paraparesis, particularly swine residing on farms in the southeastern United States.

Viral Leukoencephalomyelitis of Goats (Caprine Arthritis-Encephalomyelitis)

This disease affects goats 1 to 4 months of age and probably is caused by a lentivirus. The disease causes a perivenous demyelination and nonsuppurative granulomatous leukomyelitis. As in other viral diseases, lesions may develop anywhere in the spinal cord, producing focal or multifocal asymmetric neurologic signs. The clinical signs of this disease include a progressive paraparesis that eventually involves the thoracic limbs. More than one kid is affected in most cases. Weight loss, arthritis, pneumonitis, and a hard udder may be present in one or more animals. Neurologic signs may reflect multifocal disease, including involvement of the brain. The CSF usually contains markedly increased concentrations of mononuclear cells and modestly increased concentrations of protein; however, an eosinophilic pleocytosis is not present. EMG may indicate some LMN loss. Serologic tests (ELISA and agar gel immunodiffusion) can be helpful if positive, but many affected animals are negative. There is no effective treatment. The neurologic syndrome is permanent and may be fatal.[5]

Acute Nonprogressive Diseases, T3–L3

Spinal Cord Trauma

Spinal cord trauma, usually the result of automobile accidents, is a common neurologic injury.[12] The incidence is much greater in areas where leash laws are poorly enforced. Spinal cord trauma is more frequent in large animals when they are young but may occur in mature animals as a result of falls, trailer accidents, or overcrowding in chutes. The management of spinal cord trauma has been discussed extensively by other authors.[13–17] This section provides a concise review of the management. Veterinarians have two primary obligations. First, they must diagnose and treat shock, major abdominal or thoracic hemorrhage, visceral rupture, or ventilation abnormalities. Second, they must be able to give owners accurate prognoses for the recovery of neurologic function.

First Aid and Emergency Medical Treatment. An injury of sufficient force to produce spinal cord trauma usually results in another life-threatening injury.[12,16] Maintenance of a patent airway is of the utmost importance. The mouth is cleared of fluid or blood, the tongue is pulled forward, and the unconscious animal is intubated. Adequate ventilation is of great importance, since hypoxia aggravates CNS edema. Shock, if present, must be treated. Lactated Ringer's solution is given IV to restore vascular volume. Methylprednisolone sodium succinate is given IV at a dosage of 30 mg/kg body weight over a 10-minute period.[18] This drug is beneficial in the prevention and treatment of CNS edema and secondary reactions in the nervous tissue. Fluid therapy must be carefully monitored to prevent overhydration, which may aggravate CNS edema, but the patient must have fluid volume restored and maintained.

After providing first aid and treating shock, the veterinarian must perform a thorough physical examination. Abdominal or thoracic trauma may be difficult to appreciate immediately after an injury; therefore, visceral function must be monitored for several days. There is little benefit in successfully repairing the spinal fracture only to have the animal die several days later from a diaphragmatic hernia or a ruptured urinary bladder. However, spinal cord trauma must be treated without delay in order to improve the odds of recovery. Once circulatory problems are corrected, mannitol therapy is instituted (see Chap. 13 for details on the management of edema).

During the period of early evaluation and treatment, the animal must be restrained in order to prevent further spinal cord injury. Ani-

TABLE 7–8 Signs of Complete Spinal Cord Transection*

Spinal Cord Segments	Signs Caudal to Lesion		
	Motor	Sensory	Autonomic
C1–C4	Tetraplegia (UMN)	Anesthesia	Apnea, no micturition
C5–C6	Tetraplegia (UMN), LMN suprascapular nerve	Anesthesia, hyperesthesia—midcervical	Apnea—phrenic nerve, LMN, no micturition
C7–T2	Tetraplegia or paralegia (UMN), LMN brachial plexus	Anesthesia, hyperesthesia—brachial plexus	Diaphragmatic breathing only, no micturition
T3–L3	Paraplegia (UMN), Schiff-Sherrington syndrome	Anesthesia, hyperesthesia—segmental	Diaphragmatic, some intercostal and abdominal respiration, depending on level of lesion, no micturition
L4–S1	Paraplegia with LMN lumbosacral plexus	Anesthesia, hyperesthesia—segmental	No micturition; S1 = anal sphincter may be atonic
S1–S3	Knuckling of hind foot, paralysis of tail	Anesthesia, hyperesthesia—segmental	No micturition, sphincters atonic
Cd1–Cd5	Paralysis of tail	Anesthesia, hyperesthesia—segmental	None

* C = cervical, T = thoracic, L = lumbar, S = sacral, Cd = caudal, LMN = lower motor neuron, UMN = upper motor neuron.

mals should be transported on a rigid stretcher or a board. Movement should be discouraged, especially if vertebral fractures or luxations are suspected.

Neurologic Examination. Most spinal cord injuries are the result of vertebral fracture, vertebral luxation, or traumatic disk extrusion and are likely to produce severe permanent neurologic deficits, especially if early treatment has not been provided. The localization of the spinal cord lesion and the prognosis based on the severity of the injury are determined by the neurologic examination. The spinal column should be gently palpated for alterations in vertebral conformation, as these changes have good localizing value. The principles of lesion localization were reviewed earlier. Table 7–8 summarizes the signs of complete spinal cord transection at various levels of the cord.

The prognosis of a spinal cord injury depends on the suddenness of the injury, the duration of the compressive force, and the extent of secondary vascular responses to the injury.[13] The bottom line is reversibility. The spinal cord may be anatomically or physiologically transected. In most cases, physiologic transection is the most common cause of irreversibility. Sudden compression of the spinal cord is far worse than gradual compression. Acute experimental compression of the spinal cord with a force sufficient to produce paralysis and analgesia results in irreversible spinal cord injury if the duration of compression exceeds 4 hours. Most experimental studies documenting effective medical therapy of spinal cord trauma indicate that treatment must be given in the first hour. The key to prognosis is the *perceptual response* to noxious stimuli applied caudally to the lesion. In the absence of deep pain perception, the duration of the injury becomes the critical factor related to prognosis. The absence of deep pain perception is a very unfavorable sign, especially if the injury has been present for longer than 4 hours. Other neurologic signs that correlate with severe thoracolumbar spinal cord injury include spinal shock, crossed extensor reflexes, and the Schiff-Sherrington phenomenon. The presence of these signs does *not* indicate that the lesion is irreversible, because these signs may occur in the presence of deep pain perception.

Assuming that the skeletal lesion can be stabilized, injured animals are categorized as shown in Table 7–9.

Special Examinations. Radiographs of the spinal column are necessary if surgical treatment is contemplated. Radiographs define the precise location and type of skeletal lesion (Fig. 7–7). These findings dictate the surgical procedure needed to decompress and stabilize the

TABLE 7–9 Prognosis of Acute Spinal Cord Injuries

Group	Signs	Duration of Injury	Prognosis
Group 1	Good pain response	<24 hr	Fair to good
Group 2	No pain response	<4 hr	Poor
Group 3	No pain response	>4 hr	Grave

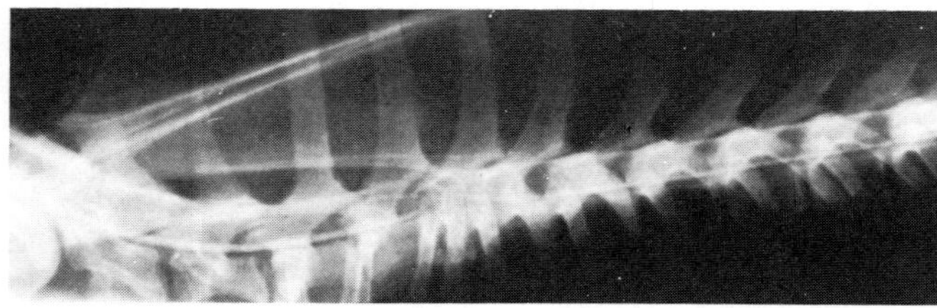

Figure 7–7 Myelogram of a dog with a compression fracture of T3. The compression of the spinal cord was not apparent on survey films.

injury. Spinal radiographs are not useful for evaluating the functional status of the spinal cord. The amount of displacement visualized on radiographs is frequently the least displacement that occurred at the time of the injury. The functional status is determined by the neurologic examination. Somatosensory-evoked potentials may be of benefit to more precisely define spinal cord integrity (see Chap. 4).

Medical Therapy. Corticosteroids are given as part of the emergency treatment for shock. Methylprednisolone sodium succinate is given in an initial dosage of 30 mg/kg, followed by a continuous infusion of 5 mg/kg/hr for 24 hours. None is given after 24 hours.[18–20] A hypertonic osmotic diuretic, such as 20% mannitol solution, should be administered immediately after hypovolemia has been corrected. Mannitol acts very quickly to reduce spinal cord edema and is indicated in addition to corticosteroids. Mannitol is given at a dosage of 0.5 g/kg body weight over the course of 30 minutes. Vomiting and severe hemolysis of red blood cells may occur if the rate of administration is too rapid. The mannitol therapy is repeated in 2 to 3 hours and then is discontinued. Dimethyl sulfoxide (DMSO) is often recommended, especially in large animals.[5] Most controlled studies do not indicate efficacy, but the literature is controversial.[21] In large animals it is used at a dosage of 1.0 g/kg, 10% DMSO in 5% dextrose, given IV.

One study of 211 dogs and cats with vertebral fractures found minimal difference between medical and surgical management.[22] Although it is clear that many vertebral fractures can be managed medically, surgery is indicated in unstable fractures.

Surgical Therapy. There are two major indications for spinal surgery in the animal with a traumatic injury: decompression and immobilization of the vertebra. The decision for decompression is based on the clinical signs. Animals with paralysis almost always need decompression and usually need stabilization. Animals with mild paresis and ataxia may need stabilization, but decompression usually is not indicated. Decompression must be performed within 4 to 6 hours on an animal with complete paralysis in order to prevent permanent damage. Animals in groups 1 and 2 in Table 7–9 should undergo early surgery. Surgery is not recommended for animals in group 3.

The decision as to the method of immobilization is based on the findings of clinical and radiographic examinations and on observations made during the operation. Flexible plates, body plates, segmental spinal instrumentation, and vertebral body pins with methylmethacrylate are the most commonly used methods and usually are superior to any form of external support.[23–27] Compressive fractures of the vertebral body and fractures of the transverse spinous processes without displacement may be stable. Fractures of the vertebral body with luxation or fractures involving several articular facets require reduction and stabilization. When decompression and stabilization are simultaneously indicated, hemilaminectomy is the favored approach for decompression, because any method of fixation can be used with this procedure. Dorsal laminectomy must be used in the lumbosacral region (Fig. 7–8). The reader is referred to other texts and the other references for in-depth descriptions of the various surgical techniques.[28]

Supportive Care and Rehabilitation. Very few animals become ambulatory during the first week after surgery following severe trauma. The majority remain paretic or paralyzed and require attentive nursing care, physical therapy, and a rehabilitation period. In general, the procedures for supportive care of the paraplegic in cases of disk disease should also be followed after spinal surgery. Animals should improve within 2 to 3 weeks, with significant improvement in a month. Failure to show improvement during this time is strongly correlated with permanent spinal cord damage; however, every clinician encounters a few dogs that regain functional use of the pelvic limbs when the initial outlook has seemed hopeless. Unfortunately, in veterinary medicine, the outcome of the case often depends on the enthusiasm and financial cooperation of the owner.

Chronic Progressive Diseases, T3–L3

Chronic progressive diseases of the T3–L3 region are characterized by insidious onset and slow progression of the neurologic signs. De-

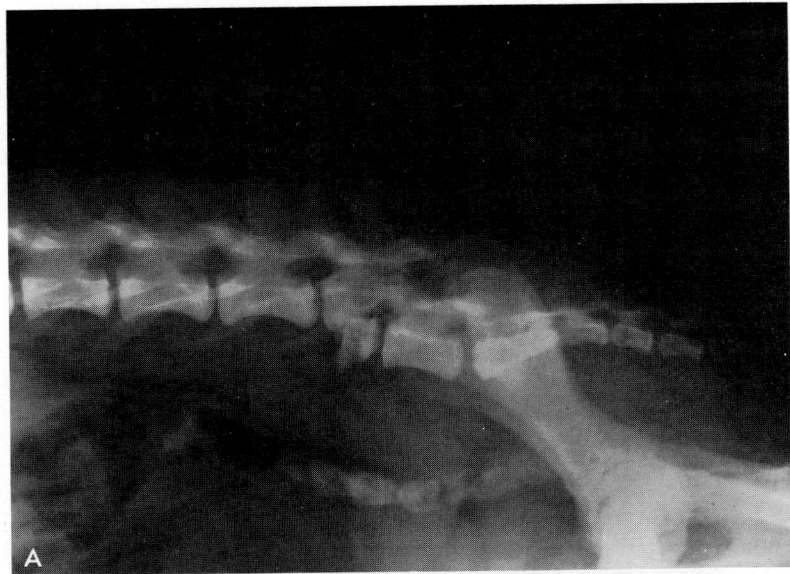

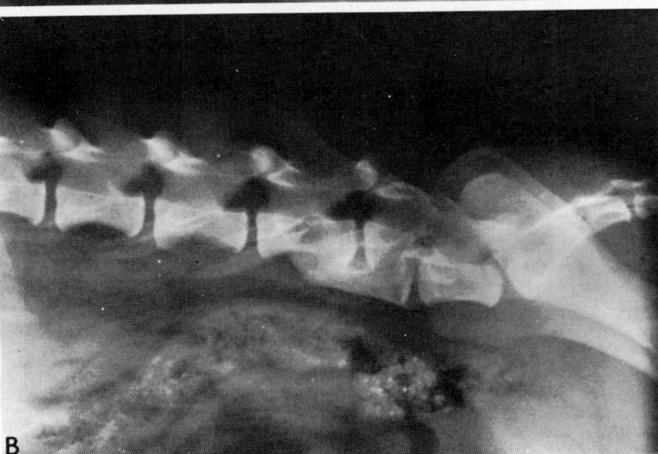

Figure 7–8 *A.* Lumbosacral lateral radiograph demonstrating a fracture of L6. These injuries entrap the spinal nerve roots forming the sciatic, pelvic, pudendal, and caudal nerves. *B.* Follow-up postsurgical radiograph of the same dog. The fracture site was decompressed and the nerves in the vertebral canal were freed from compression. A callus had bridged the fracture site, although no internal stabilization had been provided.

generative, neoplastic, and inflammatory diseases are the most important of the various etiologic categories. Although the diseases listed in the right-hand column of Tables 7–1, 7–2, and 7–3 may start in the T3–L3 spinal cord segments, progression into other regions may occur. With long-standing disease, cervical spinal cord involvement may cause tetraparesis or hemiparesis. These problems are discussed in Chapter 8.

Degenerative Myelopathy

Degenerative myelopathy is a slowly progressive degenerative disease involving primarily the long tracts of the canine thoracolumbar spinal cord. The disease was first described by Averill in 1973, and subsequent authors have reported various clinical and pathologic findings.[29–32] The disease appears to be most prevalent in older German shepherd dogs and has been termed German shepherd myelopathy and progressive myelopathy.[31,33,34] Griffiths and coworkers have termed this disorder degenerative radiculomyelopathy because of dorsal root involvement in several of their cases.[32] A degenerative myelopathy also has been described in horses. Unlike the canine disease, the equine syndrome is seen in young animals, is characterized by an acute progressive course, and involves primarily the cervical cord, although thoracolumbar lesions also occur. The equine disease is discussed in Chapter 8.

Pathologic Findings. In Averill's study, 22 dogs with progressive ataxia and paresis had diffuse degeneration of spinal cord myelin and axons in all spinal cord funiculi.[30] These changes were most extensive in the midthoracic region and were not associated with intervertebral disk extrusion, spondylosis deformans, or dural ossification. Griffiths and Duncan reported their findings in 16 dogs.[32] In addition to confirming many of Averill's observations, these authors reported extensive lesions in the lumbar dorsal columns and involvement of the dorsal nerve roots. They reported that the lesions suggested a "dying back" process of axons confined to the CNS. In another study, Braund and Vandevelde studied 14 German shepherds affected with this disease.[31] Although this study reconfirmed many of the earlier observations, it did not support the "dying back" hypothesis. Dogs with degenerative myelopathy have some cell-mediated immunologic abnormalities, and the lesions are similar in some respects to multiple sclerosis.[29,33,34] Other hypotheses include a nutritional problem, including vitamins B_{12} and E. Dogs with degenerative myelopathy were found to have decreased serum tocopherol levels, but therapy with vitamin B complex and E has not been effective. The immune hypothesis is the most attractive one at present. The predisposition of German shepherd dogs to this syndrome suggests that genetic factors may be involved in the pathogenesis.

Clinical Signs. Clinical signs generally are first recognized in affected dogs at 6 to 9 years of age, although the disease has been documented in a few 4-year-old dogs. It occurs almost exclusively in large breeds, predominantly German shepherds or shepherd dog crossbreeds. However, similar syndromes have been seen in other breeds, including a miniature poodle,[35] Siberian husky dogs,[36] and other large breeds.[37] One cat with a similar syndrome has been reported.[38] Early clinical signs include mild ataxia and paresis of the pelvic limbs. The onset is insidious, and an owner may not seek veterinary assistance for several months, believing that the dog has mild coxofemoral arthritis. The outstanding clinical sign is pelvic limb ataxia. Knuckling of the feet, dragging of the toes, and dysmetria are common signs. The pelvic limbs may cross when the animal walks, and swaying movements of the rear quarters are apparent. If forced to turn quickly, many dogs will fall in an outward direction. Clinical signs are bilateral; however, they may not be symmetric. One limb may be affected more severely than another. Urinary or fecal incontinence is uncommon. Most animals appear healthy in other respects. In chronic cases, atrophy of the caudal paraspinal and pelvic limb muscles may occur.

The neurologic examination usually suggests a lesion in spinal cord segments T3–L3. Postural reactions, such as proprioceptive positioning, hopping, placing, and the extensor postural thrust, are deficient. The degree of proprioceptive dysfunction is usually greater than the degree of motor dysfunction. Flexor (withdrawal) reflexes are normal and, in more advanced cases, may be clonic. Crossed extensor reflexes may be present. In many dogs, the knee jerk reflex is normal or exaggerated. In some dogs, the knee jerk reflex is depressed or absent, even though the leg can be extended readily at the stifle, a crossed extensor reflex may be present, and pain is perceived normally from areas innervated by the saphenous branch of the femoral nerve. It is believed that involvement of the dorsal roots of the femoral nerve may inhibit sensory impulses from stretch receptors located in the quadriceps muscle. Electrophysiologic and pathologic studies have not detected LMN abnormalities, thus confirming clinical observations that the motor reflex pathways are intact.[32] When present, this clinical finding is highly suggestive of degenerative myelopathy (radiculomyelopathy). Pain perception from the pelvic limbs is normal, and there is no evidence of hyperesthesia, a highly significant finding. Abnormalities of micturition are uncommon. Muscle atrophy develops slowly and is clinically apparent only in long-standing cases. Hyperesthesia is absent. Although mild lesions occur in the cervical spinal cord, the thoracic limbs usually retain normal function.

Diagnosis. The clinical signs and the neurologic findings suggest a slowly progressive compression of the spinal cord. In fact, this disease originally was attributed to spinal cord compression from dural ossification, Hansen type II disk protrusions, or thoracolumbar spondylosis. Degenerative myelopathy must be differentiated radiographically from type II (slow) disk protrusions and spinal neoplasia. Survey radiography and myelography should be performed to rule out the presence of compressive (potentially surgically correctable) diseases. CSF is collected at the time of myelography to help exclude the presence of inflammatory diseases. Mild increases in CSF protein concentrations are seen in some cases, especially if the fluid is collected at the lumbar subarachnoid space. Vertebral spondylosis and dural ossification are common radiographic findings in older large breed dogs. They seldom cause neurologic dysfunction, and their presence does not correlate with clinical signs or pathologic findings in dogs with degenerative myelopathy.[30] The presence of a type II disk protrusion does not rule out degenerative myelopathy, so the prognosis is guarded, especially for German shepherd dogs. Lumbosacral degenerative stenosis can usually be differentiated by the significant hyperesthesia at the lumbosacral region.

Depressed cell-mediated immune responses to concanavalin A, phytohemagglutinin P, and pokeweed mitogens occur in most affected dogs.[29] These tests are not routinely available but could be useful, especially in dogs with a positive finding on myelography, to help rule out the presence of concurrent degenerative myelopathy. MR imaging may also be useful in identifying the lesions and monitoring their progression.[29]

Treatment. Because the cause is unknown, no specific treatment is available. The animal responds poorly, if at all, to corticosteroids, nonsteroidal anti-inflammatory drugs, or B-complex vitamins. Clemmons reported some therapeutic benefit from aminocaproic acid (Amicar, Lederle), 500 mg every 8 hours given orally.[29] The proposed mechanism involves an antiprotease action that blocks the final common pathway of tissue inflammation. Progression of the degenerative process was slower in about 50% of treated dogs, and improvement occurred in some. Benefits usually occurred within 8 weeks. Intrathecal interferon therapy has also been proposed.

The owner must be warned as to the hopeless prognosis for cure; however, with supportive care, many dogs can be maintained for several months before euthanasia becomes necessary.

Type II Disk Disease

Pathophysiology. Type II disk disease occurs primarily in older (5 to 12 years of age), large breed, nonchondrodystrophoid dogs. Similar protrusions are sometimes seen in smaller dogs and in cats. [1,39,40] The pathologic change within the intervertebral disk is a fibroid degeneration and a weakening of the dorsal annulus (see Fig. 7–3).[41] Recurrent partial disk protrusion produces a dome-shaped mass that eventually becomes large enough to compress the spinal cord or to irritate meninges and nerve roots. Pain, paresis and, occasionally, paralysis develop. The spinal cord changes are those of a compressive myelopathy.

Clinical Signs. The clinical signs are similar to those of degenerative myelopathy, in that type II disk protrusions result in slowly progressive signs of ataxia and paresis. With type II disk protrusions, regional hyperesthesia in the area of the protruded disk may be present, in contrast to the lack of hyperesthesia in degenerative myelopathy. However, many of these animals are not in pain, presumably because of the slow progression of the syndrome. In addition, voluntary micturition may be affected by the compressive myelopathy, whereas micturition usually remains normal in cases of degenerative myelopathy.

Neurologic abnormalities in the pelvic limbs reflect the level of the disk protrusion and can be very similar to the findings in dogs with degenerative myelopathy or spinal neoplasia. Disk protrusions involving cord segments T3–L3 result in UMN signs, whereas protrusions involving segments caudal to L3 can produce a mixture of UMN and LMN signs. Dogs are evaluated critically for spinal pain or hyperesthesia. The cutaneous reflex may be decreased caudal to the level of the lesion. The presence of these signs has great localizing value and helps to differentiate type II disk disease from degenerative myelopathy. The response to deep pain stimuli is usually normal in both diseases.

Diagnosis. Type II disk disease is differentiated from degenerative myelopathy by radiography of the spine. Plain radiographs rarely reveal the lesion, although suggestive changes may be seen. Increased density in the vertebral canal and narrowing of the disk space are not consistently present in type II disk protrusions. Myelography is usually necessary to demonstrate the compressive nature of the disk in question (Fig. 7–9). As in cases of degenerative myelopathy, dural ossification and spondylosis are common radiographic findings. These radiographic lesions should not be construed as the cause of the dog's neurologic dysfunction.

Treatment. Early cases may respond temporarily to anti-inflammatory drugs such as corticosteroids, phenylbutazone, or salicylates; however, the signs soon recur and progressively worsen. Dogs with pain as the only clinical sign can be treated medically, but decompressive surgery with removal of the protruded disk is more satisfactory in most cases. Decompressive surgery is indicated for all dogs with paresis and ataxia. Surgery should be performed early to prevent further neurologic deterioration. The prognosis with surgery is good, in that most dogs regain normal neurologic function. All owners should be cautioned that concurrent degenerative myelopathy is always a risk, especially in German shepherds.

Neoplasia

Pathophysiology. Tumors affecting the vertebra, the meninges, the nerve roots, or the spinal cord may result in neurologic signs. These tumors are classified according to tumor type as primary, metastatic, lymphoreticular, or skeletal, and according to location as extradural, intradural-extramedullary, and intramedullary. Primary CNS tumors are classified in Table

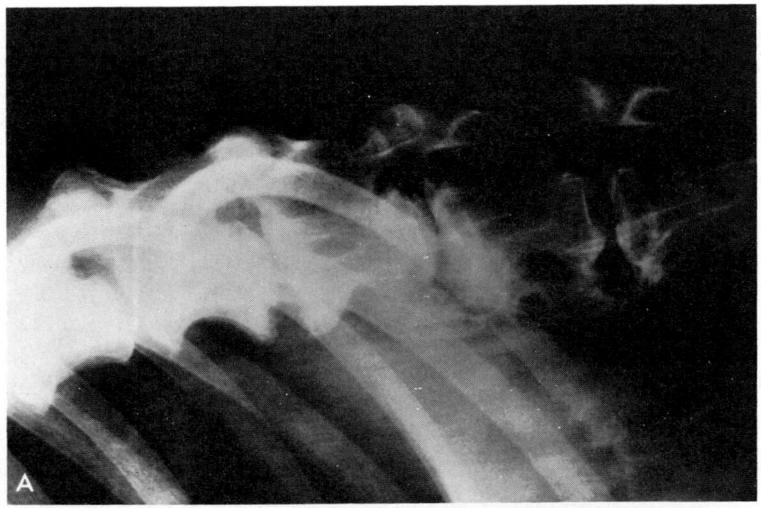

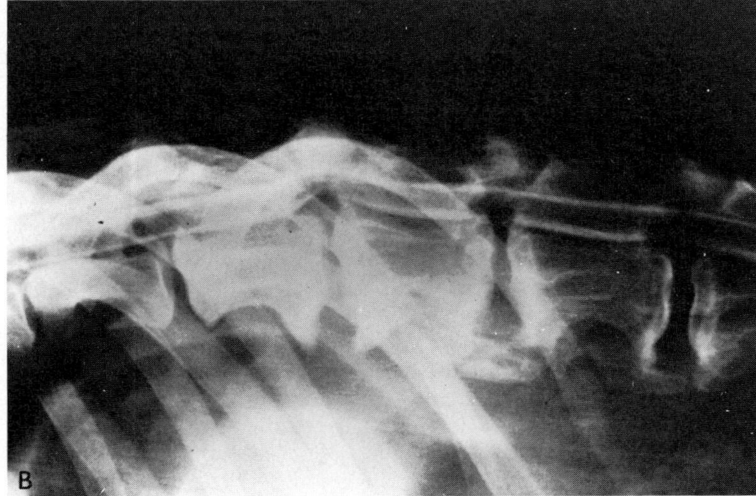

Figure 7–9 *A.* Survey lateral thoracolumbar radiograph of a dog with slowly progressive paraparesis. Note the extensive spondylosis. This radiographic finding is common in older large breed dogs; however, it is seldom a clinical problem. *B.* Myelogram of the same dog. Note the prominent extramedullary compression at T13–L1 from a type II disk protrusion. (From Kneller SK, et al: Differential diagnosis of progressive caudal paresis in an aged German shepherd dog. JAAHA 11:414, 1975. Used by permission.)

16–6. In general, the more common tumors are extradural and affect structures that house the spinal cord, such as the vertebrae or other tissues, and produce a compressive myelopathy when the mass expands on or around the cord. Most tumors slowly compress the spinal cord, producing signs similar to those of degenerative myelopathy and type II disk disease. Extradural tumors frequently cause pain, often before there is significant paresis.[42] Intradural-extramedullary tumors are usually meningiomas or nerve sheath tumors, and may be painful. A unique intradural-extramedullary, blast cell tumor is seen in young dogs, 6 months to 3 years of age, that affects the T10–L2 spinal cord segments.[43,44] Intramedullary tumors are either metastatic or primary tumors of nervous tissue. Gliomas and ependymomas are the most common.[42] Sudden onset of signs of a transverse myelopathy may be seen with intramedullary neoplasms affecting the spinal cord, presumably when blood vessels are compromised. Some tumors, such as lymphosarcoma, may embolize arteries of the spinal cord.

Skeletal (Vertebral) Tumors. Vertebral tumors may be primary or may arise from metastases. The latter case is more common. Generally, as the tumors grow into the vertebral canal, the spinal cord is compressed slowly, producing signs of a slowly progressive myelopathy. Occasionally the tumor causes considerable vertebral destruction without cord compression. These vertebrae are weakened and may fracture, resulting in acute spinal cord compression. Vertebral tumors are usually painful because of periosteal and, perhaps, meningeal irritation. Primary vertebral tumors include osteomas, osteosarcomas (Fig. 7–10), chondromas, chondrosarcomas, and plasma cell myelomas (Fig. 7–11). A variety of carcinomas and sarcomas

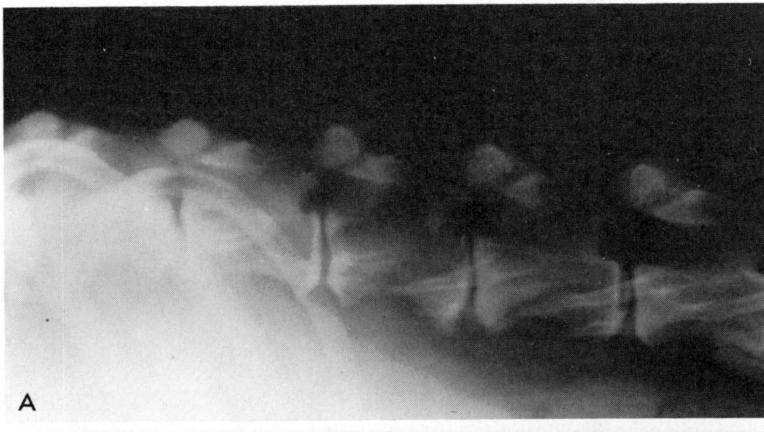

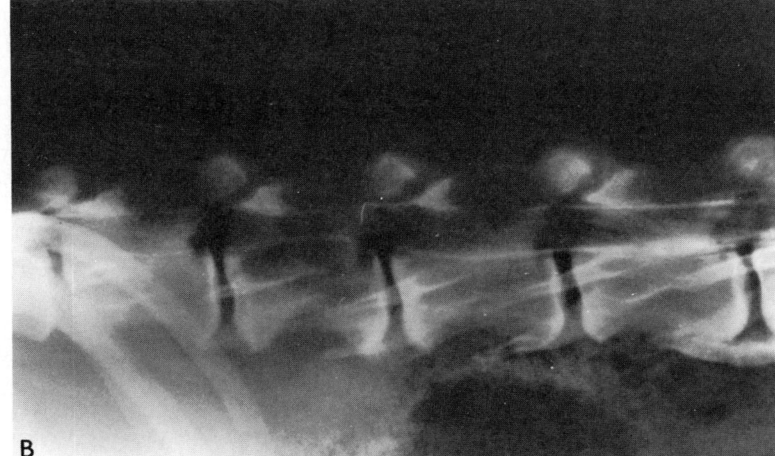

Figure 7–10 *A.* Osteogenic sarcoma of L2 in a dog with paraplegia and severe back pain. *B.* Myelogram of the thoracolumbar area of the same dog, demonstrating extradural compression at L2.

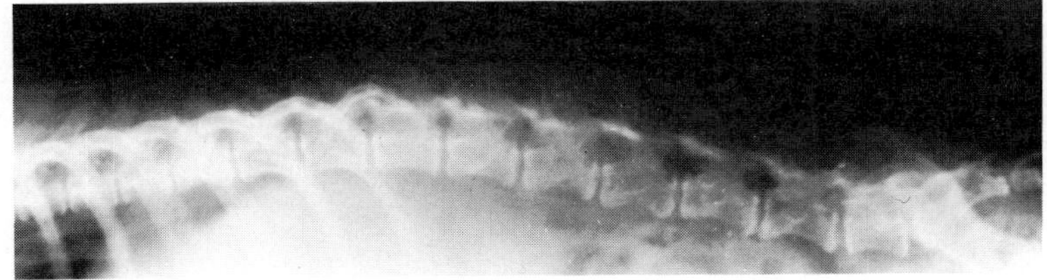

Figure 7–11 Lateral thoracolumbar radiograph demonstrating multiple areas of bone lysis in several vertebrae. These changes are characteristic of plasma cell myeloma.

metastatic to vertebrae have been reported. Survey radiographs of the spine are usually diagnostic. Treatment is usually palliative, although total vertebral removal with spinal column fixation has been advocated for certain benign tumors.

Lymphoreticular Tumors. These tumors grow in the vertebral canal and are considered epidural. They do not arise from a vertebra or from the meninges. Lymphosarcoma involving the vertebral canal is frequently encountered in cats and cattle, but is uncommon in the dog and the horse. Tumor growth within the vertebral canal produces a compressive myelopathy. Several segments of the spinal cord may be involved, but lesions in the feline and the bovine are most common in thoracolumbar segments. Spinal lymphosarcoma must be considered in any cat or in older cows with a history of progressive neurologic dysfunction of the pelvic limbs. In addition to pelvic limb ataxia and paresis, regional hyperesthesia may be present. Survey radiographs are usually normal. Myelography may reveal extensive compression, because the tumor may fill the vertebral canals of several vertebrae. In a study of 21 cases of lymphoma in the vertebral canal of cats, 85% of the 13 animals necropsied had lymphoma in other organs. Of 19 cats tested for feline leukemia virus, 16 (84.2%) were positive. CSF analysis yields variable results. The CSF is normal when the tumor is outside the meninges. In some animals the CSF may contain malignant lymphocytes and may have increased protein concentrations. In the cat, lymphosarcoma must be differentiated from the neurologic form of feline infectious peritonitis, which may also affect the thoracolumbar spinal cord and results in progressive pelvic limb paresis and ataxia. In feline infectious peritonitis, the CSF usually contains a marked increase in protein, neutrophils, and some mononuclear cells. Fluoroscopically guided percutaneous fine-needle aspiration of epidural masses is an effective method for establishing a definitive diagnosis.[45] Therapy for epidural lymphosarcoma may provide some benefit. Chemotherapy or surgical excision and chemotherapy may result in remission.[46] Treatment for intradural lymphosarcoma is usually ineffective. Corticosteroids may alleviate some of the clinical signs temporarily.

Metastatic Tumors. Malignant tumors may metastasize to the vertebra and, rarely, to the spinal cord. Neurologic signs result from spinal cord compression secondary to vertebral instability or direct compression by the neoplastic mass. Malignant mammary tumors, prostatic adenocarcinomas, and hemangiosarcomas are tumors that most frequently metastasize to a vertebra. The rare tumor, multiple myeloma, also may involve one or more vertebrae, sometimes producing multifocal signs. Spinal radiographs are usually diagnostic (see Fig. 7–11). The tumor type is confirmed by histopathology. Treatment is palliative.

Primary Tumors. Primary tumors affecting the spinal cord may be intramedullary or intradural-extramedullary.[42] Extramedullary tumors may arise from nerve roots (nerve sheath tumors) or from the meninges (meningiomas). Nerve sheath tumors, including schwannomas and neurofibromas, arise from nerve roots or peripheral nerves. They may be extradural or intradural. Early extramedullary neurofibromas result in clinical signs that are restricted to the distribution of the affected nerve root. These early signs may go undetected if nerve roots T3–L3 are affected. These nerve roots innervate the muscles of the trunk, which are difficult to examine for neurologic dysfunction. If the nerve roots forming the brachial or lumbosacral plexus are involved, neurologic signs of monoparesis develop. As these tumors grow, they follow the nerve proximally to invade or compress the spinal cord, resulting in more symmetric neurologic signs caudal to the lesion. Survey radiographs may show an enlarged intervertebral foramen, while myelography may demonstrate spinal cord compression (Fig 7–12). Many of these tumors are inoperable because the tumor either has invaded the spinal cord or involves multiple nerve roots that cannot be sacrificed at surgery. In some cases, the tumor and the affected nerve root can be removed. However, recurrence is frequent because of residual tumor cells. Amputation with complete resection of nerve roots is often the best hope for successful treatment.

Meningiomas usually grow slowly and cause progressive compression of the spinal cord. The site of the lesion may be painful. The clinical course usually resembles that of type II disk disease or degenerative myelopathy. Myelography is necessary for detection of extramedullary spinal cord compression. These lesions should be surgically explored, as many meningiomas can be completely removed if detected early.

Medullary tumors of the spinal cord are rare. Initial signs may be unilateral; however, as the tumor grows, bilateral signs develop. Myelography is helpful for differentiating extramedullary compression from intramedullary tumors (Figs. 7–10B and 7–13A). The prognosis is poor, because these tumors are generally inoperable, although newer microsurgical techniques may allow resection in some cases (Fig. 7–13B).

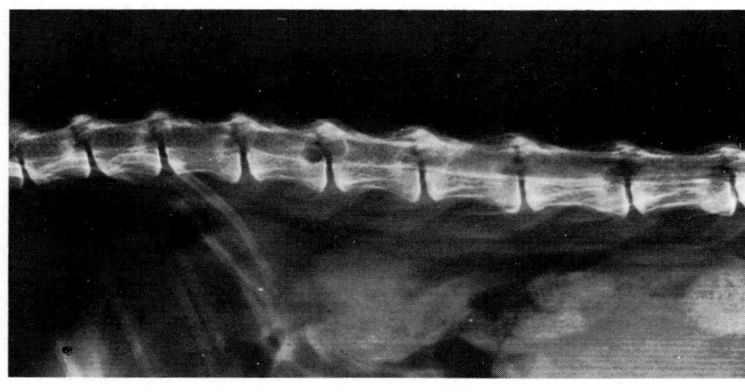

Figure 7–12 Lateral thoracolumbar myelogram of a cat with progressive paraparesis. Note the enlarged intervertebral foramen at L2–L3, suggesting a mass in this area. These changes are characteristic of nerve sheath tumors (the eventual diagnosis in this case).

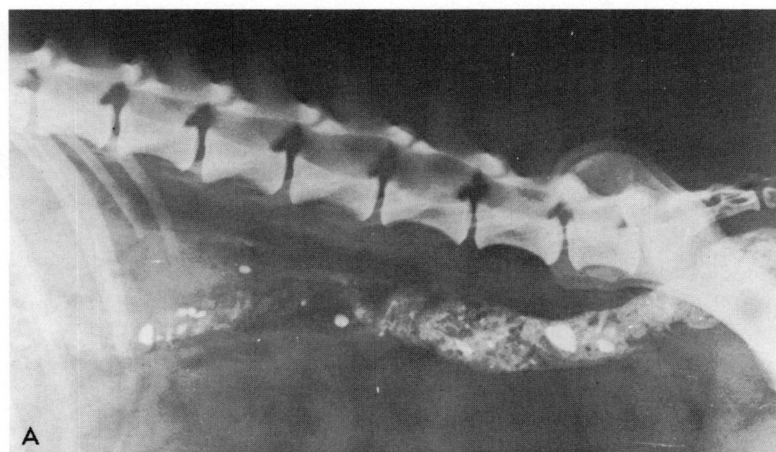

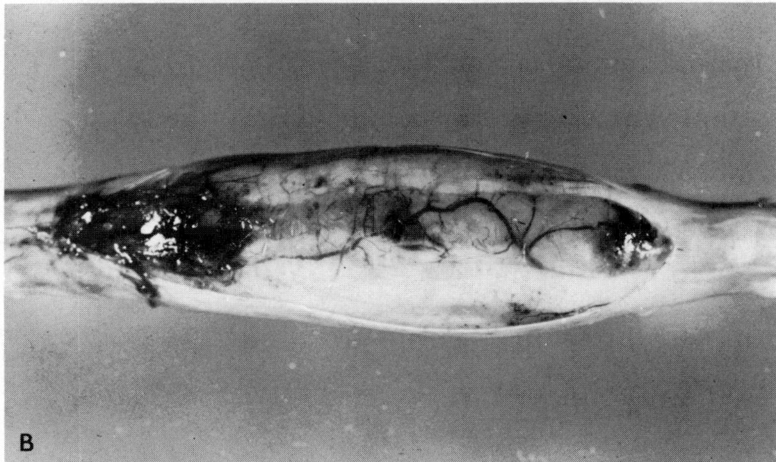

Figure 7–13 *A*. Lateral lumbar radiograph of a dog with progressive lower motor neuron paraparesis, constipation, and urinary incontinence. Note the enlarged vertebral canal of L4 and L5. These changes are characteristic of expanding intramedullary tumors. *B*. Spinal cord section from the same dog, which was affected with an intramedullary tumor. The expanding tumor produced the radiographic changes in *A*.

Spinal Dural Ossification

Dural ossification, also known as ossifying pachymeningitis, is a common radiographic or necropsy finding in middle-aged or older dogs (Fig. 7–14). Plaques of bone develop on the inner dural surface in response to an unidentified factor. The lesion is most common in large breed dogs and is often identified in association with vertebral spondylosis. The disease most commonly affects the cervical and lumbar areas. At one time, the clinical signs of degenerative myelopathy and canine wobbler syndrome were attributed to dural ossification. Later studies have demonstrated no relationship between the bony plaques and the clinical signs. The bony plaques are of little clinical importance except in rare cases in which they entrap a nerve root or cause pain. We have observed one dog with extensive dural ossification that developed clinical signs of pelvic limb paralysis following trauma. No antemortem or necropsy evidence of vertebral fracture or luxation was found. At necropsy, a large subdural hematoma was present, which apparently resulted from a fracture of a large dural bony plaque. It was believed that spinal cord compression from this hematoma produced the neurologic signs.

Rarely, large dural plaques may cause local spinal cord edema, necrosis, or fibrosis. Radiographs are useful for establishing the diagnosis in life. Myelographic evidence of compression warrants exploratory decompression of the lesion. Medical treatment is nonspecific and is directed at relief of pain. Clinicians should make every attempt to find other causes for the neurologic signs before assuming that dural ossification is the cause.

Spondylosis Deformans (Hypertrophic Spondylosis)

This noninfectious, nonseptic condition is a common finding during routine radiographic or

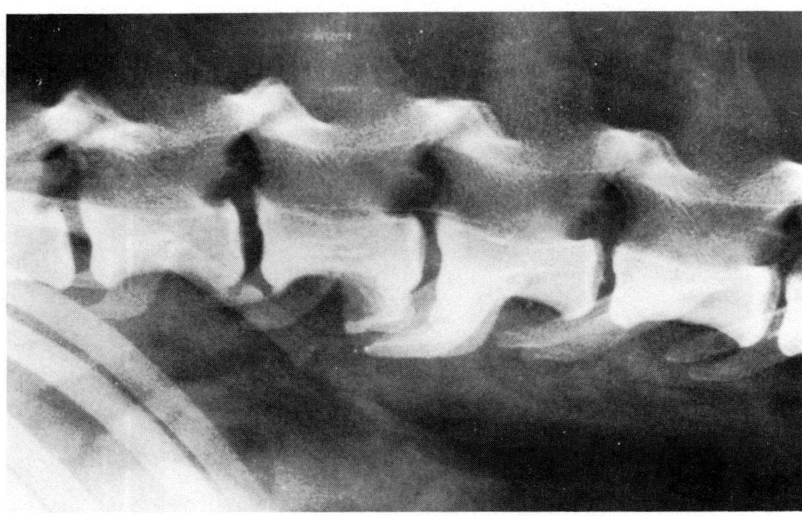

Figure 7–14 Severe spondylosis of the lumbar vertebrae and dural ossification were incidental findings in this dog. These changes seldom cause neurologic signs.

necropsy examinations. It is characterized by the formation of bony spurs and bridges at the intervertebral spaces (see Figs. 7–9A and 7–14). The term *spondylitis* originally was used to describe this condition, because investigators believed that inflammation produced the bony reaction. Later work suggested that the condition was a noninflammatory process associated with degeneration of the annulus fibrosus of the intervertebral disk.[47] The term *spondylosis* is therefore preferred. Although degeneration of the annulus may be important in the pathogenesis, nuclear degeneration and disk protrusion are not. The presence of spondylosis at a disk space is not proof of disk protrusion. The condition may be present anywhere in the spine but is most common in the caudal thoracic and caudal lumbar vertebrae. Spondylosis occurs in most species but is most frequent in dogs, bulls, and pigs.[5,48,49]

Morgan found that osteophyte formation within the spinal canal is very rare and seldom, if ever, results in spinal cord compression.[47] In addition, the osteophyte formation does not constrict spinal nerves and usually is present without detectable clinical signs. Spondylosis rarely causes neurologic signs; however, occasionally it may produce spinal pain, especially after exercise. Spondylosis is frequently present at L7–S1 in dogs and may be associated with stenosis of the vertebral canal or intervertebral foramina that produces pain and LMN signs (see Degenerative Lumbosacral Stenosis). As is true with dural ossification, clinicians must search for other causes of the neurologic signs before assuming that spondylosis is the cause. Radiographic examinations can differentiate this condition from the true inflammatory spinal disorders (osteomyelitis, diskospondylitis) that produce severe neurologic and musculoskeletal signs. Aspirin, phenylbutazone, and corticosteroids may be required in some cases to help alleviate spinal discomfort in animals with severe ankylosing spondylosis.

Multiple Cartilaginous Exostoses

Multiple cartilaginous exostoses, also known as osteochondromatosis, osteocartilaginous exostoses, and multiple osteochondroma, are a condition that occurs in dogs, cats, and horses. The disease is a benign proliferation of cartilage and bone that affects the bones formed by endochondral ossification. In addition to the appendicular skeleton, lesions may develop in the vertebral bodies or the dorsal spinous processes (Fig. 7–15A). The ribs are also commonly affected (Fig. 7–15B). A small percentage of cartilaginous exostoses may undergo malignant transformation into chondrosarcoma. Clinical evidence indicates that the condition may be inherited in the dog and horse.[50,51]

Clinical signs appear during the period of active bone growth. Pain or loss of function develops when adjacent structures are compressed or distorted by the bony lesions.[52] Vertebral involvement is frequent in the dog. Spinal cord compression with neurologic deficits caudal to the lesion is common (Fig. 7–15C). In the majority of dogs studied, progressive paraparesis was the most common neurologic finding; however, compressive lesions in the cervical spine may produce progressive tetraparesis. Radiographically, the bony exostoses are characterized as variably sized radiopaque densities with large radiolu-

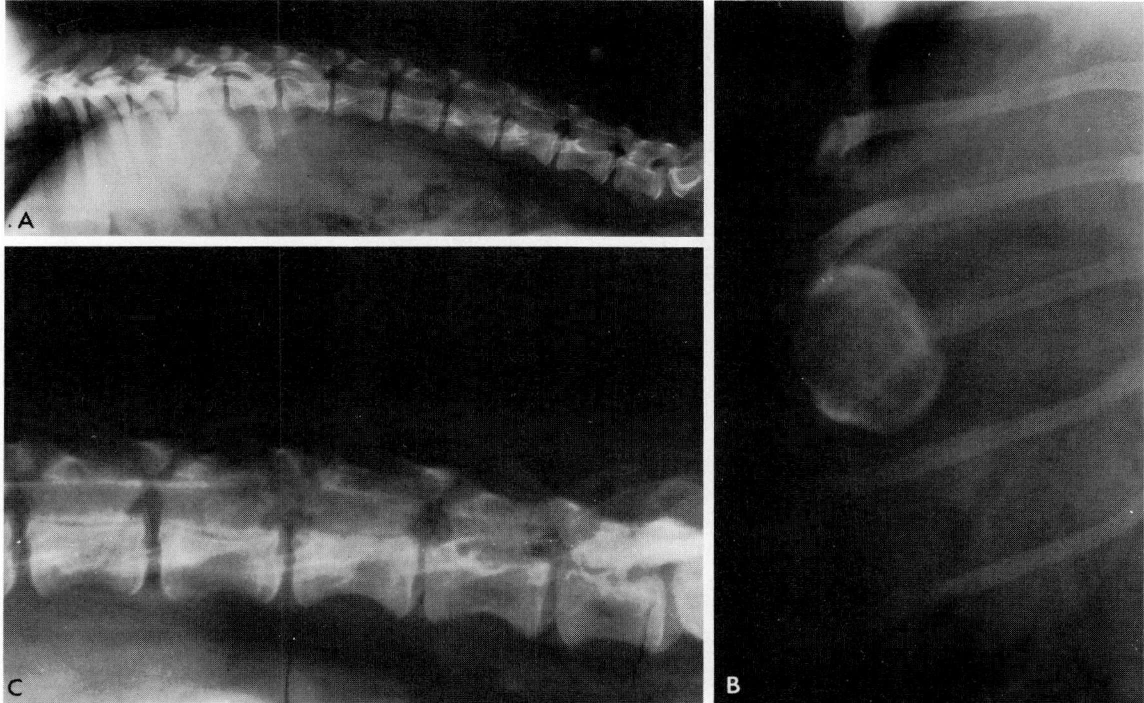

Figure 7–15 *A*. Multiple cartilaginous exostoses affecting the vertebrae of a young dog. Note the cystlike structures within the vertebrae. *B*. Radiograph of a cystlike bone lesion in the rib of the same dog. These bony, bullae-like structures are diagnostic of multiple cartilaginous exostoses. *C*. Myelogram demonstrating severe spinal cord compression from L4–L6. Occasionally, these lesions undergo malignant transformation to chondrosarcoma.

cent areas. Vertebral lesions tend to be circular in shape. Radiography provides strong supportive evidence of the diagnosis; however, a definitive diagnosis of multiple cartilaginous exostoses is based on typical biopsy findings. A microscopic examination of a tissue specimen is necessary in order to differentiate the condition from malignant vertebral neoplasia.

The exostoses apparently stop growing after physeal closure. Surgical removal of the lesion should be attempted if skeletal or neurologic dysfunction is present.

Afghan Hound Myelopathy

In 1973, Cockrell and co-workers described a demyelinating malacic spinal cord disease in related young Afghan hounds.[53] The age at onset varied from 3 to 13 months, and the clinical course was 2 to 6 weeks. Affected dogs developed progressive pelvic limb ataxia and paresis. Spinal reflexes were usually normal or exaggerated. In some dogs, mild thoracic limb deficits were detected. The disorder progressed to tetraplegia and death from respiratory failure in 2 to 6 weeks. Severe destruction of myelin with relative sparing of axons was found in the ventral, lateral, and sometimes dorsal funiculi. The lesions were prominent in spinal cord segments C5–L3. The most severe changes were found in the cranial thoracic spinal cord.

The pathogenesis is unknown, although a genetic basis may be important. de Lahunta proposes that the lesion is a primary leukodystrophy with a hereditary basis.[54] There is no effective treatment.

Diskospondylitis and Vertebral Abscess

Pathologic Findings. Diskospondylitis is an intervertebral disk infection with concurrent osteomyelitis of contiguous vertebrae (Fig. 7–16). Various causes are known, including foreign body migration and bacterial or fungal infection. In dogs, the most common causes are *Staphylococcus aureus*, *Staphylococcus intermedius*, and, occasionally, *Brucella canis*.[55] Diskospondylitis is associated with urinary tract infection and bacteremia. Infection of the intervertebral disks and the vertebrae usually occurs secondary to infection of one of these primary foci. Infrequently, infection may occur secondary to surgical fenestration of the disks. The infection may involve cervical or thoracolumbar verte-

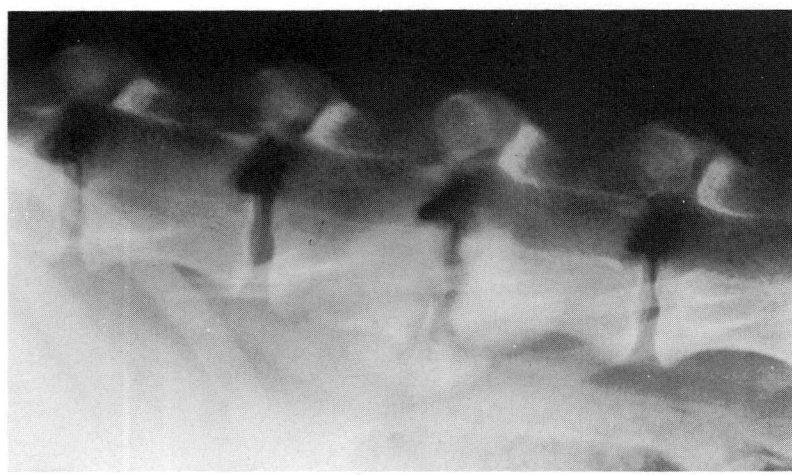

Figure 7–16 Lateral lumbar radiograph of a dog with fever, depression, and severe back pain. There is lysis at the L3–L4 disk space, with involvement of the vertebral bodies in this area. New bone production is also present. This lesion is characteristic of diskospondylitis.

brae; however, it most frequently develops in the vertebrae of the back.

Vertebral abscesses are formed primarily in young or debilitated large animals. There is often an association with omphalophlebitis (navel ill) in calves and foals, tail docking in lambs, erysipelas arthritis in swine,[56] pneumonia in cattle,[57] and enteric *Salmonella* infections in horses. The bacteria producing vertebral abscesses in foals include *Salmonella* spp., *Streptococcus* spp., *Actinobacillus equuli, Eikenella corodens,* and *Rhodococcus equi*. In adult horses, *Brucella abortus* and *Mycobacterium tuberculosis* are reported.[5] In food animals, *Corynebacterium pyogenes* is the bacterium most commonly isolated, but *Spherophorus* spp. and *Staphylococcus* spp. in cattle and streptococci and *Erysipelothrix insidiosa* in swine are also common.[5]

Neurologic signs develop from encroachment on the spinal cord or nerve roots by the expanding tissues, causing severe pain and, eventually, paresis. Destruction of the vertebrae may cause spinal instability with secondary compression of the spinal cord (Fig. 7–17). Paresis or paralysis and ataxia caudal to the lesion result from the spinal cord compression.

Clinical Signs. Diskospondylitis may affect dogs of any age but is more common in adults. In one study, the mean age was 5.1 years.[58] This disease is apparently more frequent in male dogs than in female dogs (2:1 ratio). In all animals, clinical signs may develop acutely and progress rapidly; however, the usual course is chronic and progressive. Most animals have systemic signs, including anorexia, depression, and pyrexia. In dogs, signs of urinary tract infec-

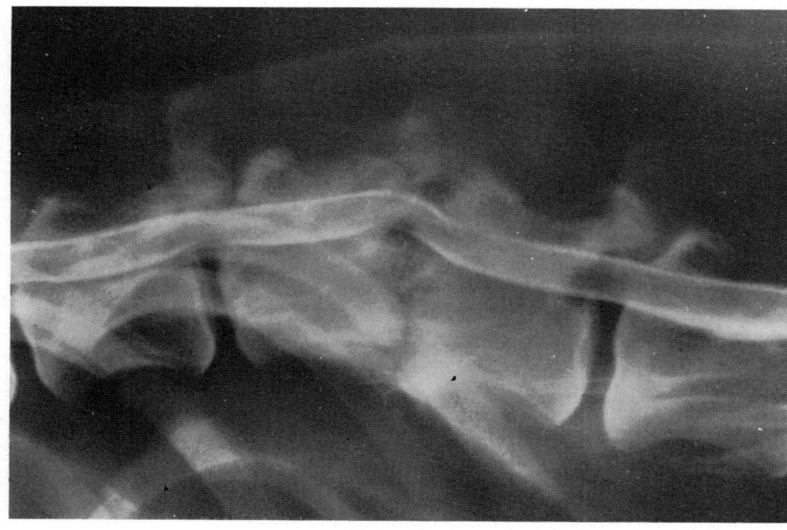

Figure 7–17 Myelogram of lumbar diskospondylitis demonstrating spinal cord compression secondary to lumbar vertebral instability. This dog had acute pelvic limb paralysis, although other signs had been present for several weeks.

tion or endocarditis-myocarditis occasionally are detected. Dogs with brucellosis may have signs suggesting this disease (orchitis, epididymitis, abortion, infertility, and so forth). Systemic signs, however, usually are not localizing to any body system.

Frequently encountered clinical signs are directly referable to the musculoskeletal and nervous systems. These signs include hyperesthesia in the area of vertebral involvement, a stiff gait, and paresis or paralysis if spinal cord compression occurs. The syndrome is quite similar to intervertebral disk disease, except that animals with diskospondylitis frequently are systemically ill and have a more chronic course of disease. Large breed dogs with type II disk disease rarely are in as much pain as those with diskospondylitis. Specific neurologic signs relate to the site of involvement. Cervical lesions may cause tetraparesis and severe neck pain. Thoracolumbar lesions cause back pain and pelvic limb paresis and ataxia.

Diskospondylitis and vertebral abscesses always are suspected in animals with fever, depression, anorexia, vertebral pain, and pelvic limb ataxia or paresis.

Diagnosis. A definitive diagnosis is made with conventional radiography of the spine. Occasionally, radiographic abnormalities are not detected in early lesions, even though typical clinical signs are present.[59] Radiographically evident lesions may lag behind the onset of clinical signs for 4 to 6 weeks. Typical radiographic findings include concentric lysis of adjacent vertebral end-plates and varying degrees of vertebral lysis and bone production (see Fig. 7–16). Vertebral bodies may be shortened, and intervertebral disk spaces may be narrowed. Severely destructive lesions may cause vertebral luxation and spinal cord compression (see Fig. 7–17). Radionuclide scintigraphy may be useful if there is a strong suspicion of diskospondylitis without vertebral lesions on survey radiographs. Radiographic changes may not be apparent for about 2 weeks after infection, whereas scintigraphy may demonstrate the lesion within 3 days.[55]

Affected dogs occasionally have leukocytosis and pyuria. Leukocytosis is more common in dogs with associated endocarditis. The CSF is usually normal, although elevations in protein concentration and mononuclear cells are occasionally encountered. Blood cultures are positive in about 75% of cases, and *Staphylococcus aureus* is the most common bacterium isolated.[59] Urine cultures also may be positive, and *S. aureus* usually is isolated in these tests as well. The tube agglutination test is usually positive in dogs affected with *Brucella canis*. Aspiration of the lesion may be accomplished with fluroscopic guidance in small animals and directly in large animals. Cultures of this material can establish a definitive diagnosis.[5,60]

Treatment. Antibiotic therapy is based on sensitivity testing of bacteria isolated from urine or blood or from infected tissues (see Chap. 5). Antibiotic therapy alone is suggested unless there is severe spinal cord compression or there is no response to therapy within 5 days. Therapy should be continued for at least 4 to 6 weeks. Compressive lesions require decompression, curettage, and stabilization in addition to long-term antibiotic therapy. Brucellosis is difficult to resolve and warrants a poor prognosis, and owners should be advised of the risk of transmission to humans (see Chap. 5). In large animals, antibiotic therapy is based on culture and sensitivity testing. In horses, surgical curettage and drainage of infected vertebrae is beneficial. Dogs that respond favorably in the first week have a good prognosis. The lesions should be monitored radiographically for several months for signs of progression.

Acute Progressive Diseases, L4–S3

The acute progressive diseases affecting the caudal lumbar and sacral spinal cord segments are listed by etiologic category in Tables 7–4, 7–5, and 7–6. Most of these diseases have been discussed in the previous sections that considered T3–L3 disorders. It must be remembered that some of these diseases initially may present as pelvic limb paresis but may progress to involve the cervical spinal cord. Tetraparesis (tetraplegia) may develop as the disease progresses (see Chap. 8).

Acute Nonprogressive Diseases, L4–S3

In this section, two diseases will be described: fibrocartilaginous embolization and lumbosacral trauma. Although fibrocartilaginous embolization can affect any spinal cord segment, it occurs most frequently in the caudal lumbar area. For this reason, we have elected to discuss it with the other L4–S3 disorders. Fibrocartilaginous embolization has a brief progressive course (a few hours) and then becomes nonprogressive. We have therefore classified it as a nonprogressive disease.

Fibrocartilaginous Embolization

Pathophysiology. Although emboli to the nervous system can come from a variety of sources, such as endocarditis, sepsis, and fat, the most common form causing spinal cord infarction is a fibrocartilaginous material. The cause of this disease is uncertain. It occurs in dogs, horses, cats, pigs, sheep, and humans.[61,62] Fibrocartilaginous material found in spinal cord arterioles and veins results in an ischemic necrotizing myelopathy (Fig. 7–18). Exactly how this material is distributed into the spinal cord circulation is not known, but several theories have been proposed. Most of these hypotheses are based on the belief that fibrocartilaginous emboli originate from the intervertebral disks. The most probable mechanism is herniation of disk material into the body of the vertebra, followed by entrance into a venous plexus and then into an arteriovenous anastomosis. The material could then enter the spinal cord in either arteries, veins, or both.[61,63]

Clinical Signs. The clinical signs develop acutely and progress rapidly within 1 to 2 hours from initial pain to unilateral or bilateral paralysis. Unilateral or asymmetric signs are common, which is explained by the frequency of unilateral branches of the central branch of the ventral spinal artery. Vigorous exercise may precede the development of signs; however, known trauma is absent. The clinical syndrome is characteristic of acute spinal cord compression from herniated intervertebral disks or vertebral fractures, except that hyperesthesia is absent. Lateralization of signs is very suggestive of fibrocartilaginous embolization, because spinal cord compression generally causes bilateral signs. The degree and character of the neurologic deficit correspond to the site and the extent of the spinal cord infarction. Larger breed dogs are affected most often. Chondrodystrophoid breeds with a predisposition for type I disk disease are affected infrequently.

Diagnosis. The key features of fibrocartilaginous embolization are a large-breed dog, acute onset, nonprogressive course (except for the first few hours), and a nonpainful, asymmetric paresis. A few animals may seem to be in pain for 1 or more days. Asymmetry is not found in every case, but is a valuable sign when present. Trauma is not in the history, but dogs are frequently reported to be exercising at the time of onset. There is no definitive antemortem diagnostic procedure for fibrocartilaginous embolization. The diagnosis is supported by evidence that rules out the presence of spinal cord compression. Survey radiography and myelography are usually negative. The myelogram may show a slight swelling of the spinal cord for the first few days. The hemogram and the biochemistries are normal. The CSF may contain a slight increase in protein.

Treatment. Therapy for fibrocartilaginous embolization is largely aimed at reducing spinal cord edema and inflammation with corticosteroids. If therapy can be administered in the first few hours after onset, the protocol described in the section on spinal cord trauma is recommended. If therapy is delayed, it is probably of no benefit. The benefit of anticoagulants is unknown, but since this is not a clotting problem there is no reason to expect it to be useful. Affected dogs should rest for 1 to 2 weeks. Improvement should be noted within a few days, but functional recovery may require several weeks. The clinical signs of complete paralysis, analgesia, or LMN involvement are associated with a very poor prognosis. Motor neurons are destroyed in the infarcted area. If this includes innervation of the limb or bladder, the deficit is likely to be permanent. Because recovery from white matter damage is more likely to occur, UMN deficits have a better prognosis.

Trauma

Pelvic fractures, caudal lumbar fractures, and lumbosacral subluxations are very common skeletal injuries in animals. Traumatic lesions in this area may involve the termination of the spinal cord or the cauda equina. These injuries

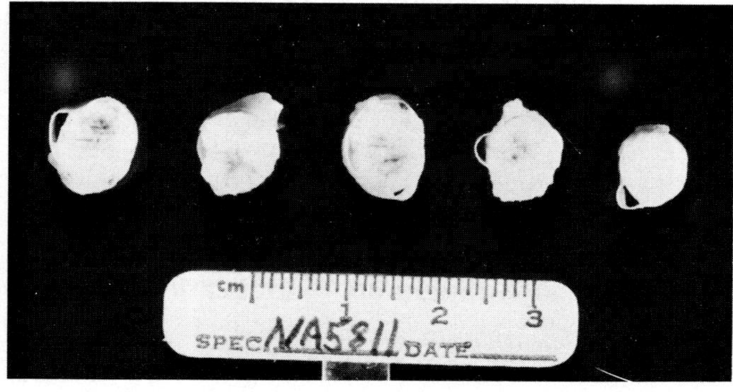

Figure 7–18 Severe lumbar spinal cord necrosis secondary to fibrocartilaginous embolization and vessel infarction. Clinical signs developed acutely in a 5-year-old Great Dane.

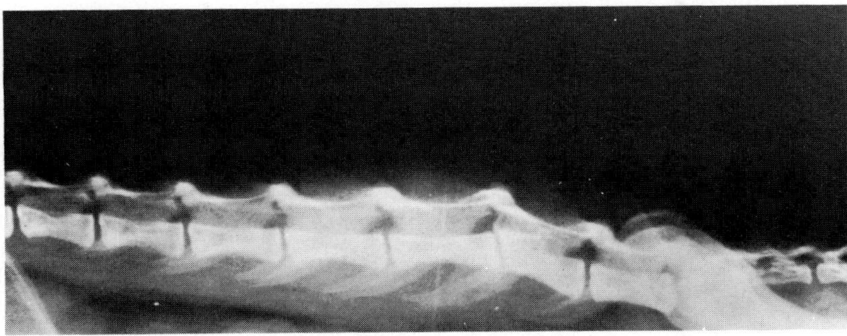

Figure 7–19 Compressive fracture of L6 produced severe paraplegia and loss of deep pain sensation caudal to the lesion. Although little displacement is appreciated radiographically, the fracture had functionally severed the spinal cord.

may compress or entrap the roots of the sciatic, pelvic, and pudendal nerves, resulting in severe neurologic dysfunction of the pelvic limbs, the urinary bladder, and the anal sphincter (Fig. 7–19). The assessment of pelvic fractures or lumbosacral subluxations must include a neurologic evaluation of the pelvic limbs, the external anal sphincter, and the urinary bladder. The prognosis for recovery is much better in animals with normal neurologic function. The diagnosis and management of sciatic nerve injury are discussed in Chapter 6.

Sacral and caudal fractures are common, especially in cats, but they also occur in dogs, horses, and cattle. The syndrome in cats is usually caused by a fracture or luxation at the sacrocaudal junction. Traction injury to the cauda equina results in loss of innervation to the tail, perineum, anal sphincter, and urinary bladder. Functional assessment of the anal sphincter affords a good indirect assessment of bladder function. However, some animals have normal anal sphincter function with no bladder function. The mechanism is not clear, but may indicate intrapelvic injury to the pelvic nerves. Animals with complete denervation to the perineum, anal sphincter, and bladder have a grave prognosis. We generally recommend medical management for 4 to 6 weeks in case the injury is only temporary (see Chap. 3 for management of neurogenic bladder).

Chronic Progressive Diseases, L4–S3

Degenerative Lumbosacral Stenosis

Compression of the cauda equina at the lumbosacral articulation has been reported in several dogs of varying ages and breeds. In several studies, older German shepherd dogs or crossbred German shepherd dogs were affected more frequently.[64,65] The condition is relatively common; it affects all breeds, although larger dogs are more commonly affected, and frequently it is not recognized because of the occurrence of other problems in the same dogs.[66–68]

Pathogenesis. Although the cause is unknown, the common initiating factor for the degenerative changes is probably abnormal motion at the lumbosacral articulations. The biomechanical abnormality causes cumulative microtrauma, resulting in replacement of damaged tissue with excessive quantities of poor quality (weaker) tissue consisting of fibrous connective tissue and osteophytes. Stresses on the annulus fibrosus lead to proliferative changes and bulging of the disk. In essence this is a Hansen type II disk degeneration with additional changes in the articulations and vertebral end-plates. Narrowing of the disk causes the intervertebral foramen to be smaller. When there are osteophytes around the foramen, the L7 spinal nerve is entrapped (Fig. 7–20). In some cases there is ventral displacement of the sacrum relative to L7, further narrowing the ver-

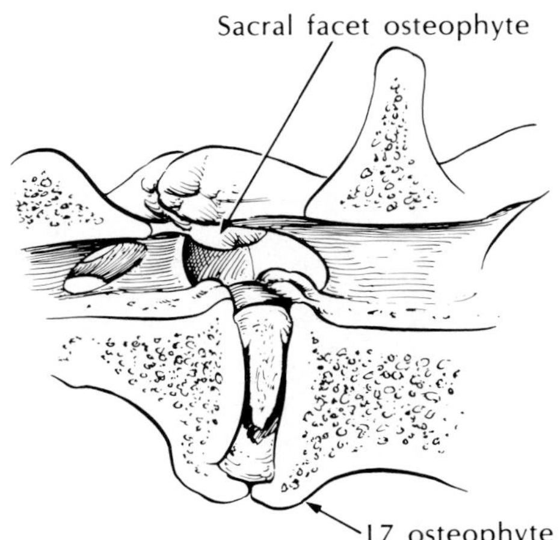

Figure 7–20 Lumbosacral degenerative stenosis. Compromise of intervertebral foramen by articular osteophytes that have formed on facet and vertebral body. (From Chambers JN: Degenerative lumbosacral stenosis in dogs. Vet Med Rep 1:166–180, 1989. Used by permission.)

tebral canal. Proliferation of the soft tissues of the joints, annulus fibrosus, and interarcuate ligament contributes to the compression. Extension of the joint causes additonal folding of these tissues, thereby increasing pressure on the nerves (Fig. 7–21). A few animals appear to have a narrow canal with shortened pedicles, suggesting a developmental stenosis similar to the cervical spondylopathy in Great Danes.

This syndrome appears to have several similarities to canine wobbler syndrome (cervical spondylopathy—see Chap. 8). Both syndromes are characterized by a narrowing of the vertebral canal as a result of subluxation or stenosis of the vertebral foramen. Altered soft tissue structures and type II disk herniations may narrow the vertebral canal further. Cervical spondylopathy results in spinal cord compression, whereas lumbosacral spondylopathy produces compression or entrapment of the cauda equina or the L7 nerve root. The high incidence in the German shepherd dog suggests a developmental predisposition, even though the clinical signs occur in older dogs.

Clinical Signs. Early clinical signs are related to lumbosacral pain. Dogs may experience difficulty rising, and at this stage, the clinical signs are easily confused with hip dysplasia. Recurring lameness of one or both pelvic limbs is common. The owner frequently reports that the dog will not jump or has difficulty going up steps. Exercise often exacerbates the signs. At this stage, various orthopedic problems, including hip dysplasia and stifle injury, are often suspected. Because most of the affected dogs also commonly have hip dysplasia, the primary problem is frequently missed. Rear limb paresis is not usual unless the condition is advanced. Then, the problem is usually weakness in the muscles innervated by the sciatic nerve, causing decreased extension of the hock. Only rarely are significant proprioceptive positioning deficits present. A few animals appear to have paresthesia in the tail or perineal region and may lick or chew the affected area. Frequently the owner may notice a less erect tail carriage.

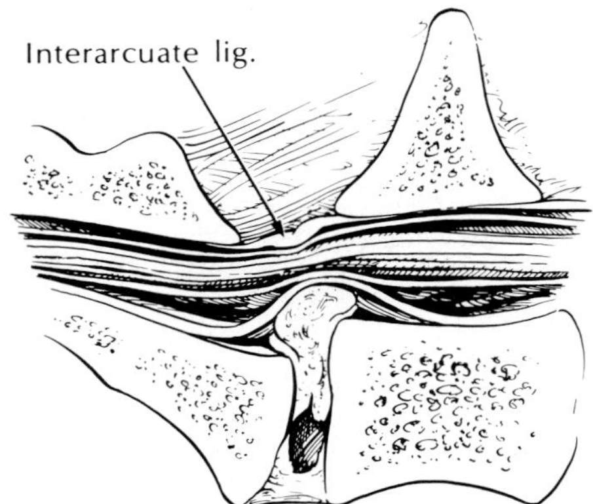

Figure 7–21 Lumbosacral degenerative stenosis. Compression of cauda equina in sagittal plane by combined effects of disk herniation and ventral folding of interarcuate ligament. Note how extension would increase the compression. (From Chambers JN: Degenerative lumbosacral stenosis in dogs. Vet Med Rep 1:166–180, 1989. Used by permission.)

Urinary and fecal incontinence are common associated clinical signs in advanced cases and result from compression of the sacral nerves. The anal sphincter may be atonic, and the perineal reflex may be weak or absent. The urinary incontinence is of the LMN type, resulting in a poor detrusor reflex and a weak urethral sphincter. The bladder usually is easily expressed.

In early cases the examination indicates a lameness, without paresis, normal to marginally slow postural reactions, and normal spinal reflexes. Some animals appear to have brisk knee jerk reflexes because of loss of resistance from the flexors innervated by the sciatic nerve. The flexion reflex is usually not weak until the condition is severe. The key to clinical diagnosis is localization of hyperesthesia in the lumbosacral region. Over 90% of affected dogs will be in pain. It is imperative that the examiner elicit pain from the lumbosacral region without causing pain from the hips. The examiner first applies pressure on the vertebral column. In contradistinction to the evaluation of most conditions, we prefer to start in the cervical region and work caudally. This establishes the dog's tolerance to deep palpation so that hyperesthesia can be recognized. The typical reaction is increasing anxiety as palpation progresses caudally, with a significant reaction when the lumbosacral area is pressed. Placing the thumbs on the midline, with the fingers on each ilium, allows the examiner direct pressure at the correct location without stressing the dog's hips. If this fails to elicit a reaction, the tail is elevated with continued pressure on the lumbosacral region. Each pelvic limb can also be extended caudally to further stress the lumbosacral articulation. Remember, extension of the lumbosacral articulation causes maximal compression and pain. Extension of the hips also may cause pain if hip dysplasia is present. However, abduction and rotation of the hips should also cause pain in hip dysplasia but not stress the lumbosacral junction. By comparing the dog's response to lumbosacral extension with the response to hip manipulation, the examiner can distinguish lumbosacral stenosis from hip dysplasia.

Diagnosis. Lumbosacral spondylopathy must be differentiated from disease syndromes with similar clinical signs. These disorders include various causes of compression, such as trauma and neoplasia, inflammatory diseases, such as diskospondylitis and abscesses, orthopedic diseases, such as arthritis, hip dysplasia, and cranial cruciate rupture, and spinal cord diseases, such as degenerative myelopathy. Localization is critical to rule out most of these diseases. Those that affect the cauda equina require additional diagnostic tests. EMG can be a valuable tool for mapping the distribution of denervation and localizing the lesion to specific nerve roots. Radiography is useful for establishing whether the skeletal lesions are compatible with stenosis, subluxation, or spondylosis. Myelography, vertebral sinus venography, epidurography, and CT are the primary diagnostic tools recommended by most authors. Our preference is epidurography and CT. Myelography is useful to help rule out concurrent disease in the spinal cord, but it is not as effective as epidurography in defining lumbosacral compression. It is imperative to take both flexed and extended lateral views during epidurography to accentuate the compression in animals with minimal change (Fig. 7–22). See Chapter 4 and the references for additional discussion and techniques.[66,68–71]

Treatment. The management of lumbosacral spondylopathy is based on an evaluation of the severity and duration of the clinical signs. Rest for 4 to 6 weeks and analgesics are recommended for dogs with an initial episode of pain only. Progression of clinical signs is a strong indication for surgery.

Dorsal laminectomy is recommended if signs continue in spite of confinement, recur as soon as exercise is allowed (the usual outcome), become progressively worse, or if significant motor deficits or urinary and fecal incontinence develop. The annulus of the disk is excised and the nucleus removed. Evidence of L7 nerve root entrapment, most readily recognized on EMG, warrants foraminotomy in addition to laminectomy. Postoperative care includes scrupulous attention to the maintenance of bladder functions if that is a problem (see Chap. 3). Exercise should be restricted for at least 6 weeks. Dogs that become active too early often have episodes of pain. Nonsteroidal analgesics may be used to reduce pain in the postoperative period. Prognosis depends on the severity and duration of signs. Dogs with pain as the only sign have an excellent prognosis for complete recovery, although they may experience episodes of discomfort after vigorous exercise. We have treated dogs that have returned to hunting following surgery. Chambers reported that 13 of 18 dogs with pain only were completely normal after surgery. Three of the remaining four dogs were substantially improved.[66] In another study, 17 of 18 dogs responded well to surgery.[65] Recovery is far less certain when LMN signs, especially with incontinence, are present before surgery.[65,66,72]

Vertebral Column Malformations

Vertebral Anomalies. Vertebral anomalies are common in dogs with a screw tail, such as the English and French bulldog and Boston terrier.[73] They are reported in other species, especially the horse.[74] Incomplete separation of the vertebral bodies, arches, or the entire vertebra is called *block vertebrae*. *Hemivertebra* is potentially of clinical significance. Failure of ossification of one half of the vertebral body may cause unilateral, dorsal, or ventral hemivertebra. Unilateral hemivertebra causes scoliosis, dorsal hemivertebra causes kyphosis, and ventral hemivertebra causes lordosis. *Butterfly vertebra* has a saggital cleft of the vertebral body. These anomalies are most common in the thoracic area and rarely cause clinical signs. Dorsal displacement of a ventral hemivertebra may induce a chronic progressive spinal cord compression. Vertebrae that have properties of two major divisions of the vertebral column are called transitional vertebrae. Cervicothoracic transitional vertebrae have transverse processes that resemble ribs. We have seen one dog that had a cervical rib that seemed to cause pain from stretching of the spinal nerve. Thoracolumbar transitional vertebrae may also have spinous processes resembling ribs, absence of a rib on one side, or the last rib may be fused like a transverse process. The major significance is in location of the correct interspace in spinal surgery, where the T13–L1 interspace is identified as a landmark. Lumbosacral transitional vertebrae may have some association with degenerative lumbosacral stenosis. The last lumbar vertebra may fuse with the first sacral vertebra bilaterally or unilaterally. Unilateral sacralization may cause deviation of the pelvis and possibly nerve root entrapment. The appearance of transverse processes on the first sacral vertebra is called lumbarization and may lead to instability.

Spinal Dysraphism. The dysraphic conditions are congenital defects that result from failure of normal closure of the neural tube. They may affect the brain or spinal cord, often with accompanying abnormalities in the surrounding bone and other tissues. Those affecting the vertebral column or the spinal cord in animals include spinal dysraphism, syringomyelia, spina

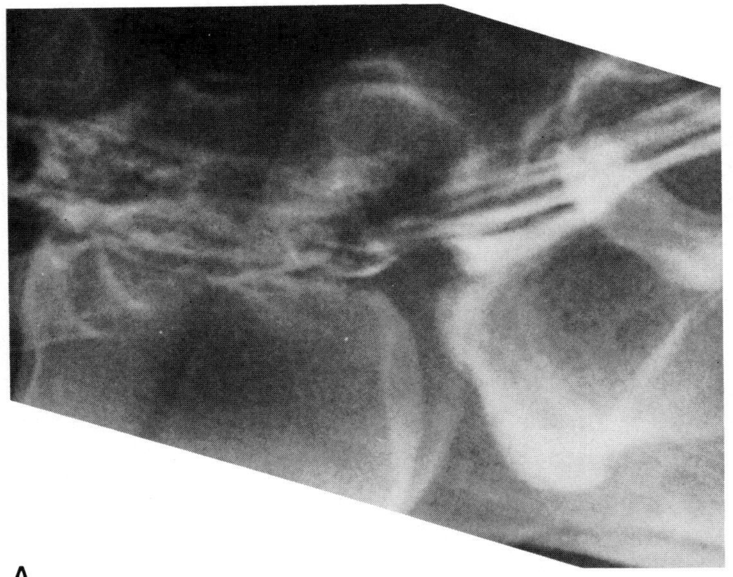

A

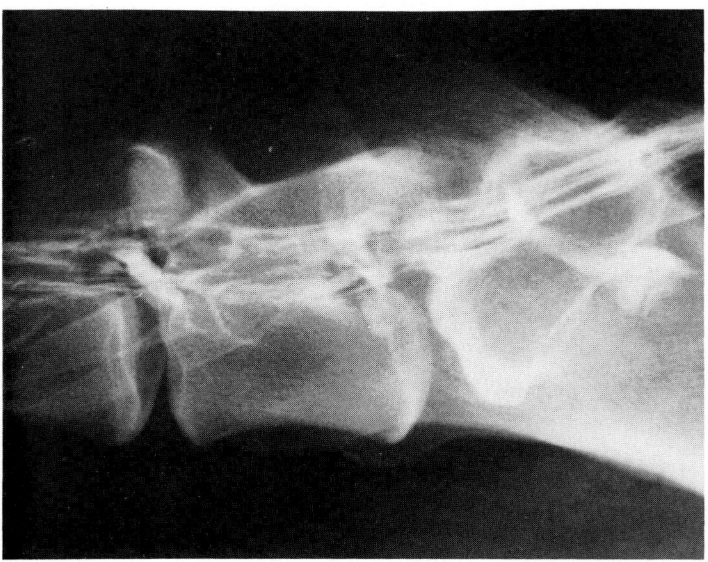

B

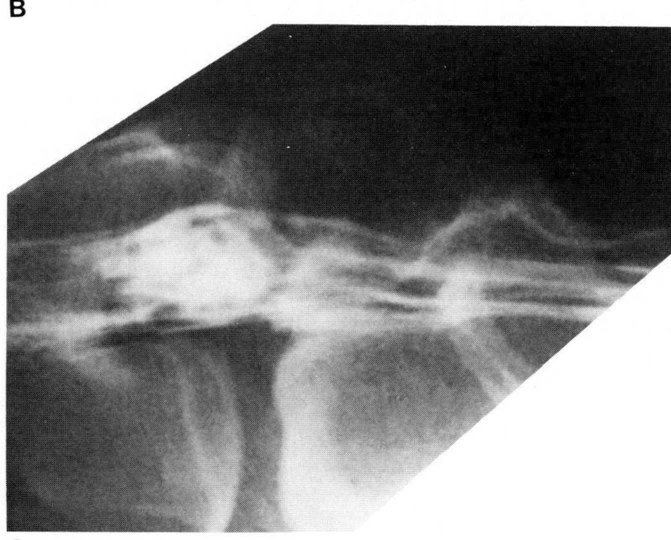

C

Figure 7–22 Degenerative lumbosacral stenosis. Lateral epidurogram view made with the legs in (*A*) dorsiflexion (extension), (*B*) neutral position, and (*C*) flexion. Lesion is most apparent in the dorsiflexion view. There is slight (less than 50%) elevation of the epidural space on the neutral view, and no compression on the flexed view. (From Selcer BA: Radiographic imaging in canine lumbrosacral disease. Vet Med Rep 1:282–290, 1989. Used by permission.)

bifida with or without myelomeningocele, and caudal vertebral hypoplasia.

Spinal dysraphism occurs in several breeds of dogs and pigs but has been documented most frequently in the weimaraner dog.[75] Changes within the spinal cord include an absence, a distention, or a duplication of the central canal. Other changes include hydromyelia, syringomyelia, and anomalies of the ventral median fissure. Fluid-filled cavitations are commonly observed in dysraphic spinal cords, and spinal dysraphism, particularly in the weimaraner breed, has been called syringomyelia. The fluid-filled cysts in the dysraphic spinal cords of weimaraner dogs probably result from abnormal vascularization that produces ischemia, degeneration, and cavitation. The thoracic spinal cord is most commonly affected. Because dysraphic lesions are the cause of the clinical signs, the term *spinal dysraphism* is preferred to the term *syringomyelia*.

The clinical signs are usually apparent at 6 to 8 weeks of age, although in mild cases, the dog may not be presented for examination until it is several months old. The classic clinical signs include a symmetric hopping gait with the pelvic limbs (bunny hopping), a crouching posture, and a wide-based stance. Proprioceptive positioning in the pelvic limbs is depressed, and the animal may occasionally knuckle over. The postural reactions are depressed. The spinal reflexes are usually normal, and exaggerated scratch reflexes may be present. Pain perception is usually intact. The neurologic signs are nonprogressive but become more obvious as the animal matures. Less common clinical signs include abnormal hair streams or hair whorls in the dorsal cervical area, kinking of the undocked tail, scoliosis, and depression of the sternum.

The diagnosis is based on the typical clinical signs and the breed involvement. The clinical signs are nearly pathognomonic in the weimaraner. Spinal radiographs and CSF analysis help eliminate the diagnosis of a treatable disease. There is no effective treatment. Because the syndrome is probably inherited in the weimaraner, owners are advised to cease breeding animals that have produced affected puppies.

Spinal Bifida. Spina bifida is the incomplete closure or fusion of the dorsal vertebral arches. In many cases it occurs in association with protrusion of the meninges (meningocele) or the spinal cord and the meninges (myelomeningocele) through the vertebral defect (Fig. 7–23). Often these meningeal or spinal cord protrusions adhere to the skin where the neural ectoderm failed to separate from the other ectodermal structures (see Fig. 7–23). These adhesions may produce a small depression or dimple in the skin at the site of attachment. In some cases this defect is open and spinal fluid leaks onto the skin, producing epidermal ulceration. Because the meninges are exposed in this situation, meningitis may develop. In most cases investigated, the caudal and some of the sacral nerves are either severely attenuated or incomplete. Associated anomalies may include myeloschisis, tethering of the distal spinal cord, and hydrocephalus.[76,77] Spina bifida may affect any vertebra but is most common in the lumbar area. This defect has been observed in the thoracic and lumbar vertebrae in a litter of kittens. Spina bifida is most common in the Manx cat and the bulldog, but can occur in all species.[76–78]

Clinical signs may be minimal or extensive, depending on the severity of the involvement of

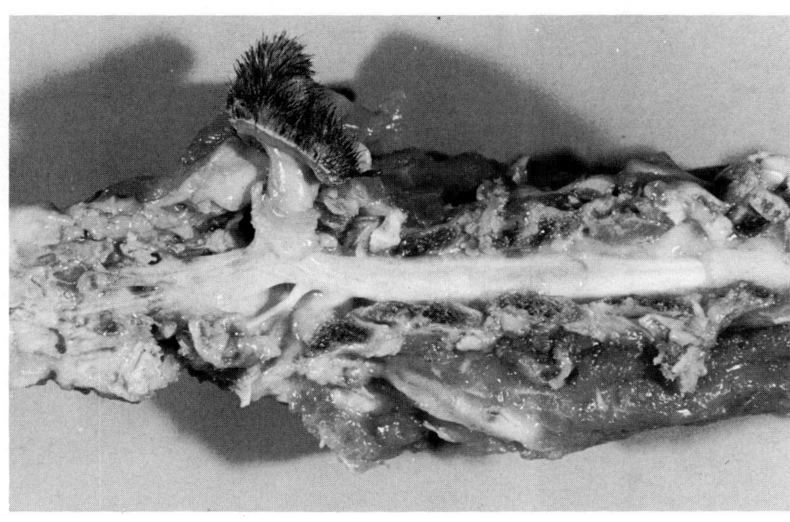

Figure 7–23 Myelomeningocele in an English bulldog puppy with spina bifida. The lesion is caused by failure of the neural ectoderm to separate from the rest of the ectoderm completely during fetal development.

the spinal cord or the cauda equina. Some animals have signs similar to those of spinal dysraphism. In the bulldog, clinical signs often are related to dysfunction in the areas innervated by the cauda equina. Mild to moderate pelvic limb ataxia and paresis may be present. Many animals have decreased innervation of the muscles supplied by the sciatic nerve. The limb may be fixed in extension, owing to the unopposed contraction of the quadriceps muscle. Affected dogs consistently have fecal and urinary incontinence and pelvic limb ataxia are usually present. Pain perception may be decreased in the perineal area and from the distal regions of the pelvic limbs. Spina bifida without myelomeningocele is not associated with any neurologic deficits.

Spina bifida is confirmed radiographically. The presence of meningocele and myelomeningocele can be determined myelographically (Fig. 7–24). There are no specific treatments available for spina bifida. Surgical correction of the tethered spinal cord has been attempted, but there was no improvement in the single case reported.[76] The extensive loss of normal nerve supply to bladder and anus makes recovery unlikely in most of these animals. Meningoceles can be closed surgically to prevent the leakage of CSF and to prevent meningeal infection.

Sacrococcygeal Hypoplasia in Manx Cats. The Manx cat has been bred selectively to have a bobtail; however, numerous spinal and neural anomalies are encountered in the breed. The Manx factor, or taillessness, is apparently inherited as an autosomal dominant trait.[78] The anomalies are caused by incomplete penetrance of the dominant genes for taillessness. In addition to coccygeal dysgenesis, sacral hypoplasia may occur. Spina bifida is also commonly encountered in this breed. Spinal cord anomalies include dysraphism, syringomyelia, meningocele, and myelomeningocele.[79]

The neurologic signs are related to abnormal development of the nerves in the cauda equina. These signs include LMN deficits to the anus, the urinary bladder, and the pelvic limbs. Urinary and fecal incontinence and fecal retention are major problems. A bunny-hopping gait is characteristic of the breed and is not considered abnormal by Manx breeders. Undoubtedly a certain degree of spinal dysraphism is present in these so-called normal cats. Severely affected cats have pelvic limb paresis or paralysis and ataxia. Primary uterine inertia has also been observed. The clinical signs are present from birth and are nonprogressive. The diagnosis is based on the breed, the clinical signs, and radiographic evidence of sacrococcygeal abnormalities (Fig. 7–25). Therapy is directed at relieving urine and fecal retention.

Neuritis of the Cauda Equina (Polyneuritis Equi)

This is a severe, slowly progressive granulomatous LMN disease that primarily affects adult horses. It is usually restricted to the sacral spinal cord nerves and nerve roots. The lesion is a demyelination with a granulomatous neuritis, and meningitis involving the sacral and caudal nerve roots. Cranial nerve involvement may also

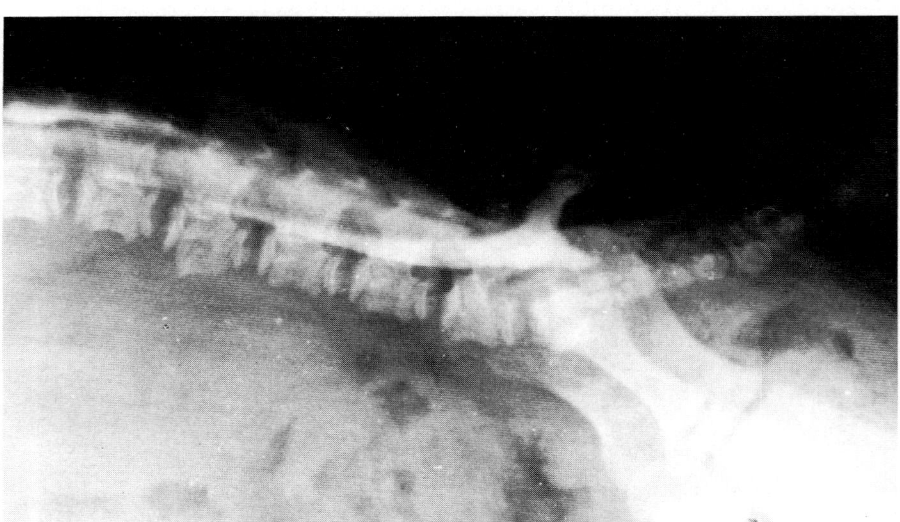

Figure 7–24 Myelogram of the puppy in Figure 7–23. Spina bifida, myeloschisis, and myelomeningocele are demonstrated.

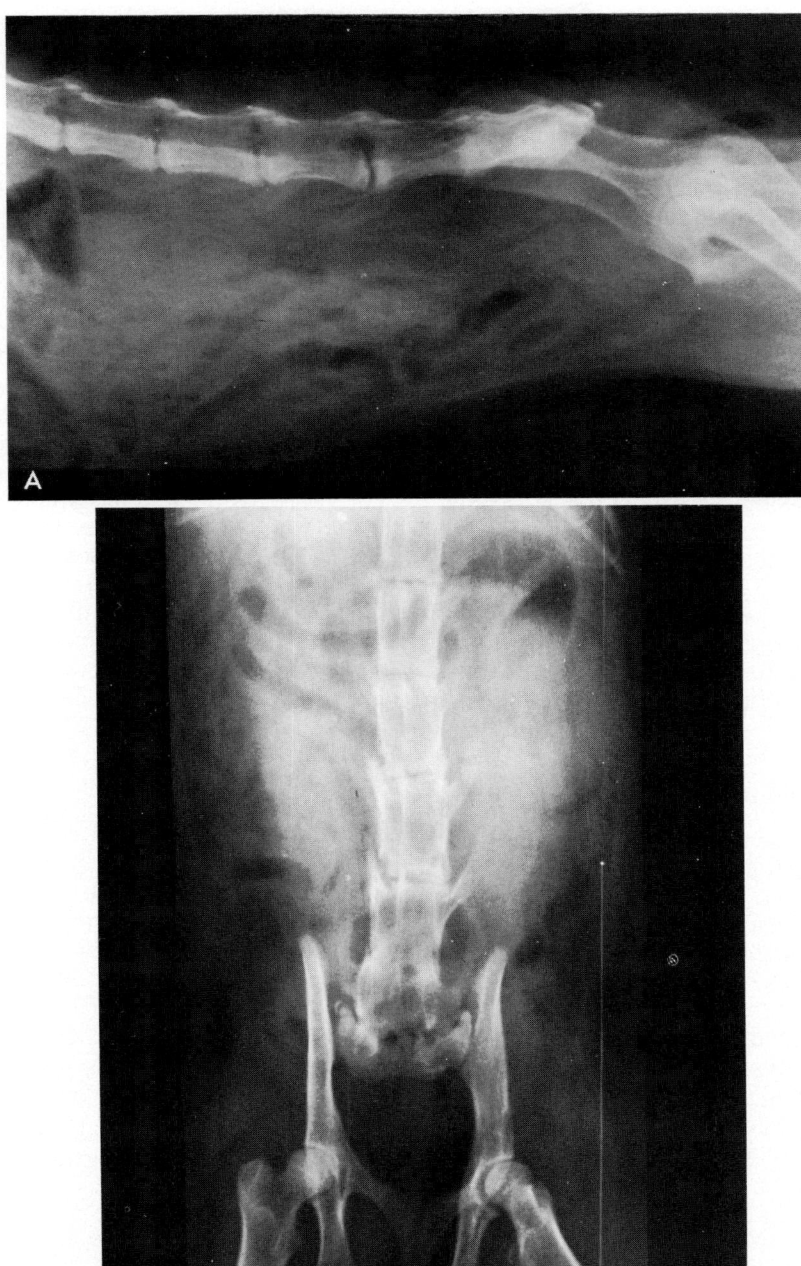

Figure 7–25 Lateral lumbosacral (*A*) and ventrodorsal (*B*) radiographs of a Manx cat with sacrocaudal abnormalities. Note the short, malformed sacrum and the absence of caudal vertebrae.

occur in some cases, hence the term polyneuritis equi.[5,80,81] The lesion resembles allergic neuritis, and the evidence suggests that this is an autoimmune polyneuritis.[82] As in coon hound paralysis and Landry-Guillain-Barré syndromes, there is likely a factor such as a virus initiating the immune reaction. A history of vaccination or respiratory illness is reported in some cases. Equine adenovirus 1 was isolated from two affected horses.[83] The etiology is unknown.

Clinical Signs. Early signs include rubbing the perineal area, urine scald, and constipation. LMN paresis or paralysis of the tail, the bladder, and the anal sphincter is found on examination. Decreased sensation in the perineal area also occurs and becomes more severe as the disease progresses. In male horses, pudendal paralysis results in a dropped penis or inability to retract the penis. Analgesia to the penis also may occur. Cranial nerves V, VII, and VIII are frequently affected. Signs such as head tilt, nystagmus, and facial paralysis may occur in some horses.

Diagnosis. If both the cauda equina and cranial nerves are affected, the diagnosis is likely. If only the cauda equina is involved, sacral fractures should be ruled out by rectal palpation and radiography. EMG and evoked potentials may be useful adjuncts if involvement of the cauda equina is in doubt. Procurement of spinal fluid at the lumbar cisternae is often diagnostic of cauda equina neuritis. Lumbosacral taps reveal moderately increased concentrations of protein (100–300 mg/dl) and cells (>100 cells/cu mm). The cytologic composition is mainly macrophages, neutrophils, and lymphocytes. Antibody to P_2 protein can be demonstrated by ELISA.[84]

Treatment. No specific treatment is known. Evacuation of the bladder and bowel may allow the animal to live for prolonged periods. However, denervation of the genital tract precludes breeding stallions.

Sorghum Cystitis and Ataxia

Neuronal fiber degeneration of the spinal cord and spinal nerves occurs in horses, cattle, and sheep that ingest sorghums, Johnson, or Sudan grass. Lesions develop primarily in the lumbar, sacral, and caudal spinal cord segments. Histopathologically these lesions are characterized by focal axonal degeneration and demyelination with associated lipid-laden macrophages. The lesions may result from chronic sublethal doses of hydrocyanic acid found in plants of the genus *Sorghum*. Production of a lathyrogenic principle (nitrile-related amino acid) has also been postulated.[85]

History. Enzootics of this disease occur in horses of all ages that graze in sorghum or Sudan grass pastures. The disease usually occurs when the plants are young and rapidly growing, but mature and second-growth pastures also have been incriminated. Apparently the toxins do not persist in cured hay or silage.

Clinical Signs. Although the signs of urinary incontinence are most noticeable in many horses, neurologic signs usually develop first. They include flaccidity of the anus and the tail and pelvic limb ataxia. Occasionally, severe LMN paralysis of the pelvic limbs develops within 24 hours after the onset of neurologic signs. In the female horse, clinical signs include continual opening and closing of the vulva, perineal paresis, and dribbling of urine. Urine scalds and thick urine deposits occur on the buttocks, the thighs, and the hocks. Male horses drip urine from a relaxed and extended penis. Urinary incontinence is intensified when the animal is forced to move suddenly. Hyporeflexia and proprioceptive deficits are detectable in the pelvic limbs. Clinical signs rarely extend to the thoracic limbs, even though brain stem and cortex lesions have been reported.

Pregnant mares may abort, and aborted foals may have severe ankylosis (arthrogryposis). Arthrogryposis also may occur in full-term foals when the dam has grazed hybrid Sudan plants.

Diagnosis. The diagnosis is suspected from the history and the clinical signs. Affected horses have a severe fibrinopurulent cystitis secondary to neurogenic urine retention. Several different bacteria have been isolated from the urine of affected horses. Some animals develop severe ascending pyelonephritis from the chronic cystitis. The sensory loss in the perineum is less than that from cauda equina neuritis or sacral fracture.[5] Ancillary diagnostic tests are of little benefit. Mild changes in the CSF are found. Protein elevations are slight (60–80 mg/dl), and the cell counts range from 5 to 10 mononuclear cells/cu mm. Urine or serum can be tested for high levels of thiocyanate, the major detoxification product of cyanide.

Treatment. No definitive treatment is known. Horses should not be allowed to graze in sorghum pastures while the plants are rapidly growing or are stunted by drought. Plants are generally safe if they are yellow in color, are more than 2 feet tall, or have formed fruiting heads. Pastures can be checked periodically to determine the amount of cyanide present when toxic forage is suspected.

Aortic Thrombosis (Ischemic Neuromyopathy)

Thromboembolism of the aorta or iliac arteries occurs with moderate frequency in cats and occasionally in dogs and horses. In cats it is associated with cardiomyopathy.[86] Saddle thrombi extend from the aorta into the iliac arteries. Vasoactive substances are believed to be involved in the pathogenesis of the ischemic changes.

Clinically the syndrome is characterized by an acute onset, with little progression. Pelvic limb pain and paralysis are common. The femoral pulse is weak or absent. The distal limbs are cool and pain sensation is absent. Distal limb muscles are affected more than proximal muscles. Although functional recovery may be possible, recurrences are possible, and the cardiomyopathy must be considered. Surgical removal of the thrombus may improve recovery, but the efficacy is controversial.

A similar syndrome is seen in performance horses. Associations with *Strongylus vulgaris* arteritis, thrombotic diseases, and cardiomyopathy have not been conclusively demonstrated.[5]

CASE HISTORIES

Case History 7A

Signalment

Canine, Saint Bernard, female, 6 years old.

History

Six days ago, the dog suddenly cried out in pain and developed paresis in the pelvic limbs. Within 2 hours she became totally paralyzed in the pelvic limbs. There was no possibility of trauma. The dog developed signs while under the owner's observation in the backyard.

Physical Examination

No abnormalities other than the neurologic problem described in the next section.

*Neurologic Examination**

A. Observation
   1. Mental status: Alert.
   2. Posture: Normal, except Gait.
   3. Gait: No voluntary movement of either pelvic limb.

B. Palpation: Hypertonus in right pelvic limb. Hypotonus in left pelvic limb.

C. Postural Reactions

Left	Reactions	Right
0	Proprioceptive positioning PL	0
+2	TL	+2
+2	Wheelbarrowing	+2
0	Hopping, PL	0
+2	Hopping, TL	+2
0	Extensor postural thrust	0
0	Hemistand-hemiwalk	0
0	Placing, tactile PL	0
+2	TL	+2
+2	Placing, visual TL	+2

D. Spinal Reflexes

Left	Reflex	Right
	Spinal Segment	
+1	Quadriceps L4–L6	+2
+2	Extensor carpi radialis C7–T1	+2
+2	Triceps C7–T1	+2
+1	Flexion, PL L5–S1	+3
+2	Flexion, TL C6–T1	+2
Absent	Crossed extensor	Present
+2	Perineal S1–S2	+2

E. Cranial Nerves

Left	Nerve + Function	Right
+2	CN II vision menace	+2
Nor.	CN II + III pupil size	Nor.
+2	Stim. left eye	+2
+2	Stim. right eye	+2
Nor.	CN II fundus	Nor.
	CN III, IV, VI	
0	Strabismus	0
0	Nystagmus	0
+2	CN V sensation	+2
+2	CN V mastication	+2
+2	CN VII facial muscles	+2
+2	Palpebral	+2
Nor.	CN IX, X swallowing	Nor.
Nor.	CN XII tongue	Nor.

F. Sensation: Location.
   Hyperesthesia: 0.
   Superficial pain: +2.
   Deep pain: +2.

Complete sections G and H before reviewing Case Summary.

G. Assessment (Anatomic diagnosis and estimation of prognosis)

H. Plan (Diagnostic)

Rule-outs *Procedure*

1.
2.
3.
4.

* *Key*: 0 = absent, +1 = decreased, +2 = normal, +3 = exaggerated, +4 = very exaggerated or clonus, PL = pelvic limb, TL = thoracic limb.

Case History 7B

Signalment

Canine, dachshund, female, 7 years old.

History

Two days ago the dog had a sudden onset of difficulty walking in the pelvic limbs and within 6 hours became paralyzed in both pelvic limbs. When the dog initially was examined, the pelvic limb reflexes were present, but pain perception was absent in both rear limbs. The thoracic limbs were normal.

Physical Examination

Urinary incontinence, hematuria, and shallow abdominal respirations. The dog cries periodically as if in pain.

*Neurologic Examination**

A. Observation
  1. Mental status: Apprehensive.
  2. Posture: Cannot maintain sternal recumbency.
  3. Gait: No voluntary movements of pelvic limbs. Short, choppy steps with thoracic limbs.

B. Palpation: Hypotonus in both pelvic limbs. Abdominal muscles are flaccid.

C. Postural Reactions

Left	Reactions	Right
0	Proprioceptive positioning PL	0
+2	TL	+2
+1 to +2	Wheelbarrowing	+1 to +2
0	Hopping, PL	0
+2	Hopping, TL	+2
0	Extensor postural thrust	0
0	Hemistand-hemiwalk	0
0	Placing, tactile PL	0
+2	TL	+2
+2	Placing, visual TL	+2

D. Spinal Reflexes

Left	Reflex	Right
0	Spinal Segment Quadriceps L4–L6	0
+2	Extensor carpi radialis C7–T1	+2
+2	Triceps C7–T1	+2
0	Flexion, PL L5–S1	0
+2	Flexion, TL C6–T1	+2
0	Crossed extensor	0
0	Perineal S1–S2	0

E. Cranial Nerves

Left	Nerve + Function	Right
+2	CN II vision menace	+2
Nor.	CN II + III pupil size	Nor.
+2	Stim. left eye	+2
+2	Stim. right eye	+2
Nor.	CN II fundus	Nor.
0	CN III, IV, VI Strabismus	0
0	Nystagmus	0
Nor.	CN V sensation	Nor.
Nor.	CN V mastication	Nor.
Nor. +2	CN VII facial muscles Palpebral	Nor. +2
Nor.	CN IX, X swallowing	Nor.
Nor.	CN XII tongue	Nor.

F. Sensation: Location.
  Hyperesthesia: Present at T2–T3.
  Superficial pain: Absent caudal to scapula.
  Deep pain: Absent caudal to scapula.

Complete sections G and H before reviewing Case Summary.

G. Assessment (Anatomic diagnosis and estimation of prognosis)

H. Plan (Diagnostic)

Rule-outs *Procedure*
1.
2.
3.
4.

* *Key*: 0 = absent, +1 = decreased, +2 = normal, +3 = exaggerated, +4 = very exaggerated or clonus, PL = pelvic limb, TL = thoracic limb.

Case History 7C

Signalment

Canine, German shepherd, female, 1½ years old.

History

Six weeks ago, the dog became lame in the right pelvic limb. Since then, paresis and ataxia have gradually developed in both pelvic limbs, more so on the right side than on the left. Three days ago the dog became completely paralyzed in both pelvic limbs.

Physical Examination

Negative except for the neurologic problem.

*Neurologic Examination**

A. Observation
   1. Mental status: Alert.
   2. Posture: See Gait.
   3. Gait: No voluntary movements in pelvic limbs; thoracic limbs normal.

B. Palpation: Muscle atrophy from TL region caudally along spine. Increased extensor tone in both pelvic limbs.

C. Postural Reactions

Left	Reactions	Right
0	Proprioceptive positioning PL	0
+2	TL	+2
+2	Wheelbarrowing	+2
0	Hopping, PL	0
+2	Hopping, TL	+2
0	Extensor postural thrust	0
0	Hemistand-hemiwalk	0
0	Placing, tactile PL	0
+2	TL	+2
+2	Placing, visual TL	+2

D. Spinal Reflexes

Left	Reflex	Right
	Spinal Segment	
+3	Quadriceps L4–L6	+3
2	Extensor carpi radialis C7–T1	+2
+2	Triceps C7–T1	+2
+2	Flexion, PL L5–S1	+2
+2	Flexion, TL C6–T1	+2
0	Crossed extensor	0
+2	Perineal S1–S2	+2

* *Key*: 0 = absent, + 1 = decreased, +2 = normal, +3 = exaggerated, +4 = very exaggerated or clonus, PL = pelvic limb, TL = thoracic limb.

E. Cranial Nerves

Left	Nerve + Function	Right
+2	CN II vision menace	+2
Nor.	CN II + III pupil size	Nor.
+2	Stim. left eye	+2
+2	Stim. right eye	+2
Nor.	CN II fundus	Nor.
	CN III, IV, VI	
0	Strabismus	0
0	Nystagmus	0
Nor.	CN V sensation	Nor.
Nor.	CN V mastication	Nor.
Nor.	CN VII facial muscles	Nor.
+2	Palpebral	+2
Nor.	CN IX, X swallowing	Nor.
Nor.	CN XII tongue	Nor.

F. Sensation: Location.
   Hyperesthesia: L2–L3.
   Superficial pain: Absent caudal to L2.
   Deep pain: Blunted caudal to L2–L3.

Complete sections G and H before reviewing Case Summary.

G. Assessment (Anatomic diagnosis and estimation of prognosis)

H. Plan Diagnostic)

Rule-outs	*Procedure*
1.	
2.	
3.	
4.	

Case History 7D

Signalment

Canine, bulldog, male, 7 weeks old.

History

Since he became ambulatory, the puppy has had a spastic, ataxic gait in the pelvic limbs. Urinary and fecal incontinence have been present for at least 2 weeks.

Physical Examination

Normal except for the neurologic problem. Urinary incontinence is present.

*Neurologic Examination**

A. Observation
   1. Mental status: Alert, responsive.
   2. Posture: See Gait.
   3. Gait: Paretic and ataxic in pelvic limbs. Wide-based stance; feet tend to slip from under the dog.

B. Palpation: No tone in anal sphincter. Small depression in lumbar area just cranial to sacrum.

C. Postural Reactions

Left	Reactions	Right
	Proprioceptive positioning	
0	PL	0
+2	TL	+2
+2	Wheelbarrowing	+2
+1	Hopping, PL	+1
+2	Hopping, TL	+2
+1	Extensor postural thrust	+1
+1	Hemistand-hemiwalk	+1
+2	Tonic neck	+2
	Placing, tactile	
0	PL	0
+2	TL	+2
	Placing, visual	
+2	TL	+2

D. Spinal Reflexes

Left	Reflex	Right
	Spinal Segment	
	Quadriceps	
+2	L4–L6	+2
	Extensor carpi radialis	
+2	C7–T1	+2
	Triceps	
+2	C7–T1	+2
	Flexion, PL	
0 to +1	L5–S1	0 to +1
	Flexion, TL	
+2	C6–T1	+2
0	Crossed extensor	0
	Perineal	
0	S1–S2	0

E. Cranial Nerves

Left	Nerve + Function	Right
+2	CN II vision menace	+2
Nor.	CN II + III pupil size	Nor.
+2	Stim. left eye	+2
+2	Stim. right eye	+2
Nor.	CN II fundus	Nor.
	CN III, IV, VI	
0	Strabismus	0
0	Nystagmus	0
+2	CN V sensation	+2
+2	CN V mastication	+2
+2	CN VII facial muscles	+2
+2	Palpebral	+2
+2	CN IX, X swallowing	+2
Nor.	CN XII tongue	Nor.

F. Sensation: Location.
   Hyperesthesia: None.
   Superficial pain: Absent in perineal area.
   Deep pain: Present but decreased in perineum and tail.

Complete sections G and H before reviewing Case Summary.

G. Assessment (Anatomic diagnosis and estimation of prognosis)

H. Plan (Diagnostic)

Rule-outs *Procedure*
1.
2.
3.
4.

Assessment 7A

Anatomic diagnosis. This dog has bilateral pelvic limb paralysis characterized by UMN signs in the right limb and LMN signs in the left limb, with no hyperesthesia. An asymmetric lesion in the midlumbar spinal cord is probably present (spinal cord segments L2–L7). The lesion has spared spinal cord sensory pathways. Acute nonprogressive diseases should be considered.

Diagnostic plan. (Rule-outs—see Tables 7–1 and 7–4):

1. Fibrocartilaginous embolization: no evidence of spinal cord compression, no hyperesthesia.
2. Intervertebral disk disease: Spinal radiography and myelography were both negative.

Therapeutic plan.

1. At 6 days after injury, it is very doubtful that corticosteroids will be beneficial.
2. Supportive care of a paraplegic.

Client education. The prognosis is poor, since the lesion is severe and there is LMN involvement. The presence of pain sensation implies that some

* *Key*: 0 = absent, +1 = decreased, +2 = normal, +3 = exaggerated, +4 = very exaggerated or clonus, PL = pelvic limb, TL = thoracic limb.

spinal cord integrity is present, however. Maintain the dog for 1 week. If there is no improvement, consider euthanasia.

Case summary.

1. Diagnosis: spinal cord infarction.
2. Result: No improvement. Euthanasia was performed.

Spinal cord hemorrhage with infarction from L2–L4.

Assessment 7B

Anatomic diagnosis. Motor examination reveals severe bilateral LMN disease in both pelvic limbs and the pudendal nerve. The symmetry of the signs suggests severe disease in segments L4–S2. The sensory examination reveals complete analgesia caudad to the shoulders. This finding suggests a severe lesion extending as far forward as T3. In addition, the LMN neurons to the abdominal and intercostal muscles are involved. Therefore, diffuse symmetric disease of the spinal cord caudad to T3 should be suspected. The history suggests lesion progression, insofar as spinal reflexes in the pelvic limbs were present 2 days ago. The lesion involves both gray and white matter throughout the spinal cord caudal to T3.

Diagnostic plan. (Rule-out—see Tables 7–1 and 7–4): Ascending—descending myelomalacia secondary to spinal cord compression.

Therapeutic plan. None.

Client education.

1. The prognosis is hopeless.
2. Recommend euthanasia.

Case summary. The diagnosis is severe ascending–descending myelomalacia secondary to a herniated disk at T13–L1.

Assessment 7C

Anatomic diagnosis. The neurologic examination reveals bilateral UMN disease to both pelvic limbs, suggesting a lesion in segment T2–L3. The clinical course suggests a progressive disease. The hyperesthesia suggests a lesion at segment L2– L3.

Diagnostic plan. (Rule-outs—see Table 7–1):

1. Type II disk disease: Spinal radiography and myelography were negative for extradural compression.
2. Neoplasia: Myelography disclosed intramedullary compression of the dye column at L1–L2.
3. Chronic meningomyelitis: CSF contained 1 WBC, 33.5 mg/dl protein.
4. Diskospondylitis: Survey radiographs were normal.

Therapeutic plan.

1. Chemotherapy, corticosteroids.
2. Exploratory laminectomy.

Client education. The prognosis is very poor. The myelogram suggests an intramedullary spinal cord tumor. These tumors are usually inoperable.

Case summary.

1. Diagnosis: Inoperable blast cell tumor at L1–L2.
2. Euthanasia was performed.

Assessment 7D

Anatomic diagnosis. LMN signs with blunted pain perception suggest a bilateral lesion in the segment L3–S2 or in the lumbosacral plexus. The urine and fecal incontinence is explained by a lesion in this region. The age and the breed suggest a developmental abnormality.

Diagnostic plan. (Rule-outs—see Table 7–4):

1. Spina bifida: Radiography of the lumbosacral area.
2. Spinal dysraphism: Myelography, EMG of the perineal muscles. A meningomyelocele was demonstrated (see Fig. 7–24).

Therapeutic plan. None.

Client education.

1. The prognosis is poor.
2. This congenital abnormality is a problem in certain lines of bulldogs.

Case summary.

1. The diagnosis was spina bifida with concurrent meningomyelocele (see Fig. 7–23).
2. Euthanasia was performed.

REFERENCES

1. Hoerlein BF: Intervertebral disk disease. In Oliver JE, Hoerlein BF, Mayhew IG: Veterinary Neurology. Philadelphia, WB Saunders, 1987, pp 321–341.
2. Griffiths I: The extensive myelopathy of intervertebral disc protrusions in dogs ("the ascending syndrome"). J Small Anim Pract 13:425–437, 1972.
3. Tarlov I, Klinger H: Spinal cord compression studies: II. Time limits for recovery after acute compression in dogs. Arch Neurol Psychiatry 71:271–290, 1954.
4. Tarlov I, Klinger H, Vitale S: Spinal cord compression studies: I. Experimental techniques to produce acute and gradual compression. Arch Neurol Psychiatry 70: 813–819, 1953.
5. Mayhew IG: Large Animal Neurology: A Handbook for Veterinary Clinicians. Philadelphia, Lea & Febiger, 1989.
6. Wright JA, Bell DA, Clayton-Jones DG: The clinical and radiologic features associated with spinal tumors in thirty dogs. J Small Anim Pract 20:461–472, 1979.
7. Ingram JT, Colter SB: How do I treat? Neurologic rhinopneumonitis in the horse. Prog Vet Neurol 1:483, 1990.
8. Beech J, Dodd DC: Toxoplasma-like encephalomyelitis in the horse. Vet Pathol 11:87–96, 1974.
9. Dorr TE, Higgins RJ, Dangler CA, et al: Protozoal myeloencephalitis in horses in California. J Am Vet Med Assoc 185:801–802, 1984.
10. Clark EG, Townsend HGG, McKenzie NT: Equine protozoal myeloencephalitis: A report of two cases from Western Canada. Can Vet J 22:140–144, 1981.
11. Fayer R, Mayhew IG, Baird JD, et al: Epidemiology of equine protozoal myeloencephalitis in North America based on histologically confirmed cases. J Vet Intern Med 4:54–57, 1990.
12. Turner WD: Fractures and fracture-luxations of the lumbar spine: A Retrospective study in the dog. J Am Anim Hosp Assoc 23:459–464, 1987.
13. Rucker NC: Management of spinal cord trauma. Prog Vet Neurol 1:397–412, 1990.
14. LeCouteur RA: Central nervous system trauma. In Kornegay JN (ed): Neurologic Disorders. New York, Churchill Livingstone, 1986, pp 147–167.

15. Collatos C, Allen D, Chambers J, et al: Surgical treatment of sacral fracture in a horse. J Am Vet Med Assoc 198:877–879, 1991.
16. Oliver JE: Neurologic emergencies in small animals. Vet Clin North Am 2:341–357, 1972.
17. Braund KG, Shores A, Brawner WR: The etiology, pathology, and pathophysiology of acute spinal cord trauma. Vet Med 85:684–691, 1990.
18. Bracken MB, Shepard MJ, Collins WF, et al: A randomized, controlled trial of methylprednisolone or naloxone in the treatment of acute spinal-cord injury. N Engl J Med 322:1405–1411, 1990.
19. Faden AI: Pharmacotherapy in spinal cord injury: A critical review of recent developments. Clin Neuropharmacol 10:193–204, 1987.
20. Hoerlein BF, Redding RW, Hoff EJ Jr, et al: Evaluation of naloxone, crocetin, thyrotropin releasing hormone, methylprednisolone, partial myelotomy, and hemilaminectomy in the treatment of acute spinal cord trauma. J Am Anim Hosp Assoc 21:67–77, 1985.
21. Hoerlein B, Redding R, Hoff E, et al: Evaluation of dexamethasone, DMSO, mannitol, and solcoseryl in acute spinal cord trauma. J Am Anim Hosp Assoc 19:216–226, 1983.
22. Selcer RR, Bubb WJ, Walker TL: Management of vertebral column fractures in dogs and cats: 211 cases (1977–1985). J Am Vet Med Assoc 198:1965–1968, 1991.
23. Hoerlein B: Methods of spinal fusion and vertebral immobilization in the dog. Am J Vet Res 17:685–709, 1956.
24. Yturraspe D, Lumb W: The use of plastic spinal plates for internal fixation of the canine spine. J Am Vet Med Assoc 161:1651–1657, 1972.
25. Blass C, Seim H: Spinal fixation in dogs using Steinmann pins and methylmethacrylate. Vet Surg 13:203–210, 1984.
26. Walter M, Smith G, Newton C: Canine lumbar spinal internal fixation techniques: A comparative biomechanical study. Vet Surg 15:191–198, 1986.
27. McAnulty J, Lenehan T, Maletz L: Modified segmental spinal instrumentation in repair of spinal fractures and luxations in dogs. Vet Surg 15:143–149, 1986.
28. Oliver JE, Hoerlein BF, Mayhew IG: Veterinary Neurology. Philadelphia, WB Saunders, 1987.
29. Clemmons RM: Degenerative myelopathy. In Kirk RW (ed): Current Veterinary Therapy. Vol X. Small Animal Practice. Philadelphia, WB Saunders, 1989, pp 830–833.
30. Averill DR: Degenerative myelopathy in the aging German shepherd dog. J Am Vet Med Assoc 162:1045–1051, 1973.
31. Braund KG, Vandevelde M: German shepherd dog myelopathy: A morphologic and morphometric study. Am J Vet Res 39:1309–1315, 1978.
32. Griffiths IR, Duncan ID: Chronic degenerative radiculomyelopathy in the dog. J Small Anim Pract 16:461–471, 1975.
33. Waxman FJ, Clemmons RM, Hinrichs DJ: Progressive myelopathy in older German shepherd dogs: II. Presence of circulating suppressor cells. J Immunol 124:1216–1222, 1980.
34. Waxman FJ, Clemmons RM, Johnson G, et al: Progressive myelopathy in older German shepherd dogs: I. Depressed response to thymus-dependent mitogens. J Immunol 124:1209–1215, 1980.
35. Matthews NS, DeLahunta A: Degenerative myelopathy in an adult miniature poodle. J Am Vet Med Assoc 186:1213–1214, 1985.
36. Bichsel P, Vandevelde M: Degenerative myelopathy in a family of Siberian Husky dogs. J Am Vet Med Assoc 183:998–1000, 1983.
37. Kornegay JN: Congenital and degenerative diseases of the central nervous system. In Kornegay JN (ed): Neurologic Disorders. New York, Churchill Livingstone, 1986, pp 109–129.
38. Mesfin GM, Kusewitt D, Parker A: Degenerative myelopathy in a cat. J Am Vet Med Assoc 176:62–64, 1980.
39. Littlewood J, Herrtage M, Palmer A: Intervertebral disc protrusion in a cat. J Small Anim Pract 25:119–127, 1984.
40. Heavner J: Intervertebral disc syndrome in the cat. J Am Vet Med Assoc 159:425–428, 1971.
41. Hansen HJ: A pathologic-anatomical study on disk degeneration in the dog. Acta Orthop Scand 1952.
42. Kornegay JN: Central nervous system neoplasia. In Kornegay JN (ed): Neurologic Disorders. New York, Churchill Livingstone, 1986, pp 79–108.
43. Ribas JL: Thoracolumbar spinal cord blastoma: A unique tumor of young dogs. J Vet Intern Med 4:127, 1990.
44. Summers BA, de Lahunta A, McEntee M, et al: A novel intradural extramedullary spinal cord tumor in your dogs. Acta Neuropathol 75:402–410, 1988.
45. Irving G, McMillan MC: Fluoroscopically guided percutaneous fine-needle aspiration biopsy of thoracolumbar spinal lesions in cats. Prog Vet Neurol 1:473–475, 1990.
46. Spodnick GJ, Berg J, Moore FM, et al: Spinal lymphoma in cats: 21 cases (1976–1989). J Am Vet Med Assoc 200:373–376, 1992.
47. Morgan J: Spondylosis deformans in the dog. Acta Orthop Scand Suppl 96:1–88, 1967.
48. Romatowski J: Spondylosis deformans in the dog. Comp Cont Educ Pract Vet 8:531–534, 1986.
49. Weisbrode S, Monke D, Dodaro S, et al: Osteochondrosis, degenerative joint disease, and vertebral osteophytosis in middle-aged bulls. J Am Vet Med Assoc 181:700–705, 1982.
50. Doige C: Multiple cartilaginous exostoses in dogs. Vet Pathol 24:276–278, 1987.
51. Shupe JL, Leone NC, Gardner EJ, et al: Hereditary multiple exostoses. Am J Pathol 104:285–288, 1981.
52. Acton CE: Spinal cord compression in young dogs due to cartilaginous exostosis. Calif Vet 41:7–26, 1987.
53. Cockrell BY, Herigstad RR, Flo GJ, et al: Myelomalacia in Afghan hounds. J Am Vet Med Assoc 162:362–365, 1973.
54. de Lahunta A: Veterinary Neuroanatomy and Clinical Neurology, 2nd ed. Philadelphia, WB Saunders, 1983.
55. Kornegay JN: Diskospondylitis revisited. In: Proceedings of the Ninth Annual Veterinary Medical Forum, New Orleans, 1991, pp 291–293.
56. Doige C: Discospondylitis in swine. Can J Comp Med 44:121–128, 1980.
57. Sherman D, Ames T: Vertebral body abscesses in cattle: A review of five cases. J Am Vet Med Assoc 188:608–611, 1986.
58. Kornegay J, Barber D: Diskospondylitis in dogs. J Am Vet Med Assoc 177:337–341, 1980.
59. Kornegay J: Diskospondylitis. In Kirk RW (ed): Current Veterinary Therapy. Vol IX. Small Animal Practice. Philadelphia, WB Saunders, 1986, pp 810–814.
60. Kornegay JN: Vertebral diseases of large breed dogs. In Kornegay JN (ed): Neurologic Disorders. New York, Churchill Livingstone, 1986, pp 197–215.
61. Penwick RC: Fibrocartilaginous embolism and ischemic myelopathy. Comp Cont Educ Pract Vet 11:287–299, 1989.
62. Johnson RC, Anderson WI, King JM: Acute pelvic limb paralysis induced by a lumbar fibrocartilaginous embolism in a sow. Cornell Vet 78:231–234, 1988.
63. Gilmore DR, de Lahunta A: Necrotizing myelopathy secondary to presumed or confirmed fibrocartilaginous embolism in 24 dogs. J Am Anim Hosp Assoc 23:373–376, 1987.
64. Oliver J, Selcer R, Simpson S: Cauda equina compres-

sion from lumbosacral malarticulation and malformation in the dog. J Am Vet Med Assoc 173:207–214, 1978.

65. Watt PR: Degenerative lumbosacral stenosis in 18 dogs. J Small Anim Pract 32:125–134, 1991.
66. Chambers JN: Degenerative lumbosacral stenosis in dogs. Vet Med Rep 1:166–180, 1989.
67. Palmer RH, Chambers JN: Canine lumbosacral diseases: Part I. Anatomy, pathophysiology, and clinical presentation. Comp Cont Educ Pract Vet 13:61–69, 1991.
68. Palmer RH, Chambers JN: Canine lumbosacral diseases: Part II. Definitive diagnosis, treatment, and prognosis. Comp Cont Educ Pract Vet 13:213–222, 1991.
69. Hathcock JT, Pechman RD, Dillon AR, et al: Comparison of three radiographic contrast procedures in the evaluation of the canine lumbosacral spinal canal. J Vet Radiol 29:4–15, 1988.
70. Selcer BA: Radiographic imaging in canine lumbosacral disease. Vet Med Rep 1:282–290, 1989.
71. Lang J: Flexion-extension myelography of the canine cauda equina. Vet Radiol 29:242–257, 1988.
72. Chambers JN, Selcer BA, Oliver JE: Results of treatment of degenerative lumbosacral stenosis in dogs by exploration and excision. Vet Comp Orthop Trauma 3:130–133, 1988.
73. Bailey CS: An embryological approach to the clinical significance of congenital vertebral and spinal cord abnormalities. J Am Anim Hosp Assoc 11:426–434, 1975.
74. Braund KG: Degenerative and developmental diseases. In Oliver JE, Hoerlein BF, Mayhew IG: Veterinary Neurology. Philadelphia, WB Saunders, 1987, pp 185–215.
75. McGrath JT: Spinal dysraphism in the dog. Pathol Vet Suppl 2:1–36, 1965.
76. Fingeroth JM, Johnson GC, Burt JK, et al: Neuroradiographic diagnosis and surgical repair of tethered cord syndrome in an English bulldog with spina bifida and myeloschisis. J Am Vet Med Assoc 194:1300–1302, 1989.
77. Wilson JW, Kurtz HJ, Leipold HW, et al: Spina bifida in the dog. Vet Pathol 16:165–179, 1979.
78. Kitchen H, Murray RE, Cockrell BY: Animal model for human disease, spina bifida, sacral dysgenesis and myelocele. Am J Pathol 68:203–206, 1972.
79. Leipold HW, Huston K, Blauch B, et al: Congenital defects of the caudal vertebral column and spinal cord in Manx cats. J Am Vet Med Assoc 164:520–523, 1974.
80. Rousseaux C, Futcher K, Clark E, et al: Cauda equina neuritis: A chronic idiopathic polyneuritis in two horses. Can Vet J 25:214–218, 1984.
81. Wright JA, Fordyce P, Edington N: Neuritis of the cauda equina in the horse. J Comp Pathol 97:667–675, 1987.
82. Cummings J, de Lahunta A, Timoney J: Neuritis in the cauda equina, a chronic idiopathic polyradiculoneuritis in the horse. Acta Neuropathol 46:17–24, 1979.
83. Edington N, Wright J, Patel J, et al: Equine adenovirus 1 isolated from cauda equina neuritis. Res Vet Sci 37:252–254, 1984.
84. Fordyce P, Edington N, Bridges G, et al: Use of an ELISA in the differential diagnosis of cauda equina neuritis and other equine neuropathies. Equine Vet J 19:55–59, 1987.
85. Osweiler GD, Carson TL, Buck WB, et al: Clinical and Diagnostic Veterinary Toxicology, 3rd ed. Dubuque, IA, Kendall/Hunt Publishing Co, 1985.
86. Braund KG: Diseases of peripheral nerves, cranial nerves, and muscle. In Oliver JE, Hoerlein BF, Mayhew IG: Veterinary Neurology. Philadelphia, WB Saunders, 1987, pp 353–392.

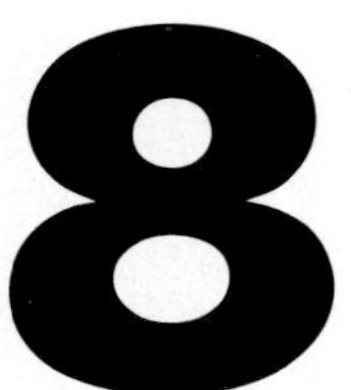

Tetraparesis, Hemiparesis, and Ataxia

Motor dysfunction of all four limbs is called *tetraparesis* or *tetraplegia* (quadriparesis, quadriplegia), depending on the severity of the motor loss. The paresis may be manifested as a gait abnormality or as postural reaction deficits. The term *hemiparesis* refers to motor dysfunction of two limbs on the same side. Ataxia is a frequently associated problem. Lesion localization has been discussed in Chapter 2 and is summarized in Figure 8–1. It will be reviewed briefly in this chapter.

Lesion Localization

Animals with tetraparesis usually have neurologic disease. Diffuse muscle or skeletal diseases may result in tetraparesis, which at times is difficult to differentiate from true neurologic lesions. In addition, tetraparesis of neurologic origin must be differentiated from generalized muscle weakness or depression associated with severe metabolic disease (e.g., adrenal insufficiency, hypoglycemia). When initially presented with a tetraparetic animal, the clinician must decide which systems are involved (nervous, musculoskeletal, or generalized metabolic disorders). The history, physical findings, and laboratory tests usually provide sufficient evidence for the practitioner to make this differentiation. In this chapter, primary consideration is given to lesions involving the nervous and musculoskeletal systems.

Neurologic lesions that produce tetraparesis may involve the cerebral cortex, the brain stem, the cervical cord, or the lower motor neurons (LMNs). Lesion localization is based on the decisions outlined in Figure 8–1. Although the motor cortex is important for the performance of learned reactions (see Chaps. 1 and 2), these areas do not maintain locomotion in domestic animals. Diffuse brain stem centers coordinate these functions, with reinforcement from the cerebral cortex. Therefore, animals with diffuse (bilateral) cerebral cortex disease usually have little or no gait abnormality. The postural reactions are generally abnormal contralateral to the lesion. Other signs of cerebral dysfunction, such as altered mental status, seizures, or blindness, may be present and may help in the localization of the lesion.

Lesions involving the brain stem and the cervical spinal cord result in an abnormal gait, because motor signals from brain stem centers to the LMNs of the spinal cord are disrupted. Tetraparesis develops if the lesion is bilateral, and hemiparesis (usually ipsilateral) occurs if the lesion is unilateral. Altered sensory function (ataxia, hypesthesia) frequently is associated with the motor dysfunction, because lesions are usually severe enough to disrupt the sensory pathways from the limbs and the body.

Lesions in the brain stem and C1–C5 spinal cord segments result in upper motor neuron (UMN) signs in the limbs. As has been explained in Chapter 2, disruption of UMN signals that inhibit the segmental spinal reflexes results in "release," or hyperactivity, of the LMNs. Brain stem and cranial cervical cord lesions are differentiated by an examination of the head, because lesions in either region can result in identical abnormalities in the limbs.

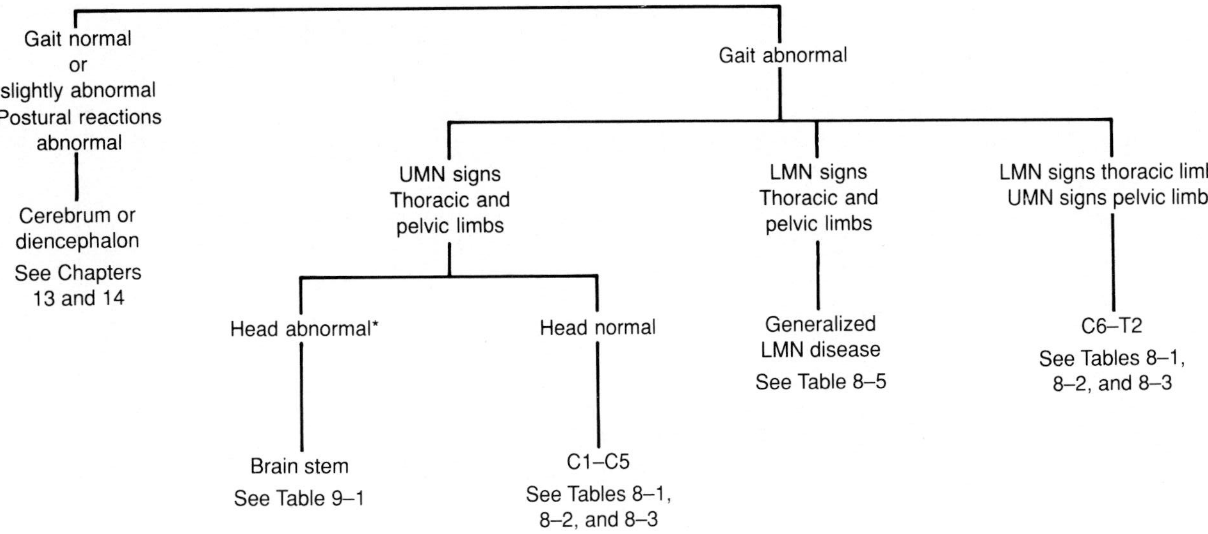

*Head involvement: one or more signs involving the head are present, e.g., head tilt, tremor of head, nystagmus, cranial nerve signs, seizures, etc.

Figure 8–1 Algorithm for the diagnosis of tetraparesis, hemiparesis, and ataxia.

The brain stem can be described as a cervical spinal cord that is modified by the presence of nuclei. Evidence of dysfunction in these nuclei indicates brain stem disease. Paresis associated with vestibular signs, altered mental status, or abnormal cranial nerve function strongly suggests a lesion in the brain stem.

Lesions involving cervical spinal segments C6–T2 result in paresis. LMN signs may be present in the thoracic limbs if the motor neurons forming the brachial plexus are injured. In addition, Horner's sign may develop if the LMNs that form the sympathetic nerve (located in segments T1–T3) are injured. UMN signs develop in the pelvic limbs because spinal pathways are disrupted as they pass through the caudal cervical spinal cord. Altered sensory function is invariably present with significant lesions in the region of C6–T2.

Animals with tetraparesis associated with diffuse LMN signs (involvement of the thoracic and the pelvic limbs) can have lesions involving the motor neurons located in the spinal cord, lesions of the axonal processes (ventral spinal root, spinal nerve, peripheral nerve), or diseases of the neuromuscular end-plate (motor end-plate). Peripheral neuropathies and motor end-plate disorders are commonly encountered in animals, whereas the neuronopathies are rare. Lesions involving the motor neurons, the ventral nerve root, or the neuromuscular end-plate do not produce sensory dysfunction. A disease that diffusely affects the peripheral nerves may cause sensory dysfunction, because most peripheral nerves contain both motor and sensory fibers. Animals with tetraparesis, LMN signs in the limbs, and normal pain perception usually have a disease involving the ventral nerve roots or the neuromuscular junction. Animals with neurologic signs that are episodic (that wax and wane with rest) usually have motor end-plate disease. A note of caution should be interjected at this point. Animals with diffuse muscle disease occasionally develop clinical signs that are strongly suggestive of diffuse LMN disease. Careful muscle palpation, laboratory tests, and biopsy are usually necessary to differentiate primary muscle disease from primary neurologic disease.

Diseases

The diseases discussed in this chapter include those that commonly affect the cervical spinal cord and those that diffusely affect the LMN system. The diseases that affect the cerebral cortex and the brain stem will be discussed in Chapters 9 through 16. As has been the style in previous chapters, this section is organized according to the anatomic location of the lesion and the course of the disease (acute versus chronic, progressive versus nonprogressive). The disorders that affect spinal cord segments C1–T2 in small animals are presented in Table 8–1. Cervical cord diseases of equids are presented in Table 8–2, and the cervical cord lesions of food animals are listed in Table 8–3. The diffuse LMN diseases are listed in Table 8–4. Each table indicates the chapter where the disease is discussed.

Acute Progressive Diseases

Cervical Disk Diseases

The pathophysiology of intervertebral disk disease was discussed in Chapter 7. Hansen type I disk protrusions in the cervical area occur most frequently in the chondrodystrophoid breeds (small poodle, dachshund, beagle, cocker spaniel) but are also encountered in certain large breed dogs, such as the Doberman pinscher. Only rarely are disk protrusions the cause of clinical signs in other species, primarily the cat and horse.[1–4] The incidence of cervical disk disease is lower than that of thoracolumbar disk disease. Approximately 14% of all disk lesions in the dog occur in the cervical area.[1] Intervertebral spaces C2–C3 and C3–C4 are most frequently involved.

Unlike thoracolumbar disk herniations, cervical disk herniations infrequently result in compressive myelopathy sufficient to cause paresis or paralysis. Although many factors may account for this finding, the larger diameter of the vertebral canal in the cervical area is probably the most important explanation. Because of the greater space surrounding the cervical cord, disk herniations in this area are less likely to result in focal compressive myelopathy. Likewise, the syndrome of ascending–descending myelomalacia rarely results from cervical disk herniation.

Clinical Signs. The most prominent sign in cervical disk protrusions is pain that arises from meningeal or nerve root irritation. The head is usually held low, and the neck may be extended rigidly. The dog may resist any attempt to move its head or neck. Occasionally, affected dogs develop a lameness of one thoracic limb. The paw may be held up intermittently as the animal stands or sits, and a slight limp may be present in the gait. A forced movement of the limb may cause considerable pain. Many of these animals have lateral extrusions of the disk causing pres-

TABLE 8–1 Small Animal C1–T2 Spinal Cord Diseases: Differential Diagnosis Based on Clinical Course and Etiologic Categories*

Etiologic Category	Acute Nonprogressive	Acute Progressive	Chronic Progressive
Degenerative	None	Type I disk disease (7, 8) Hemorrhagic myelomalacia (7)	Type II disk disease (7, 8) Cervical vertebral spondylopathy (8) Spondylosis deformans (7) Afghan hound myelopathy (7) Demyelinating diseases (8) Axonopathies and neuronopathies (8) Storage diseases (16)
Anomalous	None	None	Spinal dysraphism (7) Vertebral anomalies (7) Atlantoaxial luxation (8)
Neoplastic (7)	None	Metastatic Primary Skeletal Lymphoreticular	Primary Lymphoreticular Skeletal Metastatic
Nutritional	None	None	Hypervitaminosis A (cats) (16)
Inflammatory	None	Distemper myelitis (16) Bacterial myelitis (15) Distemper myelitis (16) Diskospondylitis (7) Protozoal myelitis (16) Mycotic myelitis (16)	Feline infectious peritonitis (16) Granulomatous meningoencephalomyelitis (16) Immune meningoencephalomyelitis (16)
Traumatic	Fractures (7) Luxations (7) Contusions (7) Intervertebral disk rupture (7)	Hemorrhagic myelomalacia (7) Intervertebral disk rupture (7)	None
Vascular	Fibrocartilaginous embolism (7) Vascular malformations (8)	None	None

* Numbers in parentheses refer to chapters in which the entities are discussed.

TABLE 8–2 Equine C1–T2 Spinal Cord Diseases: Differential Diagnosis Based on Clinical Course and Etiologic Categories*

Etiologic Category	Acute Nonprogressive	Acute Progressive	Chronic Progressive
Degenerative	None	Degenerative myeloencephalopathy (8)	Cervical spondylopathy (8) Neuronopathies (8) Demyelinating diseases (8) Axonopathies (8)
Anomalous	None	None	Vertebral anomalies (7) Occipitoatlantoaxial malformation (8) Atlantoaxial luxation (8)
Neoplastic (7)	None	Metastatic Primary Skeletal Lymphoreticular	Primary Skeletal Lymphoreticular
Nutritional	None	Degenerative myeloencephalopathy (8)	
Inflammatory	None	Herpesvirus 1 (7) Protozoal myelitis (7) Verminous migrations (7) Vertebral osteomyelitis (7) Mycotic myelitis (7)	See acute progressive
Traumatic	Fractures (7) Luxations (7)		
Vascular	Embolic myelopathy (7) Fibrocartilaginous emboli (7) Postanesthetic myelopathy		

* Numbers in parentheses refer to chapters in which the entities are discussed.

TABLE 8–3 Food Animal C1–T2 Spinal Cord Diseases: Differential Diagnosis Based on Clinical Course and Etiologic Categories*

Etiologic Category	*Acute Nonprogressive*	*Acute Progressive*	*Chronic Progressive*
Degenerative	None		Progressive ataxia of Charolais cattle – B (8) Degenerative myeloencephalopathy – B (8) Spondylosis deformans – all (7) Arthrogryposis – all (8) Demyelinating diseases – B (8) Neuronopathies – O (8)
Anomalous	None	Occipitoatlantoaxial malformations – B, O (7)	Occipitoatlantoaxial malformations – B, O (7) Vertebral anomalies – all (7)
Neoplastic (7)	None	Metastatic Primary Skeletal Lymphoreticular	Primary Lymphoreticular Skeletal Metastatic
Nutritional	None	None	Enzootic ataxia, copper deficiency – C, O (16)
Inflammatory	None	Caprine arthritis-encephalomyelitis – C (7) Bacterial myelitis – all (15) Vertebral osteomyelitis – all (7) Protozoal myelitis (16) Mycotic myelitis (16)	Visna-Maedi – O (16) Verminous migration – all (7)
Toxic	None	Selenium – P (16)	
Traumatic	Fractures (7) Luxations (7) Contusions (7)		None
Vascular	Fibrocartilaginous embolism – P (7)	None	None

* Numbers in parentheses refer to chapters in which the entities are discussed. B = bovine, C = caprine, O = ovine, P = porcine.

TABLE 8–4 Diffuse LMN Diseases

Acute Progressive Disorders
Polyradiculoneuritis
Tick paralysis
Botulism
Aminoglycoside paralysis

Chronic Progressive Disorders
Motor neuronopathies
- Spinal muscle atrophy of Brittany spaniels
- Swedish Lapland dog paralysis
- Stockard's paralysis
- Spinal muscle atrophy of pointers
- Spinal muscle atrophy of German shepherd dogs
- Spinal muscle atrophy of Rottweiler dogs
- Multisystem neuronal degenerations
- Equine motor neuron disease

Polyneuropathy (see Table 8–6)
Polymyopathy (see Table 8–7)

Episodic Progressive Disorders
Myasthenia gravis
Metabolic (polysystemic) disorders (see Chap. 16)
- Hypoglycemia
- Hyperkalemia
- Hypercalcemia
- Hypocalcemia
- Hypomagnesemia

Chronic relapsing polymyositis

sure on the spinal nerve.[5] Dogs that are in pain have a stiff, short-strided gait and may cry or whine if forced to change direction suddenly. Most dogs are reluctant to, or refuse to, descend stairs or jump. The clinical signs resulting from pain are very similar to the signs associated with bacterial meningitis.

Occasionally, a cervical disk herniation may be large enough to compress the cervical cord, and paresis and ataxia of the thoracic and pelvic limbs will result. Rarely, a massive disk blowout will produce tetraplegia. Tetraplegia with loss of deep pain sensation is not seen because respiration would be impaired with such a lesion. Disk protrusions in the cervical spinal cord may produce Horner's syndrome. Caudal cervical disk herniation may produce LMN signs in one or both thoracic limbs. The presence of neurologic signs other than pain strongly suggests spinal cord compression. Evidence of spinal cord compression is an indication for decompressive surgery.

Diagnosis. The clinical diagnosis of cervical disk disease is confirmed by radiographic examination of the cervical area (Figs. 8–2 and 8–3).

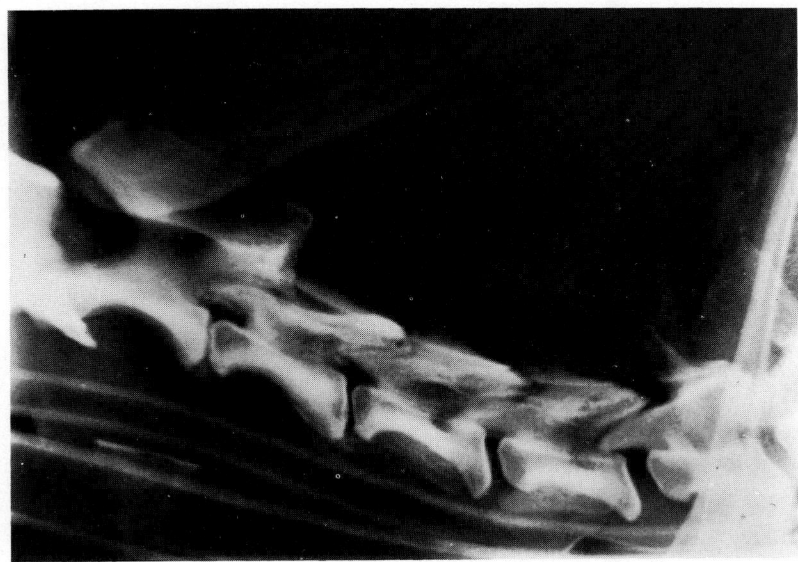

Figure 8–2 Lateral cervical radiograph of a dog with cervical disk disease. Note narrow spaces at C2–C3 and C3–C4. The condition responded to ventral fenestration.

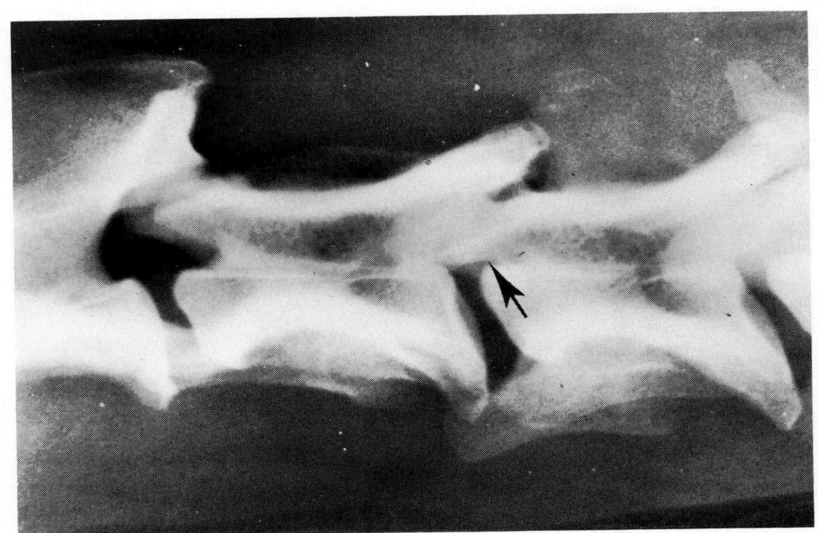

Figure 8–3 Lateral cervical radiograph showing massive disk herniation (arrow) at C3–C4. Decompressive surgery is indicated in this case.

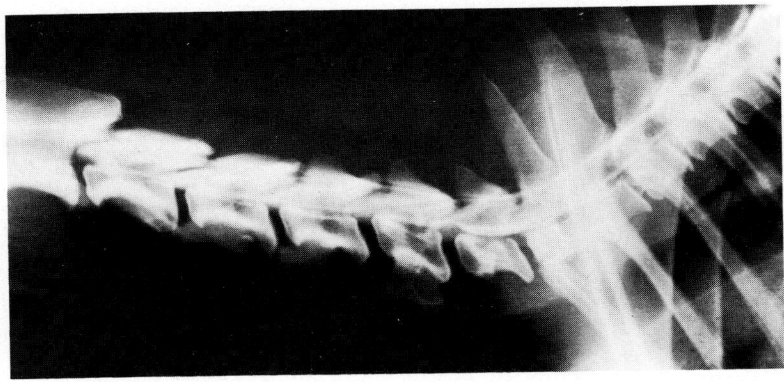

Figure 8–4 Cervical myelogram of a dog with a caudal cervical disk protrusion at C6–C7. The lesion was not visualized on survey radiographs. The condition responded to ventral decompressive surgery.

Radiographs are taken for all surgical candidates. Anesthesia is required for proper positioning when diagnostic radiographs are taken. If conventional radiographs fail to demonstrate a lesion, cerebrospinal fluid (CSF) should be obtained to rule out infectious meningomyelitis. If the spinal fluid is normal, myelography should be done to demonstrate the spinal cord compression (Fig. 8–4). Many surgeons prefer to have a myelogram for all cervical disk protrusions to define the lateralization and extent of the disk material. Dogs with an initial episode of pain may be treated medically, and in such cases conventional radiographs are not taken, since the risk of anesthesia largely outweighs the benefit of the procedure. However, the signs of cervical disk protrusion are virtually identical to those of meningitis. If the diagnosis is not clear-cut or the animal does not respond promptly to medical therapy, one should perform conventional radiography, CSF analysis, and myelography (if the CSF is normal) with the dog under anesthesia.

Treatment. Many dogs with cervical disk disease respond at least temporarily to nursing care that supports normal healing processes. Because the risk of severe, permanent neurologic dysfunction is not great, cervical disk disease is usually not considered a major neurosurgical emergency.

Many dogs with cervical disk disease are treated medically, even though the majority of these cases relapse at a later date. Fenestration of the disks at an early stage in the disease prevents recurrences in type I disk disease. Because severe herniations require decompression, and because recurrences are frequent, early fenestration is recommended. Decisions regarding medical or surgical therapy are based on the clinical signs and the chronicity of the problem.

MEDICAL THERAPY Medical therapy for cervical disk disease, like that for thoracolumbar disk herniations, should be restricted to dogs with an initial episode of neck pain. Therapy must support normal healing processes, keep the animal reasonably comfortable, and not cause serious complications. The most important part of the treatment is strict confinement to keep movement to a minimum. The more the dog moves the neck, the more disk material is extruded. Confining the dog to an airline crate is preferred. Exercise for bladder and bowel evacuation is done on a leash with a harness. Collars are avoided. If the animal is confined but still has considerable pain, mild analgesics or nonsteroidal anti-inflammatory drugs may be used (see Chap. 15). Glucocorticoids are not recommended unless the other treatments fail, because they interfere with healing and have other side effects. In addition, if there is any doubt regarding the diagnosis, corticosteroids should be avoided. Meningitis can have the same clinical presentation, and the immune suppression associated with corticosteroids could make this disease much worse. Pain relief should always be accompanied by strict confinement, as the animal may become too active when pain is relieved. The owner is instructed to maintain confinement for at least 2 weeks, regardless of how much the dog improves. If signs become worse, the dog should be reevaluated for surgery. Most dogs that are treated medically improve, only to relapse at a later date. Owners must be cautioned that medical therapy is seldom a total cure for cervical disk disease.

SURGICAL THERAPY The various forms of therapy have been reviewed extensively by Hoerlein.[1] There is general agreement that ventral fenestration is an effective procedure for dogs with recurrent cervical pain. The procedure is easy to perform and causes little postoperative reaction. This procedure will not remove disk material that has herniated into the vertebral canal. If the protrusion is large, recovery will be slow or will not occur at all.[1] A recent review comparing fenestration to decompression concluded that decompression is superior except in rates of intraoperative and postoperative complications.[6]

Dogs with persistent pain following ventral fenestration or those with paresis, paralysis, and ataxia should undergo decompressive surgery. These clinical signs indicate that the disk material is compressing the cervical cord. The inflammatory process and the compression induced by the disk material seldom resolve with medical therapy. In addition, the disk material cannot be removed by ventral fenestration. The ventral decompression technique affords nearly complete removal of the protruding mass with adequate decompression. The prognosis for functional recovery of most type I cervical disk patients following decompression is excellent. In large breed dogs with type II disk protrusions, recovery may be slow and may entail considerable physical therapy (see Cervical Spondylopathy—Management, below).

Cervical Meningomyelitis

Inflammation of the meninges by bacterial, viral, or fungal agents may produce clinical signs that are very similar to those of cervical disk disease. Cervical pain is frequent with meningitis. Involvement of the white or gray matter of the spinal cord results in paresis, paralysis, and sensory ataxia. These diseases usually are characterized by polysystemic signs and multifocal neurologic lesions. In many cases, the course becomes chronic and progressive following the acute development of neurologic signs. The diagnosis is primarily based on characteristic CSF abnormalities. These disorders will be discussed in Chapters 15 and 16.

Equine Degenerative Myeloencephalopathy

Equine degenerative myeloencephalopathy occurs in light breeds of horses. A similar disorder is seen in captive Przewalskii horses, zebras, and in a few ruminant species. It is characterized by the early onset (when the animal is 0 to 24 months old) of acute progressive symmetric ataxia and paresis. Chronic progressive forms of the disease have been described. Histopathologically, the disease is characterized by a diffuse myeloencephalopathy, with variations in the degree and extent of the lesions.[7,8] There is consistent degeneration of white matter in all spinal cord funiculi, especially in the sensory (proprioceptive) relay nuclei in the medulla oblongata and spinal cord. The lesion, a neuroaxonal dystrophy, is also seen in a syndrome of Morgan horses that appears to be familial.[9] The cause is unknown, but there is evidence that vitamin E deficiency may be one factor in the syndrome.[8,10] The disease must be differentiated clinically from cervical spondylopathy and protozoal myeloencephalitis.

Clinical Signs. Signs develop in horses that are less than 2 years of age. The signs are a symmetric UMN deficit and a general proprioceptive deficit in all four limbs; however, the clinical signs are more severe in the pelvic limbs.[7] There may be decreased cervical reflexes, such as on the slap test, and decreased cutaneous reflexes. Although the disease is progressive, tetraplegia is rare. The early onset of signs (at a mean age of 0.4 year) and the marked disparity in the gait deficit between the thoracic and pelvic limbs helps in the differentiation of equine degenerative myeloencephalopathy from focal cervical myelopathies.

Diagnosis. An antemortem diagnosis is difficult to confirm. Radiology of the cervical spine is useful for distinguishing equine degenerative myeloencephalopathy from cervical spondylopathy if rigid criteria are followed (see Cervical Spondylopathy—Diagnosis, below). Serum vitamin E concentrations should be greater than 1.5 μg/ml in normal horses.[7] Levels in affected horses may be half that or less. There are few abnormalities in the CSF of horses with equine degenerative myeloencephalopathy, a feature that is useful for differentiating this disease from protozoal encephalomyelitis.

Treatment. Vitamin E supplementation is recommended at a level of 1,000–2,000 units/day. Providing fresh green forage with an adequate vitamin E content may be better.[7] The prognosis is poor for complete resolution of signs, although they may stabilize. The possibility of a familial predisposition should be considered.

Acute Nonprogressive Diseases, C1–C5

Fibrocartilaginous Embolization

This syndrome was described in Chapter 7; however, the disease also occurs in the cervical spinal cord. The clinical signs develop acutely and progress rapidly in 1 to 2 hours from initial pain to tetraparesis or hemiparesis (if only one side of the cord is involved). The signs suggest acute cervical spinal cord compression; however, affected dogs experience much less pain than do dogs with cervical disk disease. Lesions in the caudal cervical cord frequently result in LMN signs in the thoracic limbs and UMN signs in the pelvic limbs. Lateralizing signs suggest this disease. The diagnosis and management were discussed in Chapter 7.

Cervical Spinal Cord Trauma

Traumatic compression of the cervical spinal cord, in contrast to compression of the thoracolumbar spinal cord, is more likely to cause pain with little motor dysfunction; however, extensive compression will result in motor and sensory dysfunction. Injuries cranial to C5 may produce sudden death through disruption of the respiratory pathways to the phrenic and intercostal motor neurons. Therefore, tetraplegia with loss of deep pain sensation caudal to the lesion is rare, because affected animals die of respiratory failure. The pathophysiology, the diagnosis, and the management of spinal cord trauma were discussed in Chapter 7.

Chronic Progressive Diseases, C1–C5

Atlantoaxial Subluxation

In 1967, a slowly progressive subluxation of the atlantoaxial articulation was described in ten small breed dogs.[11] The condition is seen rarely in other species.[12] Since that time, a variety of lesions involving the atlas and the axis have been reported. Most of these lesions cause dorsal displacement of the axis into the vertebral canal (Fig. 8–5A), resulting in compression of the cervical spinal cord.[13] These lesions include luxations with an intact dens, luxations with a congenital malformation of the dens (Fig. 8–5B), and fractures of the axis or the atlas. In addition, some congenital malformations involve the atlas, axis, and occipital bone. These malformations are discussed in the next section.

Pathophysiology. Disorders of the atlantoaxial articulation usually result from a congenital malformation, a traumatic fracture of the dens, or a traumatic tearing or stretching of the transverse atlantal ligament. The normal atlantoaxial articulation allows rotational movement. The dens projects from the body of the axis and is bound to the ventral arch of the atlas by a strong transverse ligament (Fig. 8–6). This at-

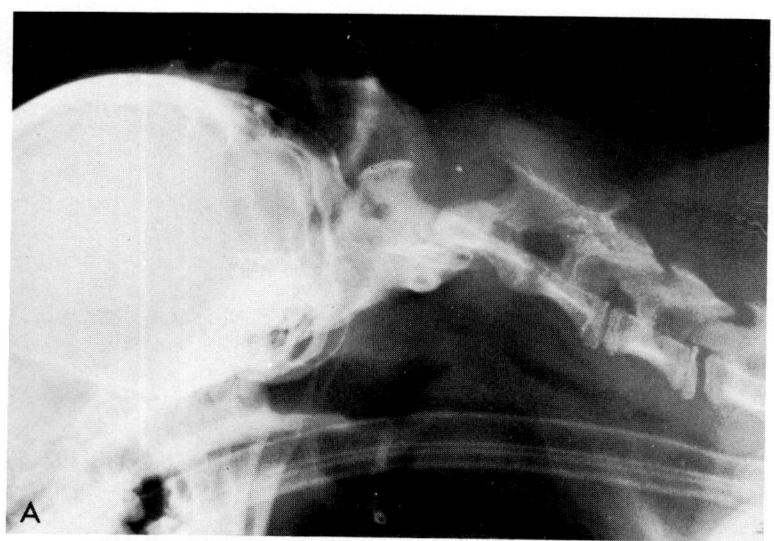

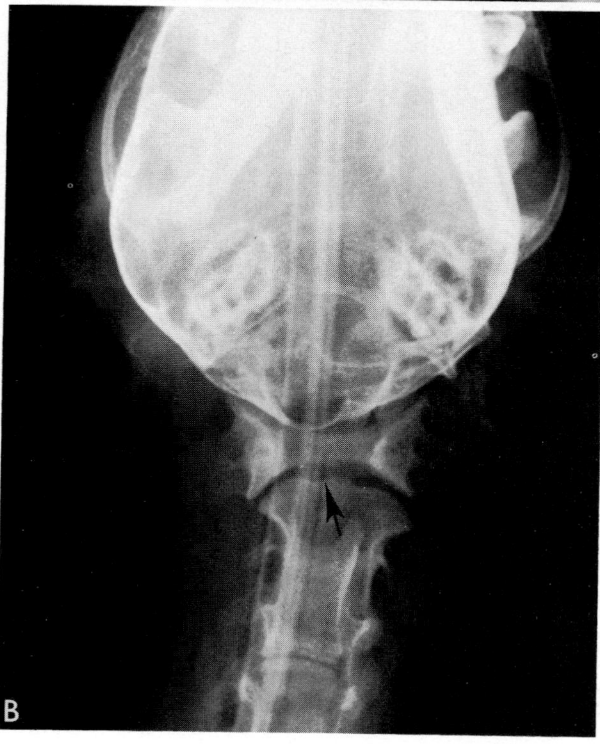

Figure 8–5 *A.* Lateral cervical radiograph of a dog with atlantoaxial luxation. Note the dorsal displacement of C2, compressing the spinal cord at this level. *B.* Ventrodorsal radiograph of the same dog. Note the absence of a normal dens (arrow). (From Oliver JE Jr, Lewis RE: Lesions of the atlas and axis in dogs. JAAHA 9:307, 1973. Used by permission.)

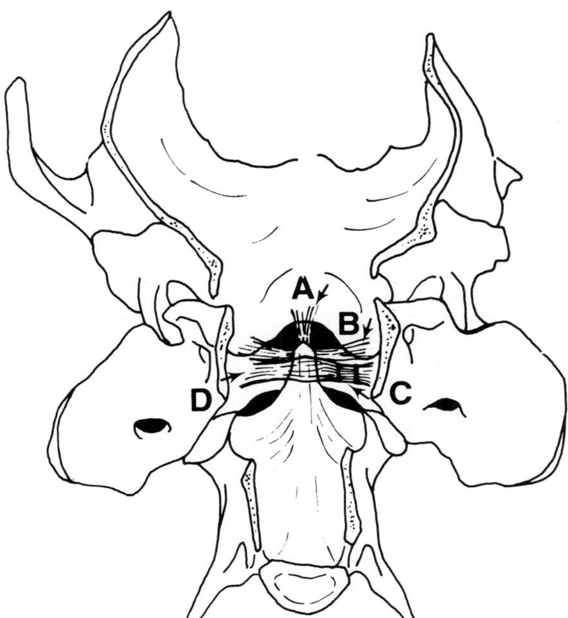

Figure 8–6 The ligamentous attachments of the dens. *A*, apical; *B*, alar; *C*, lateral; *D*, transverse atlantal. (From Oliver JE Jr, Lewis RE: Lesions of the atlas and axis in dogs. JAAHA 9:307, 1973. Used by permission.)

tachment prevents flexion between the atlas and the axis (Fig. 8–7A). Disorders of this attachment allow the axis to rotate dorsally. The spinal cord is then compressed between the axis and the dorsal arch of the atlas (Fig. 8–7B). Cervical flexion accentuates the degree of spinal cord compression.

Atlantoaxial luxation with an intact dens results from traumatic rupture of the transverse atlantal ligament or lack of development of the transverse atlantal ligament.[14] Severe spinal cord compression occurs, because the cord is pinched between the intact dens and the dorsal atlantal arch (see Fig. 8–7B). Luxations caused by a fracture or a congenital malformation of the dens usually produce less severe neurologic signs, because less compression of the spinal cord occurs. Fractures of the body of the axis produce neurologic signs similar to those of acute traumatic luxation. Neurologic signs result from acute or chronic progressive compressive myelopathy (see Chap. 7). The congenital disorders are usually more chronic with a gradual progression of neurologic signs. They occur most frequently in the toy or miniature breeds.

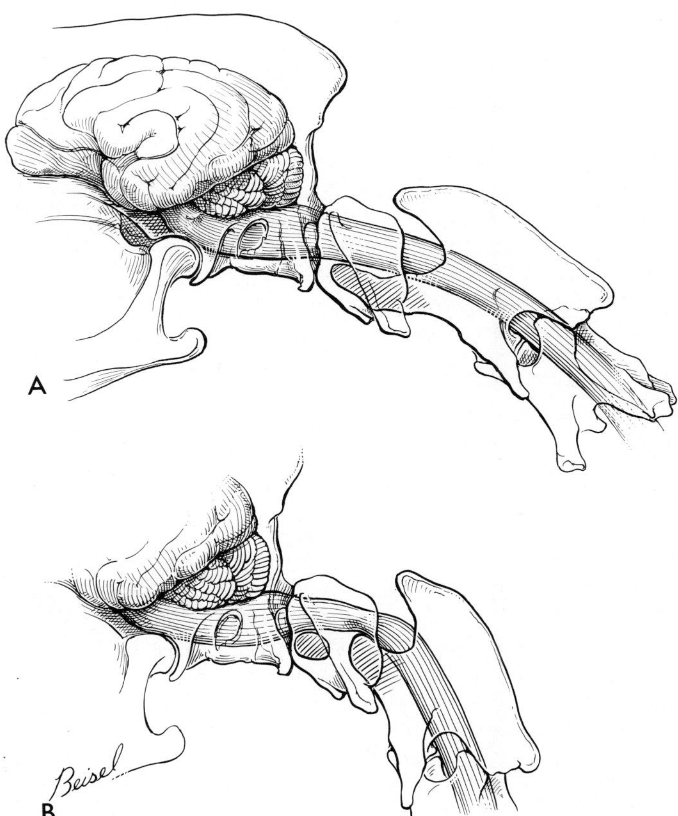

Figure 8–7 *A*. Drawing of the normal atlantoaxial articulation. *B*. Drawing of atlantoaxial luxation resulting from separation of the dens from the body of the axis. Note the dorsal displacement of the axis, compressing the spinal cord at this level.

Clinical Signs. Traumatic luxations or fractures of C1, C2 result in cervical pain, tetraparesis, and ataxia. Neurologic signs may be asymmetric. Dogs with congenital lesions usually exhibit signs during the first year of life; however, older dogs also may develop signs. Some dogs may not have clinical signs because adequate vertebral support by other fibrous and muscular structures prevents C1, C2 luxation. With age, these structures may weaken, allowing the axis to rotate dorsally and to compress the spinal cord. In the congenital form of the disorder, the initial clinical sign is usually cervical pain. The signs progress from pain to minor motor dysfunction to severe paresis or paralysis.[13,15]

The displaced axis may be palpated as a firm swelling just caudal to the occiput.[13] Flexing the neck results in severe pain and accentuates motor dysfunction. Neck flexion must be performed cautiously because it can produce severe neurologic injury. Respiratory failure occurs when these pathologic events compromise respiratory pathways. *When atlantoaxial luxation or fractures are suspected, it is vital that extension of the neck be maintained, especially during anesthesia.*[13]

Diagnosis. Atlantoaxial lesions must be suspected in all toy or miniature dogs with rostral cervical pain, neck rigidity, and paresis or paralysis. Spinal radiography is useful for demonstrating the C1, C2 malalignment. The survey spinal radiographs should be taken while the animal is awake. Anesthetized dogs do not maintain cervical muscle tension, which increases the possibility of neck flexion and severe spinal cord compression. Lateral and ventrodorsal views should be taken. If the survey films demonstrate minor displacement, a definitive diagnosis can be formulated with the aid of radiographs taken with the dog anesthetized just prior to surgical fixation.[13] Careful neck flexion may be needed to demonstrate the luxation.

Treatment. Atlantoaxial luxations and most fractures require immediate surgical immobilization. Medical management with external stabilization has been reported, but we prefer surgical stabilization. Antiedema therapy may be necessary for animals with traumatic lesions or during surgery to help control intraoperative spinal cord edema (see Chaps. 7 and 13).

Several surgical techniques have been described.[13,16–19] The techniques include simple decompression and various forms of stabilization or fusion. The surgeon can stabilize luxations with or without fracture of the dens by wiring the arch of the atlas to the dorsal spinous process of the axis (Fig. 8–8). Most surgical techniques are based on modifications of this approach, including the use of various materials instead of wire,[20,21] threading the material under the lamina of both the axis and atlas,[16] or the use of an implant.[22] Ventral stabilization with pins or screws provides the best alternative.[17] The ventral approach also allows fusion of the articulation with bone graft to potentially provide permanent fixation. However, in our experience, dorsal fixation rarely fails when done properly.

The prognosis for recovery is good if surgery is performed before irreversible spinal cord injury occurs.

Occipitoatlantoaxial Malformations (OAAM)

These congenital malformations are reported in horses, cattle, cats, and dogs.[7,23] Congenital asymmetric OAAM and asymmetric atlanto-occipital fusion are presumed to be inherited in Arabian horses.[7] Ataxia, tetraparesis, and a stiff neck may be found in neonates or in weanling foals. The abnormal cervical articulations usually can be palpated. A wide variety of anomalies are reported. Dorsal angulation of the dens is seen in dogs.[24] Fusion of the atlas to the occipital bone as part of the malformation is seen in horses, cattle, and cats.

Occipitoatlantal Luxations

Traumatic luxations of the occipitoatlantal joint are rare. They have been reported in dogs, a cat, and a goat.[25–29] In two dogs and one cat the luxations were managed by manual reduction and application of a cast with the neck in flexion. Two dogs and a goat were treated surgically. This rare injury would probably result in death of the animal in most cases, but all of these had relatively minimal neurologic deficits.

Cervical Vertebral Anomalies

Cervical vertebral malformations with or without secondary spinal cord compression occur in the cervical vertebrae as elsewhere (see Chap. 7 for a description of these anomalies). Malformations may be a component of the "wobbler" syndrome, which we call cervical spondylopathy.

Cervical Spondylopathy

The growing popularity of the giant breed dogs and the performance horses during the past 20 years is probably responsible for the increased

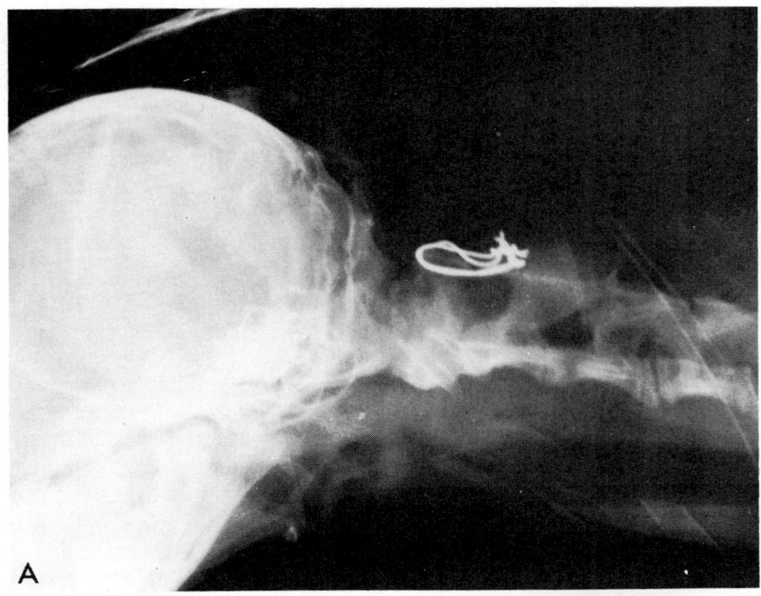

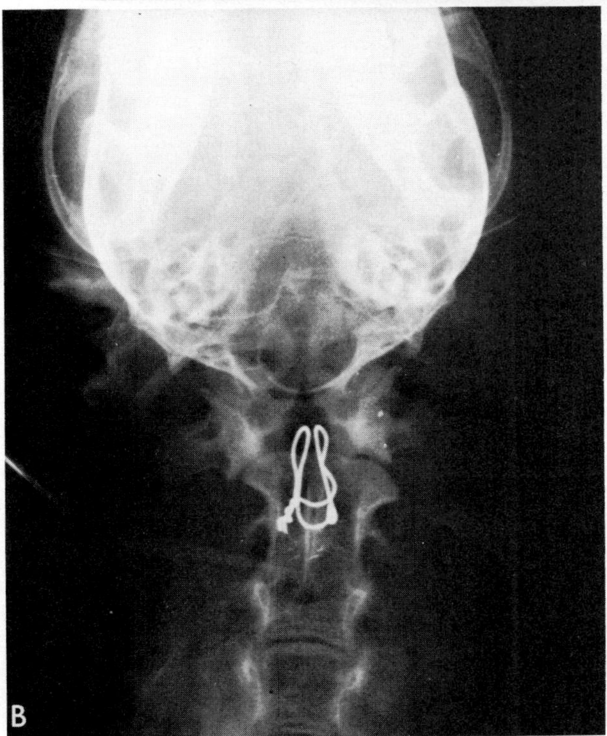

Figure 8–8 *A, B.* Lateral and ventrodorsal radiographs of a dog with atlantoaxial luxation, following reduction and wire stabilization. (From Oliver JE Jr, Lewis RE: Lesions of the atlas and axis in dogs. JAAHA 9:307, 1973.)

interest in this neurologic syndrome. The disorder appears with greater frequency in the Great Dane, the Doberman pinscher, and the Thoroughbred horse, but it has been recognized in several other breeds of dogs and horses. Controversy still exists regarding proper terminology for this syndrome. Presently, *cervical spondylopathy*, *cervical spondylomyelopathy*, *cervical vertebral malformation-malarticulation*, and *cervical vertebral stenotic myelopathy* appear to be the most useful names, encompassing the forms of the disease in all affected animals. Some investigators prefer to lump all breeds together, whereas others prefer to split the disease into separate categories for each breed. Needless to say, each group of researchers has valid reasons for its decision. Our objective is to describe the similarities and the differences in the pathology and the management of cervical spondylopathy in each affected breed.

Pathophysiology. The pathology responsible for the clinical signs in the young Great Dane, Doberman pinscher, and Thoroughbred is the basic model with which the disease in other animals is compared. In affected animals, neurologic signs develop because of progressive spinal cord compression from surrounding vertebral structures. Abnormalities of the midcervical to the caudal cervical vertebrae or their articulations, or both, are the usual lesions that are demonstrated radiographically or at necropsy. Because the exact cause is unknown, the term *cervical spondylopathy* will be used broadly to encompass the various vertebral abnormalities.

Early studies suggested that excessive mobility of the caudal cervical vertebrae was primarily responsible for the cord compression. Subsequent studies demonstrated that malformation of the cervical vertebrae resulted in stenosis of the vertebral canal.[30–34] These changes, which are more consistently present in the young Great Dane, include a narrowing and a dorsoventral flattening of the cranial vertebral foramen of C5, C6, and C7. The sixth cervical vertebra is usually most severely affected. In young Thoroughbred horses and basset hounds, these findings are more common at C3 and C4. Abnormalities in the size, shape, or position of the articular processes may be present. In some cases, hyperostosis of the articular facets may cause direct spinal cord compression. The vertebral malformation tends to lead to malarticulation and vertebral instability. Instability without severe malformation is seen in the young Doberman pinscher. Apparently, in an attempt to correct the instability, soft tissues that support and strengthen the cervical articulations proliferate. In dogs and in some horses, hypertrophy of the interarcuate ligament, the dorsal longitudinal ligament, or the dorsal annulus may produce a soft tissue compression of the spinal cord at the vertebral articulations.

In the older Doberman pinscher, degeneration and protrusion of the caudal cervical intervertebral disks are important in the development of clinical signs. The majority of the radiographic, surgical, or necropsy findings in older dogs are primarily those of type II disk disease.[32,35,36] These findings suggest that the syndrome affecting the older Doberman pinscher is different from the syndrome affecting the young Great Dane. Type II disk disease must be ruled out carefully in older Doberman pinschers that have signs suggesting cervical spondylopathy. The management and the prognosis of the two conditions are considerably different in most cases.

Although many factors, perhaps genetically controlled, may contribute to the development of cervical spondylopathy, the exact cause is unknown. Many of the large and giant breeds have been selected for their size and rapid growth. In horses, the disease occurs primarily in animals that are big for their age and breed. The very large head of certain breeds may exert an unusual force on structures that already have been genetically weakened (the midcervical to caudal cervical vertebrae). Great Danes in particular have been selected for a prancing, high-stepping gait that some consider to be a mild form of hypermetria. In selecting this gait, the breeder actually may have selected a neurologic-musculoskeletal disorder. One study of Great Danes established a relationship between excessive nutrition and several skeletal changes that also involved the cervical vertebrae.[37] Thus, nutritional factors also may be involved in the expression of clinical signs. The exact cause of the disorder awaits further classification. The vertebral pathology is quite similar in the young Great Dane and the Thoroughbred horse.

Clinical Signs. In the majority of Great Danes and horses and in some Doberman pinschers, clinical signs develop at 3 to 18 months of age. In many Dobermans, clinical signs develop later in life (3 to 8 years of age). The disease usually occurs in horses that are less than 3 years old.[7] Although most authors accept no sex predisposition, some studies report a greater incidence in males. This finding also has been noted in horses. Typical signs in dogs develop in the pelvic limbs and the pelvis as a mild lack of coordination that progresses to severe bilateral ataxia and hypermetria. The compression of ascending proprioceptive pathways is responsible for these neurologic signs. With increasing compression, the involvement of descending motor pathways produces paresis or paralysis of the UMN type. Although the site of compression is the cervical spinal cord, clinical signs are usually more severe in the pelvic limbs. Ataxia and paresis in the thoracic limbs may be pronounced in some cases but are usually detectable only by careful neurologic examination. Postural reaction deficits usually can be detected. Forcing the dog to wheelbarrow with its head extended (so that it cannot see the floor) accentuates proprioceptive deficits in the thoracic limbs. Some tetraparetic dogs and horses may have LMN signs in the thoracic limbs because of cervical gray matter involvement. Neck pain is usually absent unless the disorder is also associated with cervical disk protrusion. Extension of the neck may elicit a pain response. The signs worsen progressively, and urinary incontinence may occur as a late manifestation in dogs. In some animals, trauma may precede the development of acute signs. Deep pain responses are usually preserved. Unlike the majority of dogs, most horses have an acute onset of ataxia, paresis, and spasticity of all four limbs. After an initial period of progression, the equine disease usually stabilizes. The abnormalities of the pelvic limbs are usually one grade worse than those of the thoracic limbs.[7]

Diagnosis. The diagnosis of cervical spondylopathy is confirmed radiographically. The radiographic findings have been reported extensively and will be summarized here. The changes observed on survey radiographs include:

1. A change in shape or density, or both, of the intervertebral disk or disk space, or both (Fig. 8–9). This change is more common in the older Doberman pinscher.
2. Changes in shape or density, or both, of the articular facets (sclerosis and exostosis) (Fig. 8–10).
3. Vertebral displacement (subluxation) (Fig. 8–11). However, diagnosis of subluxation based on survey radiographs is not acceptable because of the considerable variability in normal dogs.
4. Stenosis of the vertebral canal (see Fig. 8–12).
5. Malformed or misshaped vertebral bodies (Fig. 8–12).
6. Misshapen dorsal spinous processes.[31,32,38]

Stressed (flexion, extension) survey radiographs are not useful. The range of normal variability is large, there is danger of further damaging the spinal cord, and myelography is essential for diagnosis in any case. Minor changes in spinal canal architecture, soft tissue compression, or disk protrusions are detected only on myelography. Because multiple lesions usually are present, myelography is recommended, so that the exact site or cause of the spinal cord compression can be identified (Fig. 8–13). Myelograms made with the neck extended often demonstrate soft tissue compression that may be missed if the neck is imaged in normal positions. Based on the myelographic results, rational surgical therapy can be instituted. Myelography is mandatory in the older Doberman pinscher in order to exclude disk disease as the primary cause of the neurologic signs (Fig. 8–14).

In the horse, cervical spondylopathy must be differentiated from degenerative myeloencephalopathy and protozoal myeloencephalitis. As in the dog, carefully performed cervical radiography can confirm the diagnosis, and survey radiographs can demonstrate vertebral changes. Various measurements of the sagittal diameter of the vertebral canal on neutral and flexed vertebrae have been reported.[7] However, as in the dog, myelography is necessary for an accurate assessment.

Therapy. Some dogs with mild neurologic signs improve with cage rest and mild analgesic therapy. The neurologic status usually deteriorates with resumption of normal activity. The use of corticosteroids in young, growing animals is contraindicated. The best long-term benefits are provided by surgical stabilization or decompression, or both. Abnormal vertebrae at multiple levels, as often occur in the Great Dane, are difficult to correct surgically. An extensive dorsal laminectomy is probably the best procedure. Even then, the chances of recurrent compression at adjacent spaces are great.[39–41] The type of abnormality seen in the older Doberman is more amenable to surgical correction. Although some animals will have recurrences, the prognosis is much more favorable. Currently, most surgeons use a distraction and stabilization technique or simply do a ventral decompression, but a dorsal laminectomy is still preferred by some surgeons.[36,40,42–45] The choice of techniques is based on the type of pathology and the experience of the surgeon. Regardless of the procedure used, the surgical results largely depend on the degree of spinal cord damage present at the time of surgery.

The medical therapy for equine cervical spondylopathy is similar to that for dogs. In the early stages in young horses, feeding a balanced, minimal-growth diet may result in improvement.[7] Ventral cervical fusion is indicated for horses with cord compression caused by cervical vertebral instability. Dorsal decompression is used to treat stenotic lesions that cause cord compression, irrespective of neck position.[7,46,47]

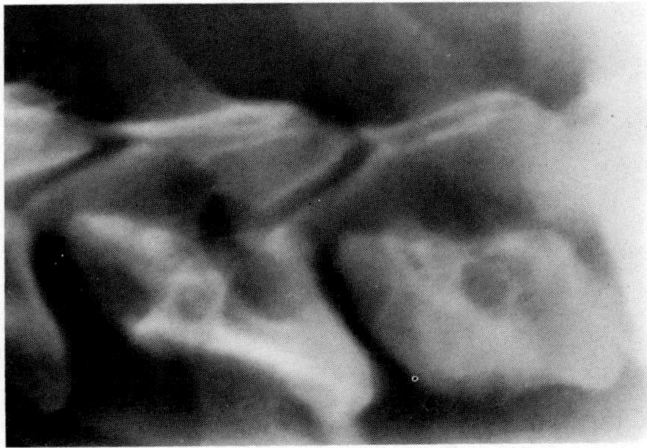

Figure 8–9 Lateral radiograph of a 6-year-old Doberman pinscher with tetraparesis and moderate caudal neck pain. The disk space at C5–C6 is narrowed, suggesting disk herniation.

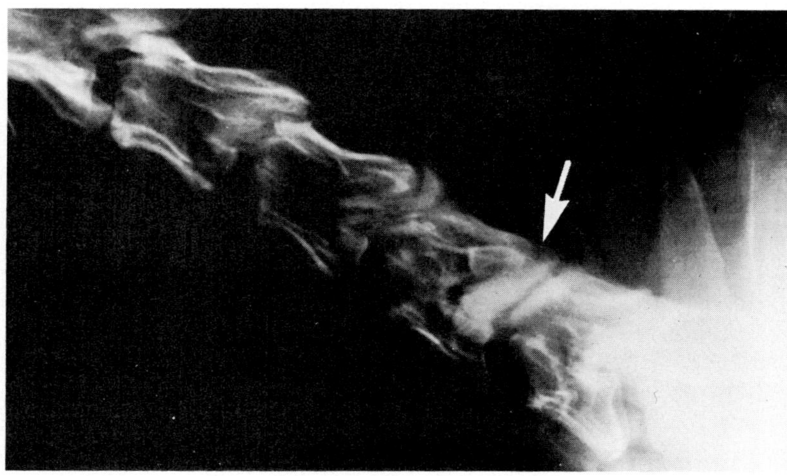

Figure 8–10 Myelogram of a 6-year-old Great Dane with tetraplegia. Note marked sclerosis and exostosis of the articular facets. The vertebral canal is extremely narrowed at C5–C6 (arrow) by the changes in the bone. Euthanasia was performed.

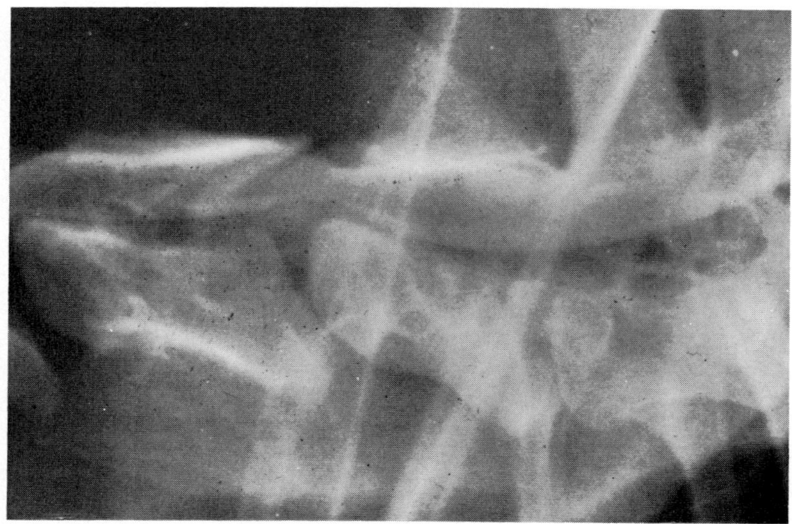

Figure 8–11 Myelogram of a 4-year-old Doberman pinscher with cervical spondylopathy. Note the subluxation of C6 and stenosis of the vertebral canal at this level.

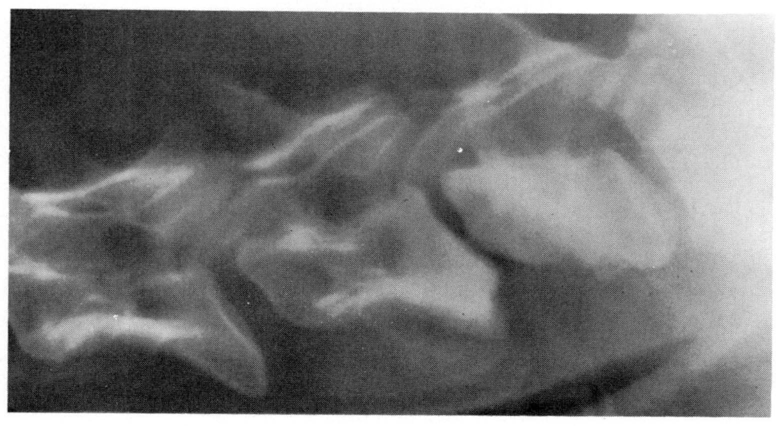

Figure 8–12 Misshaped C5 and C6 vertebrae in a 9-year-old Doberman pinscher with cervical spondylopathy.

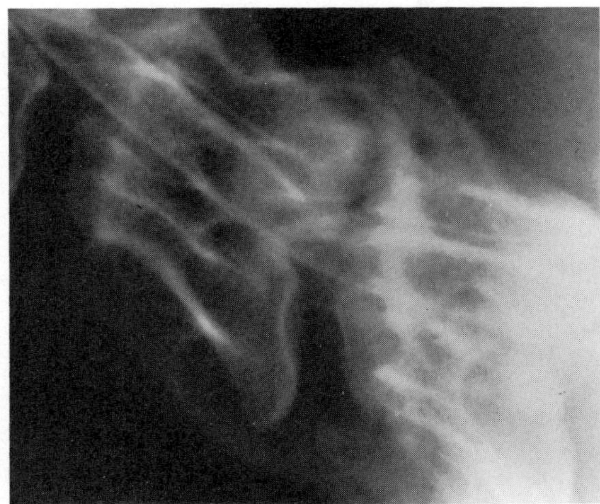

Figure 8–13 Myelogram of the cervical area with the neck extended. Note the dorsal compression of the spinal cord from ligamentous proliferation in this area. Myelograms are needed in order to demonstrate compression by soft tissues in certain cases of cervical spondylopathy.

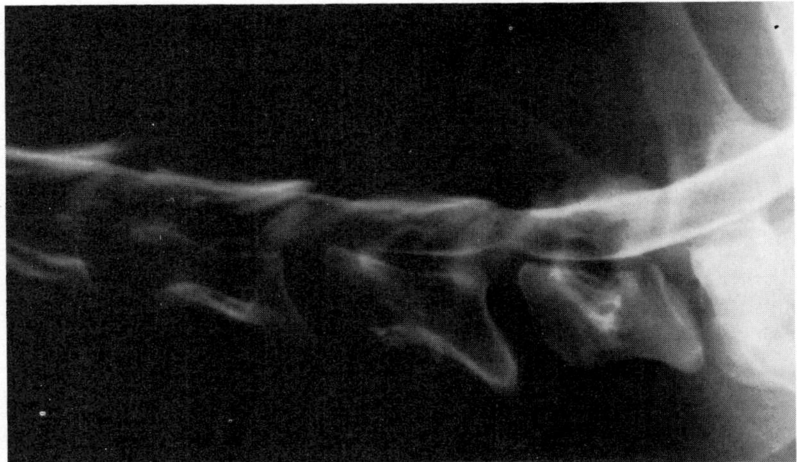

Figure 8–14 Myelogram of an adult Doberman pinscher with C6–C7 disk protrusion.

The results of surgery depend to some degree on the severity, the distribution, and the duration of cervical cord compression.

Prognosis. In general, the prognosis for full recovery is poor, especially in tetraplegic dogs. Several factors contribute to the poor recovery rates, including (1) irreparable spinal cord damage, (2) failure to provide adequate decompression or stabilization, (3) development of compression at sites adjacent to the initial lesions, and (4) postsurgical complications caused by failure to rehabilitate the recumbent large breed dog. The prognosis is better in those cases in which the clinical signs result primarily from cervical disk protrusion or herniation. Most affected animals respond to ventral decompression or distraction with stabilization. Many dogs that initially are benefited by surgery develop neurologic signs later in life because of compression at sites adjacent to the initial lesion. Certain stabilization procedures actually may increase stress forces at adjacent intervertebral sites. Owners should be warned that the surgery is difficult to perform and that the results may not be satisfactory.

In horses, the prognosis is poor without surgery. The results of ventral cervical fusion appear to be better than the results following subtotal dorsal decompression.

Diseases with Diffuse LMN Signs

Diseases that affect one or more components of the LMNs result in hyporeflexic or areflexic paresis or paralysis. Sensory function may be normal or decreased, or occasionally hyperesthesia is present. The various diseases listed in Table 8–4 can be classified as acute progressive, chronic progressive, or episodic. All are characterized by diffuse symmetric or asymmetric involvement of LMNs. The neurologic examination must be careful and thorough in these patients. In the early stages of the more chronic diseases the LMN signs are subtle. Decreased strength of the flexion reflex may be the most prominent sign.

Acute Progressive Diseases

Acute Idiopathic Polyradiculoneuritis (Coonhound Paralysis). This acute neurologic syndrome has been recognized largely in hunting dogs that have been exposed to raccoons. It also has been observed in other dogs with no raccoon exposure.[48–50] The disease is remarkably similar to acute polyneuritis in humans (Landry-Guillain-Barré syndrome).

PATHOPHYSIOLOGY An immune-mediated segmental demyelination and degeneration of axons is found in animals exposed to raccoons. Apparently, a transmissible substance in raccoon saliva produces the disease.[51] Other inflammatory neuropathies are occasionally reported in dogs and some other animals, including cats and goats.[52,53] Polyneuritis equi (cauda equina neuritis) is relatively common and is discussed in Chapter 7. Chronic polyneuropathies will be discussed separately. The Landry-Guillain-Barré syndrome in human beings has been reported to have several causes, including respiratory infections and influenza vaccinations.

The disease attacks primarily the ventral roots and the spinal nerves. Characteristic microscopic lesions include segmental demyelination, degeneration of both myelin and axons, leukocyte infiltration, secondary degeneration of the ventral horn cells, and neurogenic muscle atrophy.[54] Neurologic signs develop because motor signal transmission from the spinal cord to the muscle fibers is blocked. Pain perception is usually normal, because the dorsal root is only mildly affected in this disease. Diffuse hyperesthesia is occasionally seen.

CLINICAL SIGNS Neurologic signs develop suddenly—in some cases, 7 to 14 days following raccoon exposure. Early clinical signs include pelvic limb paresis and hyporeflexia. Ascending weakness or paralysis develops quickly. Affected dogs become tetraparetic 24 to 48 hours after the neurologic signs first develop. Spinal reflexes are severely depressed or absent. Passive flexion and extension of the limbs reveals severe hypotonus of affected muscles. Cerebral responses to painful stimuli are normal or exaggerated. Dogs with rapidly progressive disease may develop respiratory paralysis. Cranial nerve involvement is uncommon, although the animal's voice may be weak. Swallowing, the gag reflex, and the esophagus are normal. The patient remains alert, responsive, and afebrile. The disease spares the sacral and caudal nerve roots to the extent that defecation, urination, and tail mobility usually are normal. Muscle atrophy develops quickly and can be detected by direct palpation 10 to 14 days after the onset of paresis. Occasionally, the initial clinical signs are detected in the thoracic limbs and progress caudally to the pelvic limbs. The clinical course is usually 3 to 6 weeks, but is sometimes 2 to 4 months.[55] Improvement begins by the third week, and complete recovery may take 6 to 8 weeks. In patients that develop severe muscle atrophy, recovery may not be complete.

DIAGNOSIS The differential diagnosis should include tick paralysis and botulism, because these diseases produce clinical signs that are essentially identical to those of the early stages of polyradiculoneuritis. Polyradiculoneuritis should be suspected when no ticks are found on physical examination and no exposure to botulism toxin is possible. Laboratory and radiographic studies are normal. CSF collected from the lumbar subarachnoid space shows an increase in protein concentration with a normal cell count. A diagnosis of polyradiculoneuritis is supported by electromyographic (EMG) evidence of the diffuse denervation of affected muscles. These changes appear 5 to 7 days after the motor axon has been injured. EMG abnormalities include increased insertion activity, fibrillation potentials, and positive sharp waves. Evoked potentials are slightly reduced in amplitude and may be polyphasic, but are not as severely affected as in botulism and tick paralysis.[56] Nerve conduction velocities are reduced later in the course of the disease. F-waves are delayed and dispersed after paralysis has developed fully.[57] An ELISA using raccoon saliva as the antigen shows some promise as a diagnostic test.[57] Table 8–5 compares the diagnostic features of polyradiculoneuritis, tick paralysis, and botulism.

TREATMENT There is no specific treatment for polyradiculoneuritis. Despite its popularity, there is no evidence to support the use of glucocorticoid therapy, even though an immune reaction is suspected. However, no controlled trials of treatment with corticosteroids have been reported. One study in humans with a chronic inflammatory demyelinating polyradiculoneuropathy demonstrated a small but significant improvement using prednisone.[58] When corticosteroid therapy is employed, the agents should be given in immune-suppressive doses early in the course of the disease. Medication should be discontinued if adverse effects occur or no response is noted. Chronic glucocorticoid

TABLE 8–5 Diagnostic Comparison of Acute Progressive LMN Disorders

	Polyradiculoneuritis	*Tick Paralysis*	*Botulism*
History	Single case; previous exposure to raccoon in some cases	Single case—engorged tick	Multiple cases are very suggestive; access to carrion or spoiled food
Pathophysiology	Nonsuppurative nerve inflammation and demyelination	Interference with action potential release of acetylcholine and action potential production	Block of neuromuscular transmission
Cranial nerve involvement	Rare	Rare	Usual
EMG	Fibrillation potentials and positive sharp waves	No denervation	Usually no denervation
Conduction velocity	Normal to decreased	Normal to slightly decreased	Normal
Evoked potentials	Reduced	Reduced	Reduced; reduction in amplitude on repetitive stimulation
Special tests	None	None	Toxin in feces, serum, and so forth
Treatment	Supportive	Tick removal	Supportive
Recovery time	3–6 wk	24–48 hr	2–3 wk

therapy may cause urinary tract infection, muscle wasting, and delayed healing of decubital ulcers.

Supportive care consists of attentive nursing that (1) prevents decubital ulcers, (2) minimizes muscle atrophy and contractures, (3) prevents urinary tract infection, (4) prevents pneumonia, and (5) supports respiratory function. The animals should be bedded on deep straw or hay, air mattresses, sealed foam, or waterbeds. The patient should be turned frequently and kept clean. Voluntary micturition should be preserved; however, many dogs cannot produce a normal abdominal press and may fail to empty their bladders totally. Gentle manual expression of the bladder is helpful. Physical therapy consisting of muscle massage and passive manipulation of the limbs is important. Hydrotherapy is helpful for preventing muscle atrophy and contractures and for keeping the dog clean.

The prognosis for recovery is usually good. Recurrences have been observed. There is evidence that dogs having one episode are more susceptible to recurrences. The course of the illness is 3 to 6 weeks. Recovery of neurologic function is usually in the reverse order of sign development.

Botulism. For many years, this disease was suspected in dogs but never documented. Carrion eaters and some carnivores, including dogs, were thought to be resistant to botulism toxin. In 1978, Barsanti and co-workers at the University of Georgia documented an outbreak of type C botulism in foxhounds from northeastern South Carolina.[59] It has been reported in dogs in Great Britain, the European continent, and Australia.[60–63] Before a detailed description of polyradiculoneuritis was published, many hunting dogs with acute progressive LMN disease were thought to have botulism or pseudobotulism. After Cummings's report on coonhound paralysis, most dogs were thought to be affected with this disorder. Both conditions are now known to exist in dogs, and it can be difficult to make a differential diagnosis.

In large animals, botulism results from the ingestion of toxin or from the contamination of an ulcerated gastrointestinal tract with proliferating *Clostridium botulinum* spores. Outbreaks in cattle occur as a result of the ingestion of hay, ensilage, or water that has been contaminated by dead rodents, and in plastic-wrapped silage.[64] The shaker foal syndrome occurs most frequently in foals 2 to 5 weeks of age. Foals that are given highly nutritious feed develop gastrointestinal ulcers. These ulcers are colonized by *Clostridium botulinum*, which then produces the offending toxin.[65–67] Botulism can also occur from wound infection.[68]

PATHOPHYSIOLOGY Clinical signs develop when the preformed toxin of *Clostridium botulinum* is ingested. Several different strains of exotoxin-producing organisms have been identified. Types A, B, and E are the strains most commonly associated with human disease. Types C and D, found in carrion, cause most cases of botulism in birds and mammals other than human beings. All cases reported in dogs were caused by type C, and most of those in large animals were caused by type B. Botulinal toxin produces generalized neuromuscular blockade by inhibiting the release of acetylcholine from the terminals of cholinergic nerve fibers.[69] The exact mechanism is unknown. A decrease in nerve conduction velocity has been found in humans and dogs, indicating some interference with nerve transmission.[70,71]

CLINICAL SIGNS The incubation period is less than 6 days. The clinical signs are those of a progressive, symmetric, generalized LMN disorder. The severity of clinical signs varies with the amount of toxin ingested. Affected animals may develop only mild generalized weakness or tetraplegia with respiratory failure. Both cranial and spinal nerves are affected.[59,60] Facial paralysis, megaesophagus, and changes in the voice are more common than in polyradiculoneuritis. In dogs, the usual clinical course is less than 14 days.

DIAGNOSIS Botulism must be suspected in animals with acute progressive LMN disease. *Botulism is especially likely to be present in cases of multiple animal involvement.* Tick paralysis and polyradiculoneuritis are sporadic diseases involving individual animals. EMG studies may help to differentiate botulism from polyradiculoneuritis, but there is some similarity, depending on the stage of the disease. EMG findings in botulism include some spontaneous activity, including fibrillations and positive waves, and a small muscle action potential in response to a single supramaximal stimulus. Nerve conduction velocities may be normal or slightly decreased. Repetitive stimulation at slow rates (2–3 Hz) may cause a small decrement in the amplitude of the evoked potential, but we have also seen a small increment (10%–20%).

Toxin identification in the food, the carrion, the serum, the feces, or the vomitus of an affected animal is confirmatory evidence. The organism can be isolated from the viscera of clinically normal animals, and its isolation from feces therefore is insufficient for the formulation of a positive diagnosis.

TREATMENT The treatment of botulism, like that of polyradiculoneuritis, is largely supportive. To be effective, the specific antitoxin must be administered before the botulinal toxin binds to receptors at the myoneural junction. It is rarely possible to achieve this timing, because the signs usually are present before the animal is treated. Polyvalent products that contain type C antitoxin generally are not available. The efficacy of antibiotic therapy has not been proved. The prognosis for recovery is generally good, unless the dog develops severe, rapidly progressive signs. Mildly affected animals recover without therapy.[59]

Tick Paralysis. This disease has been recognized worldwide, but most in-depth reports have come from the United States and Australia. The clinical signs are similar to those of polyradiculoneuritis and botulism.

PATHOPHYSIOLOGY A neurotoxin secreted by engorged feeding female ticks either inhibits depolarization in the terminal portions of motor nerves or blocks the release of acetylcholine at the neuromuscular junction. The toxin may affect both motor and sensory nerve fibers by altering ionic fluxes that mediate action potential production.[72] In the United States, *Dermacentor andersoni* and D. *variabilis* are the primary ticks involved. In Australia, the disease is produced by *Ixodes holocyclus*, although I. *cornuatus* and I. *hirsti* are also incriminated.[73]

CLINICAL SIGNS Clinical signs develop 7 to 9 days after attachment of the tick. The earliest clinical sign is marked ataxia with rapid progression to paresis, paralysis, areflexia, and hypotonus. Early tick paralysis in dogs may have similar signs. In the United States, cranial nerve involvement is rare. Nystagmus occasionally may be observed. Death can occur from respiratory failure if the ticks are not removed. Painful stimuli normally are perceived. In Australia, affected dogs or cats develop more severe signs. Respiratory failure and autonomic signs occur with greater frequency in these animals than in those from the United States. In the Australian syndrome, clinical signs may progressively worsen, even though the ticks have been removed.[74,75] In the United States, dramatic improvement follows tick removal.

DIAGNOSIS Tick paralysis is diagnosed by the rapid improvement after tick removal. In unusual cases, EMGs can be used to differentiate this disease from acute polyradiculoneuritis.[56] EMG evidence of denervation is not found in tick paralysis. In tick paralysis, there is marked reduction in the amplitude of evoked motor potentials. Repetitive stimulation does not cause further decrement in the amplitude. Nerve conduction velocities may be slightly slower than normal, and terminal conduction times may be prolonged.[72]

TREATMENT In the United States, removal of the tick results in marked improvement within 24 hours and complete recovery within 72 hours. Animals must be examined thoroughly for ticks. The areas evaluated should include the ear canals and the interdigital spaces. Ticks are removed carefully so that the head is not left embedded in the animal's skin. The toxin probably comes from the salivary glands of the tick. Failure to remove the head may result in a worsening of the clinical signs. Insecticide solutions should be sponged over the entire dog when ticks cannot be found and tick paralysis is suspected. In Australian tick paralysis, tick removal does not prevent further progression of the disease. The use of hyperimmune dog serum has been advocated to prevent death from respiratory failure.[73] In the United States, the prognosis for complete recovery is good.

Aminoglycoside Neuropathy. The aminoglycoside antibiotics, when given parenterally, can cause neuromuscular blockade.[76] Their effects are similar to those of curare. We have observed one animal that developed severe muscle weakness and hyporeflexia following 5 days of gentamicin therapy for deep pyoderma. The clinical signs resolved within 48 hours after the drug was discontinued.

Chronic Progressive Diseases

Motor Neuronopathies. These diseases are listed in Table 8–4. As a group, they are characterized by progressive degeneration of motor neurons in the gray matter of the spinal cord and the nuclei of the brain stem. Progressive denervation of muscle fibers results in paresis, paralysis, and severe muscle atrophy. The diseases in dogs resemble the inherited spinal muscular atrophies of human beings.

BRITTANY SPANIEL SPINAL MUSCULAR ATROPHY This inherited disease was first reported in 1979 in a family of Brittany spaniel dogs in the southeastern United States.[77] The signs typically develop by the time the animal has reached 4 months of age. The characteristic signs include severe atrophy of the paraspinal and proximal pelvic girdle muscles. Affected animals walk with a crouched, waddling gait in the pelvic limbs. The involvement of the thoracic limbs is less severe. CN V, CN VII, and CN XII are involved in some dogs. The distal appendicular muscles tend to be spared. The disease is inherited as an autosomal dominant trait and has three phenotypic forms: accelerated, intermediate, and chronic. Homozygous dogs have the accelerated form. Signs are seen by 6 to 8 weeks of age, with severe paralysis developing by 3 to 4 months. Dogs with the chronic form may live for several years. Pathologic studies have established that degeneration of motor neurons produces the clinical signs. However, some dogs have relatively normal numbers of neurons, although the neurons are smaller than normal. These neurons may be dysfunctional.[78,79] The condition is nearly identical to juvenile spinal muscular atrophy of children. There is no effective known treatment.

HEREDITARY NEURONAL ABIOTROPHY OF THE SWEDISH LAPLAND DOG Dogs with this disorder develop paralysis at 5 to 7 weeks of age and within 2 weeks become tetraparetic.[80] There is no predilection for more severe involvement of the pelvic limbs, and weakness and atrophy are most conspicuous in the distal muscles. The disease shows little tendency to progress after the initial 2 weeks. The disease may be inherited as an autosomal recessive trait. There is no known effective treatment.

ROTTWEILER SPINAL MUSCULAR ATROPHY This disease is similar to the Brittany spaniel disease. Accumulation of neurofilaments is not seen in the Rottweiler. Megaesophagus was present in both pups studied. Both pups were euthanized by 8 weeks of age because of severe tetraplegia. The mode of inheritance is not known.[81,82]

POINTER SPINAL MUSCULAR ATROPHY Another disease similar to Brittany spaniel spinal muscular atrophy is reported in pointer dogs. It is believed to be inherited as an autosomal recessive trait. Inclusions found in motor neurons suggest that this may be a storage disease.[83–85]

GERMAN SHEPHERD SPINAL MUSCULAR ATROPHY Two German shepherd pups developed a focal degeneration of motor neurons in the brachial plexus region of the spinal cord. Denervation of thoracic limb muscles caused weakness and atrophy. The lesions resemble other spinal muscular atrophies, but were localized.[86]

EQUINE MOTOR NEURON DISEASE A spontaneous motor neuron disease was seen in ten horses in the northeastern United States. The horses were of various breeds and ages. The cause is not known. Lesions are similar to those of the other spinal muscular atrophies.[87]

STOCKARD'S PARALYSIS This is a paraplegic syndrome that affects the offspring of Great Dane–bloodhound or Great Dane–Saint Bernard matings.[88] There is a predilection for pelvic limb involvement. Signs of pelvic limb paresis develop when the animal is 11 to 14 weeks of age and progressively worsen for a few days. Thereafter the signs remain rather constant. There is preferential involvement of the distal muscles of the limbs.

MULTISYSTEM NEURONAL DEGENERATIONS A progressive neuronopathy occurs in 4- to 7-month-old cairn terriers. Pelvic limb paresis progresses to tetraplegia in weeks to months. The lesions are characterized by chromatolysis in spinal and brain stem neurons. Some degeneration is found in the peripheral nerves. A hereditary basis is assumed but not proven.[89,90] Four cocker spaniels had neuronal degeneration of multiple areas of the brain, causing a syndrome of behavioral changes, ataxia, dysmetria, and normal spinal reflexes. Pedigree analysis suggested a hereditary cause.[91]

Polyneuropathy. These diseases are listed in Table 8–6. They are recognized more frequently in dogs now than a few years ago, but they are relatively uncommon in other species. The chronic neuropathies have an insidious onset and progress slowly over several months. At-

TABLE 8–6 Causes of Polyneuropathy*

Congenital or Hereditary (See appendices for complete list by species and breed)
- Peripheral neuropathies (motor or sensory)
  - Progressive axonopathy in boxer dogs
  - Giant axonal neuropathy in German shepherd dogs
  - Neurofibrillary accumulations
  - Hypertrophic neuropathy in Tibetan mastiff dogs
  - Sensory neuropathy in long-haired dachshunds, pointers, golden retriever, Doberman pinscher, Siberian husky, whippet, Scottish terrier
  - Storage diseases (e.g., sphingomyelinosis in the cat, globoid leukodystrophy in cairn and West Highland white terriers; see Chap. 16)
  - Demyelinating diseases (e.g., globoid cell leukodystrophy in the dog; see Chap. 16)
  - Laryngeal paralysis in horses, Siberian husky, Bouvier des Flandres dog (see Chap. 10)

Metabolic
- Endocrine
  - Hypoglycemia
  - Beta cell tumor
  - Hyperglycemia
  - Diabetes mellitus
  - Hypothyroidism
- Metabolic defects
  - Hyperchylomicronemia in cats
  - Hyperoxaluria in cats
- Kangaroo gait in ewes

Neoplastic
- Paraneoplastic neuropathies

Nutritional
- Copper deficiency in lambs and kids

Idiopathic
- Distal denervating disease in dogs
- Neurofibrillary accumulations
- Dysautonomia in cats and dogs (see Chap. 10)
- Distal symmetric polyneuropathy in dogs
- Stringhalt in horses (see Chap. 11)

Inflammatory and Immune
- Acute polyradiculoneuritis
- Coonhound paralysis
- Idiopathic
- Chronic polyneuritis
- Ganglioradiculoneuritis
- Brachial plexus neuritis (see Chap. 6)
- Neuritis of the cauda equina in horses (see Chap. 7)
- Protozoal polyradiculoneuritis

Toxic (Including Drugs)
- Aminoglycosides
- Heavy metals
  - Lead
  - Mercury
  - Thallium
  - Copper, antimony, zinc
- Organophosphate compounds
- Industrial
  - Trichlorethylene
  - *N*-hexane
  - Acrylamide

Vascular
- Ischemic neuromyopathy (see Chap. 7)
- Aortoiliac thrombosis (see Chap. 7)

* All have a chronic progressive course except acute idiopathic polyneuritis, vascular neuropathies, and aminoglycoside toxicity.

tacks of the disease may be disrupted by periods of spontaneous improvement. A definitive diagnosis of the cause of chronic polyneuropathy is often elusive. Better diagnostic techniques, especially electrophysiologic tests and histopathologic assessment of muscle and nerve biopsies, have contributed to a greater understanding of this problem.[92–96]

CHRONIC IDIOPATHIC POLYNEURITIS This syndrome affects mature dogs primarily. Signs of lameness, muscle atrophy, paresis, and eventually paralysis develop slowly over several months. The neurologic findings vary with the stage of the illness. Postural reactions, spinal reflexes, and muscle strength are decreased. CN V and CN VII may be involved. Hypalgesia may occur later in the disease, when sensory nerves become involved. The clinical course varies from several months to years. This disease can resemble primary muscle disorders.

The diagnosis is made by biopsy of the muscles and nerves. EMG and nerve conduction velocity studies are useful but do not provide evidence of an inflammatory reaction. Pathologic studies of affected dogs suggest that nonsuppurative inflammation, perhaps with an immune basis, is responsible for the disease.[97,98] The dorsal root ganglia and cranial nerves are affected in some cases, causing sensory deficits; this condition has been called *ganglioradiculitis*.[99] Some patients benefit from corticosteroid therapy, but relapse and slow progression of the disease is the most common course. Because of the waxing-waning character of the natural disease, the benefit of corticosteroids is not proven.

DEGENERATIVE HEREDITARY NEUROPATHIES The hereditary neuropathies are rare diseases, with a chronic progressive course.

Progressive Axonopathy of Boxer Dogs. This disease is usually apparent by 2 to 3 months of age.[100,101] It begins as a pelvic limb ataxia that progresses to involve the thoracic limbs. Postural reactions are abnormal, muscle tone and spinal reflexes are decreased, and ocular tremor or head bobbing may be present. The clinical signs tend to stabilize after 1 to 2 years, and the animals can lead a reasonably normal life. Axonal swellings are seen in the nerve roots, with distal atrophy of the axons. Demyelination and remyelination are present, probably secondary to the axon changes.[92] Progressive axonopathy is inherited as an autosomal recessive trait. It has been reported only in the United Kingdom.

Giant Axonal Neuropathy of German Shepherd Dogs. Axons of both the central and peripheral nervous systems are affected in a disease reported in one family of German shepherd dogs in the United Kingdom.[92,102,103] It is believed to be inherited as an autosomal recessive trait. Swollen axons are found in the distal portions of long tracts and peripheral nerves. The pelvic limb nerves are more severely affected than the thoracic limb nerves. Swellings containing disoriented neurofilaments are multifocal along the course of a single fiber. Both sensory and motor fibers are affected. Signs begin at 14 to 16 months of age. Proprioceptive deficits are noted first, and signs progress over several months' time. Regurgitation because of megaesophagus is seen at about 18 months. Pain sensation may be reduced before 2 years of age.

Neurofibrillary Accumulations. Accumulation of neurofilaments in neurons causes a generalized LMN weakness that progresses to tetraplegia. It has been reported in pigs, a cat, and a collie pup.[104–106] The cause is unknown.

Hypertrophic Neuropathy of Tibetan Mastiff Dogs. Tibetan mastiff pups developed generalized weakness and decreased reflexes at 7 to 12 weeks of age. They became tetraplegic within 3 weeks of onset. Nerve conduction velocities were decreased. The primary lesion was demyelination of peripheral nerves, with little axonal degeneration. An autosomal recessive inheritance is suggested.[107] A similar syndrome was seen in one mongrel dog.[108]

DISTAL SYMMETRIC POLYNEUROPATHY This disease of dogs is characterized by degeneration of the distal axons of peripheral nerves, often only in the intramuscular branches. It is common in the United Kingdom, but not elsewhere.[92,109] Signs develop in 1 to 4 weeks. Tetraparesis varies in severity, the neck muscles may be weak, but cranial nerves and pain sensation are not affected. Biopsy of the more proximal portions of the nerve may be normal, but muscle biopsy with examination of intramuscular nerve fibers often demonstrates distal nerve degeneration. Most of the dogs recovered. There was no evidence of breed or age predisposition. A distal neuropathy has also been seen in Doberman pinschers.[110] Initial signs are of pelvic limb weakness. Typically, in affected dogs one pelvic limb is flexed while standing. Eventually both pelvic limbs are affected so that the dog alternately flexes each limb. All four limbs are affected over a period of years. The dogs are 2 to 5 years old at onset and the disease progresses slowly for at least 5 years. Distal neuropathy has also been seen in Rottweilers.

SENSORY NEUROPATHIES Hereditary sensory neuropathies occur in long-haired dachshunds and pointer dogs.[111,112] Sensory neuropathies of unknown cause have also been reported in various other dogs.[113–115] In the dachshund, abnormalities of proprioception, pain sensation, and urinary function begin as early as 8 weeks of age. Paresis and muscular atrophy are not seen. The animals described with this disease were severely incontinent by the age of 1.5 years. EMG and motor nerve conduction velocities were normal. There was severe depletion of both large myelinated and unmyelinated fibers. No treatment is known, and an inherited basis is presumed. In the pointer, the syndrome is characterized by self-mutilation. The dogs lick and chew the feet to the point of digital amputation. Pain sensation is reduced distally. Signs begin at about 4 months of age. The primary sensory neurons in the dorsal root ganglia are depleted, and there is a reduction in substance P in the ganglia.[116] The condition is hereditary, and there is no treatment. The cause of the sensory neuropathy in the other reported cases is unknown.

HYPOTHYROID NEUROPATHY Hypothyroidism is one of the more common causes of polyneuropathy in dogs in our clinic. Complete studies have not been published, but the documentation is convincing.[117] The disease may manifest as a generalized LMN disorder or as a variety of cranial nerve deficits. In most animals both cranial and spinal peripheral nerves are affected. The early stages are often missed because the signs are mild. Only with EMG examination is the generalized nature of the problem appreciated. Further confounding the diagnosis, many of the affected animals are not obviously hypothyroid, based on activity level, skin condition, and body weight. Presenting complaints include weakness, intermittent lameness, and signs of the affected cranial nerves (most frequently CN VII, VIII, IX, and X; see Chaps. 9 and 10). EMG examination must include sampling of all parts of the body. An animal with signs of pelvic limb weakness may have evidence of denervation in facial muscles and muscles of the thoracic limb. The diagnosis of hypothyroidism is currently made by finding low thyroxine (T_4) levels after stimulation of the thyroid gland with thyroid-stimulating hormone. Baseline T_4 levels are not adequate to substantiate a diagnosis.[118] Confirmation of degenerative change in the nerve must be made by biopsy. Muscle abnormalities may also be present.[119] Most animals treated with levothyroxine improve dramatically. The rate and degree of recovery depend on the severity of the denervation when treatment is started. Most animals appear better in the first week, but actual improvement of motor function usually takes several months. Animals with severe, generalized denervation have not done well. Some dogs with hypothyroidism and a polyneuropathy have not responded. In these dogs a mononuclear infiltration in the nerves was discovered on biopsy or necropsy, suggesting an inflammatory response. It is not clear whether the inflammation is primary or secondary to the degenerative change, but the lack of such a response in most cases suggests that it is a primary inflammation. One of the primary causes of hypothyroidism is an immune-mediated thyroiditis; therefore the inflammation may be a manifestation of the systemic immune disease.

NEUROPATHY WITH DIABETES MELLITUS Peripheral neuropathy has been documented in association with diabetes mellitus in both cats and dogs.[120–123] Both demyelination and axonal degeneration may be seen. Abnormal EMG and nerve conduction velocities were found in several dogs with diabetes mellitus that had no evidence of LMN disease. Sensory nerves are often more severely affected than motor nerves in human diabetics, and sensory nerve conduction was delayed in these dogs.[124] Improvement should occur if the diabetes can be regulated.

HYPOGLYCEMIC NEUROPATHY Beta cell tumors produce a profound hypoglycemia that affects the metabolism of the CNS, causing seizures, behavioral abnormalities, and other cortical signs (see Chaps. 13 and 14). A rare complication is a polyneuropathy.[125] Clinical signs are subtle, but the weakness associated with the syndrome may be related to peripheral neuropathy in addition to the central disorder.

HYPERCHYLOMICRONEMIA IN CATS Cats with a hereditary hyperlipemic syndrome may have masses around the spinal, cranial, and distal peripheral nerves.[126] The masses are organizing hematomas with large amounts of lipid that compress the nerves. A similar problem is possible in the miniature Schnauzer.

HYPEROXALURIA IN CATS A hereditary renal failure from deposition of oxalate crystals in the kidney is a newly described disease.[92] Paresis with reduced reflexes from a polyneuropathy is associated with the disease, but the cause of the nerve pathology is not known.

KANGAROO GAIT IN EWES A polyneuropathy in lactating ewes that primarily affects the radial nerve has been reported in the United Kingdom and New Zealand.[127,128] It is not clear whether this is a true polyneuropathy, since lesions outside of the brachial plexus are minimal. Most ewes recover.

PARANEOPLASTIC NEUROPATHIES Neoplasms can cause a variety of systemic abnormalities not related to the tumor mass. Collectively these are called paraneoplastic disorders. Polyneuropathies associated with neoplasia have been reported in dogs. The pathogenesis is not known. Hypotheses include (1) the release of toxic principles from the tumor, (2) alterations in homeostasis, (3) a decrease in specific factors or nutrients, and (4) secondary reactive factors produced by the host in response to the tumor.[94] Both demyelination and axonal degeneration may be seen. Most reported cases had mild signs of neuropathy.[129,130]

PROTOZOAL POLYRADICULONEURITIS *Neospora caninum* and *Toxoplasma gondii* can cause inflammation of the peripheral nerves, muscles, or CNS. *Neospora* is the likely causative agent in many cases thought to be toxoplasmosis. In the peripheral nervous system, the spinal nerve roots are more severely affected. The syndrome is usually seen in young dogs.[131] Serologic tests establish the diagnosis (see Chap. 16). Early treatment may be beneficial, but if muscle contracture is present, recovery is unlikely.

TOXIC NEUROPATHIES Table 8–6 lists some of the toxic substances capable of causing a neuropathy. None of these are common. Chronic organophosphate toxicity can cause a degeneration of peripheral nerves. Affected animals usually develop signs of pelvic limb paresis that may eventually progress to tetraparesis. Heavy metals, such as lead, cause neuropathies in rare cases.

Diffuse Muscle Disorders. Diseased muscles are usually weak. Muscle pain (myalgia), failure of muscles to relax (myotonia), and sudden muscle contraction (cramp) also suggest muscle disease. Myopathies include disorders characterized by a weakness that does not have neurogenic causes. A myopathy may be a result of inflammation (myositis) or degeneration. Inflammatory muscle disease is usually an immune-mediated disorder that causes weakness and muscular pain. Degenerative diseases are either acquired or congenital. Nutritional, endocrine, metabolic, and vascular diseases may cause the acquired forms of muscle diseases. Most of the congenital diseases are inherited. Muscular dystrophies are progressive degenerative myopathies that are genetically determined. The signs of diffuse muscle disease are very similar to those of diffuse polyneuropathies. Because of ambiguities in the diagnosis, increasing attention has been given to three laboratory aids: serum enzyme levels, EMG and nerve conduction velocity studies, and muscle biopsy.[132,133] A classification of animal myopathies is presented in Table 8–7. These diseases will be discussed briefly in subsequent sections of this chapter.

POLYMYOSITIS Polymyositis is classified as diffuse muscle inflammation of infectious or noninfectious origin (see Table 8–7).[133] Infectious polymyositis is rare but may be seen with toxoplasmosis, neosporosis, or leptospirosis. Clostridial infections are relatively common in large animals but usually affect only one limb. Inflammations of noninfectious origin appear to be the result of cell-mediated immunity.[132] Polymyositis may occur in association with systemic lupus erythematosus, as a paraneoplastic syndrome, and with some drugs, notably trimethoprim-sulfadiazine in Doberman pinschers, and D-penicillamine in human beings.[132,133] The most common clinical signs include muscle pain, weakness, a stilted gait, and fever. Less frequent signs include muscle atrophy, depression, anorexia, weight loss, and voice change.[134,135] Regurgitation may develop in dogs that have diseased esophageal muscles and megaesophagus. Signs may be episodic—characterized by acute attacks followed by periods of spontaneous remission. Other dogs have chronic progressive signs. The clinical signs resemble those of chronic polyneuritis or myasthenic syndromes. The acute, painful episodes must be differentiated from meningitis and skeletal diseases.

TABLE 8–7 Causes of Polymyopathy in Animals

Inflammatory
Infectious
Toxoplasma gondii
Neospora caninum
Leptospira icterohaemmorrhagiae
Clostridium spp.
Hepatozoan canis
Microfilariasis
Noninfectious
Idiopathic polymyositis
Masticatory myositis
Systemic lupus erythematosus–polymyositis
Eosinophilic myositis
Dermatomyositis in collie and border collie dogs
Extraocular myositis
Paraneoplastic thymoma associated
Drug-induced
Trimethoprim-sulfadiazine
D-Penicillamine
Degenerative
Inherited
Muscular dystrophy in Labrador retriever, golden retriever, Bouvier des Flandres dog, Samoyed, Rottweiler, Irish terrier, domestic cats, merino sheep
Mitochondrial myopathy in Sussex spaniel, Clumber spaniel
Myotonic myopathy in Chow Chow, Staffordshire terrier, Great Dane, Rhodesian ridgeback, Cavalier King Charles spaniel, golden retriever, goats, Shropshire lambs, (various horses, inheritance not proven) (see Chap. 11)
Myopathy of Pietrain pigs (Creeper)
Phosphofructokinase deficiency in springer spaniels
Nutritional (white muscle disease)
Vitamin E deficiency
Selenium deficiency
Endocrine
Hyperadrenocorticism (steroid myopathy)
Hypothyroidism
Hypokalemia
Hyperkalemia
Periodic paralyses
Metabolic
Exertional rhabdomyolysis
Malignant hyperthermia
Postanesthetic myopathy (large animals)
Vascular
Ischemic neuromyopathy (see Chap. 7)

A definitive diagnosis of polymyositis is based on (1) evidence of muscle pain or weakness, (2) elevations in the concentrations of serum muscle enzymes (creatine kinase [CK], lactic dehydrogenase, serum glutamic oxalotransaminase), (3) EMG abnormalities, and (4) histopathologic evidence of muscle necrosis and inflammation.[134] A probable diagnosis can be made when three of these four findings are present. There appears to be little correlation between muscle enzyme concentrations and either the severity of clinical signs or the degree of muscle necrosis or inflammation seen on biopsy.[134] EMG changes include fibrillation potentials, positive sharp waves, polyphasic motor unit potentials, motor unit potentials of decreased duration, complex repetitive discharges, and increased insertional activity. The fading of evoked motor unit potentials, reversed with neostigmine, has been reported.[134] Pathologic changes may include muscle fiber necrosis, muscle regeneration, and variable fiber size and hyaline fibers. Inflammatory cells include lymphocytes and some neutrophils. Eosinophilic inflammation has been reported.[135] Serologic tests for toxoplasmosis and neosporosis should be included in the diagnostic plan.

Idiopathic polymyositis should be treated with prednisone, 2.0 mg/kg/day, until remission is achieved. Alternate-day glucocorticoid therapy then is instituted to maintain remission. Dogs with megaesophagus may develop aspiration pneumonia. Management of these cases is difficult, and the prognosis for regaining normal esophageal function is poor.

MASTICATORY MUSCLE MYOSITIS An inflammation affecting primarily the muscles of mastication is seen more commonly than polymyositis in dogs. In some cases the other muscles of the body are affected, producing a generalized polymyositis. In the acute stages of masticatory myositis the temporal and masseter muscles are firm, swollen, and painful. The selective involvement is due to a difference in histochemical and biochemical properties of the masticatory muscles. Antibodies are produced against specific myofibrillar proteins. It is possible that the autoimmune reaction is initiated by a bacterial antigen.[133] The diagnosis and treatment are the same as for polymyositis. The prognosis is guarded, and relapses are common. A bilateral myositis of the extraocular muscles has also been reported.[136]

DERMATOMYOSITIS Collies and Shetland sheepdogs have an inherited inflammatory skin and muscle disease.[137,138] The dermatitis is most severe on the ears, face, tail, and distal extremities. The myositis is often subclinical, but atrophy, weakness, and EMG changes may be seen. An autosomal dominant inherited immune-mediated pathogenesis is suspected.[138]

MUSCULAR DYSTROPHIES The muscular dystrophies are inherited primary myopathies characterized by progressive degeneration of skeletal muscle. Affected breeds are listed in Table 8–7. The X-linked muscular dystrophies are similar to Duchenne muscular dystrophy in human beings and have been reported in the golden retriever, Irish terrier, Samoyed, Rottweiler, and domestic cats.[133,139–141] Clinical signs may be seen as early as 6 weeks of age. Stilted gait, trismus, atrophy of muscles, stunted growth, and drooling develop early and progress in severity. Signs often stabilize after 6 months of age in the golden retriever.[142] The Labrador retriever has an autosomal recessive muscular dystrophy. Signs are similar to those in the golden retriever, with an onset at about 8 to 12 weeks of age and stabilization by about 1 year.[143–145] The Bouvier des Flandres dog has a later onset, around 2 years of age. In the reported cases the esophagus was affected, causing regurgitation.[146,147] Degeneration of the pharyngeal and esophageal muscles with normal nerves was found in ten Bouviers with dysphagia.[148] The muscular dystrophy of Merino sheep is inherited as an autosomal recessive trait. Signs develop at 3 to 4 weeks of age and are similar to the canine diseases.[149,150] Skeletal muscle changes in the muscular dystrophies include degeneration, mineralization, and mild to moderate phagocytic reaction. Prolonged complex repetitive discharges and a few fibrillations and positive sharp waves have been found on EMG examination. Serum CK levels are greatly increased in the X-linked muscular dystrophies, but are less significant in the others. There is no treatment for the muscular dystrophies.

OTHER INHERITED MUSCLE DISEASES Several rare inherited metabolic disorders affect muscle function. Examples include deficiency of phosphofructokinase in English springer spaniels, a debrancher enzyme deficiency in German shepherd dogs, and glycogen storage diseases in dogs and cats.[133,151,152] Mitochondrial myopathies are reported in Clumber and Sussex spaniels.[151]

MYOPATHY OF PIETRAIN PIGS (CREEPER) This is an autosomal recessive inherited trait in Pietrain pigs beginning at about 3 weeks of age. Progressive muscular weakness leads to permanent recumbency by 12 weeks. Atrophy of type I myofibers was prominent in proximal muscles. There is no treatment.[7,153]

MYOTONIC MYOPATHIES A contraction of muscle that persists after the cessation of voluntary effort or stimulation is called myotonia (if generalized) or a cramp (if localized). Myotonic myopathies are discussed in Chapter 11.

NUTRITIONAL MYOPATHIES (WHITE MUSCLE DISEASE) White muscle disease is a degenerative myopathy of many species that is caused by a dietary deficiency of α-tocopherol or selenium.[7] It occurs most frequently in calves and lambs, less frequently in pigs, and rarely in other large animals, cats and dogs. Two forms of the disease exist. An acute form is characterized by sudden death resulting from cardiac muscle degeneration during exertion or exercise. The second form is marked by a gradual onset of tetraparesis in calves 2 weeks of age or older. Lambs develop similar signs and are affected when they are 10 days to 2 months of age. Lambs may have a stiff gait and tetraparesis. Muscles may be swollen and painful. Foals may have painful areas around the base of the tail, beneath the mane, and the tongue and submandibular tissues. Other diseases linked to a selenium deficiency include mulberry heart disease in baby pigs, white muscle disease in foals, the equine tying-up syndrome, and retained placenta in cattle.

The diagnosis is based on clinical signs, biopsy of affected muscles, quantitation of glutathione peroxidase levels, and the animal's response to therapy.[154] In the skeletal form of the disease, muscle degeneration is characterized by symmetric grayish or white streaks in groups of skeletal muscle. Selenium and vitamin E preparations are very beneficial if the signs are severe. Diets should be corrected if selenium deficiencies are found. Selenium can be highly toxic if it is used at high concentrations.

STEROID-INDUCED MYOPATHY This muscle disease is caused by exogenous or endogenous glucocorticoids. It is observed in both spontaneous and iatrogenic Cushing's disease.[155,156] Dogs with steroid-induced myopathy develop muscle atrophy and weakness. The muscle changes may be subclinical, but some develop an associated myotonia-like syndrome.[157,158] High-frequency discharges that do not wax and wane are typical EMG findings. The exact biochemical cause of steroid-induced myopathy is not known. Disturbances of calcium metabolism have been suggested. Myopathic changes include fiber atrophy, necrosis, regeneration, and increased muscle fat and connective tissue. Withdrawal of exogenous steroids or suppression of endogenous steroids may benefit many dogs greatly. Dogs with severe disease may not improve even after plasma steroid levels are decreased. Even in dogs that improve with appropriate therapy, high-frequency discharges can be detected in muscles several years after remission has been achieved.[155]

Splayleg, a muscular weakness in newborn pigs, has been postulated to be a congenital form of glucocorticoid myopathy resulting from stress and hormonal imbalance in the sow.[159]

HYPOTHYROID MYOPATHY Weakness and some degenerative changes have been seen in some hypothyroid dogs.[119,151] These changes are less common than the neuropathy previously described. Varied neonatal musculoskeletal abnormalities, including ruptured tendons, angular limb deformities, forelimb contracture, and mandibular prognathism, have been found in foals with hypothyroidism.[160]

EXERTIONAL RHABDOMYOLYSIS This disorder of racing greyhounds and horses, also known as Monday morning disease, tying-up, and paralytic myoglobinuria, develops from local muscle ischemia.[7,94,161] A similar syndrome in exotic animals is called capture syndrome. Altered glycogen storage, electrolyte abnormalities, including hypokalemia, and other factors seem to be the initiating cause. The final event appears to be muscle swelling and necrosis.

Horses may become stiff and painful after exercise, or may suddenly stop while exercising. Myoglobinuria is often seen. The muscles are painful and swollen on palpation. Increased serum muscle enzyme levels are common. Muscle atrophy may be a complication on recovery. Gannon has categorized the clinical signs in dogs as hyperacute, acute, and subacute.[161] Factors that tend to lead to the syndrome include (1) a lack of physical fitness, (2) excitement prior to racing, (3) hot and humid conditions, and (4) excessive frequency of running. In the more acute forms of the disease, clinical signs are observed during the race. The most severe signs include generalized muscle pain, hyperpnea, and heavy myoglobinuria. Death may occur within 48 hours. Recumbent horses usually die.[7] In the milder (subacute) form of the disease, muscle pain is confined to the longissimus thoracis muscle and may not be apparent for 24 to 72 hours after the race. Myoglobinuria is rarely observed in subacute exertional rhabdomyolysis.

The hyperacute and acute forms of the disease are treated in a similar fashion. Intravenous (IV) fluids are given to treat or to prevent hypovolemic shock and to aid in the renal excretion of myoglobin. Sodium bicarbonate is added to the fluid to combat muscle acidosis and to help prevent the precipitation of myoglobin in renal tubules. The patient is cooled to help remove excess heat. Other treatments to be considered include anabolic steroids, oral sodium bicarbonate, B vitamins, and analgesics.

The prophylactic therapy that should be contemplated includes (1) installation of air conditioning in kennels, (2) reduction of the body temperature with cool-water baths before racing, (3) administration of oral bicarbonate-glucose solutions prior to kenneling for the race, (4) alkalinization of the urine with sodium bicarbonate or potassium citrate, (5) administration of oral potassium supplement, and (6) decreasing the frequency of racing.[161] Recommendations are similar for horses. Sodium bicarbonate added to the diet may be beneficial. The sodium may be the important factor. Deficiencies of vitamin E or selenium have not been demonstrated.[7]

MALIGNANT HYPERTHERMIA Also called the porcine stress syndrome, malignant hyperthermia is rarely seen in dogs, cats, or horses.[7,94] It is apparently a heritable trait in Pietrain, Poland China, and Landrace breeds. Following stress, such as anesthesia, hot weather, exercise, or restraint, pigs exhibit stiffness, reluctance to move, and difficult respiration. Sudden death may occur. A hypersensitive calcium-release mechanism causing high levels of myoplasmic calcium apparently initiates the increased muscle activity and hyperthermia. Muscles are pale, soft, and exudative on necropsy. A halothane test is available to detect susceptible pigs. Dantrolene sodium may be helpful, but death usually results. Reducing stress and selective breeding are recommended for prevention.[7]

POSTANESTHETIC MYOPATHY Heavy, large animals have pain and swelling of groups of muscle following long anesthesia. Nerves may be affected as well. The condition is caused, at least in part, by a compartment syndrome of affected muscles. Prolonged recumbency causes increased pressure in the muscle, with subsequent ischemia and necrosis. Treatment includes supporting the animal in a sling, administering IV fluids and electrolytes, and providing analgesics for relief of pain. Massage and passive manipulation of the limbs help increase blood flow and reduce the risk of decubital ulcers. The prognosis is good if the horse is standing. Recumbent animals may have severe muscle atrophy. Preventive measures include careful padding, elevating the uppermost limb, and avoiding hypotension during anesthesia.[7]

HYPOKALEMIC MYOPATHY Potassium depletion can occur in any species, causing muscle weakness. The general principles are discussed in Chapter 16. Since 1984, a generalized polymyopathy of cats has been characterized.[162–165] Affected cats have signs of muscular weakness—cervical ventroflexion, exercise intolerance, a stiff gait, and in some cases muscle pain on palpation. Tiring and lethargy may be observed before obvious weakness is noticed. Initially, muscle cell hyperpolarization increases refractoriness to depolarization. Eventually the cell membrane becomes more permeable to sodium, causing a sudden hypopolarization and severe weakness. The condition is apparently caused by chronic renal dysfunction with excessive potassium loss. Hypokalemia induces further renal dysfunction, establishing a vicious cycle of renal dysfunction and hypokalemia. In addition, some diets were low in potassium, although these diets have subsequently been corrected. Acidification of the urine, as is often done for management of urinary calculi, also accelerates potassium excretion. The diagnosis is based on the clinical signs, serum potassium levels (<3.0 mEq/L), increased serum CK levels, and assessment of renal function. Cats with muscle weakness are treated with oral potassium gluconate. The initial dosage is 5.0–8.0 mEq/day in divided doses.[163,166] Severe weakness may require IV fluids with potassium supplementation.

Episodic Progressive Diseases

Diseases in which episodes of weakness are interspersed with periods of normality are perplexing, because many different body systems may be involved. Episodic weakness usually

TABLE 8–8 Episodic Progressive Diseases

Diseases	*Diagnostic Tests*
Metabolic Disorders (see also Chap. 16)	
Hyperkalemia	Serum potassium levels, electrocardiogram (ECG)
Adrenal insufficiency	Plasma cortisol levels
Severe acidosis	Blood gases and pH
Severe renal failure	Blood urea nitrogen levels, urinalysis
Hypokalemia	Serum potassium levels
Chronic renal failure	Serum potassium levels, blood urea nitrogen levels, urinalysis
Hypocalcemia	Serum calcium and phosphorus levels
Hypoparathyroidism	Serum parathyroid hormone (PTH) assays
Hypercalcemia	Serum calcium levels
Primary hyperparathyroidism	Serum PTH assay, parathyroid mass
Pseudohypoparathyroidism	Evidence of lymphosarcoma or myeloma
Hypoglycemia	Fasting blood glucose levels
Functional beta cell tumor	Amended glucose insulin ratio
Glycogen storage disease	Glucagon response test
Adrenal insufficiency	Plasma cortisol levels
Cardiovascular Disorders (see Chap. 14)	
Arrhythmias	ECG
Conduction disturbances	ECG
Congestive heart failure	ECG, thoracic radiographs, auscultation
Dirofilariasis	Thoracic radiographs, Knott test
Respiratory Disorders	Auscultation, thoracic radiographs
Neuromuscular Disorders	
Myasthenia gravis	Repetitive nerve stimulation, anticholinesterase test, antibodies against acetylcholine receptors
Polymyositis	Serum muscle enzyme levels, muscle biopsy, EMG
Inherited myopathies	See Table 8–7
Narcolepsy	See Chapter 14

results from cardiovascular, metabolic, or neuromuscular diseases (Table 8–8). The primary neuromuscular disorder is myasthenia gravis, which will be discussed in this section. Some of the neuropathies and myopathies discussed previously may manifest as episodic weakness in the early stages. The endocrine-metabolic causes will be discussed in Chapter 16.

Myasthenia Gravis

PATHOPHYSIOLOGY Myasthenia gravis is a disease involving the motor end-plate that results in progressive loss of muscle strength with exercise. The basic defect is a reduction of available acetylcholine receptors (AChR) at neuromuscular junctions, which is caused by autoimmune attack.[133,167,168] Human myasthenic muscles have a 70% to 90% reduction in the number of AChR per motor end-plate. The decreased number of available receptors reduces the probability that acetylcholine molecules will react with muscle receptor sites. The safety margin of neuromuscular transmission is greatly reduced in myasthenia gravis. With repeated nerve stimulations of the motor end-plate, severe muscle weakness results. In human beings and animals, myasthenia gravis has been associated with several thymic disorders and other autoimmune diseases.[168–170] The inciting antigen is known, and radioimmunoassay tests for serum are available for diagnosis. Decreased muscle AChR and antibodies fixed to AChR have been documented in dogs. Myasthenia gravis occurs in dogs and cats, but has not been documented in large animals.[7]

Congenital myasthenia gravis is a rare disease with no antibodies to AChR. It has been documented in springer spaniels, Jack Russell terriers, smooth fox terriers, Samoyeds, Gammel Dansk honsehund, and cats.[168,171,172] The congenital form is caused by a depletion of AChR, or, in the case of the Gammel Dansk honsehund, by a presynaptic abnormality. The condition is inherited as an autosomal recessive trait in the two terrier breeds and the Gammel Dansk honsehund.[172,173]

CLINICAL SIGNS The neurologic examination is normal when the animal is rested. With exercise, muscle weakness becomes progressively worse. This phenomenon is most apparent in the appendicular muscles. Animals become fatigued, develop a shortened stride, and then lie down to rest. Strength returns with rest. Ptosis of the upper eyelids and drooping of the lips occur in some dogs with weak facial muscles. Sialosis, regurgitation of food, and dysphagia develop in a high percentage of cases. Megaesophagus is common, because the esophagus of the dog contains a considerable amount of striated muscle. Aspiration pneumonia occurs in many dogs with megaesophagus. Some dogs with idiopathic megaesophagus or laryngeal paralysis without generalized muscle weakness have myasthenia gravis. German shepherd dogs and golden retrievers were overrepresented in a review of 152 cases with megaesophagus.[174] Thymoma is found in a small portion of cases.

DIAGNOSIS Formulation of the diagnosis is aided by the exclusion of cardiovascular and metabolic diseases with appropriate laboratory or electrophysiologic tests. Exercise-induced weakness, a decremental response to repetitive nerve stimulation, and a positive response to anticholinesterase drugs support the diagnosis. Definitive diagnosis is made by detection of AChR antibody or immune complexes on the neuromuscular junction.[167]

EMG findings are usually normal in myasthenia gravis, although variability in amplitude of motor units and occasional fibrillations may be seen. Repetitive nerve stimulation at 3 Hz does not cause any decrement in the amplitude or area of the evoked muscle action potential in normal animals.[175] In myasthenia gravis, the response will decrease by at least 10% in the first ten responses. However, definitive studies on large numbers of myasthenic dogs have not been reported. Based on studies in human beings, the decrement is maximal in the first two responses. Any decrement is suspicious, and the results are sufficiently variable as to make a definitive rule difficult. At least two muscles should show a decrement.[176] The muscle should be kept warm during the test. If a decrement is demonstrated, administration of edrophonium chloride at a dose of 1–10 mg IV should cause a normal response for a few minutes. Although the decremental response is abnormal in most myasthenics, both false positive and false negative results may occur. Single fiber EMG analysis of "jitter" is reported to have the greatest accuracy in identifying myasthenia gravis.[176]

In field testing, the diagnosis of myasthenia gravis has been supported by the administration of edrophonium or neostigmine. The patient is exercised until weakness develops. Edrophonium or neostigmine is given by parenteral injection. The patient is then exercised again and is watched for evidence of increased strength and endurance. Care must be exercised both in the performance and in the interpretation of the test results. The anticholinesterase drugs may cause excessive muscle depolarization (cholinergic crisis), vomiting, salivation, and defecation. In addition, these drugs may improve the strength of dogs with primary muscle disease (polymyositis). A definitive diagnosis must be based on serologic techniques.

Serum autoantibodies to AChR provide the strongest evidence for a diagnosis. About 15% of dogs that had typical signs of myasthenia gravis and were seronegative had positive immune complexes at the neuromuscular junction.[167]

TREATMENT Once the diagnosis has been confirmed, initial therapy consists of the administration of anticholinesterase agents. Pyridostigmine bromide, 0.5–3.0 mg/kg per os, is given as needed to control the clinical signs. If the results are not satisfactory, one should consider the addition of glucocorticoids, such as prednisone, at a dosage of 0.50–1.0 mg/kg/day. This dosage can be increased to 1.0–2.0 mg/kg/day after a few days. Once remission is achieved, the patient is continued on alternate-day steroid therapy at a dosage of 2.0 mg/kg. The dosage of anticholinesterase drugs is gradually decreased and, if possible, eliminated. Drastic changes in the therapy should not occur. Thymectomy should be considered for those dogs that respond poorly to medical therapy.[168] Other forms of immune suppressive therapy, such as cyclosporine, may be of benefit.[177,178] Some dogs with myasthenia-like syndromes improve spontaneously, or the condition resolves after several weeks. In human patients, in contrast, the disease tends to get progressively worse with time. The prognosis is poor for dogs with megaesophagus. The esophageal dilation is permanent in many dogs, although this abnormality has been reported to resolve with anticholinesterase therapy.

HYPERKALEMIC PERIODIC PARALYSIS Episodic weakness and muscle trembling occurs in Quarter Horses, possibly as an inherited trait.[7,179,180] Episodes last minutes to hours and may be precipitated by exercise. Horses are normal between episodes. The signs vary from mild muscle tremors to complete recumbency. Blood samples taken during an episode show hemoconcentration and hyperkalemia. The serum potassium concentration is very high—5.0–11.7 mEq/L in one study.[179] Other parameters are not remarkable. Complex repetitive discharges were found in horses during periods of normal behavior. Treatment of acute episodes is by IV administration of sodium bicarbonate, dextrose, or calcium solutions. Diuretic therapy may lessen the frequency and severity of attacks. A similar syndrome has been reported in one dog.[181]

CASE HISTORIES

Case History 8A

Signalment

Canine, mixed breed, male, 6 months old.

History

An acute onset of tetraparesis progressed rapidly to total paralysis. The dog has been paralyzed for 24 hours.

Physical Examination

Nothing significant found except for the neurologic problems.

*Neurologic Examination**

A. Observation
   1. Mental status: Alert.
   2. Posture: Recumbent.
   3. Gait: The dog cannot support weight or maintain sternal recumbency. Tetraplegia. The dog can wag his tail.

B. Palpation: The limbs have decreased muscle tone and strength.

C. Postural Reactions

Left	Reactions	Right
0	Proprioceptive positioning PL	0
0	TL	0
0	Wheelbarrowing	0
0	Hopping, PL	0
0	Hopping, TL	0
0	Extensor postural thrust	0
0	Hemistand-hemiwalk	0
0	Placing, tactile PL	0
0	TL	0
0	Placing, visual TL	0

D. Spinal Reflexes

Left	Reflex Spinal Segment	Right
0	Quadriceps L4–L6	0
+1	Extensor carpi radialis C7–T1	+1

* *Key*: 0 = absent, +1 = decreased, +2 = normal, +3 = exaggerated, +4 = very exaggerated or clonus, PL = pelvic limb, TL = thoracic limb.

0 to +1	Flexion, PL L5–S1	0 to +1
0 to +1	Flexion, TL C6–T1	0 to +1
0	Crossed extensor	0
+2	Perineal S1–S2	+2

E. Cranial Nerves

Left	Nerve + Function	Right
+2	CN II vision menace	+2
Nor.	CN II, III pupil size	Nor.
+2	Stim. left eye	+2
+2	Stim. right eye	+2
Nor.	CN II fundus	Nor.
	CN III, IV, VI	
0	Strabismus	0
0	Nystagmus	0
+2	CN V sensation	+2
Nor.	CN V mastication	Nor.
Nor.	CN VII facial muscles	Nor.
+2	Palpebral	+2
+2	CN IX, X swallowing	+2
Nor.	CN XII tongue	Nor.

F. Sensation: Location.
Hyperesthesia: None.
Superficial pain: +2.
Deep pain: +2.

Complete sections G and H before reviewing Case Summary.

G. Assessment (Anatomic diagnosis and estimation of prognosis)

H. Plan (Diagnostic)

Rule-outs	*Procedure*
1.	
2.	
3.	
4.	

Case History 8B

Signalment

Canine, miniature schnauzer, male, 6 years old.

History

The dog had a sudden onset of falling to the right with paresis of both pelvic limbs and paralysis of the right thoracic limb. No previous trauma. The signs began 7 days ago.

Physical Examination

Negative except for the neurologic problem.

*Neurologic Examination**

A. Observation
1. Mental status: Alert.
2. Posture: Lateral recumbency.
3. Gait: The dog can stand if assisted for a short period of time. He knuckles severely on the right limbs.

B. Palpation: Atrophy of the right supraspinatus, deltoid, and triceps muscles.

C. Postural Reactions

Left	Reactions	Right
	Proprioceptive positioning	
+2	PL	0
+2	TL	+1
+2	Wheelbarrowing	+1
+2	Hopping, PL	0
+2	Hopping, TL	+1
+2	Extensor postural thrust	0
+2	Hemistand-hemiwalk	0
	Placing, tactile	
+2	PL	0
+2	TL	+1
	Placing, visual	
+2	TL	+1

D. Spinal Reflexes

Left	Reflex	Right
	Spinal Segment	
+2	Quadriceps L4–L6	+3
+2	Extensor carpi radialis C7–T1	+1
+2	Flexion, PL L5–S1	+2
+2	Flexion, TL C6–T1	+1
0	Crossed extensor	Present
+2	Perineal S1–S2	+2

E. Cranial Nerves

Left	Nerve + Function	Right
+2	CN II vision menace	+2
Nor.	CN II, III pupil size	Nor.
+2	Stim. left eye	+2

* *Key*: 0 = absent, +1 = decreased, +2 = normal, +3 = exaggerated, +4 = very exaggerated or clonus, PL = pelvic limb, TL = thoracic limb.

+2	Stim. right eye	+2
Nor.	CN II fundus	Nor.
	CN III, IV, VI	
0	Strabismus	0
0	Nystagmus	0
Nor.	CN V sensation	Nor.
+2	CN V mastication	+2
Nor.	CN VII facial muscles	Nor.
+2	Palpebral	+2
Nor.	CN IX, X swallowing	Nor.
+2	CN XII tongue	+2

F. Sensation: Location.
   Hyperesthesia: None.
   Superficial pain: +2.
   Deep pain: +2.

Complete sections G and H before reviewing Case Summary.

G. Assessment (Anatomic diagnosis and estimation of prognosis)

H. Plan (Diagnostic)

Rule-outs *Procedure*
1.
2.
3.
4.

Case History 8C

Signalment

Canine, miniature poodle, male, 11 years old.

History

One month ago lameness developed in the left thoracic limb, progressing to both thoracic limbs within 7 days. Two weeks later the dog developed ataxia of both pelvic limbs; 1 week ago he developed severe paresis of both pelvic limbs. The dog does not wag his tail.

Physical Examination

Grade IV/VI holosystolic mitral murmur. Fluid lung sounds. Severe periodontal disease.

*Neurologic Examination**

A. Observation
   1. Mental status: Alert.
   2. Posture: Recumbent (sternal).
   3. Gait: Tetraparesis.

B. Palpation: Extensor rigidity of thoracic limbs. Hypertonus of pelvic limbs.

C. Postural Reactions

Left	Reactions	Right
	Proprioceptive positioning	
0	PL	0
0	TL	0
0	Wheelbarrowing	0
0	Hopping, PL	0 to +1
0	Hopping, TL	0 to +1
0	Extensor postural thrust	0
0	Hemistand-hemiwalk	0
	Placing, tactile	
0	PL	0
0	TL	0
	Placing, visual	
0	TL	0

D. Spinal Reflexes

Left	Reflex	Right
	Spinal Segment	
	Quadriceps	
+2	L4–L6	+3
	Extensor carpi radialis	
+2	C7–T1	+3
	Flexion, PL	
+2	L5–S1	+2
	Flexion, TL	
+2	C6–T1	+2
0	Crossed extensor	0
	Perineal	
+2	S1–S2	+2

E. Cranial Nerves

Left	Nerve + Function	Right
+2	CN II vision menace	+2
Nor.	CN II, III pupil size	Nor.
+2	Stim. left eye	+2
+2	Stim. right eye	+2
Nor.	CN II fundus	Nor.
	CN III, IV, VI	
0	Strabismus	0
0	Nystagmus	0
Nor.	CN V mastication	Nor.
Nor.	CN VII facial muscles	Nor.
+2	Palpebral	+2
Nor.	CN IX, X swallowing	Nor.
Nor.	CN XII tongue	Nor.

* *Key*: 0 = absent, +1 = decreased, +2 = normal, +3 = exaggerated, +4 = very exaggerated or clonus, PL = pelvic limb, TL = thoracic limb.

F. Sensation: Location.
 Hyperesthesia: Moderate on palpation of cervical area.
 Superficial pain: Good.
 Deep pain: Good.

Complete sections G and H before reviewing Case Summary.

G. Assessment (Anatomic diagnosis and estimation of prognosis)

H. Plan (Diagnostic)

Rule-outs	*Procedure*
1.	
2.	
3.	
4.	

Case History 8D

Signalment

Canine, toy poodle, male, 1 year old.

History

Five weeks ago the dog experienced severe pain and could not walk up or down stairs. The head was slightly flexed, and the neck was stiff. One week ago the dog bumped his head, cried out in pain, fell down, and became stiff. He cries out when the head is moved.

Physical Examination

Negative except for 5% dehydration and the neurologic problem.

*Neurologic Examination**

A. Observation
 1. Mental status: Alert; cries out if manipulated.
 2. Posture: Lateral recumbency. Neck is slightly extended and rigid.
 3. Gait: Severe tetraparesis.

B. Palpation: The thoracic limbs are in extensor rigidity. Open fontanelle.

C. Postural Reactions

Left	Reactions	Right
+1	Proprioceptive positioning PL	+1
+1 to +2	TL	+1 to +2
+1	Wheelbarrowing	+1
+1	Hopping, PL	+1
+1	Hopping, TL	+1
+1	Extensor postural thrust	+1
+1	Hemistand-hemiwalk	+1
0	Placing, tactile PL	0
+1	TL	+1
+1	Placing, visual TL	+1

D. Spinal Reflexes

Left	Reflex Spinal Segment	Right
+3	Quadriceps L4–L6	+3
+3	Extensor carpi radialis C7–T1	+3
+2	Flexion, PL L5–S1	+2
+2	Flexion, TL C6–T1	+2
0	Crossed extensor	0
+2	Perineal S1–S2	+2

E. Cranial Nerves

Left	Nerve + Function	Right
+2	CN II vision menace	+2
Nor.	CN II, III pupil size	Nor.
+2	Stim. left eye	+2
+2	Stim. right eye	+2
Nor.	CN II fundus	Nor.
	CN III, IV, VI	
0	Strabismus	0
0	Nystagmus	0
Nor.	CN V sensation	Nor.
Nor.	CN V mastication	Nor.
Nor.	CN VII facial muscles	Nor.
+2	Palpebral	+2
Nor.	CN IX, X swallowing	Nor.
Nor.	CN XII tongue	Nor.

F. Sensation: Location.
 Hyperesthesia: Cervical. Resists movement, painful on palpation of cranial cervical area.
 Superficial pain: Good.
 Deep pain: Good.

Complete sections G and H before reviewing Case Summary.

G. Assessment (Anatomic diagnosis and estimation of prognosis)

* *Key*: 0 = absent, +1 = decreased, +2 = normal, +3 = exaggerated, +4 = very exaggerated or clonus, PL = pelvic limb, TL = thoracic limb.

H. Plan (Diagnostic)

Rule-outs	*Procedure*
1.	
2.	
3.	
4.	

Case History 8E

Signalment

Canine, Doberman pinscher, male, 8 years old.

History

For several months the dog has had knuckling, ataxia, and paresis in the pelvic limbs. He occasionally knuckles on the thoracic limbs. He has been treated with intramuscular injections of corticosteroids that gave temporary improvement. He recently developed paralysis of the right pelvic limb.

Physical Examination

Negative except for the neurologic signs described below.

*Neurologic Examination**

A. Observation
   1. Mental status: Alert.
   2. Posture: Ambulatory.
   3. Gait: Paraparesis and ataxia. Occasionally knuckles on the thoracic limbs.

B. Palpation: Stiff neck. Muscle atrophy is severe in the right pelvic limb below the stifle. Abrasions are present on the dorsal surface of the right pelvic foot.

C. Postural Reactions

Left	Reactions	Right
0	Proprioceptive positioning PL	0
+2	TL	+2
Knuckles	Wheelbarrowing	Knuckles
+1	Hopping, PL	0
+2	Hopping, TL	+2
+1	Extensor postural thrust	+1
+1	Hemistand-hemiwalk	+1
+1	Placing, tactile PL	0
+2	TL	+2
+2	Placing, visual TL	+2

* *Key*: 0 = absent, +1 = decreased, +2 = normal, +3 = exaggerated, +4 = very exaggerated or clonus, PL = pelvic limb, TL = thoracic limb.

D. Spinal Reflexes

Left	Reflex	Right
	Spinal Segment	
+3	Quadriceps L4–L6	+3
+3	Extensor carpi radialis C7–T1	+3
+2	Flexion, PL L5–S1	0; flexes at hip
+2	Flexion, TL C6–T1	+2
0	Crossed extensor	0
+2	Perineal S1–S2	+2

E. Cranial Nerves

Left	Nerve + Function	Right
+2	CN II vision menace	+2
Nor.	CN II, III pupil size	Nor.
+2	Stim. left eye	+2
+2	Stim. right eye	+2
Nor.	CN II fundus	Nor.
	CN III, IV, VI	
0	Strabismus	0
0	Nystagmus	0
Nor.	CN V sensation	Nor.
Nor.	CN V mastication	Nor.
Nor.	CN VII facial muscles	Nor.
+2	Palpebral	+2
Nor.	CN IX, X swallowing	Nor.
Nor.	CN XII tongue	Nor.

F. Sensation: Location.
   Hyperesthesia: Mild in midcervical area.
   Superficial pain: Good, but absent in right pelvic foot.
   Deep pain: Good, except absent in right pelvic foot.

Complete sections G and H before reviewing Case Summary.

G. Assessment (Anatomic diagnosis and estimation of prognosis)

H. Plan (Diagnostic)

Rule-outs	*Procedure*
1.	
2.	
3.	
4.	

Assessment 8A

Anatomic diagnosis. Generalized LMN signs are present, and pain perception is preserved. Generalized neuropathy or motor end-plate disease should be suspected.

Diagnostic plan (Rule-outs):

1. Tick paralysis: Examine for ticks (present).
2. Botulism: History, EMGs, toxin analysis.
3. Polyradiculoneuritis: EMGs.
4. Other polyneuropathies.

Therapeutic plan:

1. Remove ticks.
2. Support the dog with attentive nursing care.

Client education. The prognosis is good.

Case summary. Tick paralysis was diagnosed. The ticks were removed, and the dog improved within 24 hours and was normal in 36 hours. This is a typical recovery for tick paralysis.

Assessment 8B

Anatomic diagnosis. This dog has a right hemiparesis with a normal left thoracic limb and a nearly normal left pelvic limb. The right hemiparesis is characterized by LMN signs in the thoracic limb and UMN signs in the pelvic limb. The lesion is most likely C6–T2.

Diagnostic plan (Rule-outs):

1. Trauma: History, cervical radiography (negative).
2. Cervical disk disease: Myelography (negative).
3. Myelitis: CSF examination (negative).
4. Cervical spinal cord infarction: Supported by negative diagnostic tests.

Therapeutic plan:

1. Prescribe cage rest, prevent decubital sores, perform hydrotherapy.
2. Corticosteroid therapy is of questionable value at this stage of the spinal cord infarction.

Client education. The prognosis is poor, because of LMN signs to the right thoracic limb. The tracts frequently recover, but neurons do not.

Case summary. A severe hemorrhagic vascular lesion on the right (C7–C8, C8–T1) was diagnosed. The dog did not improve, and euthanasia was performed. Necropsy confirmed the presence of the lesion. The cause of the infarction was not found.

Assessment 8C

Anatomic diagnosis. The dog has UMN tetraparesis with no evidence of brain stem disease. This finding localizes the lesion to the segment C1–C5.

Diagnostic plan (Rule-outs). The disease is acutely progressive in course, and there is hyperesthesia in the cervical area.

1. Cervical disk disease: radiology (disk herniation at C2–C3), myelography demonstrated significant compression of the spinal cord.
2. Cervical neoplasia. Myelography (negative).
3. Cervical myelitis. CSF analysis (protein 35 mg/dl, 2 WBC, not indicative of inflammatory disease).

Therapeutic plan. Although this dog has other medical problems, surgery was done because of the severity of signs and a compression of the spinal cord on myelography.

Client education. The prognosis is fair to poor. If the dog were in excellent health, the prognosis would be good.

Case summary. Cervical disk disease was diagnosed. The dog did well in surgery and went home significantly improved.

Assessment 8D

Anatomic diagnosis. Severe tetraparesis is present with UMN signs in all four limbs. Cervical pain and the absence of brain stem signs localize the lesion to the segment C1 – C5.

Diagnostic plan (Rule-outs). The dog has hyperesthesia in the cranial cervical region and is a toy breed, but is very young for disk disease. Inflammatory disease is a possibility, but atlantoaxial luxation should be ruled out before any manipulation of the neck is done.

1. Atlantoaxial subluxation: Cervical radiography (atlantoaxial subluxation is present).
2. Cervical disk: Myelography (not performed).
3. Meningomyelitis: CSF examination (not performed).

Therapeutic plan. Surgical stabilization.

Client education. The prognosis is fair to good.

Case summary. Atlantoaxial subluxation was diagnosed. Following surgery, the patient recovered.

Assessment 8E

Anatomic diagnosis. Two lesions must be present to explain the clinical findings in this case. LMN disease and hypalgesia are present in the right pelvic limb, suggesting a selective sciatic nerve injury (probably a needle injury from intramuscular injections). The other neurologic signs suggest a midcervical lesion.

Diagnostic plan (Rule-outs):

1. Cervical spondylopathy: Cervical radiography and myelography (negative).
2. Cervical disk: Type II compression of the spinal cord at C5–C6.
3. Cervical myelitis: CSF analysis (normal).
4. Injection neuritis: EMG (denervation potentials in the flexors of the stifle and all muscles below the stifle).

Therapeutic plan:

1. Ventral cervical decompression or distraction and stabilization of C5–C6.
2. Physical therapy and a boot for the right pelvic limb.

Client education. The prognosis is very guarded.

Case summary. Cervical disk compression and sciatic neuritis were diagnosed. The UMN deficits improved so that gait was nearly normal. The right pelvic limb improved more than 50% in the first 4 months following surgery.

REFERENCES

1. Hoerlein BF: Intervertebral disk disease. In Oliver JE, Hoerlein BF, Mayhew IG (eds): Veterinary Neurology. Philadelphia, WB Saunders, 1987, pp 321–341.
2. Stadler P, Van den Berg SS, Tustin RC: Servikale intervertebrale diskus prolaps in 'n perd. J South Afr Vet Assoc 59:31–32, 1987.
3. Foss R, Genetzky R, Riedesel E, et al: Cervical intervertebral disc protrusion in two horses. Can Vet J 24:188–191, 1983.
4. Nixon A, Stashak T, Ingram J, et al: Cervical intervertebral disk protrusion in a horse. Vet Surg 13:154–158, 1984.
5. Felts J, Prata R: Cervical disk disease in the dog: Intraforaminal and lateral extrusions. J Am Anim Hosp Assoc 19:755–760, 1983.
6. Fry TR, Johnson AL, Hungerford L, et al: Surgical treatment of cervical disc herniations in ambulatory dogs: Ventral decompression vs. fenestration, 111 cases (1980–1988). Prog Vet Neurol 2:165–173, 1991.
7. Mayhew IG: Large Animal Neurology: A Handbook for Veterinary Clinicians. Philadelphia, Lea & Febiger, 1989.
8. Mayhew I, Brown C, Stowe H, et al: Equine degenerative myeloencephalopathy: A vitamin E deficiency that may be familial. J Vet Intern Med 1:45–50, 1987.
9. Beech J, Haskind M: Genetic studies of neuraxonal dystrophy in the Morgan. Am J Vet Res 48:109–113, 1987.
10. Blythe LL, Craig AM, Lassen ED, et al: Serially determined plasma α-tocopherol concentrations and results of the oral vitamin E absorption test in clinically normal horses and in horses with degenerative myeloencephalopathy. Am J Vet Res 52:908–911, 1991.
11. Bailey CS: An embryological approach to the clinical significance of congenital vertebral and spinal cord abnormalities. J Am Anim Hosp Assoc 11:426–434, 1975.
12. Shelton SB, Bellah J, Chrisman C, et al: Hypoplasia of the odontoid process and secondary atlantoaxial luxation in a Siamese cat. Prog Vet Neurol 2:209–211, 1991.
13. Oliver JE, Lewis RE: Lesions of the atlas and axis in dogs. J Am Anim Hosp Assoc 9:304–313, 1973.
14. Watson AG, de Lahunta A: Atlantoaxial subluxation and absence of transverse ligament of the atlas in a dog. J Am Vet Med Assoc 195:235–237, 1989.
15. Geary JC, Oliver JE, Hoerlein BF: Atlanto-axial subluxation in the canine. J Small Anim Pract 8:577–582, 1967.
16. Cook JR, Oliver JE: Atlantoaxial luxation in the dog. Comp Cont Educ Pract Vet 3:242–252, 1981.
17. Sorjonen DC, Shires PK: Atlantoaxial instability: A ventral surgical technique for decompression, fixation and fusion. Vet Surg 10:22–29, 1981.
18. Owen RAR, Maxie LLS: Repair of fractured dens of the axis in a foal. J Am Vet Med Assoc 173:854–856, 1978.
19. Nixon AJ, Stashak TS: Laminectomy for relief of atlantoaxial subluxation in four horses. J Am Vet Med Assoc 193:677–682, 1988.
20. Chambers JN, Betts CW, Oliver JE: The use of nonmetallic suture material for stabilization of atlantoaxial subluxation. J Am Anim Hosp Assoc 13:602–604, 1977.
21. LeCouteur RA, McKeown D, Johnson J, et al: Stabilization of atlantoaxial subluxation in the dog, using the nuchal ligament. J Am Vet Med Assoc 177:1011–1017, 1980.
22. Kishigami M: Application of an atlantoaxial retractor for atlantoaxial subluxation in the cat and dog. J Am Anim Hosp Assoc 20:413–419, 1984.
23. Jaggy A, Hutto VL, Roberts RE, et al: Occipitoatlantoaxial malformation with atlantoaxial subluxation in a cat. J Small Anim Pract 32:366–372, 1991.
24. Parker AJ, Park RD, Cusick PK: Abnormal odontoid process angulation in a dog. Vet Rec 93:559–561, 1973.
25. DeCamp CE, Schirmer RG, Stickle RL: Traumatic atlantooccipital subluxation in a dog. J Am Anim Hosp Assoc 27:415–418, 1991.
26. Lappin MR, Dow S: Traumatic atlanto-occipital luxation in a cat. Vet Surg 12:30–32, 1983.
27. Greenwood KM, Oliver JE: Traumatic atlanto-occipital dislocation in two dogs. J Am Vet Med Assoc 173:1324–1327, 1978.
28. Crane SW: Surgical management of traumatic atlanto-occipital instability in a dog. Vet Surg 7:39–42, 1978.
29. Sorjonen DC, Powe TA, West M, et al: Ventral surgical fixation and fusion for atlanto-occipital subluxation in a goat. Vet Surg 12:127–129, 1983.
30. Powers B, Stashak T, Nixon A, et al: Pathology of the vertebral column of horses with cervical static stenosis. Vet Pathol 23:392–399, 1986.
31. Trotter E: Canine wobbler syndrome. In Kirk RW: Current Veterinary Therapy, IX. Philadelphia, WB Saunders, 1986, pp 806–810.
32. Chambers J, Betts C: Caudal cervical spondylopathy in the dog: A review of 20 clinical cases and the literature. J Am Anim Hosp Assoc 13:571–576, 1977.
33. Selcer R, Oliver J: Cervical spondylopathy: Wobbler syndrome in dogs. J Am Anim Hosp Assoc 11:175–179, 1975.
34. Fraser H, Palmer A: Equine inco-ordination and wobbler disease of young horses. Vet Rec 80:338–355, 1967.
35. Lewis DG: Cervical spondylomyelopathy ('wobbler' syndrome) in the dog: A study based on 224 cases. J Small Anim Pract 30:657–665, 1989.
36. Seim HB: Wobbler syndrome in the Doberman pinscher. In Kirk RW (ed): Current Veterinary Therapy, X. Philadelphia, WB Saunders, 1989, pp 858–862.
37. Hedhammer A, Wu FM, Krook L, et al: Overnutrition and skeletal disease: An experimental study in growing Great Dane dogs. Cornell Vet 64:1–160, 1974.
38. VanGundy T: Canine wobbler syndrome: Part I. Pathophysiology and diagnosis. Comp Cont Educ Pract Vet 11:144–158, 1989.
39. Lyman RL, Seim HB: Viewpoint: Wobbler syndrome. Prog Vet Neurol 2:143–150, 1991.
40. Bruecker KA, Seim HB III, Withrow SJ: Clinical evaluation of three surgical methods for treatment of caudal cervical spondylomyelopathy of dogs. Vet Surg 18:197–203, 1989.
41. Lyman R: Continuous dorsal laminectomy for the treatment of caudal cervical vertebral instability and malformation. In: Proceedings of the 13th Annual Kal-Kan Symposium, Columbus, OH, 1989, pp 13–16.
42. McKee WM, Lavelle RB, Richardson JL, et al: Vertebral distraction-fusion for cervical spondylopathy using a screw and double washer technique. J Small Anim Pract 31:22–27, 1990.
43. Bruecker KA, Seim HB, Blass CE: Caudal cervical spondylomyelopathy: Decompression by linear traction and stabilization with Steinmann pins and polymethyl methacrylate. J Am Anim Hosp Assoc 25:677–683, 1989.
44. Van Gundy T: Canine wobbler syndrome: Part II. Treatment. Comp Cont Educ Pract Vet 11:269–284, 1989.
45. Ellison GW, Seim HB, Clemmons RM: Distracted spinal fusion for management of caudal cervical spondylomyelopathy in large-breed dogs. J Am Vet Med Assoc 193:447–453, 1988.
46. Wagner P, Grant B, Bagby G, et al: Evaluation of cervi-

cal spinal fusion as a treatment in the equine wobbler syndrome. Vet Surg 8:84–88, 1979.
47. Nixon AJ: Surgical management of equine cervical vertebral malformation. Prog Vet Neurol 2:183–195, 1991.
48. Northington J, Brown M: Acute canine idiopathic polyneuropathy: A Guillain-Barré-like syndrome in dogs. J Neurol Sci 56:259–272, 1982.
49. Northington J, Brown M, Farnbach G, et al: Acute idiopathic polyneuropathy in the dog. J Am Vet Med Assoc 179:375–379, 1981.
50. Vandevelde M, Oettli P, Fatzer R, et al: Polyradikuloneuritis beim Hund: Klinische, histologische und ultrastrukturelle Beobachtungen. Schweiz Arch Tierheilkd 123:207–217, 1981.
51. Holmes D, Schultz R, Cummings J, et al: Experimental coonhound paralysis: Animal model of Guillain-Barré syndrome. Neurology 29:1186–1187, 1979.
52. Luttgen PJ: Polyradiculoneuritis in a cat. In: Proceedings of an ACVIM Forum, San Diego, 1987, p 842.
53. MacLachlan N, Gribble D, East N: Polyradiculoneuritis in a goat. J Am Vet Med Assoc 180:166–167, 1982.
54. Cummings J, de Lahunta A, Holmes D, et al: Coonhound paralysis: Further clinical studies and electron microscopic observations. Acta Neuropathol 57:167–178, 1982.
55. Duncan I: Polyradiculoneuritis: Coonhound paralysis revisited. In: Proceedings of an ACVIM Forum, San Diego, 1987, pp 334–337.
56. Chrisman C: Differentiation of tick paralysis and acute idiopathic polyradiculoneuritis in the dog using electromyography. J Am Anim Hosp Assoc 11:455–458, 1975.
57. Cuddon PA: Electrophysiological and immunological evaluation in coonhound paralysis. In: Proceedings of the Eighth Ann Veterinary Medical Forum, Washington, DC, 1990, pp 1009–1012.
58. Dyck P, O'Brien P, Oviatt K, et al: Prednisone improves chronic inflammatory demyelinating polyradiculoneuropathy more than no treatment. Ann Neurol 11:136–141, 1982.
59. Barsanti J, Walser M, Hathaway C, et al: Type C botulism in American foxhounds. J Am Vet Med Assoc 172: 809–814, 1978.
60. Cornelissen J, Haagsma J, van Nes J: Type C botulism in five dogs. J Am Anim Hosp Assoc 21:401–404, 1985.
61. Farrow B, Murrel W, Revington M, et al: Type C botulism in young dogs. Aust Vet J 60:374–377, 1983.
62. Darke P, Robert T, Smart J, et al: Suspected botulism in foxhounds. Vet Rec 99:98–99, 1976.
63. Marlow G, Smart JL: Botulism in foxhounds. Vet Rec 111:242, 1982.
64. Ricketts SW, Greet TRC, Glyn PJ, et al: Thirteen cases of botulism in horses fed big bale silage. Equine Vet J 16: 515–518, 1984.
65. Swerczek T: Toxicoinfectious botulism in foals and adult horses. J Am Vet Med Assoc 176:217–220, 1980.
66. Swerczek T: Experimentally induced toxicoinfectious botulism in horses and foals. Am J Vet Res 41:348–350, 1980.
67. Kelly AP, Jones RT, Gillick JC, et al: Outbreak of botulism in horses. Equine Vet J 16:519–521, 1984.
68. Bernard W, Divers TJ, Whitlock TH, et al: Botulism as a sequel to open castration in a horse. J Am Vet Med Assoc 191:73–74, 1987.
69. Kao I, Drachman D, Price D: Botulinum toxin: Mechanism of presynaptic blockade. Science 193:1256–1258, 1976.
70. van Nes J, van der Most van Spijk D: Electrophysiology evidence of peripheral nerve dysfunction in six dogs with botulism type C. Res Vet Sci 40:372–376, 1986.
71. Oh S: Botulism: Electrophysiological studies. Ann Neurol 1:481–485, 1976.
72. Swift TR, Ignacio OJ: Tick paralysis: Electrophysiologic studies. Neurology 25:1130–1133, 1975.
73. Ilkiw JE: Tick paralysis in Australia. In Kirk RW (ed): Current Veterinary Therapy, VIII. Philadelphia, WB Saunders, 1983, pp 691–693.
74. Farrow BRH: Tick paralysis and botulism. In: Proceedings of the Sixth Annual Veterinary Medical Forum, Washington, DC, 1988, pp 61–63.
75. Ilkiw J, Turner D: Infestation in the dog by the paralysis tick *Ixodes holocyclus*: 2. Blood-gas and pH, haematological and biochemical findings. Aust Vet J 64:139–142, 1987.
76. Osweiler GD, Carlson TL, Buck WB, et al: Clinical and Diagnostic Veterinary Toxicology, 3rd ed. Dubuque, IA, Kendall/Hunt Publishing Co, 1985.
77. Lorenz MD, Cork LC, Griffin JW, et al: Hereditary muscular atrophy in Brittany spaniels: Clinical manifestations. J Am Vet Med Assoc 175:833–839, 1979.
78. Cork LC, Griffin JW, Choy C, et al: Pathology of motor neurons in accelerated hereditary canine spinal muscular atrophy. Lab Invest 46:89–99, 1982.
79. Cork LC, Troncoso JC, Klavano GG, et al: Neurofilamentous abnormalities in motor neurons in spontaneously occurring animal disorders. J Neuropathol Exp Neurol 47:420–431, 1988.
80. Sandefeldt E, Cummings JF, de Lahunta A, et al: Hereditary neuronal abiotrophy in the Swedish Lapland dog. Cornell Vet 63:1–71, 1973.
81. Shell L, Jortner B, Leib M: Spinal muscular atrophy in two Rottweiler littermates. J Am Vet Med Assoc 190: 878–880, 1987.
82. Shell L, Jortner B, Leib M: Familial motor neuron disease in Rottweiler dogs: Neuropathologic studies. Vet Pathol 24:135–139, 1987.
83. Inada S, Yamauchi C, Igata A, et al: Canine storage disease characterized by hereditary progressive neurogenic muscular atrophy: Breeding experiments and clinical manifestation. Am J Vet Res 47:2294–2299, 1986.
84. Izumo S, Ikuta F, Igata A, et al: Morphological study on the hereditary neurogenic amyotrophic dogs: Accumulation of lipid compound-like structures in the lower motor neuron. Acta Neuropathol 61:270–276, 1983.
85. Inada S, Sakamoto H, Haruta K, et al: A clinical study on hereditary progressive neurogenic muscular atrophy in pointer dogs. Jpn J Vet Sci 40:539–547, 1978.
86. Cummings JF, George C, de Lahunta A, et al: Focal spinal muscular atrophy in two German shepherd pups. Acta Neuropathol 79:113–116, 1989.
87. Cummings JF, de Lahunta A, George C, et al: Equine motor neuron disease: A preliminary report. Cornell Vet 80:357–379, 1990.
88. Stockard C: An hereditary lethal factor for localized motor and preganglionic neurons. Am J Anat 59:1–53, 1936.
89. Palmer AC, Blakmore WF: A progressive neuronopathy in the young cairn terrier. J Small Anim Pract 30:101–106, 1989.
90. Cummings JF, de Lahunta A, Moore JJ: Multisystemic chromatolytic neuronal degeneration in a cairn terrier pup. Cornell Vet 78:301–314, 1988.
91. Jaggy A, Vandevelde M: Multisystem neuronal degeneration in cocker spaniels. J Vet Intern Med 2:117–120, 1988.
92. Duncan ID: Peripheral neuropathy in the dog and cat. Prog Vet Neurol 2:111–128, 1991.
93. Duncan I: Etiology and classification of peripheral neuropathies. In: Proceedings of an ACVIM Forum, San Diego, 1987, pp 325–329.

94. Braund KG: Diseases of the peripheral nerves, cranial nerves, and muscle. In Oliver JE, Hoerlein BF, Mayhew IG (eds): Veterinary Neurology. Philadelphia, WB Saunders, 1987, pp 353–392.
95. Braund KG: Nerve and muscle biopsy techniques. Prog Vet Neurol 2:35–56, 1991.
96. Shelton GD: Diagnosis and treatment of disorders of peripheral nerve, muscle, and neuromuscular junction. In: Proceedings of the 13th Annual Kal-Kan Symposium, Columbus, OH, 1989, pp 7–11.
97. Cummings J, de Lahunta A: Chronic relapsing polyradiculoneuritis in a dog: A clinical, light- and electron-microscopic study. Acta Neuropathol 28:191–204, 1974.
98. Bichsel P, Oliver J Jr, Tyler D, et al: Chronic polyneuritis in a Rottweiler. J Am Vet Med Assoc 191:991–994, 1987.
99. Cummings J, de Lahunta A, Mitchell W: Ganglioradiculitis in the dog: A clinical, light- and electron-microscopic study. Acta Neuropathol 60:29–39, 1983.
100. Griffiths IR: Progressive axonopathy: An inherited neuropathy of boxer dogs. I. Further studies of the clinical and electrophysiological features. J Small Anim Pract 26:381–392, 1985.
101. Griffiths IR, Duncan ID, Barker J: A progressive axonopathy of boxer dogs affecting the central and peripheral nervous system. J Small Anim Pract 21:29–43, 1980.
102. Duncan ID, Griffiths IR: Canine giant axonal neuropathy: Some aspects of its clinical, pathological and comparative features. J Small Anim Pract 22:491–501, 1981.
103. Griffiths IR, Duncan ID, McCulloch M, et al: Further studies of the central nervous system in canine giant axonal neuropathy. Neuropathol Appl Neurobiol 6: 421–432, 1980.
104. Higgins RJ, Rings DM, Fenner WR, et al: Spontaneous lower motor neuron disease with neurofibrillary accumulation in young pigs. Acta Neuropathol 59:288–294, 1983.
105. de Lahunta A, Shively GN: Neurofibrillary accumulation in a puppy. Cornell Vet 65:240–247, 1975.
106. Vandevelde M, Greene C, Hoff E: Lower motor neuron disease with accumulation of neurofilaments in a cat. Vet Pathol 13:428–435, 1976.
107. Cooper BJ, de Lahunta A, Cummings JF, et al: Canine inherited hypertrophic neuropathy: Clinical and electrodiagnostic studies. Am J Vet Res 45:1172–1177, 1984.
108. Cummings J, de Lahunta A: Hypertrophic neuropathy in a dog. Acta Neuropathol 20:325–336, 1974.
109. Griffiths I, Duncan I: Distal denervating disease: A degenerative neuropathy of the distal motor axon in dogs. J Small Anim Pract 20:579–592, 1979.
110. Chrisman CL: Distal polyneuropathy of doberman pinschers. In: Proceedings of the Third Annual Medical Forum, ACVIM, San Diego, 1985.
111. Cummings JF, de Lahunta A, Braund KG, et al: Animal model of human disease: Hereditary sensory neuropathy. Nociceptive loss and acral mutilation in pointer dogs: Canine hereditary sensory neuropathy. Am J Pathol 112:136–138, 1983.
112. Duncan ID, Griffiths IR, Munz M: The pathology of a sensory neuropathy affecting long haired dachshund dogs. Acta Neuropathol 58:141–151, 1982.
113. Wouda W, Vandevelde M, Oettli P, et al: Sensory neuronopathy in dogs: A study of four cases. J Comp Pathol 93:437–450, 1983.
114. Wheeler SJ: Sensory neuropathy in a border collie puppy. J Small Anim Pract 28:281–289, 1987.
115. Nes J: Electrophysiological evidence of sensory nerve dysfunction in 10 dogs with acral lick dermatitis. J Am Anim Hosp Assoc 22:157–160, 1986.
116. Cummings JF, de Lahunta A, Simpson ST, et al: Reduced substance P-like immunoreactivity in hereditary sensory neuropathy of pointer dogs. Acta Neuropathol 63:33–40, 1984.
117. Jaggy A: Neurologic manifestations of hypothyroidism to dogs. In: Proceedings of the Eighth Annual Veterinary Medical Forum, Washington, DC, 1990, pp 1037–1040.
118. Ferguson DC: Diagnosis of canine hypothyroidism. Vet Med Rep 3:172–177, 1991.
119. Indrieri R, Whalen L, Cardinet G, et al: Neuromuscular abnormalities associated with hypothyroidism and lymphocytic thyroiditis in three dogs. J Am Vet Med Assoc 190:544–548, 1987.
120. Wolff A: Neuropathy associated with transient diabetes mellitus in 2 cats. Mod Vet Pract 65:726–728, 1984.
121. Kramek B, Moise S, Cooper B, et al: Neuropathy associated with diabetes mellitus in the cat. J Am Vet Med Assoc 184:42–45, 1984.
122. Johnson C, Kittleson M, Indrieri R: Peripheral neuropathy and hypotension in a diabetic dog. J Am Vet Med Assoc 183:1007–1009, 1983.
123. Katherman A, Braund K: Polyneuropathy associated with diabetes mellitus in a dog. J Am Vet Med Assoc 182:522–524, 1983.
124. Steiss J, Orsher A, Bowen J: Electrodiagnostic analysis of peripheral neuropathy in dogs with diabetes mellitus. Am J Vet Res 42:2061–2064, 1981.
125. Braund KG, Steiss JE, Amling KA, et al: Insulinoma and subclinical peripheral neuropathy in two dogs. J Vet Int Med 1:86–90, 1987.
126. Jones B, Johnstone A, Cahill J, et al: Peripheral neuropathy in cats with inherited primary hyperchylomicronaemia. Vet Rec 119:268–272, 1986.
127. O'Toole D, Wells GAH, Green RB, et al: Radial and tibial nerve pathology of two lactating ewes with kangaroo gait. J Comp Pathol 100:245–258, 1989.
128. Duffell S, Wells G, Winkler C: 'Kangaroo gait' in ewes: A peripheral neuropathy. Vet Rec 118:296–298, 1986.
129. Braund K, McGuire J, Amling K, et al: Peripheral neuropathy associated with malignant neoplasms in dogs. Vet Pathol 24:16–21, 1987.
130. Presthus J, Teige J: Peripheral neuropathy associated with lymphosarcoma in a dog. J Small Anim Pract 27: 463–469, 1986.
131. Greene CE: Infectious Diseases of the Dog and Cat. Philadelphia, WB Saunders, 1990.
132. Shelton GD: Differential diagnosis of muscle diseases in companion animals. Prog Vet Neurol 2:27–33, 1991.
133. Shelton G, Cardinet H: Pathophysiologic basis of canine muscle disorders. J Vet Intern Med 1:36–44, 1987.
134. Kornegay JN, Gorgacz EJ, Dawe DL, et al: Polymyositis in dogs. J Am Vet Med Assoc 176:431–438, 1980.
135. Smith MO: Idiopathic myositides in dogs. Semin Vet Med Surg 4:156–160, 1989.
136. Carpenter JL, Schmidt GM, Moore FM, et al: Canine bilateral extraocular polymyositis. Vet Pathol 26:510–512, 1989.
137. Hargis AM, Haupt KH, Prieur DJ, et al: A skin disorder in three shetland sheepdogs: Comparison with familial canine dermatomyositis of collies. Comp Cont Educ Pract Vet 7:306–315, 1985.
138. Haupt KH, Prieur DJ, Moore MP, et al: Familial canine dermatomyositis: Clinical, electrodiagnostic, and genetic studies. Am J Vet Res 46:1861–1869, 1985.
139. Carpenter JL, Hoffman EP, Romanul FCA, et al: Feline muscular dystrophy with dystrophin deficiency. Am J Pathol 135:909–919, 1989.

140. Valentine BA, Kornegay JN, Cooper BJ: Clinical electromyographic studies of canine X-linked muscular dystrophy. Am J Vet Res 50:2145–2148, 1989.
141. Wentink GH, van der Linde-Sipman JS, Meijer AEF, et al: Myopathy with a possible recessive X-linked inheritance in a litter of Irish terriers. Vet Pathol 9:328–349, 1972.
142. Kornegay JN: Golden retriever muscular dystrophy. In: Proceedings of the Sixth Annual Veterinary Medical Forum, Washington, DC, 1988, pp 470–471.
143. Kramer JW, Hegreberg GA, Hamilton MJ: Inheritance of a neuromuscular disorder of Labrador retriever dogs. J Am Vet Med Assoc 179:380–381, 1981.
144. McKerrell R, Braund K: Hereditary myopathy in Labrador retrievers: Clinical variations. J Small Anim Pract 28:479–489, 1987.
145. Braund KG: Labrador retriever myopathy. In: Proceedings of the Sixth Annual Veterinary Medical Forum, Washington, DC, 1988, pp 85–87.
146. Braund KG, Steinberg HS: Degenerative myopathy of Bouvier des Flandres: In Proceedings of the Seventh Annual Veterinary Medical Forum, San Diego, 1989, pp 995–998.
147. Braund KG, Steinberg HS, Mehta JR, et al: Investigating a degenerative polymyopathy in four related Bouvier des Flandres dogs. Vet Med 85:558–570, 1990.
148. Peeters ME, Haagen AJ V-V, Goedegebuure SA, et al: Dysphagia in Bouviers associated with muscular dystrophy: Evaluation of 24 cases. Vet Q 13:65–73, 1991.
149. Richards RB, Lewer RP, Passmore IK, et al: Ovine congenital progressive muscular dystrophy: Mode of inheritance. Aust Vet J 65:93–94, 1988.
150. Richards R, Passmore I, Bretag A, et al: Ovine congenital progressive muscular dystrophy: Clinical syndrome and distribution of lesions. Aust Vet J 63:396–401, 1986.
151. LeCouteur RA, Dow SW, Sisson AF: Metabolic and endocrine myopathies of dogs and cats. Semin Vet Med Surg 4:146–155, 1989.
152. Giger U, Argov Z: Metabolic myopathy in phosphofructokinase deficient English springer spaniels. In: Proceedings of an ACVIM Forum, San Diego, 1987, p 912.
153. Wells GAH, Pinsent PJN, Todd JN: A progressive, familial myopathy of the Pietrain pig: The clinical syndrome. Vet Rec 106:556–558, 1980.
154. Roneus B: Glutathione peroxidase and selenium in the blood of healthy horses and foals affected by muscular dystrophy. Nord Vet Med 34:350–353, 1982.
155. Greene CE, Lorenz MD, Munnell JF, et al: Myopathy associated with hyperadrenocorticism in the dog. J Am Vet Med Assoc 174:1310–1315, 1979.
156. Braund KG, Dillon AR, Mikeal RL: Experimental investigation of glucocorticoid-induced myopathy in the dog. Exp Neurol 68:50–71, 1980.
157. Braund KG, Dillon AR, Mikeal RL, et al: Subclinical myopathy associated with hyperadrenocorticism in the dog. Vet Pathol 17:134–148, 1980.
158. Duncan ID, Griffiths IR, Nash AS: Myotonia in canine Cushing's disease. Vet Rec 100:30–31, 1977.
159. Jirmanova I: The splayleg disease: A form of congenital glucocorticoid myopathy? Vet Res Commun 6:91–101, 1983.
160. McLaughlin B, Doige C, McLaughlin P: Thyroid hormone levels in foals with congenital musculoskeletal lesions. Can Vet J 27:264–267, 1986.
161. Gannon JR: Exertional rhabdomyolysis (myoglobinuria) in the racing greyhound. In Kirk RW (ed): Current Veterinary Therapy, VII. Philadelphia, WB Saunders, 1980, p 783.
162. Schunk KL: Feline polymyopathy. In: Proceedings of an ACVIM Forum, 1984, Washington, DC, pp 197–200.
163. Dow SW, LeCouteur RA, Fettman MJ, et al: Potassium depletion in cats: Hypokalemic polymyopathy. J Am Vet Med Assoc 191:1563–1568, 1987.
164. Dow SW, Fettman MJ, LeCouteur RA, et al: Potassium depletion in cats: Renal and dietary influences. J Am Vet Med Assoc 191:1569–1575, 1987.
165. Dow SW, Fettman MJ, Curtis CR, et al: Hypokalemia in cats: 186 cases (1984–1987). J Am Vet Med Assoc 194: 1604–1608, 1989.
166. Dow SW: Potassium depletion in cats. In: Proceedings of the Sixth Annual Veterinary Medical Forum, Washington, DC, 1988, pp 33–35.
167. Shelton GD: Disorders of neuromuscular transmission. Semin Vet Med Surg 4:126–132, 1989.
168. Wheeler SJ: Disorders of the neuromuscular junction. Prog Vet Neurol 2:129–135, 1991.
169. O'Dair HA, Holt PE, Pearson GR, et al: Acquired immune-mediated myasthenia gravis in a cat associated with a cystic thymus. J Small Anim Pract 32:198–202, 1991.
170. Scott-Moncrieff JC, Cook JR Jr, Lantz GC: Acquired myasthenia gravis in a cat with thymoma. J Am Vet Med Assoc 196:1291–1293, 1990.
171. Joseph RJ, Carrillo JM, Lennon VA: Myasthenia gravis in the cat. J Vet Intern Med 2:75–79, 1988.
172. Flagstad A, Trojaborg W, Gammeltoft S: Congenital myasthenic syndrome in the dog breed Gammel Dansk Honsehund: Clinical, electrophysiological, pharmacological and immunological comparison with acquired myasthenia gravis. Acta Vet Scand 30:89–102, 1989.
173. Wallace ME, Plamer AC: Recessive mode of inheritance in myasthenia gravis in the Jack Russell terrier. Vet Rec 114:350, 1984.
174. Shelton SD, Willard MD, Cardinet GH, et al: Acquired myasthenia gravis: Selective involvement of esophageal, pharyngeal, and facial muscles. J Vet Intern Med 4:281–284, 1990.
175. Sims MH, McLean RA: Use of repetitive nerve stimulation to assess neuromuscular function in dogs: A test protocol for suspected myasthenia gravis. Prog Vet Neurol 1:311–319, 1990.
176. Kimura J: Electrodiagnosis in Diseases of Nerve and Muscle: Principles and Practice, 2nd ed. Philadelphia, FA Davis, 1989.
177. Tindall RS, Rollins JA, Phillips JT et al: Preliminary results of a double-blind, randomized, placebo-controlled trial of cyclosporine in myasthenia gravis. N Engl J Med 316:719–724, 1987.
178. Bartges JW, Klausner JS, Bostwick EF, et al: Clinical remission following plasmapheresis and corticosteroid treatment in a dog with acquired myasthenia gravis. J Am Vet Med Assoc 196:1276–1278, 1990.
179. Spier SJ, Carlson GP, Holliday TA, et al: Hyperkalemic periodic paralysis in horses. J Am Vet Med Assoc 197: 1009–1017, 1990.
180. Cox JH, DeBowes RM: Episodic weakness caused by hyperkalemic periodic paralysis in horses. Comp Cont Educ Pract Vet 12:83–89, 1990.
181. Jezyk PF: Hyperkalemic periodic paralysis in a dog. J Am Anim Hosp Assoc 18:977–980, 1982.

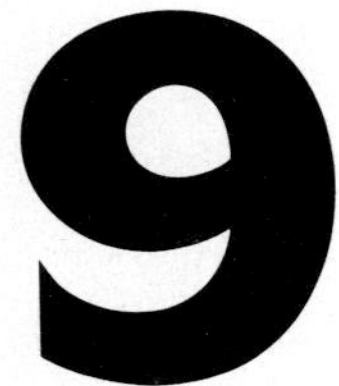

Ataxia of the Head and the Limbs

Ataxia is a lack of coordination that may be present without spasticity, paresis, or involuntary movements. When present, the associated signs, such as paresis, are important localizing features. Ataxia is characterized by a broad-based stance and uncoordinated movements of the head, the trunk, or the limbs. Lesion localization of ataxic animals has been discussed in Chapter 2 and is summarized in Figure 9–1. A brief review is presented in this chapter.

Lesion Localization

Ataxia is a sign of specific sensory dysfunction. For clinical purposes, it can be classified in three major categories: sensory, vestibular, and cerebellar. Clinical signs result when a disease interferes with the recognition or coordination of position changes involving the head, the trunk, or the limbs. Key neurologic signs that are useful for localizing the lesion may be observed. Figure 9–2 is an algorithm for the formulation of a differential diagnosis of ataxia. This algorithm is largely based on a few key differential signs. For example, abnormal movements of the head or the eyes indicate that the lesion is not in the spinal cord but rather in the vestibular system, the brain stem, or the cerebellum.

Sensory Ataxia

Loss of proprioceptive signals from the limbs and, in some cases, the trunk produces sensory ataxia. For the purpose of localization, abnormalities of proprioception in the limbs are interpreted in exactly the same way as motor dysfunction (see Chaps. 2, 7, and 8). For example, loss of proprioception in the pelvic limbs with normal proprioception in the thoracic limbs indicates a lesion caudal to T3 involving the sensory long tracts, spinal nerves, or peripheral nerves. Further localization is achieved by examining the spinal reflexes and segmental pain responses. Sensory ataxia is frequently associated with motor dysfunction (paresis).

Vestibular Ataxia

The vestibular system detects linear acceleration and rotational movements of the head. This system does not initiate motor activity; however, its sensory input is used to modify and coordinate movement. The vestibular system primarily controls the muscles that are involved in maintaining equilibrium, positioning the head, and regulating eye movements. Sensory receptors are located in the inner ear in the vestibular labyrinth. Two kinds of receptors are present: maculae in the utriculi and sacculi and cristae in the semicircular canals. The maculae are arranged approximately at right angles to each other. They function to detect head position with respect to gravity and linear acceleration and help to maintain equilibrium. The cristae in the semicircular canals detect the onset of angular or rotational acceleration. These receptors predict loss of balance and maintain equilibrium. Input to the brain is by way of CN

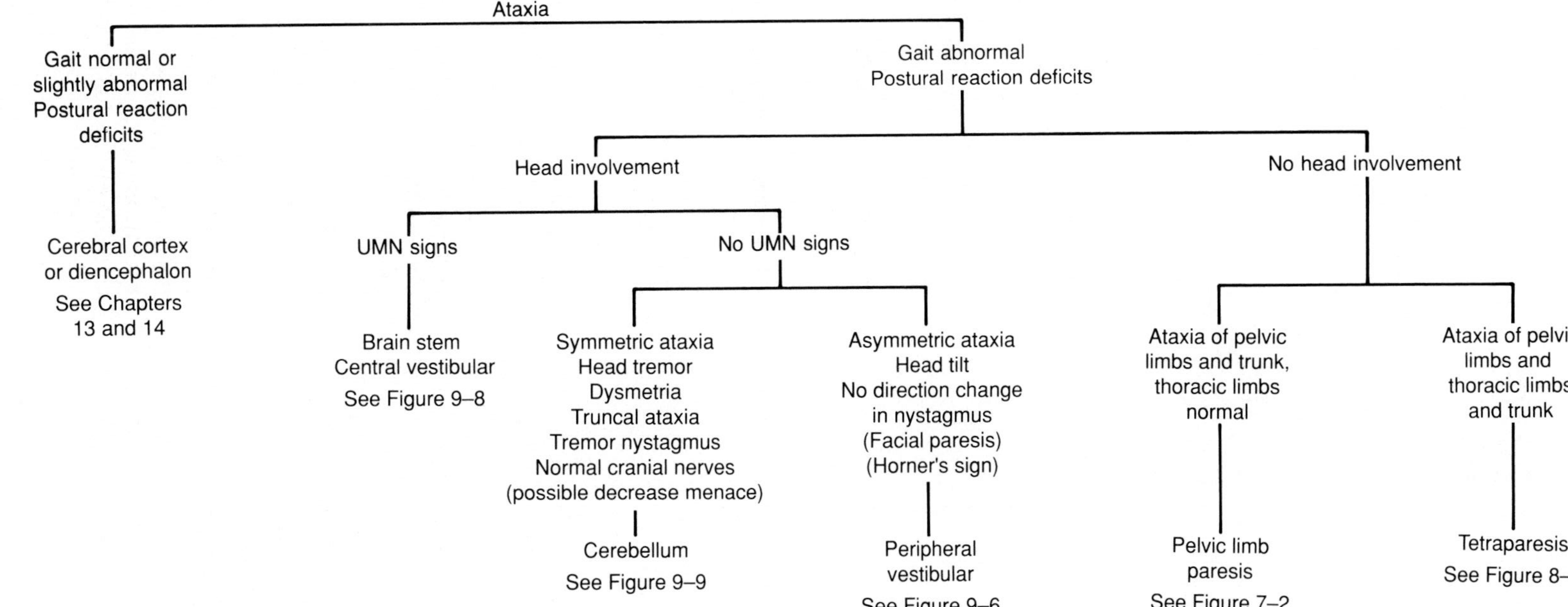

Figure 9–1 Algorithm for the diagnosis of ataxia based on gait, head involvement, and motor function of the limbs.

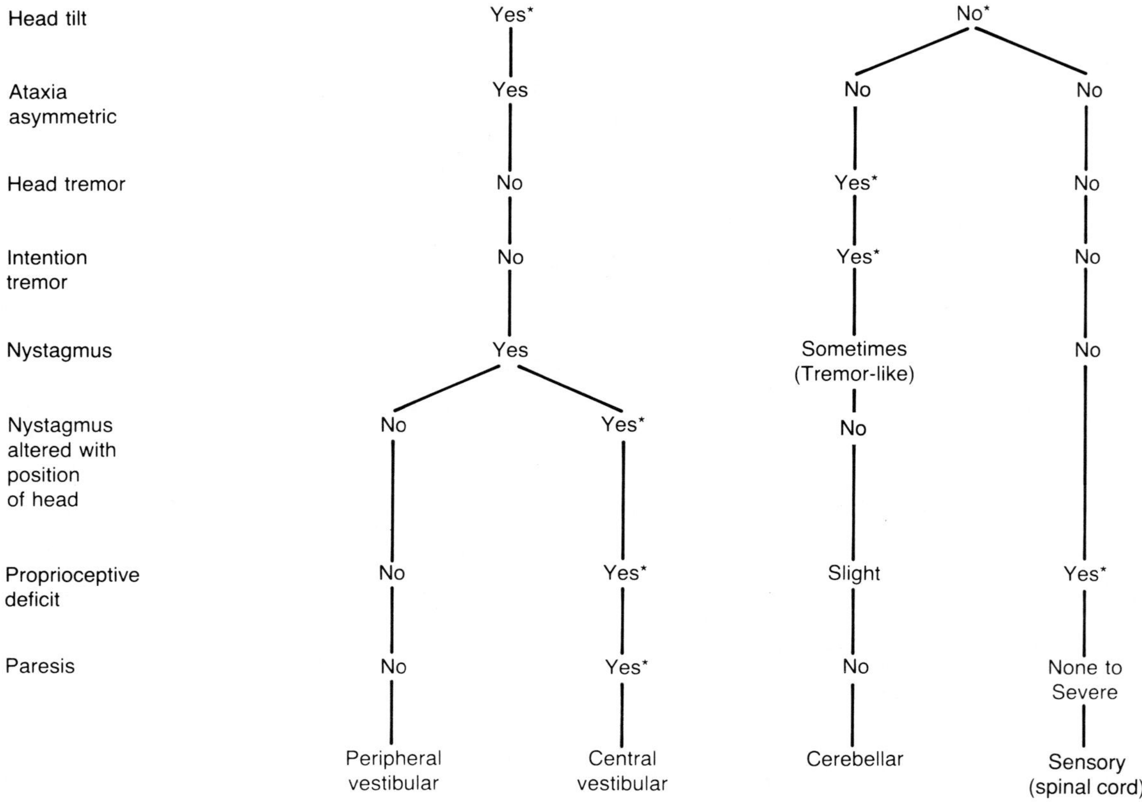

*Key differential signs. Lesion in the brain stem can cause central vestibular, cerebellar and sensory signs.

Figure 9–2 Algorithm for the diagnosis of ataxia resulting from vestibular, cerebellar, or spinal cord disease.

VIII (vestibular division). The cell bodies of the vestibular nerve are in a ganglion in the petrosal bone. The nerve terminates in one of four vestibular nuclei or in the cerebellum. Pathways from the vestibular nuclei project to other brain stem centers, to the cerebellum, to the cerebral cortex, and to the spinal cord. Projections to the nuclei of nerves controlling eye movements travel by way of the medial longitudinal fasciculus (MLF) in the brain stem.

This system controls normal physiologic nystagmus, and it can be demonstrated in the normal animal by moving the animal's head from side to side or up and down. When this control mechanism is disrupted, nystagmus occurs independently of head movement (pathologic nystagmus). Projections to the emetic center in the brain stem are important in the development of motion sickness (visual-vestibular sensory dissociation). The vestibular apparatus works in close association with the cerebellum to maintain balance and coordination. Pathways project from the vestibular nuclei through the cerebellar peduncles to several cerebellar centers. Vestibular impulses reach the cerebral cortex and inform the animal of its position during movement. Vestibular information is transmitted to the somatic muscles via the vestibulospinal tracts. These pathways are important for the regulation of the antigravity muscles of the limbs and the trunk. Most important, the vestibulospinal tracts stimulate the ipsilateral extensor muscles. Unilateral vestibular lesions cause animals to fall toward the side of the lesion. Animals actually are forced to fall in this direction, because extensor tone on the contralateral side is not antagonized by extensor muscle tone on the ipsilateral side. (Extensor tone is lost because of the lesion.)

On the basis of a neurologic examination, vestibular ataxia can be localized to peripheral vestibular disease or central vestibular (brain stem) disease. A head tilt indicates vestibular system disease. In most cases the head will tilt toward the side of the lesion. The ataxia is often asymmetric unless bilateral lesions are present. The animal usually falls or drifts toward the side of the lesion. Turning in tight circles is usually a vestibular sign, although exceptions have been observed. The movement is usually toward the side of the lesion, but movement in the opposite direction has been observed with central vestibular lesions. *Signs of paresis or proprioceptive deficit associated with a head tilt indicate central vestibular disease.* Paresis in central vestibular disease is caused by injury of the motor tracts that project through the brain stem. Thus, a major way of differentiating central and peripheral vestibular disease is to evaluate the animal critically for evidence of motor dysfunction or sensory ataxia. Careful assessment of postural reactions is the key to recognizing these deficits.

Nystagmus may be present in central or peripheral vestibular disease. In peripheral vestibular disease, the nystagmus may be horizontal or rotatory, with the quick phase directed away from the side of the lesion. With a central vestibular lesion, the nystagmus may be similar to that described for peripheral lesions; however, nystagmus that changes direction with alterations in head position or that is vertical in direction strongly suggests a central vestibular lesion. Facial and sympathetic nerve function may be impaired in cases of either peripheral or central vestibular diseases. The facial nerve exits the brain stem in close association with the vestibular nerve and separates from it in the petrosal bone. It does not cross through the middle ear.[1] The sympathetic nerve courses through the middle ear in dogs and cats and is often affected in otitis media. Brain stem lesions affecting the sympathetic pathways must be severe and other signs are obvious. Dysfunction of other cranial nerves associated with head tilt indicates a central vestibular lesion with extension to other areas of the brain stem. Physiologic nystagmus may be depressed or absent with vestibular lesions. Caloric tests and assessment of postrotatory nystagmus are difficult to perform and interpret and are usually not needed in the evaluation of vestibular disease.

Paradoxical vestibular disease is evidenced by one or more vestibular signs (e.g., head tilt, nystagmus) that are in the direction opposite the other localizing signs. These signs generally are caused by lesions near the cerebellar peduncles.[2] Bilateral vestibular disease does not cause a head tilt. The animal often walks in a crouched position, tends to avoid sudden movements, and exhibits a characteristic side-to-side swaying of the head. Vestibular eye movements are absent.

Cerebellar Ataxia

The cerebellum functions as a major coordinator of motor activity. It compares the intent of motor activity with the performance required to complete the activity. The cerebellum receives its sensory input through three paired peduncles. The caudal cerebellar peduncles carry sensory fibers from the vestibular system, the basal nuclei, and the spinal cord. The middle cerebellar peduncle carries information from the cerebral cortex by way of brain stem centers. Cerebellar output to the cerebral cortex, the brain stem, and the spinal cord travels through the rostral and caudal cerebellar peduncles. A disease of the cerebellum or its peduncles results in characteristic clinical signs. The cerebellum performs below the level of consciousness to control muscle movements accurately, to assist in maintaining equilibrium, and to control posture.

Most diseases affecting the cerebellum are relatively slow in onset. The most common clinical signs described relate to these diseases. Because the cerebellum does not initiate motor activity, paresis is not a sign of cerebellar dysfunction. Symmetric ataxia characterized by a hypermetric, base-wide gait, truncal ataxia, a head tremor, and an intention tremor is very suggestive of cerebellar disease. The head tremor is most obvious when the animal attempts a purposeful movement such as eating or drinking. Unlike vestibular disorders, cerebellar dysfunction rarely produces head tilt or circling. Nystagmus, when present, is tremor-like (rapid eye flutter). A deficient menace response has been observed in animals with diffuse cerebellar disease. Behavior and level of consciousness are not affected by cerebellar lesions.

Acute cerebellar dysfunction has a different clinical picture. The animal has what has been called decerebellate posture: opisthotonus, tonic extension of the thoracic limbs, and clonic movements of the pelvic limbs. The pelvic limbs may also be extended if the ventral aspect of the rostral lobe is affected. Spinal reflexes may be exaggerated in the early stages.[2] Rigidity decreases after a few days, and the other signs of chronic lesions, including tremor and ataxia develop over a period of several weeks to months.

Diseases that involve the caudal brain stem may cause a combination of signs suggesting both central vestibular and cerebellar dysfunction. These signs develop because of the close anatomic location of cerebellar pathways to the brain stem in the area of the pons. The flocculonodular lobes of the cerebellum are important in vestibular reactions. Lesions of these lobes cause vestibular signs, often paradoxical, as described in the discussion of vestibular signs. Because they are anatomically and functionally related to the vestibular system, we will consider signs arising from their dysfunction as part of the central vestibular syndrome.

Diseases

The diseases discussed in this chapter include those that commonly affect the brain stem, the cerebellum, and the peripheral vestibular system. The disorders that produce sensory ataxia have been presented in Chapters 7 and 8 and will not be repeated here. Diseases with involuntary movement as the primary sign (e.g., tremor, spasticity) are discussed in Chapter 11. As in previous chapters, this section is organized according to the anatomic location of the lesion and the course of the disease (acute versus chronic, progressive versus nonprogressive).

Peripheral Vestibular Diseases

A diagnostic approach to peripheral vestibular disorders is outlined in Figure 9–3. Using otoscopic and radiographic examinations of the ear canal and the osseous bulla, the clinician must decide if abnormalities exist. If no lesions are detected, a search is made for evidence of ototoxic drugs. If these agents have not been administered, the patient's history is used to place the condition in one of two categories: chronic progressive or acute nonprogressive disorders. If the initial otoscopic or radiographic examination is positive, the disorder is classified as inflammatory or noninflammatory, based on results of myringotomy, cytology, and culture and sensitivity testing. Certain inflammatory and neoplastic diseases can fall into either broad category, depending on the propensity of the disease to produce grossly visible or radiographically detectable lesions.

Otitis Media-Interna

The most common cause of peripheral vestibular disease in dogs and cats is an inner ear infection that has progressed from the middle ear. Of 83 cases of peripheral vestibular disease in the dog, 49% were attributed to infection.[3] Otitis media-interna is also common in food animals, but not in horses.[4] Otitis externa caused by bacteria is the most common cause of otitis media in small animals. Otitis media-interna may develop in animals with no historical or physical evidence of otitis externa, especially in large an-

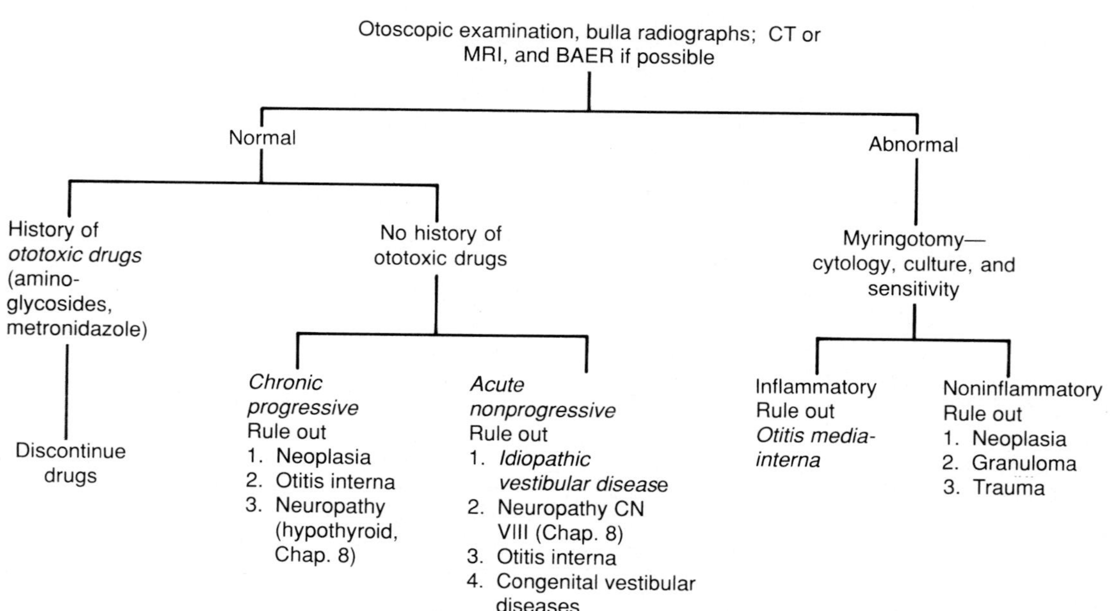

Figure 9–3 Algorithm for the diagnosis of peripheral vestibular disease. Italics indicate clinically most important diseases.

imals. In these cases, retrograde infection through the auditory tube from the pharynx or hematogenous infection is suspected. Extension of guttural pouch mycosis in horses is a rare cause of vestibular signs. In most cases the infection is caused by bacteria, although yeast and fungal organisms occasionally are encountered. The causative bacteria in small animals include staphylococci, *Proteus* spp., *Pseudomonas* spp., and *Escherichia coli*. The last three organisms are usually secondary invaders. In horses, *Streptococcus* spp., *Actinobacillus* spp., and *Staphylococcus* spp. are most frequent. Lambs and cattle more often have *Pasteurella* spp., *Streptococcus* spp., or *Corynebacterium* spp.[5] *Streptococcus* spp. are most likely in swine.[6] Breeds of dogs that are predisposed to chronic otitis externa (cocker spaniels, poodles, German shepherds, and so forth) or animals with chronic *Otodectes* infection are at increased risk for the development of otitis media-interna. Occasionally, otic foreign bodies (such as grass awns) are found as the underlying etiology. In areas where foxtail awns or spear grass is endemic, otic foreign bodies are a significant cause of otitis externa with progression to otitis media-interna. Recurrent episodes are not uncommon.

Clinical Signs. The clinical signs of otitis media-interna were described at the beginning of this chapter. It is important to recognize that several of these clinical signs (head tilt, head shaking, aural pain, inflammatory discharge) also are associated with primary otitis externa. Torticollis, circling, ataxia, positional ventral strabismus, and nystagmus are specific neurologic signs that are suggestive of otitis interna *if the patient has no demonstrable paresis*. Unilateral facial nerve paralysis is common because the inflammatory process often extends to the facial nerve as it passes through the petrosal bone. Otitis media, with no involvement of the inner ear, will not cause a facial paralysis. A complete or partial Horner's sign also can be seen on the affected side if there is involvement of the sympathetic nerve in the middle ear. Since the sympathetic nerves do not enter the middle ear in large animals, Horner's sign is not seen with otitis media-interna in these species.

Otitis media can be detected by direct otoscopic examination of the tympanic membrane. If purulent otitis externa is present, the external ear is cultured for bacteria and the ear then is cleaned gently but thoroughly. Deep sedation or anesthesia aids in critical otoscopic examination. The tympanic membrane is examined carefully for hyperemia, edema, hemorrhage, and erosion. Fluid in the middle ear makes the tympanic membrane appear opaque and produces bulging of the membrane into the external auditory canal.

Diagnosis. The diagnosis of otitis media-interna is confirmed by otoscopic examination and skull radiography. If the tympanic membrane is ruptured or eroded, fluid is aspirated gently from the middle ear for cytologic and bacteriologic examination. If the tympanic membrane is intact but abnormal, myringotomy is performed. In our opinion, this procedure should be done with the animal under general anesthesia and only after the external ear canal has been cleaned and dried thoroughly. Myringotomy can be performed with a 3-inch, 18- to 20-gauge spinal needle or with a sterile myringotomy knife. Aspiration of the middle ear may produce a small quantity of fluid for evaluation. If not, 0.25 to 0.5 ml of sterile saline is injected and then aspirated. The fluid is examined for cells and bacteria, and cultured.

Radiographic examination of the skull is a valuable aid in the diagnosis and prognosis of chronic otitis media-interna. Radiographic projections include lateral, dorsoventral, open-mouth, and oblique views of each tympanic bulla. Positive findings include fluid density in the bulla and exostosis, sclerosis, or erosion of the bulla (Fig. 9–4). Lysis of the bulla or surrounding structures is more often associated with neoplasia. Stress fractures of the petrosal bone and periosteal proliferative changes around the bulla and hyoid bones may be seen in horses.[7–9] Unfortunately, normal radiographs do not rule out middle ear disease.[10] It is not rare to have a positive finding on otoscopic examination that is not confirmed on radiographs. Computed tomography (CT) or magnetic resonance (MR) imaging is valuable, if available.

Treatment. The medical treatment of otitis media-interna consists of long-term systemic antibiotics chosen on the basis of positive culture and sensitivity examinations. Penicillinase-resistant penicillins, cephalosporins, and chloramphenicol are good initial antibiotics. Long-term chloramphenicol therapy is used with caution in cats because of its propensity to cause anorexia, depression, weight loss, and occasional blood dyscrasia. We prefer to use long-term bactericidal antibiotic therapy. In chronic cases, therapy for 6 to 8 weeks is recommended. Therapy with systemic aminoglycosides must be performed with caution, because ototoxic signs are masked by the existing disease. Topical therapy with antibiotics and corticosteroids instilled in the external ear canal, although beneficial for cases of otitis externa, rarely reaches the middle ear and therefore is seldom useful for resolving the inner ear infection. In addition,

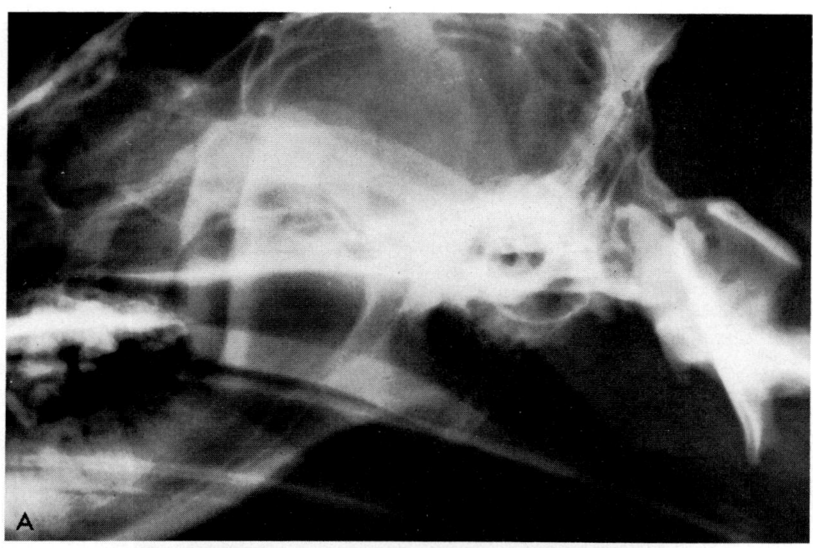

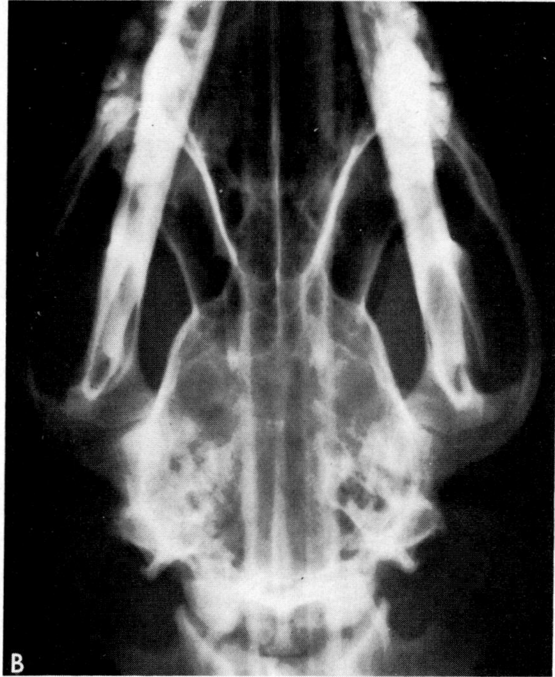

Figure 9–4 *A*. Lateral skull radiograph of a dog with severe otitis media-interna. Note the proliferative bony reaction of the osseous bulla. *B*. Ventrodorsal skull radiograph of the same dog. Note the opacity of the right tympanic bulla. A bulla osteotomy was performed to curette the diseased bone and to establish drainage from the middle ear.

ototoxic agents can penetrate into the inner ear from the middle ear. Therefore, ototoxic agents should be avoided. Unfortunately, this excludes most of the common topical medications (see Ototoxicity, below).[11]

In chronic disease involving the middle ear and the bulla, surgical debridement and drainage often are needed in order to resolve the infection. Various techniques have been described; however, we prefer the ventral bulla osteotomy because it affords the best visibility and exposure for biopsy, debridement, and drainage. Following surgery, drains are left in place for 10 days, and medical therapy is followed as described previously. Nasopharyngeal polyps of the middle ear may result in recurrent infections and must be removed.[12]

Therapy for otitis media-interna must resolve the infection and prevent its extension into the brain stem. The prognosis for recovery depends on several factors: (1) the resistance of the organism, (2) the chronicity of disease, (3) the extent of the bone involvement, and (4) the reversibility of the neurologic damage. In chronic otitis interna, neurologic deficits may be permanent; however, most animals soon compensate for their vestibular deficits. Facial paralysis is usually permanent, and the resulting keratoconjunctivitis sicca requires long-term therapy with artificial tears.

Idiopathic Vestibular Diseases

Feline Vestibular Syndrome. An acute nonprogressive vestibular disturbance has been recognized in cats. The cause is unknown. The disease occurs sporadically and is not associated with other infectious feline diseases. The incidence seems to be higher in July and August in the northeastern United States, although these observations have not been substantiated in the southern United States.[13] The syndrome has been termed *lizard poisoning* in some areas and is believed to be related to the ingestion of blue-tailed lizards. However, these lizards are not present in the Northeast, where the incidence of disease seems high. A review of 75 cases included two necropsies. One cat had hemorrhage in the labyrinth on the affected side. The other cat had a mild nonsuppurative leptomeningitis, but no lesions directly involving the vestibular system.[13]

CLINICAL SIGNS Clinical signs develop acutely and are usually unilateral, although bilateral involvement has been observed. Signs of otitis externa are lacking, and affected cats are usually healthy in all other respects. There appears to be no sex, breed, or age predilection. Cats with unilateral disease develop severe head tilt, disorientation, falling, rolling, and nystagmus. In bilateral disease, affected cats have little head tilt but are unable to move because of severe disorientation. The head may swing in wide excursions from side to side. The cat usually remains in a crouched posture with the limbs widely abducted. It may cry out as if extremely frightened. Nystagmus may not be present; however, vestibular eye movements are depressed bilaterally.

DIAGNOSIS The diagnosis is based on the clinical signs and the absence of evidence supporting a diagnosis of bacterial otitis externa, otitis media, or otitis interna.

TREATMENT No specific therapy is available. Affected cats spontaneously improve within 72 hours and are usually normal in 2 to 3 weeks. Antimotion drugs do not benefit the vestibular signs. Sedation may be necessary during the acute phase of the disease in order to suppress crying or thrashing about. Although bacteria are not incriminated in the pathogenesis of this disease, antibiotics should be considered in cases in which differentiation from acute bacterial otitis media-interna is difficult. The prognosis for recovery is excellent. Residual vestibular dysfunction is uncommon.

Canine Vestibular Syndrome. Idiopathic acute vestibular syndromes are recognized in older dogs. In a review of 83 cases of peripheral vestibular disease, 39% were considered to be idiopathic.[3] The disease is not associated with any known infectious agent. The syndrome has been diagnosed erroneously as a stroke, even though the signs are those of a peripheral vestibular disturbance.

CLINICAL SIGNS Signs develop acutely and on occasion may be preceded by vomiting and nausea. The signs are similar to those described in the section on the feline syndrome.

DIAGNOSIS The diagnosis is based on the clinical signs and the absence of evidence supporting a diagnosis of bacterial otitis media-interna, or other disease. We have recognized an increasing number of dogs with peripheral vestibular disease that are hypothyroid and recover with thyroid supplementation. Because the idiopathic disease is usually self-limiting, it is difficult to prove cause and effect. See the discussion of hypothyroidism in Chapter 8.

TREATMENT No specific therapy is available. Dogs spontaneously improve in 72 hours and are usually normal in 7 to 10 days. Head tilt may persist in some cases but usually does not interfere with function.

Congenital Vestibular Syndromes

Congenital vestibular syndromes occur sporadically in litters of purebred dogs and cats. They have been reported in beagle, German shepherd, Doberman pinscher, cocker spaniel, smooth fox terrier, Akita, and rarely other dogs. Affected Siamese, Burmese, and Tonkanese cats also have been identified.[14–18] Vestibular signs develop from the time of birth until the animal is several weeks of age. Deafness may accompany the vestibular disease and may be unilateral or bilateral. The pathogenesis of the lesion is unknown. Histologic examination has been negative in most cases. We have seen one Doberman puppy that had degenerating axons in the cochlear nerve. Some animals gradually improve, whereas others have persistent head tilt and are deaf. No effective therapy is known.

The pendular nystagmus of Siamese cats is caused by an abnormality of the visual pathways, not vestibular disease (see Chap. 12). A pendular nystagmus of Holstein and Jersey cattle with no other clinical signs could be a similar syndrome.[4]

Neoplastic Diseases

Primary tumors initially may cause peripheral vestibular dysfunction if the tumor originates from or compresses the vestibular nerve. Neurofibromas rarely develop in this nerve; however, when present, a slowly progressive course of vestibular disease evolves over several months. Eventually this tumor grows into the brain stem, and central vestibular signs become apparent. Tumors of the osseous bullae or the labyrinth (fibrosarcomas, chondrosarcomas, osteosarcomas) may destroy structures in the inner ear. Unlike neurofibromas, these tumors are recognized easily with skull radiography.

Ototoxicity

A large variety of drugs have been found to cause ototoxicity, affecting vestibular function, hearing, or both. The majority of the agents initially cause damage to the receptors and eventually a degeneration of the nerve. Toxicity can occur from either systemic or topical therapy. Topical application is probably safe if the tympanic membrane is intact. Ototoxic agents are listed in Table 9–1.[11]

The aminoglycoside antibiotics are most frequently incriminated in ototoxic problems. The signs may be unilateral or bilateral. High doses of these drugs, prolonged therapy (over 14 days), or use in patients with impaired renal function are factors that contribute to ototoxicity. Patients receiving these drugs are monitored closely for signs of renal toxicity and ototoxicity. In patients with decreased renal function, dosages are reduced or the drugs are replaced by other nontoxic antibiotics. Vestibular signs usually improve once the offending antibiotics are discontinued; however, deafness may be permanent.

TABLE 9–1 Ototoxic Drugs and Chemicals[11]

Antibiotics	*Antineoplastics*
Aminoglycosides	Cisplatin
Streptomycin	Nitrogen mustard
Dihydrostreptomycin	*Diuretics*
Gentamicin	Bumetanide
Neomycin	Ethacrynic acid
Kanamycin	Furosemide
Amikacin	*Heavy Metals*
Tobramycin	Arsenic
Other	Lead
Polymixin B	Mercury
Minocycline	*Miscellaneous*
Erythromycin	Ceruminolytic agents
Vancomycin	Detergents
Chloramphenicol	Quinine
Antiseptics	Propylene glycol
Ethanol	Salicylates
Iodine and iodophors	
Benzalkonium chloride	
Chlorhexidine	
Centrimide	
Benzethonium chloride	

Central Vestibular Diseases

A diagnostic approach to central vestibular (brain stem) disorders is outlined in Table 9–2. Of the various categories listed, the chronic degenerative and inflammatory conditions are most important. These disorders produce multifocal neurologic lesions and systemic signs. They will be discussed as a group in Chapter 16. The localization of lesions to the caudal brain stem has been discussed previously.

Cerebellar Diseases

A diagnostic approach to cerebellar disorders is outlined in Table 9–3. Of the categories listed, the chronic degenerative conditions, malformations, and inflammatory conditions are most important. Those diseases likely to produce multifocal neurologic lesions will be discussed in Chapter 16. Idiopathic cerebellitis, a disease that is characterized by a tremor, is discussed in Chapter 11. Disorders that are confined to the cerebellum will be discussed in the following sections. These conditions are largely congenital, in which the abnormality occurs during gestation or prior to normal ambulation. In a review of congenital cerebellar diseases, de Lahunta grouped these disorders in three categories: (1) in utero or neonatal viral infections, (2) malformations of genetic or unknown causes, and (3) degenerative diseases, referred to as *abiotrophies*.[19] Tables 9–4 and 9–5 list the congenital disorders occurring in animals. The appendix also has these diseases listed by breed and species.

Neonatal Syndromes

Clinical signs are present at birth or in the early postnatal period prior to normal ambulation. These syndromes are characterized by symmetric signs and a nonprogressive course.

Viral Infection

FELINE PARVOVIRUS The parvovirus responsible for feline infectious enteritis (panleukopenia) can produce a variety of cerebellar malformations, including cerebellar hypoplasia. In utero or perinatal infection of the brain ad-

TABLE 9–2 Etiology of Central Vestibular (Brain Stem) Disease*

Etiologic Category	*Acute Nonprogressive*	*Acute Progressive*	*Chronic Progressive*
Degenerative			Storage diseases (16) Neuronopathies (16) Demyelinating diseases (16)
Anomalous			Hydrocephalus (13)
Metabolic		Hypoglycemia (16)	
Neoplastic (16)		Metastatic	Primary: Meningioma Medulloblastoma Glioma Choroid plexus papilloma Epidermoid cyst
Inflammatory (16)		Viral: Distemper Equine encephalomyelitis Neuritis of the cauda equina Bacterial: Listeriosis Various bacteria Rickettsial Protozoal	Viral: Distemper Feline coronavirus Bacterial Protozoal Mycotic Granulomatous meningoencephalitis
Toxic (16)		Lead Hexachlorophene	Lead Hexachlorophene
Traumatic (13)	Head injury		
Vascular (13)	Hemorrhage Infarction		

* Numbers in parentheses refer to chapters in which entities are discussed.

TABLE 9–3 Etiology of Cerebellar Disease*

Etiologic Category	*Acute Nonprogressive*	*Acute Progressive*	*Chronic Progressive*
Degenerative			Abiotrophies Neuroaxonal dystrophies Demyelinating diseases (16) Storage diseases (16) Spongiform encephalopathies (11)
Anomalous	Malformations (cerebellar hypoplasia) Dysmyelinogenesis (11)		
Neoplastic (16)		Metastatic	Primary: Medulloblastoma Choroid plexus papilloma Epidermoid cyst Gliomas Meningiomas
Nutritional (16)		Thiamine	
Inflammatory (16)	Idiopathic cerebellitis (11)	Viral: Distemper Feline coronavirus Scrapie Louping ill Protozoal Rickettsial Granulomatous meningoencephalitis	Viral: Distemper Feline coronavirus Protozoal Mycotic Granulomatous meningoencephalitis
Toxic (16)			Lead Hexachlorophene Organophosphates Plants
Traumatic (13)	Head injury		
Vascular (13)	Infarction, septic emboli Hemorrhage		

* Numbers in parentheses refer to chapters in which the entities are discussed.

TABLE 9–4 Congenital Cerebellar Diseases in Dogs and Cats

	Diseases	Inherited	References
Neonatal Syndromes			
Viral infections			
Dogs	Canine herpesvirus	No	19,23
Cats	Feline panleukopenia, cerebellar hypoplasia	No	20, 21, 22, 26
Malformations	Cerebellar hypoplasia (dysplasia) with lissencephaly		
Dogs	Wire-haired fox terriers	Possible	19, 26
	Irish setters	Possible	19, 26
	Cerebellar hypoplasia		
	Chow chows	Autosomal recessive (?)	27
	Miniature poodle	Unknown	48, 49
	Various breeds	Single cases	29, 31, 50
Abiotrophies			
Dogs	Beagles	Multiple litters	19
	Labrador retrievers	One litter	69
	Samoyeds	Multiple litters	19
	Irish setters	Autosomal recessive	23
	Bull mastiffs, with hydrocephalus	Autosomal recessive	51
	Australian kelpie	Unknown	23
Cats	Olivopontocerebellar atrophy	Unknown	15, 19
Postnatal Syndromes			
Abiotrophies			
Dogs	Kerry blue terriers	Autosomal recessive	33, 34, 35
	Rough-coated collies	Autosomal recessive	39
	Border collies	Multiple litters	52
	Cairn terriers	Single case	53
	Cocker spaniels	Single case	54
	Gordon setters	Autosomal recessive	36, 37, 38, 55
	Airedale terriers	Multiple litters	56
	Finnish harriers	Multiple litters	57
	Bern running dogs	Possible	19, 51
	Bernese mountain dog	Multiple litters	32
	Brittany spaniels	Multiple litters	58
	Clumber spaniel	Multiple litters	32
	Akita	Multiple litters	32
	Miniature poodle	Single case	26
	Miniature schnauzer x beagle	Single case	59
	Beagle	Multiple litters	23, 59
	Fox terrier	Single case	32
	Labrador retriever	Single case	19
	Golden retriever	Single case	19
	Great Dane	Single case	19
	Mixed breed	Single case	32

versely affects the development of the cerebellum. Destruction of the external germinal layer produces hypoplasia of the granular cell layer. Growing Purkinje neurons also may be destroyed. The destruction may be so severe that the size of the cerebellar cortex is grossly reduced (hence the term *cerebellar hypoplasia*) (Fig. 9–5). The resulting lesions are permanent.[20–22]

Symmetric nonprogressive cerebellar signs are present in affected kittens at the time of ambulation. There are no systemic signs of panleukopenia. Kittens that are infected with the virus after 2 weeks of age rarely develop neurologic signs, even though the systemic signs may be severe. In addition to the virulent virus, a modified live vaccine virus also may produce this syndrome. Pregnant queens and kittens less than 3 weeks old should be given killed virus vaccines. There is no effective therapy for this disease. Some kittens can function as pets; however, many have incapacitating disease, and euthanasia should be performed in these instances.

CANINE HERPESVIRUS This viral agent affects puppies less than 2 weeks of age. The disease is characterized by generalized systemic signs, including sudden death. Rarely, puppies survive the systemic effects of the virus and develop a residual cerebellar ataxia. This form of cerebellar disease should be suspected in puppies that survive systemic herpes infection. The cerebellar signs are nonprogressive.[19,23]

BOVINE VIRUS DIARRHEA Fetal calves infected with this virus between 100 and 200 days of gestation develop severe cerebellar degeneration and atrophy. Ocular lesions include retinal

TABLE 9–5 Congenital Cerebellar Diseases in Large Animals

	Diseases	*Inherited*	*References*
Neonatal Syndromes			
Viral infections			
Cattle	Bovine virus diarrhea		19, 24, 60
	Akabane virus		19
	Bluetongue virus		19
Sheep	Akabane virus		19
	Bluetongue virus		19
Swine	Hog cholera virus		19, 61
Malformations			
Cattle	Hereford — cerebellar hypoplasia and polymicrogyria	Autosomal recessive	4, 19
	Short horn — cerebellar hypoplasia	Autosomal recessive	4, 19
	Ayrshire, Angus and other breeds — cerebellar hypoplasia	Suspected	4, 62
Sheep	Various malformations		19
Abiotrophies			
Cattle	Hereford	Probable	19
Sheep	Welsh mountain	Autosomal recessive	19
	Corriedale	Autosomal recessive	19
Swine	Saddleback x large white	Probable	63
Postnatal Syndromes			
Abiotrophies			
Horses	Arabian	Recessive inheritance (?)	19, 64
	Gotland pony	Autosomal recessive	19, 65
	Oldenburg	Unknown	4
	Thoroughbred	Single case	66
Cattle	Holstein Fresian	Recessive (?)	19, 40
	Polled Hereford	Probable	67
	Angus	Probable	32
Sheep	Merino	Unknown	68
Swine	Yorkshire	Recessive (?)	19

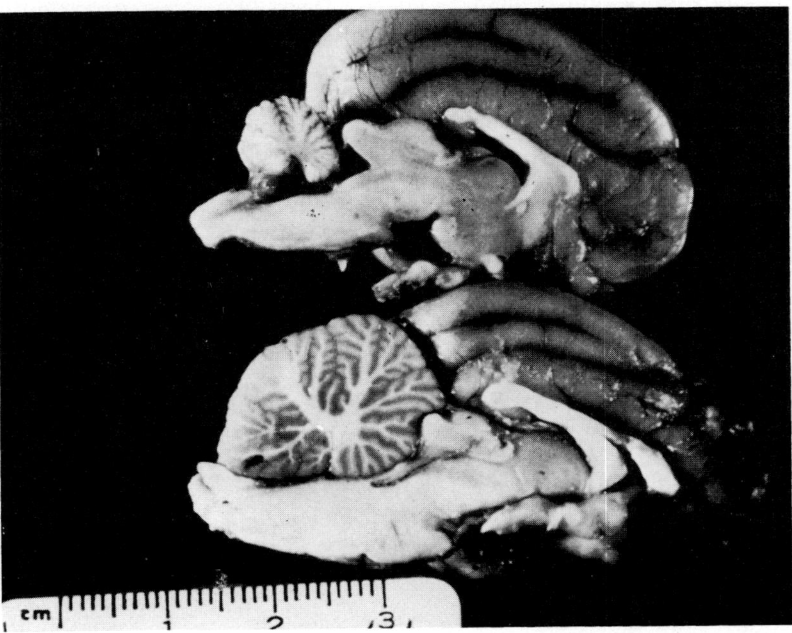

Figure 9–5 Cerebellar hypoplasia in a kitten affected in utero with panleukopenia virus. Note the small cerebellum, compared with that of a normal cat.

atrophy, optic neuritis, cataracts, and microphthalmia with retinal dysplasia. At birth, affected calves have symmetric nonprogressive cerebellar signs. A few calves may show an improved ability to ambulate as they compensate for the cerebellar disease. No treatment is known. The disease can be prevented by vaccinating appropriately.[4,24,25]

AKABANE VIRUS This virus produces severe destruction of germinal cells in the brains of fetal lambs and calves. It has been observed in Australia, Japan, and Israel. The clinical signs are related to the cerebral and cerebellar lesions.[4,19]

BLUETONGUE VIRUS This virus produces severe destruction of germinal cells in the brains of fetal lambs and calves. Hydranencephaly and cerebellar atrophy are the usual lesions. Lambs develop the most severe lesions when infected at 50 to 58 days of gestation.[4,19]

HOG CHOLERA VIRUS Hog cholera vaccine virus, when administered to susceptible pregnant sows, produces numerous lesions in fetal pigs, including lesions in the cerebellum. The clinical signs are those of a diffuse whole body tremor (see Chap. 11, Demyelinating Diseases).

Malformation. Dysplasia of the cerebrum and the cerebellum has been reported in wirehaired fox terriers and Irish setters.[19,26] The clinical signs are nonprogressive. Generalized seizures developed in one dog after 1 year of age and were associated with lissencephaly. The cerebellum is symmetrically small as a result of abnormal development of the cerebellar cortex. The cause is unknown, but a genetic mode is suspected.

A microscopic cerebellar hypoplasia has been reported in chow chow puppies.[27] Cerebellar ataxia was present at birth and persisted as the puppies developed. The clinical signs resulted from a depletion of Purkinje neurons and granular cells. An autosomal recessive mode of inheritance was suspected. This syndrome should not be confused with a similar syndrome in chow chow puppies that results from dysmyelinogenesis. The latter syndrome tends to improve as the age of the dog increases (see Chap. 11).

Cerebellar hypoplasia is also seen in most species in single cases. Dogs often have a selective loss of the caudal vermis, similar to the Dandy-Walker syndrome in human beings. Some of these animals have hydrocephalus.[4,23,28–31]

Abiotrophies. These neonatal syndromes are characterized by degenerative changes that affect Purkinje neurons primarily and result in clinical signs at the time of ambulation. The disease has been studied most extensively in the beagle and Samoyed breeds.[19] Severe ataxia, tremor, and dysmetria are the predominant signs. Microscopic lesions include swollen axons and diffuse absence of Purkinje neurons. Irish setters also have a neonatal syndrome, but it is more severe. The animals are blind and nonambulatory. Severe loss of Purkinje neurons, including degeneration of those remaining, is seen histologically. Swollen axons and proliferation of astrocytes are also present.

Postnatal Syndromes: Abiotrophies

The term *abiotrophy* denotes premature death of neurons, presumably from abnormal metabolic processes within the cell. The term implies a lack of the intrinsic biologic activity that is necessary for cell vitality and function.[32] After a variable period of normal neurologic function, cerebellar signs develop and may progress slowly or rapidly. Microscopic lesions are most profound in the Purkinje neurons. Occasionally, lesions are found in granular cells, cerebellar medullary nuclei, and brain stem nuclei.[19] These diseases have been studied most extensively in Kerry blue terriers and Gordon setters in the United States and in rough-coated collies in Australia. Other affected breeds are listed in Table 9–4.

Kerry Blue Terrier Abiotrophy. This syndrome was reported in 1968 in a study involving nine dogs from New York and California.[33] Since then, additional dogs have been evaluated.[34,35] Puppies develop a progressive cerebellar disorder at 9 to 16 weeks of age. The earliest signs include stiffness of the pelvic limbs and a mild head tremor. These signs progress to severe dysmetria (hypermetria). Most animals are unable to stand by 10 to 12 months of age. Progressive cerebellar cortical degeneration with loss of Purkinje cells has been demonstrated. Degenerative lesions also have been observed in the olivary nuclei, the substantia nigra, and the caudate nucleus. An autosomal recessive inheritance has been proposed.

Gordon Setter Abiotrophy. This syndrome has been studied in dogs from several states.[36–38] The clinical sign is a slowly progressive cerebellar ataxia that develops when the dog is 6 to 24 months of age. The ataxia worsens but does not prevent the dog from standing. Early signs include mild thoracic limb stiffness, hypermetria, and stumbling. The signs progress slowly and at times even appear static. Necropsy studies have established a diffuse degeneration of neurons in the cerebellar cortex. The accumulated evidence suggests an autosomal recessive mode of inheritance.

Rough-Coated Collie Abiotrophy. This autosomal recessive inherited disease has been documented in rough-coated collies in Australia.[39] The signs develop when the animal is 4 to 12 weeks of age and progress fairly rapidly for 1 to 4 weeks. In addition to cerebellar cortical degeneration, lesions also occur in cerebellar and brain stem nuclei.

Arabian Horse Abiotrophy. Signs of cerebellar ataxia may occur from 1 to 6 months of age.[4,19] The signs may progress rapidly and then stabilize, or they may progress slowly. Most affected foals can walk but have a symmetric spasticity of all four limbs and head tremor. The menace reaction may be absent. Nystagmus and opisthotonos are absent. A hereditary basis is suspected. A similar syndrome has been described in Gotland ponies and Oldenberg foals.

Holstein-Friesian Cattle Abiotrophy. Acute cerebellar ataxia has been noted in Holstein cattle, beginning when the animals are 3 to 8 months of age.[40] The signs initially are rapidly progressive and then become static or slowly progressive. The neck is extended with the ears retracted. Head tremors are common. Dorsomedial strabismus and nystagmus may be present. The menace reaction is often absent. A recessive inheritance is suspected.

Yorkshire Swine Abiotrophy. Acute pelvic limb stiffness and cerebellar ataxia have been observed in Yorkshire pigs that are from 1 to 5 weeks of age.[19] The clinical signs progress over a few days. A recessive inheritance is suspected.

Neuroaxonal Dystrophy. This abiotrophy affects neurons of multiple systems, including the cerebellum and associated pathways. Signs may be primarily cerebellar in origin in some dogs (Rottweiler, collie, Chihuahua) and domestic cats. Similar lesions, predominantly in the spinal cord, are seen in the German shepherd, boxer, Suffolk sheep, and Morgan horses (see Chap. 8). The neurons degenerate with prominent axonal swellings called spheroids. The age of onset was 5 weeks in the cats, 7 weeks in Chihuahuas, 2 to 4 months in collies, and 1 to 2 years in Rottweilers. All have signs of a cerebellar ataxia with tremor. An autosomal recessive inheritance is suspected.[32,41]

Occipital Dysplasia

An enlargement of the foramen magnum and congenital shortening of C1, most often seen in toy breed dogs has been called occipital dysplasia.[42,43] Concomitant hydrocephalus has been observed. In severe cases the cerebellum and the brain stem are exposed, making these structures vulnerable to compression. The clinical signs reported included cranial neck pain, personality change, and cerebellar ataxia. Many dogs remain asymptomatic. Often, the clinical signs are more related to the hydrocephalus. The diagnosis was confirmed by radiographs of the skull and the cervical vertebrae. Other causes of the signs should be pursued, as many normal animals have an enlarged foramen magnum.[44] Marked variation in the shape of the foramen magnum was found in a study of 48 beagle skulls. No impairment of function could be attributed to the change. No brain or spinal cord anomalies were found. An apparent correlation of the larger opening and brachycephalic skulls was noted.[45]

Neoplasia

Primary and secondary tumors may affect the cerebellum. Medulloblastomas selectively arise in the cerebellum in all species, and are most likely to occur in younger animals.[23] Choroid plexus papillomas may occur in any part of the ventricular system but are most common in the fourth ventricle. Gliomas and meningiomas may occur in the caudal fossa affecting the cerebellum, but they are more frequent in the rostral fossa.

Signs of cerebellar neoplasia are usually typical of a slowly progressive cerebellar disorder. However, acute exacerbation of signs may follow hemorrhage or obstruction of cerebrospinal fluid (CSF) flow with secondary increased intracranial pressure.

The diagnosis should be made with CT or MR imaging. Spinal puncture for CSF analysis is contraindicated because of the risk of herniation. Surgical resection of these tumors is difficult because of limited exposure, but debulking and radiation therapy or chemotherapy provides an alternative to euthanasia.

Miscellaneous Ataxias

Plant-Induced Ataxias

A number of plants in different parts of the world cause ataxia, tremors, tetany, and other signs related, at least in part, to cerebellar involvement. Table 16–25 lists some of the more common ones. For a complete discussion, a toxicology book should be consulted.[46]

Ergotism (Dallis Grass Staggers). This is an acute disorder of the nervous system that is seen in cattle (and, rarely, in horses) that ingest Dallis grass or rye infected with the fungus *Clavi-*

ceps paspali. The sclerotium of this fungus develops in the seed head of Dallis grass and is present in highest concentrations during wet summers. Toxic fungal alkaloids, found primarily in the mature sclerotia, produce the neurologic signs. A similar syndrome has been described in cattle grazing in Bermuda grass pastures in Louisiana.

Affected animals have an uncoordinated gait when stimulated. Tremors, twitching, and dysmetria are apparent. Affected animals are bright and alert and gradually recover when removed from toxic pastures. Severely affected animals may develop extensor rigidity, opisthotonos, and clonic convulsions. The treatment consists of removing cattle from affected pastures. Control of the disorder is achieved by grazing cattle on pastures before the seed heads develop or by mowing affected pastures to remove the seed heads.

Similar syndromes are seen following grazing on ryegrass and Bermuda grass.[47]

CASE HISTORIES

Case History 9A

Signalment

Canine, spitz, female, 3 years old.

History

The owner reported severe lack of coordination and loss of balance since the dog was 6 weeks old. The signs have been nonprogressive.

Physical Examination

Negative except for the neurologic problem.

*Neurologic Examination**

A. Observation
   1. Mental status: Alert.
   2. Posture: Severe symmetric trunkal ataxia. Head tremors. No head tilt or circling.
   3. Gait: Severe hypermetria and ataxia. Wide-based stance. Intention tremors of the head and the body.

B. Palpation

C. Postural Reactions

Left	Reactions	Right
+2	Proprioceptive positioning PL	+2
+2	TL	+2
Dysmetric	Wheelbarrowing	Dysmetric
+2	Hopping, PL	+2
+2	Hopping, TL	+2
+2	Extensor postural thrust	+2
+1 to +2	Hemistand-hemiwalk	+1 to +2
Hypermetric	Placing, tactile PL	Hypermetric
Hypermetric	TL	Hypermetric
Hypermetric	Placing, visual TL	Hypermetric

* *Key*: 0 = absent, +1 = decreased, +2 = normal, +3 = exaggerated, +4 = very exaggerated or clonus, PL = pelvic limb, TL = thoracic limb.

D. Spinal Reflexes

Left	Reflex	Right
+2 to +3	Spinal Segment Quadriceps L4–L6	+2 to +3
+2	Extensor carpi radialis C7–T1	+2
+2	Triceps C7–T1	+2
+2	Flexion, PL L5–S1	+2
+2	Flexion, TL C6–T1	+2
0	Crossed extensor	0
+2	Perineal S1–S2	+2

E. Cranial Nerves

Left	Nerve + Function	Right
+2	CN II vision menace	+2
Nor.	CN II, III pupil size	Nor.
+2	Stim. left eye	+2
+2	Stim. right eye	+2
Nor.	CN II fundus	Nor.
	CN III, IV, VI	
0	Strabismus	0
0	Nystagmus	0
Nor.	CN V sensation	Nor.
Nor.	CN V mastication	Nor.
Nor.	CN VII facial muscles	Nor.
+2	Palpebral	+2
Nor.	CN IX, X swallowing	Nor.
Nor.	CN XII tongue	Nor.

F. Sensation: Location.
   Hyperesthesia: None.

Superficial pain: Normal.
Deep pain: Normal.

Complete sections G and H before reviewing Case Summary.

G. Assessment (Anatomic diagnosis and estimation of prognosis)

H. Plan (Diagnostic)

Rule-outs	*Procedure*
1.	
2.	
3.	
4.	

Case History 9B

Signalment

Canine, Pekingese, male, 2 years old.

History

Progressive lack of coordination and falling from side to side in the past 72 hours. The head swings from side to side and bobs up and down. There is no history of trauma, and no other clinical signs are present.

Physical Examination

Normal except for the neurologic problem.

*Neurologic Examination**

A. Observation
1. Mental status: Alert, hyperventilating.
2. Posture: Sternal recumbency, rolls to right, extreme head tilt to right.
3. Gait: Cannot stand. Moderate truncal and severe head ataxia. Head drop is present. Severe dysmetria of limbs.

B. Palpation: Negative.

C. Postural Reactions

Left	Reactions	Right
+1 to +2	Proprioceptive positioning PL	0 to +1
0 to +1	TL	+1
+2	Wheelbarrowing	+1
+1	Hopping, PL	0
+1 to +2	Hopping, TL	+1
+1	Extensor postural thrust	0
0	Hemistand-hemiwalk	0
0	Placing, tactile PL	0
+1	TL	0 to +1
+1	Placing, visual TL	0 to +1

* *Key*: 0 = absent, +1 = decreased, +2 = normal, +3 = exaggerated, +4 = very exaggerated or clonus, PL = pelvic limb, TL = thoracic limb.

D. Spinal Reflexes

Left	Reflex Spinal Segment	Right
+3	Quadriceps L4–L6	+4
+3	Extensor carpi radialis C7–T1	+3
+3	Triceps C7–T1	+3
+3	Flexion, PL L5–S1	+3
+2	Flexion, TL C6–T1	+2
0	Crossed extensor	Present
+2	Perineal S1–S2	+2

E. Cranial Nerves

Left	Nerve + Function	Right
+2	CN II vision menace	+2
Nor.	CN II, III pupil size	Nor.
+2	Stim. left eye	+2
+2	Stim. right eye	+2
Nor.	CN II fundus	Nor.
0 Positional-left	CN III, IV, VI Strabismus Nystagmus	0 Positional-left
Nor.	CN V sensation	Nor.
Nor.	CN V mastication	Nor.
Nor. +2	CN VII facial muscles Palpebral	Nor. +2
Nor.	CN IX, X swallowing	Nor.
Nor.	CN XII tongue	Nor.

F. Sensation: Location.
Hyperesthesia: None.
Superficial pain: Good.
Deep pain: Good.

Complete sections G and H before reviewing Case Summary.

G. Assessment (Anatomic diagnosis and estimation of prognosis)

H. Plan (Diagnostic)

Rule-outs	*Procedure*
1.	
2.	
3.	
4.	

Case History 9C

Signalment

Feline, domestic, male, 6 months old.

History

The cat has been ill for 10 days. He is depressed, confused, and ataxic, and sleeps most of the time. He has gotten progressively worse.

Physical Examination

The cat is dehydrated, thin, and extremely depressed. Temperature: 102.5°F.

*Neurologic Examination**

A. Observation
   1. Mental status: Depressed, stuporous, grinds teeth when aroused.
   2. Posture: Recumbent, slight head tilt.
   3. Gait: Tetraparesis. Falls to left and right when forced to stand. Front legs are extended.

B. Palpation: Hypertonus of thoracic limbs.

C. Postural Reactions

Left	Reactions	Right
+1	Proprioceptive positioning PL	+1
0 to +1	TL	0 to +1
+1	Wheelbarrowing	+1
+1	Hopping, PL	+1
+1	Hopping, TL	+1
+1	Extensor postural thrust	+1
0	Hemistand-hemiwalk	0
+1 to +2	Placing, tactile PL	+1 to +2
+1	TL	+1
+1	Placing, visual TL	+1

D. Spinal Reflexes

Left	Reflex	Right
	Spinal Segment	
+3	Quadriceps L4–L6	+3
+2	Extensor carpi radialis C7–T1	+2
+2	Triceps C7–T1	+2
+3	Flexion, PL L5–S1	+3
+3	Flexion, TL C6–T1	+3
Present	Crossed extensor	0
+2	Perineal S1–S2	+2

* *Key*: 0 = absent, +1 = decreased, +2 = normal, +3 = exaggerated, +4 = very exaggerated or clonus, PL = pelvic limb, TL = thoracic limb.

E. Cranial Nerves

Left	Nerve + Function	Right
+2	CN II vision menace	
Nor.	CN II, III pupil size	Nor.
+2	Stim. left eye	+2
+2	Stim. right eye	+2
Nor.	CN II fundus	Nor.
0 Rotatory	CN III, IV, VI Strabismus Nystagmus	0 Rotatory
Nor.	CN V sensation	Nor.
Nor.	CN V mastication	Nor.
Nor. +2	CN VII facial muscles Palpebral	Nor. +2
Nor.	CN IX, X swallowing	Nor.
Nor.	CN XII tongue	Nor.

F. Sensation: Location.
   Hyperesthesia: None.
   Superficial pain: Good.
   Deep pain: Good.

Complete sections G and H before reviewing Case Summary.

G. Assessment (Anatomic diagnosis and estimation of prognosis)

H. Plan (Diagnostic)

Rule-outs *Procedure*
1.
2.
3.
4.

Case History 9D

Signalment

Feline, domestic, female, 2 years old.

History

The cat developed acute ataxia and lack of coordination. The head tilts to the right and the cat circles right. Appetite is good. There is no history of previous ear infection.

Physical Examination

Otic examination is negative.

*Neurologic Examination**

A. Observation
   1. Mental status: Alert.
   2. Posture: Circles to the right, head tilts to the right, falls to the right.
   3. Gait: Asymmetric ataxia. The cat drifts and falls to the right.

B. Palpation: Negative.

C. Postural Reactions

Left	Reactions	Right
	Proprioceptive positioning	
+2	PL	+2
+2	TL	+2
+2	Wheelbarrowing	Dysmetria
+2	Hopping, PL	+2
+2	Extensor postural thrust	+2
Ataxia	Hemistand-hemiwalk	Ataxia
	Placing, tactile	
+2	PL	+2
+2	TL	+2
	Placing, visual	
+2	TL	+2

D. Spinal Reflexes

Left	Reflex	Right
	Spinal Segment	
	Quadriceps	
+2	L4–L6	+2
	Extensor carpi radialis	
+2	C7–T1	+2
	Triceps	
+2	C7–T1	+2
	Flexion, PL	
+2	L5–S1	+2
	Flexion, TL	
+2	C6–T1	+2
0	Crossed extensor	0
	Perineal	
+2	S1–S2	+2

E. Cranial Nerves

Left	Nerve + Function	Right
+2	CN II vision menace	+2
Nor.	CN II, III pupil size	Nor.
+2	Stim. left eye	+2
+2	Stim. right eye	+2
Nor.	CN II fundus	Nor.
0	CN III, IV, VI Strabismus	Ventrolateral when head is elevated
Horizontal-left	Nystagmus	Horizontal-left
Nor.	CN V sensation	Nor.
Nor.	CN V mastication	Nor.
Nor.	CN VII facial muscles	Nor.
+2	Palpebral	+2
Nor.	CN IX, X swallowing	Nor.
Nor.	CN XII tongue	Nor.

* *Key*: 0 = absent, +1 = decreased, +2 = normal, +3 = exaggerated, +4 = very exaggerated or clonus, PL = pelvic limb, TL = thoracic limb.

F. Sensation: Location.
   Hyperesthesia: None.
   Superficial pain: Normal.
   Deep pain: Normal.

Complete sections G and H before reviewing Case Summary.

G. Assessment (Anatomic diagnosis and estimation of prognosis)

H. Plan (Diagnostic)

Rule-outs	*Procedure*
1.	
2.	
3.	
4.	

Assessment 9A

Anatomic diagnosis. The dog has generalized symmetric ataxia associated with head tremor and intention tremor. No paresis, cranial nerve dysfunction, or vestibular signs are present. The signs are related to generalized cerebellar disease. A congenital or early postnatal syndrome is suspected, because the signs began at an early age. The signs have been nonprogressive, which tends to rule out abiotrophies, storage diseases, and inflammation. A good choice for the diagnosis would be cerebellar hypoplasia.

Diagnostic plan (Rule-outs):

1. Cerebellar hypoplasia: There is no noninvasive method available (histopathology).
2. Cerebellar abiotrophy: history, histopathology.
3. Inflammation—CSF analysis (if early in course). This method probably is not useful at this time.

Therapeutic plan. None. The disease is untreatable.

Client education. The dog will not improve but can function as a pet in her current condition. The dog should not be bred, because the disease may be hereditary in this breed.

Case summary. The presumptive diagnosis was cerebellar hypoplasia. A follow-up was not recorded.

Assessment 9B

Anatomic diagnosis. Both cerebellar (head drop, head ataxia, truncal ataxia) and vestibular (head tilt, rolling, nystagmus) signs are present. Because the dog has motor deficits associated with the vestibular signs, central vestibular (brain stem) disease probably is present. A lesion or a disease involving the cerebellar-medullary junction could cause both cerebellar and central vestibular signs. The progressive course suggests inflammation, neoplasia, or degeneration.

Diagnostic plan (Rule-outs):

1. Encephalitis: CSF examination (WBCs 380, 88% lymphocytes, 12% neutrophils; protein 120 mg/dl), CSF culture (negative), conjunctival smear—fluorescent antibody titer for distemper (negative).
2. Neoplasia: CT (negative).
3. Degeneration: Check complete blood cell (CBC) count and profile (normal) for evidence of polysystemic disease.

Therapeutic plan. Antibiotics, although they are unlikely to be beneficial.

Client education. The prognosis is guarded, since it is most likely that a viral infection is present. Distemper encephalitis is a strong possibility.

Case summary. The diagnosis was nonsuppurative encephalitis of unknown etiology. The dog recovered in 6 weeks.

Assessment 9C

Anatomic diagnosis. The predominant signs are those of central vestibular disease (vestibular signs plus postural reaction abnormalities = brain stem disease). The severe depression and altered mental attitude could be of cerebral or brain stem origin. The multifocal progressive features suggest inflammation or degeneration.

Diagnostic plan (Rule-outs):

1. Infectious diseases, including feline infectious peritonitis (FIP), bacterial, fungal, protozoal, or viral agents: CSF analysis (WBCs 200, 90% segmented neutrophils, 10% lymphocytes; protein 120 mg/dl), electron microscopy (negative), culture (negative), fundus examination (negative).
2. Thiamine deficiency: Response to thiamine therapy.

Therapeutic plan:

1. Intramuscular thiamine: No response
2. Antibiotics were given IV for 5 days, with continued progression of the disease.

Client education. The prognosis is poor.

Case summary. Noneffusive FIP was diagnosed. The diagnosis was confirmed by necropsy study.

Assessment 9D

Anatomic diagnosis. The circling, head tilt, asymmetric ataxia, and spontaneous nystagmus with the quick left phase suggest a right vestibular lesion. The positional strabismus in the right eye also suggests a right vestibular lesion. The absence of paresis localizes the lesion to the right peripheral vestibular system.

Diagnostic plan (Rule-outs):

1. Acute bacterial otitis media-interna: Otoscopic examination (negative), skull radiography (negative), CBC and chemistries (normal).
2. Trauma: History, physical examination, and radiography.
3. Feline vestibular syndrome: Exclude diagnostic plan Nos. 1 and 2.

Therapeutic plan. Although otitis media-interna is unlikely, one still could choose to treat the cat with the appropriate antibiotics, just to be safe. In this case the cat was treated with chloramphenicol for 10 days.

Client education. Feline vestibular syndrome is a disease of unknown cause and no specific therapy is known. Recovery usually takes 3 to 6 weeks.

Case summary. The cat recovered in 3 weeks. The presumptive diagnosis was feline vestibular syndrome.

REFERENCES

1. Little CJL: Otitis media in the dog: A review. Vet Ann 29: 183–188, 1989.
2. Holliday T: Clinical signs of acute and chronic experimental lesions of the cerebellum. Vet Sci Commun 3: 259–278, 1980.
3. Schunk KL, Averill DR: Peripheral vestibular syndrome in the dog: A review of 83 cases. J Am Vet Med Assoc 182:1354–1357, 1983.
4. Mayhew IG: Large Animal Neurology: A Handbook for Veterinary Clinicians. Philadelphia, Lea & Febiger, 1989.
5. Jensen R, Maki LR, Lauerman LH, et al: Cause and pathogenesis of middle ear infection in young feedlot cattle. J Am Vet Med Assoc 182:967–972, 1983.
6. Olson LD: Gross and microscopic lesions of middle and inner ear infections in swine. Am J Vet Res 42:1433–1440, 1981.
7. Geiser DR, Henton JR, Held JP: Tympanic bulla, petrous temporal bone, and hyoid apparatus disease in horses. Comp Cont Educ Pract Vet 10:740–756, 1988.
8. Power HT, Watrous BJ, de Lahunta A: Facial and vestibulocochlear nerve disease in six horses. J Am Vet Med Assoc 183:1076–1080, 1983.
9. Blythe LL, Watrous BJ, Schmitz JA, et al: Vestibular syndrome associated with temporohyoid joint fusion and temporal bone fracture in three horses. J Am Vet Med Assoc 185:775–781, 1984.
10. Remedios AM, Fowler JD, Pharr JW: A comparison of radiographic versus surgical diagnosis of otitis media. J Am Anim Hosp Assoc 27:183–188, 1991.
11. Mansfield PD: Ototoxicity in dogs and cats. Comp Cont Educ Pract Vet 12:332–337, 1990.
12. Stanton ME, Wheaton LG, Render JA, et al: Pharyngeal polyps in two feline siblings. J Am Vet Med Assoc 186: 1311–1313, 1985.
13. Burke EE, Moise NS, de Lahunta A, et al: Review of idiopathic feline vestibular syndrome in 75 cats. J Am Vet Med Assoc 187:941–943, 1985.
14. Schunk KL: Diseases of the vestibular system. Prog Vet Neurol 1:247–254, 1990.

15. de Lahunta A: Veterinary Neuroanatomy and Clinical Neurology, 2nd ed. Philadelphia, WB Saunders, 1983.
16. Chrisman CL: Problems in Small Animal Neurology, 2nd ed. Philadelphia, Lea & Febiger, 1991.
17. Lee M: Congential vestibular disease in a German shepherd dog. Vet Rec 113:571, 1983.
18. Forbes S, Cook JR: Congenital peripheral vestibular disease attributed to lymphocytic labyrinthitis in two related litters of doberman pinscher pups. J Am Vet Med Assoc 198:447–449, 1991.
19. de Lahunta A: Comparative cerebellar disease in domestic animals. Comp Cont Educ Pract Vet 2:8–19, 1980.
20. Csiza C, de Lahunta A, Scott F, et al: Spontaneous feline ataxia. Cornell Vet 62:300–322, 1972.
21. Herndon R, Margolis G, Kilham L: The synaptic organization of the malformed cerebellum induced by perinatal infection with the feline panleukopenia virus (PLV). J Neuropathol Exp Neurol 30:196–205, 1971.
22. Carpenter M, Harter D: A study of congenital feline cerebellar malformations: An anatomic and physiologic evaluation of agenetic defects. J Comp Neurol 105:51–94, 1956.
23. Kornegay JN: Ataxia of the head and limbs: Cerebellar diseases in dogs and cats. Prog Vet Neurol 1:255–274, 1990.
24. Wilson T, de Lahunta A, Confer L: Cerebellar degeneration in dairy calves: Clinical, pathologic, and serologic features of an epizootic caused by bovine viral diarrhea virus. J Am Vet Med Assoc 183:544–545, 1983.
25. Kornegay J: Diskospondylitis. In Kirk RW, (ed): Current Veterinary Therapy. IX. Small Animal Practice. Philadelphia, WB Saunders, 1986, pp 810–814.
26. Kornegay JN: Congenital cerebellar diseases of dogs and cats. In Kirk RW: Current Veterinary Therapy, X. Philadelphia, WB Saunders, 1989, pp 838–841.
27. Knecht C, Lamar C, Schaible R, et al: Cerebellar hypoplasia in chow chows. J Am Anim Hosp Assoc 15:51–53, 1979.
28. O'Sullivan B, McPhee C: Cerebellar hypoplasia of genetic origin in calves. Aust Vet J 51:469–471, 1975.
29. Harari J, Miller D, Padgett G, et al: Cerebellar agenesis in two canine littermates. J Am Vet Med Assoc 182:622–623, 1983.
30. Duncan I: Congenital tremor and abnormalities of myelination. In: Proceedings of the Fifth Annual Veterinary Medical Forum, San Diego, 1987, pp 869–873.
31. Kornegay J: Cerebellar vermian hypoplasia in dogs. Vet Pathol 23:374–379, 1986.
32. de Lahunta A: Abiotrophy in domestic animals: A review. Can J Vet Res 54:65–76, 1990.
33. de Lahunta A, Averill DR: Hereditary cerebellar cortical and extrapyramidal nuclear abiotrophy in Kerry Blue terriers. J Am Vet Med Assoc 168:1119–1124, 1976.
34. Montgomery D, Storts R: Hereditary striatonigral and cerebello-olivary degeneration of the Kerry Blue terrier: II. Ultrastructural lesions in the caudate nucleus and cerebellar cortex. J Neuropathol Exp Neurol 43:263–275, 1984.
35. Montgomery D, Storts R: Hereditary striatonigral and cerebello-olivary degeneration of the Kerry blue terrier. Vet Pathol 20:143–159, 1983.
36. de Lahunta A, Fenner WR, Indrieri RJ, et al: Hereditary cerebellar cortical abiotrophy in the Gordon setter. J Am Vet Med Assoc 177:538–541, 1980.
37. Cork LC, Troncoso JC, Price DL: Canine inherited ataxia. Ann Neurol 9:492–499, 1981.
38. Steinberg S, Troncoso J, Cork L, et al: Clinical features of inherited cerebellar degeneration in Gordon setters. J Am Vet Med Assoc 179:886–890, 1981.
39. Hartley WJ, Barker JSF, Wanner RA, et al: Inherited cerebellar degeneration in the rough coated collie. Aust Vet Pract 8:79–85, 1978.
40. White ME, Whitlock RH, de Lahunta A: A cerebellar abiotrophy of calves. Cornell Vet 65:476–491, 1975.
41. Clark RG, Hartley WJ, Burgess GS, et al: Suspected neuroaxonal dystrophy in collie sheep dogs. NZ Vet J 30: 102–103, 1982.
42. Parker AJ, Park RD: Occipital dysplasia in the dog. J Am Anim Hosp Assoc 10:520–525, 1974.
43. Bardens JW: Congenital malformations of the foramen magnum in dogs. Southwest Vet 18:295–298, 1965.
44. Evans HE, Christensen GC: Miller's Anatomy of the Dog. Philadelphia, WB Saunders, 1979.
45. Watson AG, de Lahunta A, Evans HE: Dorsal notch of foramen magnum due to incomplete ossification of supraoccipital bone in dogs. J Small Anim Pract 30:666–673, 1989.
46. Osweiler GD, Carson TL, Buck WB, et al: Clinical and Diagnostic Veterinary Toxicology, 3rd ed. Dubuque, IA, Kendall/Hunt Publishing Co, 1985.
47. Galey FD, Tracy ML, Craigmill AL, et al: Staggers induced by consumption of perennial ryegrass in cattle and sheep from northern California. J Am Vet Med Assoc 199:466–470, 1991.
48. Oliver JE, Geary JC: Cerebellar anomalies: Two cases. Vet Med Small Anim Clin 60:697, 1965.
49. Kay WJ, Budelovich GN: Cerebellar hypoplasia and agenesis in the dog. J Neuropathol Exp Neurol 29:156, 1970.
50. Pass DA, Howell JM, Thompson RR: Cerebellar malformation in two dogs and a sheep. Vet Pathol 18:405–407, 1981.
51. Carmichael S, Griffiths IR, Harvey MJA: Familial cerebellar ataxia with hydrocephalus in bull mastiffs. Vet Rec 112:354–358, 1983.
52. Gill JM, Hewland ML: Cerebellar degeneration in the border collie. NZ Vet J 8:170, 1980.
53. Cummings JF, de Lahunta A, Gasteiger EL: Multisystemic chromatolytic neuronal degeneration in Cairn terriers. J Vet Intern Med 5:91–94, 1991.
54. Jaggy A, Vandevelde M: Multisystem neuronal degeneration in cocker spaniels. J Vet Intern Med 2:117–120, 1988.
55. Troncoso JC, Cork LC, Price DL: Canine inherited ataxia: Ultrastructural observations. J Neuropathol Exp Neurol 44:165–175, 1985.
56. Cordy DR, Snelbaker HA: Cerebellar hypoplasia and degeneration in a family of Airedale dogs. J Neuropathol Exp Neurol 11:324–328, 1952.
57. Tontitila P, Lindberg LA: ETT fall av cerebellar ataxi hos finsk stovare. Svoman Elainlaakarilehti 77:135, 1971.
58. LeCouteur RA, Kornegay JN, Higgins RJ: Late onset progressive cerebellar degeneration of Brittany spaniel dogs. In Proceedings of the Sixth Annual Veterinary Medical Forum, Washington, DC, 1988, pp 657–658.
59. Chrisman CL, Spencer CP, Crane SW, et al: Late-onset cerebellar degeneration in a dog. J Am Vet Med Assoc 182:717–720, 1983.
60. Kahrs RF, Scott FW, de Lahunta A: Congenital cerebellar hypoplasia and ocular defects in calves following bovine viral diarrhea-mucosal disease infection in pregnant cattle. J Am Vet Med Assoc 156:1443–1450, 1970.
61. Emmerson JL, Delez AL: Cerebellar hypoplasia, hypomyelinogenesis and congenital tremors of pigs associated with prenatal hog cholera vaccination of sows. J Am Vet Med Assoc 147:47–54, 1965.
62. Edmonds L, Crenshaw D, Selby LA: Micrognathia and cerebellar hypoplasia in an Aberdeen Angus herd. J Hered 64:62–64, 1973.
63. Kidd A, Done J, Wrathall A, et al: A new genetically-

determined congenital nervous disorder in pigs. Br Vet J 142:275–285, 1986.

64. Palmer AC, Blakemore WF, Cook WR, et al: Cerebellar hypoplasia and degeneration in the young Arab horse: Clinical and neuropathological features. Vet Rec 93:62–66, 1973.
65. Bjorck G, Everz KE, Hansen HJ, et al: Congenital cerebellar ataxia in the Gotland pony breed. Zentralbl Veterinarmed 20:341–354, 1973.
66. Poss M, Young S: Dysplastic disease of the cerebellum of an adult horse. Acta Neuropathol 75:209–211, 1987.
67. Whittington RJ, Morton AG, Kennedy DJ: Cerebellar abiotrophy in crossbred cattle. Aust Vet J 66:12–15, 1989.
68. Harper P, Duncan D, Plant J, et al: Cerebellar abiotrophy and segmental axonopathy: Two syndromes of progressive ataxia of Merino sheep. Aust Vet J 63:18–21, 1986.
69. Perille AL, Baer K, Joseph RJ, et al: Postnatal cerebellar cortical degeneration in Labrador retriever puppies. Can Vet J 32:619–621, 1991.

10

Disorders of the Face, Tongue, Esophagus, Larynx, and Hearing

Lesion Localization

The problems described in this chapter result from dysfunction of cranial nerves V, VII, VIII (cochlear), IX, X, and XII. Disorders of CN VIII (vestibular) are discussed in Chapter 9, and disorders of the cranial nerves associated with vision and the eyes are discussed in Chapter 12. The localization of cranial nerve lesions was presented in Chapters 1 and 2 and will be reviewed briefly in this chapter (see Table 2–5 and Fig. 1–23).

Injury to cranial nerves may be peripheral (nerve fibers) or central (neurons in the brain stem). Differentiation is based on the results of a careful neurologic examination. Peripheral cranial nerve disorders are characterized by specific nerve deficits with no evidence of appendicular paresis.

Cranial nerve dysfunction resulting from brain stem lesions is characterized by multiple cranial nerve involvement and, more important, by specific brain stem signs (paresis, central vestibular disease, depression, and so forth). Occasionally, the generalized lower motor neuron (LMN) diseases produce cranial nerve signs. These diseases usually are recognized because of LMN signs in the limbs. In some cases, electromyography (EMG) is needed to establish the generalized nature of the neuropathy.

CN V (Trigeminal Nerve)

Anatomy

The motor neurons of CN V are located in the pons near the rostral cerebellar peduncles. The motor fibers are distributed to the muscles of mastication by the mandibular branch of CN V. Sensation to the surface of the head is supplied by CN V through its divisions. The ophthalmic nerve innervates the dorsal eyelids and the cornea, and the maxillary division provides sensation to the ventral eyelids, the face, and the nasal area. The ophthalmic nerve is the sensory arc of the corneal reflex. The ophthalmic and maxillary nerves are the sensory arcs of the commonly performed palpebral reflex. The mandibular nerve provides sensation to the lower jaw. The cell bodies of these sensory neurons are located in the trigeminal ganglia. The trigeminal nerve enters the pons just rostral to the origin of the facial and vestibulocochlear nerves. The sensory axons of the trigeminal nerve course caudally through the medulla in the spinal tract of the trigeminal nerve. This tract continues caudally into the first cervical segment. Nerve fibers within this tract synapse on neurons that are located in nuclei distributed along its course.

The anatomic distribution of pain fibers in CN V is of considerable importance in the location of lesions involving the trigeminal nerve. Lesions in the medulla involving the spinal tract of CN V result in ipsilateral loss of facial sensation but no impairment of the masticatory muscles. Loss of both sensory and motor function of the trigeminal nerve usually results from pontine lesions or extramedullary disorders that affect both motor and sensory neurons or fibers. Loss of motor function with no sensory impairment is associated with discrete lesions in the trigeminal motor nucleus located in the pons.

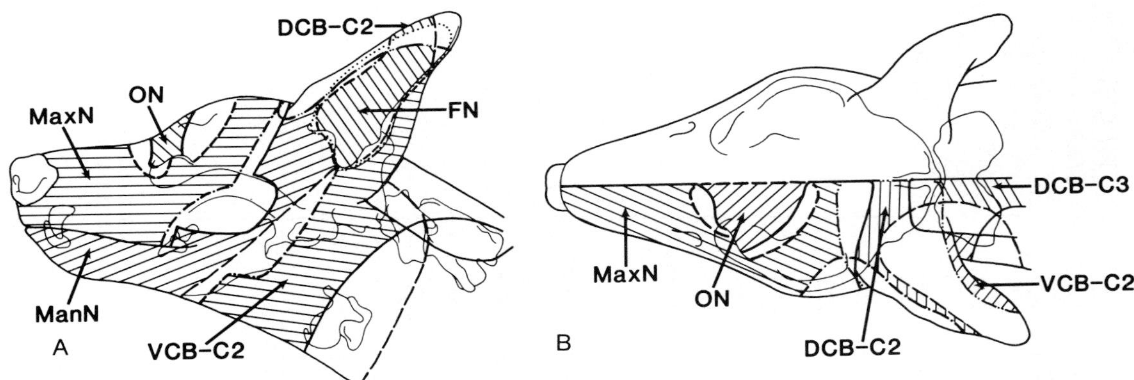

Figure 10–1 Areas of cutaneous innervation of the head that are supplied by one nerve (autonomous zones). DCB-C2 = dorsal cutaneous branch of the second cervical nerve; VCB-C2 = ventral cutaneous branch of the second cervical nerve; DCB-C3 = dorsal cutaneous branch of the third cervical nerve; FN = facial nerve; MaxN = maxillary nerve, CN V; ManN = mandibular nerve, CN V; ON = ophthalmic nerve, CN V. *A.* Lateral; *B,* dorsal view. (From Whalen LR, Kitchell RL: Electrophysiologic studies of the cutaneous nerves of the head of the dog. Am J Vet Res 44:615, 1983. Used by permission.)

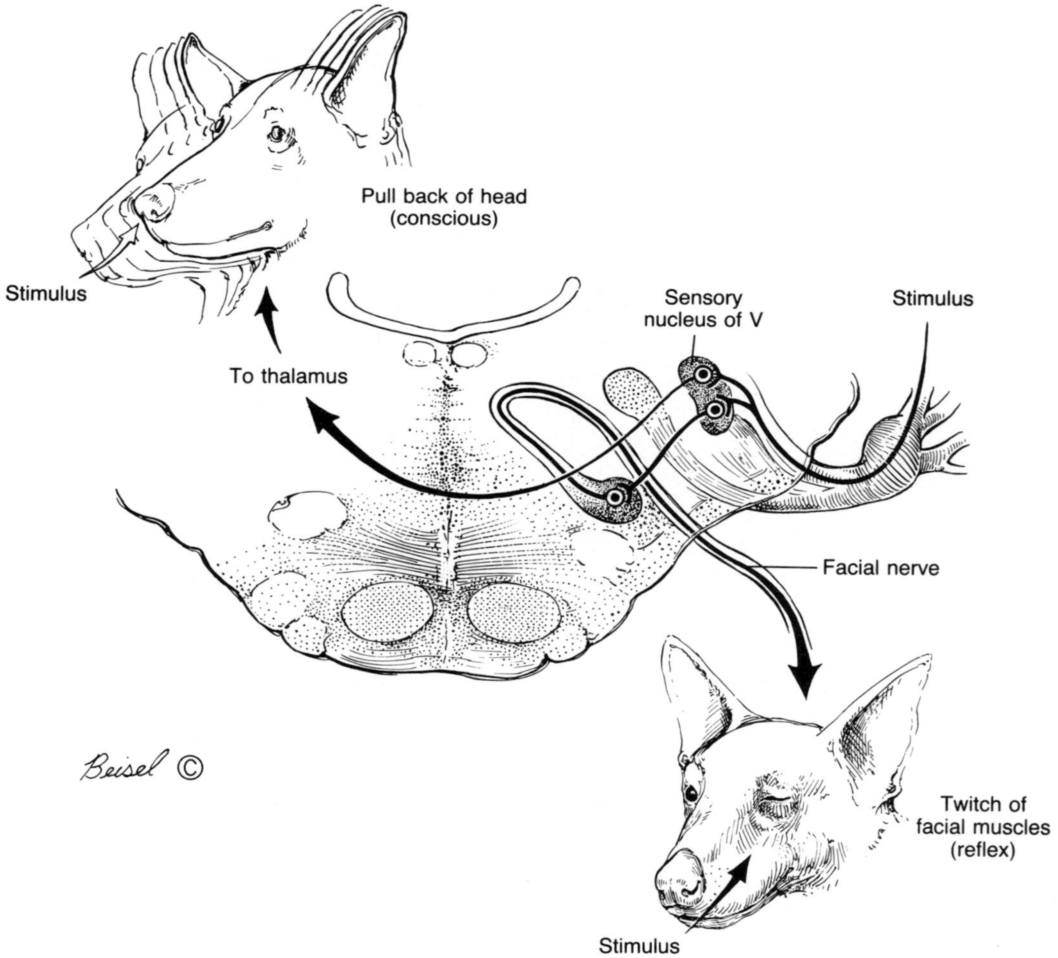

Figure 10–2 Reflex and conscious pain perception pathways of the trigeminal nerve (CN V). (From Greene CE, Oliver JE: Neurologic examination. In Ettinger SJ (ed): Textbook of Veterinary Internal Medicine, 2nd ed. Philadelphia, WB Saunders, 1983. Used by permission.)

Clinical Signs

For the reasons just described, sensation may be lost ipsilaterally to the lesion. In addition, diminished corneal and palpebral reflexes may be observed as a result of interference with the sensory arcs of these reflexes. The pinna of the dog (and probably other species) is innervated by the facial nerve on the concave surface and by branches of C2 on the convex surface, not by the trigeminal nerve (Fig. 10–1).[1,2] Diminished conscious reaction to facial stimulation can also be caused by lesions of the somatosensory cerebral cortex. The animal has decreased sensation, but it is usually not totally absent. Palpebral and corneal reflexes are normal if the lesion is cortical (Fig. 10–2). Bilateral involvement of motor nerves results in a dropped jaw that cannot be closed voluntarily (mandibular paralysis). The jaw muscles are atonic and become atrophic if the paralysis persists for longer than 7 days. Unilateral motor lesions are difficult to detect until specific muscle atrophy develops.

CN VII (Facial Nerve)

Anatomy

The facial nerve innervates the muscles of facial expression. The neurons are located in the facial nuclei of the rostral medulla (Fig. 10–3). Nerve fibers leave the facial nuclei and course dorsomedially and around the abducent nucleus. The fibers leave the ventrolateral surface of the medulla ventral to CN VIII. The facial nerve enters the petrosal bone through the internal acoustic meatus on the dorsal side of the vestibulocochlear nerve. It emerges from the skull through the stylomastoid foramen to innervate the muscles of facial expression. A disease involving the inner ear may extend to the facial nerve, resulting in an ipsilateral facial palsy. The facial nerve is the main motor path-

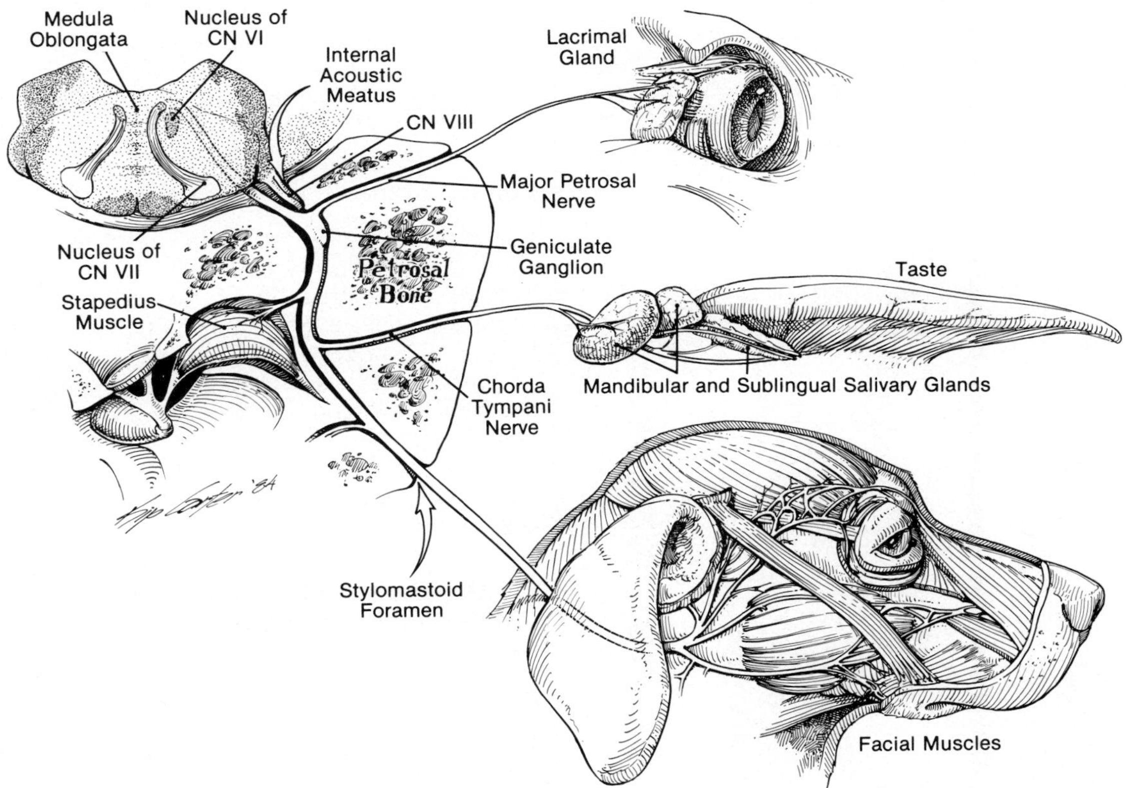

Figure 10–3 The facial nerve originates in the medulla oblongata and enters the internal acoustic meatus of the petrosal bone with the vestibulocochlear nerve (CN VIII). Branches include nerves to the lacrimal glands, stapedius muscle, mandibular and sublingual salivary glands, and sensory fibers for taste. The major component exits the stylomastoid foramen and innervates the muscles of facial expression. Testing for function of the various branches can localize the site of the lesion in facial paralysis.

way for the corneal and palpebral reflexes. Lesions of the UMN to the facial nucleus may cause abnormal facial expression without loss of facial reflexes.[3]

Clinical Signs

Lesions of CN VII result in ipsilateral facial paresis or paralysis. The lip may droop on the affected side, and food or saliva may fall from that side of the mouth. The nasal philtrum may be deviated to the normal side. Drooping of the ear may be observed in animals with erect ears (Fig. 10–4). The palpebral fissure may be wider than normal and may fail to close on elicitation of the palpebral or the corneal reflex. Exposure keratitis is a common sequela of facial nerve injury in the dog. It is especially prevalent in breeds that tend to have ectropion or exophthalmic globes.

Vestibular signs associated with facial paresis or paralysis are very commonly observed. These clinical findings are explained by the close anatomic relationship of the facial nerve to the vestibular nerve at the brain stem and in the course of these nerves into the petrosal bone. It is extremely important to differentiate these two locations because of the difference in prognosis and therapy. Lesions at the brain stem result in central vestibular disease, whereas lesions in the petrosal bone cause peripheral vestibular disease. See Chapter 9 for a discussion of these disorders.

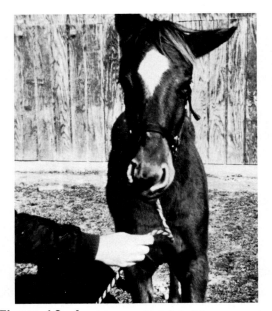

Figure 10–4 A horse with left facial nerve paralysis. Note the drooped ear and deviation of the nose to the right.

CN VIII (Cochlear Nerve)

Anatomy

The vestibular branch of CN VIII was discussed in Chapter 9. The tympanic membrane separates the external ear from the middle ear. The auditory ossicles transmit vibrations from air entering the external ear across the middle ear to the oval window of the inner ear. The wave form is transmitted to the perilymph in the inner ear, moving the basilar membrane containing the hair cells of the spiral organ. Movement of the hair cells causes release of transmitter, activating the cochlear nerve. The bipolar cell bodies of the cochlear nerve form the spiral ganglion in the petrosal bone. The axons extend proximally to join the vestibular neurons in the internal acoustic meatus. They enter the brain stem at the junction of the medulla and pons, terminating on the cochlear nuclei. The central pathway is bilateral and multisynaptic, projecting to the medial geniculate nucleus of the thalamus. Other axons project to several brain stem nuclei and the caudal colliculus in the midbrain. The conscious perception of sound is served by the projection from the geniculate nucleus to the temporal lobe of the cerebral cortex. Although the pathway has significant bilateral components, the cortical projection is largely from the contralateral ear.[4]

Clinical Signs

Deafness can be caused by failure of the conduction system, for example with fusion of the ossicles or obstruction of the external ear. These changes generally cause a partial loss of hearing, but rarely a total loss. Lesions of the cochlear nerve or the receptors cause complete deafness. Unilateral deafness is difficult to recognize clinically without electrophysiologic tests. Central lesions rarely cause clinically detectable hearing loss. Tests for hearing were discussed in Chapters 1 and 4.

CN IX (Glossopharyngeal Nerve), CN X (Vagus Nerve), and CN XI (Accessory Nerve)

Anatomy

These cranial nerves will be discussed as a group, because their nerve fibers originate from the same medullary nuclei and because they interact to control pharyngeal and laryngeal motor activity. These nerves originate in the nucleus ambiguus, located in the medulla. The rostral two thirds of the nucleus ambiguus is involved in swallowing by means of motor impulses through the glossopharyngeal and vagus nerves. The caudal nucleus ambiguus controls the laryngeal and esophageal muscles through the accessory and vagus nerves and its branches (recurrent laryngeal nerves).

Clinical Signs

Dysphagia is the primary clinical sign of lesions involving the rostral nucleus ambiguus or its nerves (glossopharyngeal, vagus). The gag reflex is absent or depressed. Inspiratory dyspnea from laryngeal paralysis is the primary clinical sign of lesions involving the caudal nucleus ambiguus or its nerves (vagus, recurrent laryngeal). Regurgitation is the primary sign of megaesophagus.

CN XII (Hypoglossal Nerve)

Anatomy

This nerve originates from cell bodies located in the medulla. The hypoglossal nerve exits the medulla at a site just caudal to the accessory nerve. It innervates the muscles of the tongue.

Clinical Signs

Paresis or paralysis of the tongue is the main clinical sign of bilateral lesions. Affected animals cannot prehend food or water. With unilateral lesions, the tongue, when protruded, tends to deviate toward the side of the lesion. Atrophy of the tongue may be severe (Fig. 10–5).

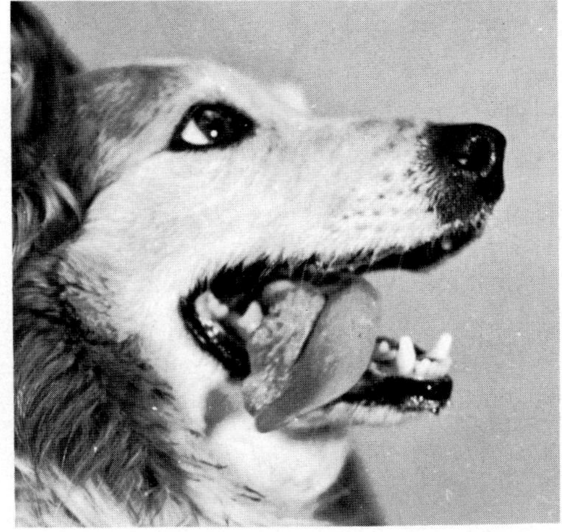

Figure 10–5 A right hypoglossal nerve injury in a dog hit by a car 4 years previously. Notice the atrophy of the right side of the tongue. When it is protruded, the tongue deviates to the injured side. The dog submerges its muzzle to drink.

Diseases

Mandibular Paralysis (CN V)

An idiopathic trigeminal neuritis that results in sudden onset of bilateral paralysis of the masticatory muscles has been observed in dogs and cats.[4,5] Most dogs and cats recover in 2 to 3 weeks. Extensive bilateral nonsuppurative inflammation, demyelination, and some axonal degeneration of all portions of the trigeminal nerve and the ganglion with no brain stem lesions have been observed at necropsy.[4]

Clinical Signs

The onset of clinical signs is acute or subacute. The jaw hangs open, and the mouth cannot be closed voluntarily. The dog cannot prehend food and has difficulty drinking water. Mild dysphagia may be present. Dehydration and drooling saliva are associated signs. Horner's syndrome is seen in some dogs. Affected dogs are alert and responsive and have no other detectable neurologic deficits. Sensation to the face appears to be normal. The clinical signs are suggestive of bulbar paralysis, which is observed with rabies. Clinicians should be extremely cautious in examining these dogs until they have accumulated sufficient evidence to rule out rabies. A diagnosis is based on the clinical signs and the absence of other brain stem signs. The disease should not be confused with masticatory myositis. In the latter disease, the mouth is closed, and the animal resents having its jaw moved or manipulated. Pain may be associated with muscle palpation.

Treatment

There is no definitive treatment. Affected animals are supported with fluid therapy and enteral caloric support. Pharyngostomy or gastrotomy tubes may be beneficial. The clinician should exercise caution to avoid aspiration pneumonia, especially in dysphagic animals. Performing frequent physical therapy by opening and closing the mouth helps to delay muscle atrophy. The recovery is usually complete in 2 to 3 weeks. Multiple episodes may occur in the same dog. The prognosis is good.

Abnormal Facial Sensation

Hyperesthesia of the face is a common problem in human beings, but it is rarely observed in animals. We have seen one cat with unilateral facial hyperesthesia. There were excoriations on the face, apparently self-inflicted. A nonsuppurative meningoencephalitis, including involvement of the trigeminal nerve and ganglion, was found on necropsy.

Hypesthesia is seen with many causes of trigeminal nerve damage. One case of bilateral sensory loss with normal motor function has been reported in a dog.[6] The condition was nonprogressive for 18 months. There was neuronal loss in the ganglia and axonal loss in the nerve and spinal tract of the fifth nerve. No cause could be found. Decreased facial sensation with normal palpebral reflexes indicates a lesion of the sensory cortex or in the pathways from the sensory nucleus of CN V to the cerebrum.

Facial Paralysis

As was stated previously, the most common disease producing facial nerve injury is otitis media-interna (see Chap. 9). Polyneuropathies also can affect the facial nerve (see Chap. 8).

Idiopathic Facial Paralysis

This disease occurs in the absence of otitis media-interna. The cause is unknown; however, the clinical signs are similar to those of human facial neuritis (Bell's palsy), which has no known etiology.[7] Undoubtedly, many cases are caused by viral inflammation, with herpes zoster and herpes simplex viruses suspected.[8] Swelling of the nerve in the petrosal bone causes compression and ischemia, presumably leading to degenerative change.

In a study of 95 cases of facial paralysis in dogs and cats, the condition was judged to be idiopathic because of lack of any other findings in 74.7% of dogs and 25% of cats.[8] Otitis media-interna was the most frequently associated disease in dogs. Hypothyroidism was found in some cases. In dogs, the cocker spaniel has an increased incidence of facial paralysis.[8,9] Cocker spaniels are also at greater risk for otitis media-interna than the general canine population. Biopsy of facial nerves in two cases showed nerve fiber degeneration and loss of large-diameter myelinated fibers.[9]

Clinical Signs. The onset of facial paralysis is sudden and the distribution is usually unilateral. There is no clinical evidence of vestibular disease or otitis media-interna. Affected animals are nonfebrile and have no polysystemic signs. The course is variable; however, the clinical signs are maximal in 7 days. Recovery takes 3 to 6 weeks. Exposure keratitis is a common problem that results from improper lubrication of the cornea.

Diagnosis. All possible causes should be ruled out before the diagnosis of idiopathic facial paralysis is made. Otitis media-interna is the most common problem; therefore, a thorough otoscopic examination and radiography of the bulla should be performed. Hypothyroidism is commonly associated with facial paralysis in our clinic, so a thyroid-stimulating hormone (TSH) response test is highly recommended. EMG of the face and other muscles helps to rule out polyneuropathy.

Treatment. No specific treatment is known. The treatment of Bell's palsy in humans is controversial. Corticosteroids have a beneficial effect if given early.[7] The administration of steroids in moderate or severe cases of facial paralysis when there are no illnesses that might be exacerbated by their use is recommended. The prognosis for recovery with or without therapy is good. If tear production is decreased, artificial tears should be prescribed.

Hemifacial Spasm

This syndrome is rarely observed in dogs or cats. In human beings, the cause is usually pressure on the nerve by tortuous vessels in the caudal fossa.[7] It has been reported in dogs with otitis media and a degenerative lesion of the medulla.[10,11] The signs include blepharospasm, elevation of the ear, deviation of the nose to the affected side, and wrinkling or displacement of the upper lip (Fig. 10–6). Ipsilateral Horner's syndrome has been reported.[10] Facial neuritis

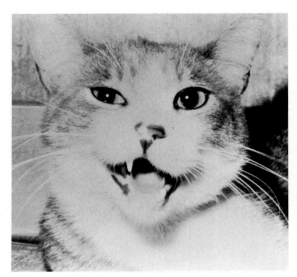

Figure 10–6 A cat with right hemifacial spasm. Note the deviation of the nose and the wrinkling of the right upper lip. There is narrowing of the right palpebral fissure.

resulting from trauma or from inflammation in the middle ear is thought to be the cause of the syndrome. It may precede signs of facial paralysis. Spasm must be differentiated from contractures secondary to denervation. Contractures result from denervation atrophy and fibrosis of the muscle, so that the muscle is fixed in contraction.

Hemifacial spasm also may occur as a UMN sign involving the facial nerve. Lesions that isolate the facial nuclear motor neurons from UMN control could result in hemifacial spasm caused by the loss of inhibitory interneuronal activity. The palpebral reflex may be hyperactive, in that spasm of the eyelids may be observed when the reflex is elicited. This form of hemifacial spasm is associated with other brain stem neurologic signs.[4]

The diagnosis and treatment are the same as those described for facial nerve paralysis.

Facial Nerve Trauma

Injury to one or more branches of the facial nerve can occur in all species. The most common causes are recumbency and tight halters in large animals.[3,12] Closed injury to the facial nerve causes varying degrees of neurapraxia and axonotmesis. Neurapraxias usually show signs of recovery in two weeks or less. Axonotmesis requires regrowth of the axon from the site of injury at an approximate rate of 1 inch a month.

Deafness

Most of the information on deafness in animals is in cats and dogs. Deafness can be acquired or congenital.

Acquired Deafness

Older animals often have some degree of hearing loss. Loss of cells in the spiral ganglion appears to be the primary cause.[13] Some attempts have been made to fit dogs with hearing aids. Generally, it is difficult to train dogs to wear them.

Some polyneuropathies affect the cochlear nerve, especially hypothyroid neuropathy. Severe hypoxia may also cause damage to the cochlear nerve or receptors. Neoplasms and trauma may cause deafness in rare cases. Toxic agents and drugs cause progressive cochlear damage (see Table 9–1). Common agents include aminoglycoside antibiotics, salicylates, loop diuretics (such as furosemide), and topically applied antiseptics (such as chlorhexidine and cetrimide).[14,15] Severe infections of the middle ear may cause conduction problems, but toxins reaching the inner ear produce receptor or nerve degeneration.

Congenital Deafness

Animals with congenital deafness have varying degrees of abnormal development of the spiral organ of the cochlea.[16] Cases in large animals have been recognized infrequently, but Mayhew describes a Paint gelding with blanched brown patches that was deaf.[3] Small animals with reported hereditary deafness are listed in Table 10–1. Deafness is associated with the merle or piebald gene where large amounts of white are

TABLE 10–1 Hereditary Deafness in Dogs and Cats: Sources of Additional Information

Breed	*Reference*
*Canine**	
Akita	17
American staffordshire	17
Australian heeler	61
Australian shepherd	61, 62
Beagle	4
Border collies	62
Boston terrier	61
Boxer	61
Bull terrier	62
Catahoula	17
Cocker spaniels	61
Collie	63, 64
Dalmatian	63, 65–68
Dappled dachshund	17
Doberman pinscher	69
Dogo Argentino	17
English bulldog	61
English setter	61, 70
Fox terriers	71
Great Dane	64
Great Pyrenees	17
Maltese	17
Miniature poodle	17
Mongrel	17
Norwegian dunkerhound	4, 65
Old English sheepdog	61
Papillon	17
Pointer	72
Rhodesian ridgeback	17
Scottish terrier	71
Sealyham terrier	73
Shetland sheepdog	61
Shropshire terrier	62
Walker foxhound	73
West Highland white terrier	17
Feline	
White, blue eye	55–60

From Oliver JE: Deafness. In Lorenz MD, Cornelius LM (eds): Small Animal Medical Diagnosis, 2nd ed. Philadelphia, JB Lippincott, 1993. Used by permission.
* Associated with white or merle color gene.

present. Apparently, the absence of melanocytes in the stria vascularis of the cochlea is associated with the degenerative change.[17] These animals are deaf at birth, but the owner usually does not notice until the animal is 8 to 10 weeks of age. Animals with a known predisposition for congenital deafness, such as the Dalmatian, may be tested with brain stem auditory–evoked potentials at about 5 to 6 weeks of age. Some of the breed groups are actively promoting auditory testing in an effort to reduce the incidence of this hereditary condition. There is no treatment for congenital deafness.

Laryngeal Paralysis

Unilateral and bilateral paresis or paralysis of the laryngeal muscles have been reported in dogs, cats, and horses. Unilateral paralysis results in moderate inspiratory dyspnea and inspiratory noise. Bilateral paralysis results in episodes of gagging, cyanosis, severe inspiratory dyspnea, and collapse. The intrinsic muscles of the larynx are innervated by the recurrent laryngeal nerves, which are branches of the vagus nerve. An injury to these nerve fibers or their cell bodies, which are located in the caudal nucleus ambiguus, results in the clinical signs. Laryngeal paralysis may be acquired or may occur as a congenital problem, which accounted for 21% to 30% of the cases reported in two studies.[18,19] A hereditary laryngeal paralysis occurs in the Bouvier des Flandres dog and Siberian husky. Idiopathic laryngeal paralysis of horses is a frequent problem.

Hereditary Laryngeal Paralysis in the Bouvier des Flandres

Laryngeal paralysis in Bouviers des Flandres dogs is inherited as an autosomal dominant trait and results in bilateral partial destruction of the innervation of the larynx. The disease results from progressive degeneration of neurons within the nucleus ambiguus with subsequent wallerian degeneration throughout the length of the laryngeal nerves. In a few dogs, bilateral cranial tibial muscle denervation is observed.[4,20,21] A similar syndrome has been identified in Siberian husky and husky crosses.[22]

Clinical Signs. The onset of recognizable clinical signs occurs at 4 to 6 months of age. The chief signs include decreasing endurance and noisy breathing. Severe respiratory distress associated with cyanosis or regurgitation occurs in more severely affected dogs. The signs are progressive. Laryngeal stridor, pharyngitis, and tonsillitis are consistent physical findings.

Diagnosis. Laryngoscopy usually reveals unilateral or bilateral immobility of the vocal folds. In a study of 105 affected Bouviers des Flandres, 28 dogs had bilateral immobility, 71 had immobility of the left vocal fold and moderate abduction of the right on inspiration, 3 had slight motion of both vocal folds, and 3 had abduction of both vocal folds on inspiration.[20]

An EMG examination reveals a varying pattern of denervation of the abductor muscles on both sides. The EMG findings are usually in agreement with the laryngoscopic findings. Normal motor unit potentials frequently are found in muscles with denervation activity. A histologic examination of the affected muscles reveals changes that are characteristic of denervation atrophy.

Three dogs had bilateral cranial tibial muscle denervation, which resulted in a dropped foot.

In experimental studies, evidence of laryngeal dysfunction can be established when the animal is as young as 12 weeks of age with laryngoscopy or, more specifically, with EMG. Normal abduction or adduction, or both, can be observed, even though EMG findings clearly indicate the presence of denervation.

Treatment. There is no effective cure. Because the disease is inherited as an autosomal dominant trait, it can be eradicated through selective breeding programs.

Acquired Laryngeal Paralysis in Dogs and Cats

Laryngeal paralysis has been associated with chronic polyneuropathy (see Chap. 8), injury to the vagus nerve during neck surgery, lead and organophosphate toxicity, or retropharyngeal infection (discussed under Dysphagia).[3,19,23–25]

In our clinic, hypothyroidism is the most frequently associated cause of a polyneuropathy with concurrent laryngeal paralysis. It is infrequently associated with polyradiculoneuritis (coonhound paralysis). Cases of chronic progressive neuropathy often have laryngeal paralysis. EMG can confirm the involvement of laryngeal muscles and determine if other muscles are affected.[20,24]

If a cause for the neuropathy, such as hypothyroidism, is found, it is treated. Many animals will require surgical correction of the obstructed airway because of severe inspiratory dyspnea. Several surgical techniques are used.[18,19,26–28]

Equine Laryngeal Paralysis

Idiopathic laryngeal paralysis is frequent in young, mature Thoroughbred, hunter types, and draft horses.[29–31] It is more prevalent in males than in females. Long necks and larger size have been suggested as correlating with laryngeal paralysis. Hereditability has not been substantiated as yet.

Pathologically, the disease is an axonal degeneration with demyelination and regeneration occurring. It has been characterized as a distal axonopathy that preferentially affects the longest and largest fibers. Nerves of the limbs and axons of the long fiber tracts of the central nervous system (CNS) are involved in some animals.[29,32] Numerous causes of distal axonopathy are known (see Chap. 8). Generally they involve energy-dependent metabolic disorders, antioxidant deficiency at the cell membrane, or filamentous neuropathies.[29] Neurofilaments are not involved in the equine disease, so it is likely to be one of the other problems. A distal axonopathy involving metabolic mechanisms may explain the population of affected animals. Larger performance horses have longer nerves and greater energy requirements.

Diagnosis is by endoscopic examination of the paralyzed vocal folds. The slap test demonstrates poor adduction of the vocal fold. The test is performed by slapping the horse behind the withers on the right side, which should cause an adduction of the left arytenoid cartilage.[3] Palpation of the muscles of the larynx can usually detect unilateral atrophy.[33] EMG is also useful.[34]

Surgical treatment is effective in better than half of the cases.[3,35–37]

Dysphagia

Ingestion of food includes prehension, bolus formation, initiation of swallowing reflex, contractions of the pharynx to propel the food aborally, relaxation of the upper esophageal sphincter, passage of the bolus, closure of the sphincter, and relaxation of the sphincter. Prehension includes function of the lips (CN VII), jaw (CN V), and tongue (CN XII). Inability to swallow is caused by lesions of the glossopharyngeal or vagus nerves or of the rostral two thirds of the nucleus ambiguus in the medulla oblongata.[4] The vagus nerve apparently is the most important.[38] Partial lesions cause choking and gagging.

Dysphagia is a common problem in large animals and frequently results from nonneurologic disorders, such as pharyngitis, obstructive choke in the esophagus, and abscesses.[3,39,40] Inability to prehend food or to propel food or water into the pharynx with the tongue may be confused with the inability to swallow. Prehension and bolus formation are functions of the facial muscles (CN VII) and the tongue (CN XII). Abnormality of these functions may also occur with forebrain diseases. The neurologic causes of dysphagia include polyneuropathies (see Chap. 8), botulism (Chap. 8), rabies (Chap. 16), other infectious diseases such as listeriosis and protozoal encephalitis (Chap. 16), guttural pouch infections in horses, nigropallidal encephalomalacia in horses, and idiopathic cricopharyngeal achalasia in dogs.

Guttural Pouch Infections

Infections of the guttural pouch, usually by *Aspergillus* spp. or *Streptococcus equi*, may cause dysphagia, epistaxis, nasal discharge, and pain. Horner's syndrome, laryngeal paresis, and facial paresis may be present. The infection tends to localize in the dorsal wall of the guttural pouch close to the course of the glossopharyngeal nerve, the pharyngeal branch of the vagus nerve, and the internal carotid artery with the closely associated sympathetic nerves.[3,4]

Diagnosis is made by endoscopy, radiography, and culture of material from the pouch. Treatment with topical antifungal agents has not been successful. Surgical removal or cauterization of lesions and blocking the internal carotid artery are reported to be effective. Mycotic infections have a worse prognosis than bacterial infections.[3,4]

Nigropallidal Encephalomalacia

This disease is characterized by the sudden onset of functional impairment of the muscles that are supplied by motor fibers of CN V, CN VII, and CN XII. It was first described in horses from northern California and southern Oregon that were grazed on pastures containing large quantities of yellow star thistle.[41] Because of the typical clinical signs and the association with yellow star thistle, the disease also is called "chewing disease" and yellow star thistle poisoning. The disease also has been reported in horses from Colorado and Utah that were grazed on pastures containing abundant Russian knapweed, a plant related to yellow star thistle.[42,43] Although the specific factor or toxin has not been identified, necrosis and malacia develop in the brain stem in the region of the globus pallidus and the substantia nigra. The disease occurs in the western United States and in Australia, where the offending plants are endemic. The lesion is a bilateral symmetric necrosis of the substantia nigra and pallidum, both components of the extrapyramidal system.

Clinical Signs. Affected horses range in age from 4 months to 10 years. In general, younger horses are affected more often. Foals that are nursed by clinically normal mares have been affected. Conversely, affected mares have continued to nurse normal foals. A prominent feature of this disease is the sudden onset of inability to eat and drink. The ability to prehend food or water is partially or totally lost. The mouth is held partially open, the lips are retracted, and rhythmic tongue movements and purposeless chewing motions are apparent. The movements of the lips and tongue are similar to the "pill-rolling" movements of humans with Parkinson's disease. Affected horses assume a drowsy pose and have a fixed facial expression. The facial muscles are hypertonic. Flaccidity of facial muscles and gait impairment do not develop. Food or water that is placed in the posterior pharynx can be swallowed. The clinical signs suggest specific UMN dysfunction of CN V, CN VII, and CN XII. Complete recovery has not been reported, although some horses may improve with time. The cause of death in most horses has been starvation or aspiration pneumonia.

Diagnosis. Because no specific tests are available, the diagnosis is based on the history and the clinical signs. The disease must be differentiated from rabies, equine encephalomyelitis, brain stem abscess, and hematoma. The facial hypertonicity and the lack of ataxia or paresis differentiate nigropallidal encephalomalacia from these diseases.

Treatment. No specific treatment is known. Feeding affected horses by tube will prolong life while one waits to see if improvement will occur. The prognosis is poor. Horses should not be allowed to graze on pastures in which the offending plants are abundant.

Glossopharyngeal Neuralgia

One case of a brain stem tumor causing a sensory and autonomic syndrome associated with the glossopharyngeal nerve has been reported.[44] A 7-year-old male miniature poodle had cervical pain that was unresponsive to confinement and medication. Episodes of syncope and seizures were associated with pharyngeal stimulation. Bradycardia, cyanosis, weak pulse pressure, and small pupils were observed. Dysphagia was observed with eating, but not with drinking. Palpation of the pharyngeal area also induced the episodes. There were no EMG or cerebrospinal fluid (CSF) abnormalities. Computed tomography (CT) demonstrated a mass in the brain stem, presumed to be a tumor. Necropsy was not performed. The syndrome is apparently caused by activation of the brain stem cardiovascular centers.

Cricopharyngeal Achalasia

The cricopharyngeal muscle forms a sphincter around the proximal esophagus. Relaxation of this muscle is part of the swallowing reflex. Failure of relaxation is seen as an acquired or congenital condition, especially in cocker spaniels and springer spaniels. Attempts to swallow result in gagging, coughing, and sneezing. The diagnosis is made by barium swallow examination. Treatment entails resection of the dorsal portion of the cricopharyngeus muscle.[45]

Megaesophagus

Megaesophagus is common in the dog, infrequent in the cat, and rare in large animals. The canine esophagus has striated muscle throughout its length that is innervated by the vagus nerve. Esophageal paralysis and dilation are common in generalized neuropathies and myopathies, including myasthenia gravis and hypothyroidism (see Chap. 8). Megaesophagus is reported as an inherited disease in miniature schnauzers and wire-haired fox terriers.[46,47] An increased prevalence is reported in Great Danes, German shepherds, and Irish setters.[48] Congenital megaesophagus has been reported in litters of Newfoundlands, Shar Peis, and Siamese cats.[49–51]

Regurgitation is the primary sign of megaesophagus. The diagnosis is made radiographically. EMG of the esophageal muscles can be done by passing a stomach tube to define the cervical esophageal wall. The examination should include representative muscles of the limbs and face to rule out neuropathies and myopathies. If a primary disease is found it is treated appropriately. Symptomatic management of megaesophagus entails feeding the animal with the head elevated. Aspiration pneumonia is a common complication. The prognosis for functional recovery is poor in many cases.

Hypoglossal Paralysis

Paralysis of the tongue usually results from diseases affecting the medulla. It has been observed with neoplastic, granulomatous, viral, and bacterial inflammations of the caudal brain stem. It is a common sign in bulbar paralysis from rabies. The tongue is often affected in generalized neuropathies (see Chap. 8). Specific inflammatory disease of the hypoglossal nerve has not been reported.

Dysautonomia

Feline dysautonomia, also called the Key-Gaskell syndrome, affects cats worldwide. Except for isolated cases, the majority of reports are from the United Kingdom and Scandinavia.[52,53] The clinical signs include depression, anorexia, reduced production of tears and saliva, bradycardia, dilated pupils with normal vision, megaesophagus, and, less commonly, fecal and urinary incontinence. Most of the signs can be attributed to loss of parasympathetic innervation, but some sympathetic abnormality is also seen. Somatic innervation may be affected—for example, anal sphincter function—but paresis is not a feature of the disease.

The etiology of this condition is unknown. Pathologically, both the sympathetic and parasympathetic neurons are vacuolated, both centrally and in the ganglia. Ultrastructurally, the rough endoplasmic reticulum and the Golgi apparatus are disrupted. The incidence peaked in the United Kingdom in 1982–1984 and seems to be decreasing in recent years. Several of the cases reported in the United States occurred in animals imported from the United Kingdom.

A similar condition in horses is called grass sickness.[53] It is also prevalent in the United Kingdom, but has been seen in various European countries. A few isolated cases of dysautonomia have been reported in dogs.[54]

Treatment of affected cats is directed at correcting fluid and electrolyte problems, maintaining nutrition, and assisting bowel and bladder evacuation. Management is difficult and often extends over several months. The more severely affected cats have a very poor prognosis because the signs cannot be effectively managed.

CASE HISTORIES

Case History 10A

Signalment

Canine, poodle, male, 8 years old.

History

Right head tilt of 10 days duration. The dog fell downstairs 1 week prior to developing signs. A severe ocular discharge in the right eye is present.

Physical Examination

Exposure keratitis of the right eye.

*Neurologic Examination**

A. Observation
  1. Mental status: Alert.
  2. Posture: Right head tilt.
  3. Gait: The dog drifts to the right and falls if he turns quickly.

B. Palpation: Negative.

C. Postural Reactions

Left	Reactions	Right
+2	Proprioceptive positioning PL	+2
+2	TL	+2
+2	Wheelbarrowing	
+2	Hopping, PL	+2
+2	Hopping, TL	+2
+2	Extensor postural thrust	+2
+2	Hemistand-hemiwalk	+2
+2	Placing, tactile PL	+2
+2	TL	+2
+2	Placing, visual TL	+2

D. Spinal Reflexes

Left	Reflex Spinal Segment	Right
+2	Quadriceps L4–L6	+2
+2	Extensor carpi radialis C7–T1	+2
+2	Triceps C7–T1	+2
+2	Flexion, PL L5–S1	+2
+2	Flexion, TL C6–T1	+2
0	Crossed extensor	0
+2	Perineal S1–S2	+2

E. Cranial Nerves

Left	Nerve + Function	Right
+2	CN II vision menace	+2
Nor.	CN II, III pupil size	Nor.
+2	Stim. left eye	+2

* *Key*: 0 = absent, +1 = decreased, +2 = normal, +3 = exaggerated, +4 = very exaggerated or clonus, PL = pelvic limb, PT = thoracic limb.

+2	Stim. right eye	+2
Nor.	CN II fundus	Nor.
0	CN III, IV, VI Strabismus	Positional, ventral
Present	Nystagmus	Present
+2	CN V sensation	+2
+2	CN V mastication	+2
Nor. +2	CN VII facial muscles Palpebral	Paralyzed 0
Nor.	CN IX, X swallowing	Nor.
Nor.	CN XII tongue	Nor.

F. Sensation: Location.
 Hyperesthesia: None.
 Superficial pain: Good.
 Deep pain: Good.

Complete sections G and H before reviewing Case Summary.

G. Assessment (Anatomic diagnosis and estimation of prognosis)

H. Plan (Diagnostic)

Rule-outs *Procedure*
1.
2.
3.
4.

Case History 10B

Signalment

Canine, English setter, female, 7 years old.

History

"Throwing up" shortly after eating for last week. Owner reports the dog will not run with her any more.

Physical Examination

The dog is very thin and mildly dehydrated.

*Neurologic Examination**

A. Observation
 1. Mental status: Alert.
 2. Posture: Pelvic limbs seem slightly more flexed than usual, especially at hocks.
 3. Gait: Slight tendency to sway a little on turns.

B. Palpation: Some generalized loss of muscle mass and body fat.

C. Postural Reactions

Left	Reactions	Right
+2	Proprioceptive positioning PL	+2
+2	TL	+2
+2	Wheelbarrowing	+2
+2	Hopping, PL	+2
+2	Hopping, TL	+2
+2	Extensor postural thrust	+2
+2	Hemistand-hemiwalk	+2
+2	Placing, tactile PL	+2
+2	TL	+2
+2	Placing, visual TL	+2

D. Spinal Reflexes

Left	Reflex	Right
+1	Spinal Segment Quadriceps L4–L6	+1
+2	Extensor carpi radialis C7–T1	+2
+1	Flexion, PL L5–S1	+1
+2	Flexion, TL C6–T1	+2
0	Crossed extensor	0
+2	Perineal S1–S2	+2

E. Cranial Nerves

Left	Nerve + Function	Right
+2	CN II vision menace	0
Nor.	CN II, III pupil size	Nor.
+2	Stim. left eye	+2
+2	Stim. right eye	+2
Nor.	CN II fundus	Nor.
0	CN III, IV, VI Strabismus	0
0	Nystagmus	0
+2	CN V sensation	+2
+2	CN V mastication	+2
+1	CN VII facial muscles	+1
+1	Palpebral	+1
+2	CN IX, X swallowing	+2
+2	CN XII tongue	+2

* *Key*: 0 = absent, +1 = decreased, +2 = normal, +3 = exaggerated, +4 = very exaggerated or clonus, PL = pelvic limb, PT = thoracic limb.

F. Sensation: Location.
   Hyperesthesia: None.
   Superficial pain: Good.
   Deep pain: Good.

Complete sections G and H before reviewing Case Summary.

G. Assessment (Anatomic diagnosis and estimation of prognosis)

H. Plan (Diagnostic)

Rule-outs	*Procedure*
1.	
2.	
3.	
4.	

Case History 10C

Signalment

Canine, poodle, male, 6 years old.

History

Sudden onset of inability to close the mouth. The jaw hangs open. The dog cannot prehend food but can lap water. No other signs have been observed.

Physical Examination

Negative except for the neurologic signs.

*Neurologic Examination**

A. Observation
   1. Mental status: Alert.
   2. Posture: Normal.
   3. Gait: Normal.

B. Palpation: Lower jaw hangs open. Hypotonus of masticatory muscles.

C. Postural Reactions

Left	Reactions	Right
+2	Proprioceptive positioning PL	+2
+2	TL	+2
+2	Wheelbarrowing	+2
+2	Hopping, PL	+2
+2	Hopping, TL	+2
+2	Extensor postural thrust	+2
+2	Hemistand-hemiwalk	+2
+2	Placing, tactile PL	+2
+2	TL	+2
+2	Placing, visual TL	+2

* *Key*: 0 = absent, +1 = decreased, +2 = normal, +3 = exaggerated, +4 = very exaggerated or clonus, PL = pelvic limb, PT = thoracic limb.

D. Spinal Reflexes

Left	Reflex	Right
	Spinal Segment	
+2	Quadriceps L4–L6	+2
+2	Extensor carpi radialis C7–T1	+2
+2	Triceps C7–T1	+2
+2	Flexion, PL L5–S1	+2
+2	Flexion, TL C6–T1	+2
+2	Crossed extensor	+2
+2	Perineal S1–S2	+2

E. Cranial Nerves

Left	Nerve + Function	Right
+2	CN II vision menace	+2
+2	CN II, III pupil size	+2
+2	Stim. left eye	+2
+2	Stim. right eye	+2
Normal	CN II fundus	Normal
0	CN III, IV, VI Strabismus	0
0	Nystagmus	0
+2	CN V sensation	+2
Paralysis	CN V mastication	Paralysis
+2 +2	CN VII facial muscles Palpebral	+2 +2
+2	CN IX, X swallowing	+2
+2	CN XII tongue	+2

F. Sensation: Location.
   Hyperesthesia: None.
   Superficial pain: Good.
   Deep pain: Good.

Complete sections G and H before reviewing Case Summary.

G. Assessment (Anatomic diagnosis and estimation of prognosis)

H. Plan (Diagnostic)

Rule-outs	*Procedure*
1.	
2.	
3.	
4.	

Assessment 10A

Anatomic diagnosis. Two major findings are important in the localization of this lesion. Vestibular signs with no paresis strongly suggest a right peripheral vestibular disease. Facial paralysis on the right side probably has occurred secondary to the peripheral vestibular disorder.

Diagnostic plan (Rule-outs):

1. Otitis media-interna: Otoscopic examination (negative), skull radiography (negative).
2. Geriatric vestibular syndrome: diagnosis of exclusion.
3. Facial nerve paralysis: EMG.

Therapeutic plan:

1. Treat the exposure keratitis of the right eye.
2. Chloramphenicol, 50 mg/kg t.i.d. for 10 days.

Client education. The prognosis is good.

Case summary. Otitis media-interna with facial paralysis was suspected. The dog recovered following therapy. The facial paralysis persisted.

Assessment 10B

Anatomic diagnosis. "Throwing up" may be either vomiting or regurgitation. Careful questioning reveals that it occurs within a few minutes of eating and the food is an undigested bolus. These findings suggest regurgitation. A major cause of regurgitation is megaesophagus. Other findings indicate slightly reduced strength in the limbs and reduced flexion reflexes. There is also reduced facial nerve response. No single lesion could account for these signs. The likely explanation is polyneuropathy or polymyopathy.

Diagnostic plan (Rule-outs):

1. Polymyopathy: CPK (normal), EMG (see 2).
2. Polyneuropathy: Definitive diagnosis requires EMG and biopsy. EMG showed fibrillations and positive waves in all distal muscles of limbs and face, and some areas of abnormality in the paravertebral muscles. Radiography of the chest revealed megaesophagus with no evidence of pneumonia or metastases. Causes of polyneuropathy include endocrine, toxic, and immune diseases. There was no history of toxic exposure. A TSH stimulation test disclosed T_4 values of 1.0 μg/dl and 1.4 μg/dl before and after.

Therapeutic plan. Levothyroxine was prescribed. The dog was fed soft food in an elevated position and was monitored carefully for signs of pneumonia.

Client education. The prognosis is guarded because of the megaesophagus.

Case summary. The dog began to improve after 3 weeks of treatment. At a recheck 6 months later, the megaesophagus could not be seen on radiographs.

Assessment 10C

Anatomic diagnosis. The neurologic findings localize the lesion to bilateral involvement of the motor division of CN V. (Normal facial sensation and palpebral reflex suggest clinically normal function of the sensory fibers of CN V.) Since the lesion is rather specific for motor neurons and is bilateral, involvement of the peripheral nerves is unlikely. (The peripheral nerves have both motor and sensory fibers.) The lesion therefore most likely affects both motor nuclei of CN V. One disease that causes these lesions is clinically recognized: idiopathic mandibular paralysis.

Diagnostic plan (Rule-outs):

1. Mandibular nerve paralysis: EMG of masticatory muscles (diffuse evidence of denervation 7 days after the onset of the signs).
2. Temporal, masseter myositis: History and physical examination (negative for pain; the jaw is open rather than closed; the muscles are hypotonic rather than firm), muscle biopsy (not done in this case).
3. Rabies: Clinical history and course of the disease. *Rabies always is considered when bulbar signs are present.*
4. Trauma: Skull radiography (negative).

Therapeutic plan. Support hydration and nutrition with tube feedings.

Client education. The disease is of unknown etiology. Recovery takes 3 to 6 weeks and is usually complete. No specific therapy is known.

Case summary. A uneventful recovery occurred in 4 weeks. A second episode was recorded 6 months later. A complete recovery again occurred in 4 weeks.

REFERENCES

1. Whalen LR, Kitchell RL: Electrophysiologic studies of the cutaneous nerves of the head of the dog. Am J Vet Res 44:615–627, 1983.
2. Whalen LR, Kitchell RL: Electrophysiologic and behavioral studies of the cutaneous nerves of the concave surface of the pinna and the external ear canal of the dog. Am J Vet Res 44:628–634, 1983.
3. Mayhew IG: Large Animal Neurology: A Handbook for Veterinary Clinicians. Philadelphia, Lea & Febiger, 1989.
4. de Lahunta A: Veterinary Neuroanatomy and Clinical Neurology, 2nd ed. Philadelphia, WB Saunders, 1983.
5. Hoelzle RJ: Idiopathic trigeminal neuropathy in a dog. Vet Med Small Anim Clin 58:345, 1983.
6. Carmichael S, Griffiths IR: Case of isolated sensory trigeminal neuropathy in a dog. Vet Rec 109:280–282, 1981.
7. Asbury AK, McKhann GM, McDonald WI: Diseases of the Nervous System. Philadelphia, Ardmore Medical Books, 1986.
8. Kern TJ, Erb HN: Facial neuropathy in dogs and cats: 95 cases (1975–1985). J Am Vet Med Assoc 191:1604–1609, 1987.
9. Braund KG, Luttgen PJ, Sorjonen DC, et al: Idiopathic facial paralysis in the dog. Vet Rec 105:297–299, 1979.
10. Roberts SR, Vainisi SJ: Hemifacial spasm in dogs. J Am Vet Med Assoc 150:381–385, 1967.
11. Parker AJ, Cusick PK, Park RD, et al: Hemifacial spasm in a dog. Vet Rec 93:514–516, 1973.
12. Renegar WR: Auriculopalpebral nerve paralysis follow-

ing prolonged anesthesia in a dog. J Am Vet Med Assoc 174:1007–1009, 1979.
13. Knowles K: Reduction of spiral ganglion neurons in the aging canine with hearing loss. In: Proceedings of the Eighth Annual Veterinary Medical Forum, Washington, DC, 1990, pp 105–108.
14. Sims MH: Hearing loss in small animals: Occurrence and diagnosis. In Kirk, RW (ed): Current Veterinary Therapy X. Philadelphia, WB Saunders, 1989.
15. Mansfield PD: Ototoxicity in dogs and cats. Comp Cont Educ Pract Vet 12:332–337, 1990.
16. Oliver JE: Deafness. In Lorenz MD, Cornelius LM (eds): Small Animal Medical Diagnosis, 2nd ed. Philadelphia, JB Lippincott, 1993.
17. Strain GM: Congenital deafness in dogs and cats. Comp Cont Educ Pract Vet 13:245–253, 1991.
18. Harvey CI, O'Brien JA: Treatment of laryngeal paralysis in dogs by partial laryngectomy. J Am Anim Hosp Assoc 18:551–556, 1982.
19. Greenfield CL: Canine laryngeal paralysis. Comp Cont Educ Pract Vet 10:1011–1020, 1987.
20. Haagen AJ V-V, Hartman W, Goedegebuure SA: Spontaneous laryngeal paralysis in young Bouviers. J Am Anim Hosp Assoc 14:714–720, 1978.
21. Venker-van Haagen AJ, Bouw J, Hartman W: Hereditary transmission of laryngeal paralysis in young Bouviers. J Am Anim Hosp Assoc 17:75–76, 1981.
22. Hendricks JC, O'Brien JA: Inherited laryngeal paralysis in Siberian husky crosses. In: Proceedings of the Third Annual Veterinary Medical Forum 3:143, 1985.
23. Gaver CE, Amis TC, LeCouteur RA: Laryngeal paralysis in dogs: A review of 23 cases. J Am Vet Med Assoc 186:377–380, 1985.
24. Braund KG, Steinberg S, Shores A, et al: Laryngeal paralysis in immature and mature dogs as one sign of a diffuse polyneuropathy. J Am Vet Med Assoc 194:1735–1740, 1989.
25. Hardie EM, Kolata RJ, Stone EA, et al: Laryngeal paralysis in three cats. J Am Vet Med Assoc 179:879–882, 1981.
26. Smith M, Gourley I, Kurpershoek C, et al: Evaluation of a modified castellated laryngofissure for alleviation of upper airway obstruction in dogs with laryngeal paralysis. J Am Vet Med Assoc 188:1279–1283, 1986.
27. Greenfield CL, Walshaw R, Kumar K, et al: Neuromuscular pedicle graft for restoration of arytenoid abductor function in dogs with experimentally induced laryngeal hemiplegia. Am J Vet Res 49:1360–1366, 1988.
28. Payne JT, Martin RA, Rigg DL: Abductor muscle prosthesis for correction of laryngeal paralysis in 10 dogs and one cat. J Am Anim Hosp Assoc 26:599–604, 1990.
29. Cahill JI, Goulder B: The pathogenesis of equine laryngeal hemiplegia: A review. NZ Vet J 35:82–90, 1987.
30. Bohanon TC, Beard WL, Robertson JT: Laryngeal hemiplegia in draft horses: A review of 27 cases. Vet Surg 19:456–459, 1990.
31. Goulden BE, Anderson LJ, Cahill JI: Roaring in Clydesdales. NZ Vet J 33:73–76, 1985.
32. Cahill JI, Goulden B: Equine laryngeal hemiplegia: Part I. A light microscopic study of peripheral nerves. NZ Vet J 34:161–169, 1986.
33. Cook WR: Diagnosis and grading of hereditary recurrent laryngeal neuropathy in the horse. Equine Vet Sci 8:432–455, 1988.
34. Moore MP, Andrews F, Reed SM, et al: Electromyographic evaluation of horses with laryngeal hemiplegia. Equine Vet Sci 8:424–427, 1988.
35. Ducharme NG, Horney FD, Partlow GD, et al: Attempts to restore abduction of the paralyzed equine arytenoid cartilage: I. Nerve-muscle pedicle transplants. Can J Vet Res 53:202–209, 1989.
36. Fulton IC, Derksen FJ, Stick JA, et al: Treatment of left laryngeal hemiplegia in standardbreds, using a nerve muscle pedicle graft. Am J Vet Res 52:1461–1467, 1991.
37. Tulleners EP, Harrison IW, Raker CW: Management of arytenoid chondropathy and failed laryngoplasty in horses: 75 cases (1879–1985). J Am Vet Med Assoc 192:670–675, 1988.
38. Venker-van Haagen A, Hartman W, Wolvekamp W: Contributions of the glossopharyngeal nerve and the pharyngeal branch of the vagus nerve to the swallowing process in dogs. Am J Vet Res 47:1300–1307, 1986.
39. Greet T: Dysphagia in the horse. In Pract 11:256–262, 1989.
40. Baum KH, Halpern NE, Banish LD, et al: Dysphagia in horses: The differential diagnosis. Part II. Comp Cont Educ Pract Vet 10:1405–1410, 1988.
41. Fowler ME: Nigropallidal encephalomalacia in the horse. J Am Vet Med Assoc 147:607–616, 1965.
42. Young S, Brown WW, Klinger B: Nigropallidal encephalomalacia in horses caused by ingestion of weeds of the genus *Centaurea*. J Am Vet Med Assoc 157:1602–1605, 1970.
43. Larson KA, Young S: Nigropallidal encephalomalacia in horses in Colorado. J Am Vet Med Assoc 156:626–628, 1970.
44. Shores A, Vaughn DM, Holland M, et al: Glossopharyngeal neuralgia syndrome in a dog. J Am Anim Hosp Assoc 27:101–104, 1991.
45. Morgan RV: Handbook of Small Animal Practice. New York, Churchill Livingstone, 1988.
46. Osborne CA, Clifford DH, Jessen C: Hereditary esophageal achalasia in dogs. J Am Vet Med Assoc 151:572–581, 1967.
47. Cox VS, Wallace LJ, Anderson VE, et al: Hereditary esophageal dysfunction in the miniature schnauzer dog. Am J Vet Res 41:326–330, 1980.
48. Strombeck DR: Pathophysiology of esophageal motility disorders in the dog and cat. Vet Clin North Am 8:229–244, 1978.
49. Guilford WG: Megaesophagus in the dog and cat. Semin Vet Med Surg 5:37–45, 1990.
50. Knowles KE, O'Brien DP, Amann JF: Congenital idiopathic megaesophagus in a litter of Chinese shar peis: Clinical, electrodiagnostic, and pathological findings. J Am Anim Hosp Assoc 26:313–318, 1990.
51. Schwartz A, Ravin CE, Greenspan RH, et al: Congenital neuromuscular esophageal disease in a litter of Newfoundland puppies. J Vet Radiol 17:101–105, 1976.
52. Sharp NJH: Feline dysautonomia. Semin Vet Med Surg 5:67–71, 1990.
53. Edney ATB, Gaskell CJ, Sharp NJH: Feline dysautonomia. J Small Anim Pract 28:333–416, 1987.
54. Wise LA, Lappin MR: Canine dysautonomia. Semin Vet Med Surg 5:72–74, 1990.
55. Creel D, Conlee JW, Parks TN: Auditory brainstem anomalies in albino cats: I. Evoked potential studies. Brain Res 260:1–9, 1983.
56. Delack JB: Hereditary deafness in the white cat. Comp Cont Educ Pract Vet 6:609–616, 1984.
57. Elverland HH, Mair IWS: Hereditary deafness in the cat. Acta Otolaryngol 90:360–369, 1980.
58. Rebillard G, Rebillard M, Carlier E, et al: Histo-physiological relationships in the deaf white cat auditory system. Acta Otolaryngol 82:48–56, 1976.
59. Bosher SK, Hallpike CS: Observations on the histologic features, development, and pathogenesis of the inner ear degeneration of the deaf white cat. Proc R Soc (Biol) Series B 162:147–170, 1965.
60. Wolff D: Three generations of deaf white cats. J Hered 33:39–43, 1942.
61. Hayes HM, Wilson GP, Fenner WR, et al: Canine congen-

ital deafness: Epidemiologic study of 272 cases. J Am Anim Hosp Assoc 17:473, 1981.
62. Igarashi M, Alford B, Cohn A, et al: Inner ear anomalies in dogs. Ann Otol 81:249–255, 1972.
63. Lurie M: The membranous labyrinth in the congenitally deaf collie and Dalmatian dog. Laryngoscope 58:279–287, 1948.
64. Gwin RM, Wyman M, Lim DJ, et al: Multiple ocular defects associated with partial albinism and deafness in the dog. J Am Anim Hosp Assoc 17:401–408, 1981.
65. Hudson W, Ruben R: Hereditary deafness in the Dalmatian dog. Arch Otol 75:213–219, 1962.
66. Johnsson L, Hawkins J, Muraski A, et al: Vascular anatomy and pathology of the cochlea in Dalmatian dogs. In Darin de Lorenzo AJ (ed): Vascular Disorders and Hearing Defects. University Park, Md, University Park Press, 1973.
67. Suga F, Hattler K: Physiological and histopathological correlates of hereditary deafness in animals. Laryngoscope 80:80–104, 1970.
68. Marshall A: Use of brain stem auditory-evoked response to evaluate deafness in a group of Dalmation dogs. J Am Vet Med Assoc 188:718–722, 1986.
69. Wilkes M, Palmer A: Congenital deafness in Dobermanns. Vet Rec 118:218, 1986.
70. Sims MH, Shull-Selcer E: Electrodiagnostic evaluation of deafness in two English setter littermates. J Am Vet Med Assoc 187:398–404, 1985.
71. Erickson F, Leipold HW, McKinley J: Congenital defects in dogs: Part 2. Canine Pract 14:51–61, 1977.
72. Steinberg SA, Klein E, Killens R, et al: Inherited deafness among nervous pointer dogs. In: Proceedings of the Seventh Annual Veterinary Med Forum, San Diego, 1989, pp 953–956.
73. Adams EW: Hereditary deafness in a family of foxhounds. J Am Vet Med Assoc 128:302–303, 1956.

11

Disorders of Involuntary Movement

Problems to be discussed in this chapter have some form of involuntary movement as the most prominent clinical sign. Some movement disorders also have other clinical signs that may be more obvious, and they will be mentioned with reference to other chapters, where they are discussed in detail.

Movement disorders are of two kinds, those with negative defects and those with positive defects (Table 11–1).[1] A negative defect refers to a movement that cannot be performed, as in paresis or paralysis. These have been discussed in Chapters 6–8. A positive defect is an involuntary movement such as seizure, ataxia, tremor, or an abnormal posture. Seizures are discussed in Chapter 14 and ataxias are discussed in Chapter 9. Disorders of involuntary movement can be further classified as those having increased muscle tone as the primary defect and those characterized by repetitive movements.

Movement disorders in which muscle tone is increased include tetanus and tetany, spasticity, myotonia, and opisthotonos. Those characterized by repetitive movements include tremor, myoclonus, and several abnormal movements seen primarily in nonhuman primates and human beings, such as athetosis, chorea, and ballism.

Tetanus is "a state of sustained muscular contraction without periods of relaxation caused by repetitive stimulation of the motor nerve trunk at frequencies so high that individual muscle twitches are fused and cannot be distinguished from one another; called also tonic spasm and tetany."[2] In clinical medicine, the term *tetanus* is generally reserved for the disease caused by *Clostridium tetani* toxin. *Tetany* is generally used to describe a similar condition, but characterized by intermittent tonic muscular contractions. Tetany is frequently caused by hypocalcemia, but may be seen in a variety of conditions.

Spasticity is a motor disorder characterized by a velocity-dependent increase in tonic stretch reflexes ("muscle tone") with exaggerated myotatic reflexes, resulting from hyperexcitability of the stretch reflex.[2] It is often associated with damage to the upper motor neurons. *Opisthotonos* is a posture with the head and neck severely extended and the back arched in an exaggerated lordotic position. It is generally accompanied by increased extensor tone in the limbs.

Myotonia is a sustained contraction of muscles caused by a primary defect in the muscle membrane. Both congenital and acquired forms are described in animals.

Tremor is an involuntary trembling or quivering that may occur at rest or during movement. Resting tremors are unusual in domestic animals. Most tremors occurring with movement are associated with diseases of the cerebellum and its related pathways.

Myoclonus denotes repetitive, rhythmic contractions of a portion of a muscle, an entire muscle, or a group of muscles. It may be restricted to one area or may occur synchronously or asynchronously in several areas.[2] The primary example is canine myoclonus following canine distemper viral infection.

TABLE 11–1 Disorders of Movement*

Negative Defects
Paresis-paralysis (6–8, 10)
Cataplexy (14)

Positive Defects
Gait abnormalities
  Ataxia, dysmetria (8–9)
  Circling, compulsive walking (9, 13, 16)
Seizures (14)
Involuntary movements
  Increased muscle tone
    Tetanus, tetany (11)
    Spasticity, opisthotonos (7–9, 11, 13)
  Repetitive movements
    Tremor (11, 9)
    Myoclonus (11)
    Other adventitious movements (11)

* Numbers in parentheses refer to chapters in which the disorders are discussed.

A number of other involuntary movement disorders are described in human beings and nonhuman primates. Most of these have not been reproduced in quadrupeds, even with experimental lesions in areas thought to cause the disorder in primates. *Chorea* is the contraction of random muscles throughout the body, occurring at random times and for random durations.[3] Canine distemper myoclonus was called chorea for many years, but it does not fit the definition. *Dystonia* is contraction of muscles, either focal or generalized, often including antagonist muscles that contract simultaneously. The movements in man are frequently described as twisting on the long axis of the body part. *Athetosis* is a slow, writhing movement of the fingers, sometimes described as "pill-rolling" movements in humans. The movements of the lips in horses with nigropallidal encephalomalacia caused by a plant toxin have been compared to athetosis. The comparison is interesting because the fingers of primates are the primary prehensile organ, with fine motor control, as are the lips of horses. A related movement disorder has been produced in cats with lesions in the caudate nucleus. The cats had slow kneading movements of the paws of the thoracic limb.[4] *Ballismus* denotes wild, large-amplitude, irregular limb movements. It is frequently on one side of the body and is then referred to as hemiballismus. Ballismus is apparently related to chorea, as human patients often have ballismus following a stroke, which then gradually changes to chorea over days.[3] Some of the movements seen in dogs with hypomyelination are almost suggestive of ballismus, but they tend to be more rhythmic and are called myoclonus.

Lesion Localization

Increased Muscle Tone

The disorders of increased muscle tone, including tetanus, tetany, and spasticity, are caused by imbalance of facilitation and inhibition on the lower motor neuron (LMN). The firing pattern of an individual LMN is determined by synaptic connections from the primary peripheral afferents, descending pathways from the brain, and local interneuron connections. Loss of adequate facilitation causes decreased muscle tone and reflexes. Loss of the inhibitory control causes increased firing of the LMN and intermittent or continuous contraction of the muscles it innervates. Each of the disorders of importance has a specific pathogenesis.

Tetanus and Tetany

Tetanus is caused by the toxin produced by *Clostridium tetani*. The bacterial spores are very resistant and can persist in the environment for long periods. Bacteria gain access to the animal's tissues through open wounds, proliferate, and produce the toxin. The toxin ascends to the spinal cord through the axons of peripheral nerves. From the LMN, the toxin invades the inhibitory interneurons and blocks the release of the inhibitory neurotransmitters glycine and γ-aminobutyric acid (GABA).[5] Glycine is the transmitter for primary inhibitory interneurons and for the Renshaw cells, which mediate recurrent inhibition; GABA is the inhibitory transmitter for descending pathways. Strychnine also blocks glycine, but it acts at the receptor.[6] The result is uninhibited firing of the LMN, a decrease in long latency reflexes, and an increase in short latency reflexes.

Tetany is generally similar to tetanus, but with intermittent relaxation of the muscles. The most common forms are caused by abnormalities in electrolytes, principally decreased serum calcium or magnesium levels. The blood calcium level may vary considerably because the abnormality is specifically related to a decrease in ionized calcium below 2.5 mg/dl.[7] For example, in hypoproteinemia, low total calcium levels are associated with hypoalbuminemia, since albumin is the primary binding protein for calcium. Ionized calcium levels may be normal, and clinical signs of hypocalcemia do not occur. Calcium is necessary for release of neurotransmitters and for excitation-contraction coupling in muscle. Magnesium has the opposite effect on the synapse, blocking the release of the transmitter. Hypocalcemia and hypomagnesemia can cause either tetany or weakness, apparently depending on the degree and rate of development of the decrease in the ionic form. Hypocalcemia is caused by increased loss of calcium in milk, decreased absorption from the intestinal tract in renal disease and in the presence of oxalates and ethylene glycol, and from the saponification of fat in acute pancreatitis. Hypoparathyroidism (decreased parathormone production) causes decreased calcium by increasing renal excretion and urinary loss, reducing gastrointestinal (GI) absorption, and decreasing reabsorption of calcium from the bones. Hypomagnesemia is caused by inadequate intake, usually in large animals feeding on fresh green pastures that are low in magnesium content.

Myotonia

Myotonia is characterized by sustained contraction of muscle fibers caused by repetitive depolarization of their cell membranes. Muscle relaxation is delayed after a voluntary or evoked contraction.[8] The congenital myotonia of goats has been studied most extensively. The defect is a lowered muscle membrane permeability to chloride. One of the characteristic clinical signs is "dimpling" of the muscle after percussion, which reflects the prolonged contraction of the small group of muscle fibers excited by the stimulus. There is no evidence of LMN or UMN involvement in these animals. They have normal postural reactions within the limitations of the prolonged contractions of the muscles.

Spasticity and Opisthotonos

Spasticity is generally related to UMN deficits, with reduced inhibition of the extensor motor neurons. The term is also used for some poorly defined syndromes, such as spastic paresis of cattle and Scotty cramp in dogs. These diseases may result from a primary defect in neurotransmitters. With UMN disease there is paresis or paralysis, increased myotatic reflexes, and sometimes abnormal reflexes, such as crossed extensor and extensor toe reflexes. Lesion localization for UMN disease is described in Chapter 2. Lesions of the rostral brain stem (midbrain, rostral pons) produce a posture called *decerebrate rigidity*. All four limbs are extended with increased extensor tone. Forced flexion of the limb causes increased resistance to a point, then abrupt loss of resistance and flexion, the clasp-knife reflex. If the rostral lobe of the cerebellum is also damaged, the head and neck are extended dorsally in a posture called *opisthotonos*.[9] Acute lesions of the cerebellum without damage to the brain stem cause a posture termed *decerebellate rigidity* that is similar to decerebrate posture, but the pelvic limbs are flexed and uncoordinated movements occur.

Repetitive Movements

Tremor

Tremor may occur only with movements or may be present at rest. Most of the tremor syndromes in domestic animals are associated with movement. The lesion causing tremor is usually either in the cerebellum or associated with diffuse abnormality of myelin. Tremors may also be a component of tetany. The classic tremor syndromes of human beings associated with extrapyramidal system abnormality are not seen in domestic animals.

Cerebellar tremor is called an intention tremor because it progresses in severity as the animal initiates movement. The tremor subsides as the animal relaxes. Tremor is one manifestation of the abnormal control of the rate, range, and force of the movements. Dysmetria is similar, but the movement is of greater amplitude. The head must be affected to localize the lesion to the cerebellum because similar signs in the limbs can be caused by lesions in the pathways mediating these functions. A simple test entails giving the animal food or water. The animal with cerebellar disease will have tremors or dysmetria of the head as it tries to eat or drink.

Tremor in animals with myelin disease is usually worse than in those with cerebellar disease. The tremor is often accompanied with myoclonus, is more persistent at rest, and may even be present during light sleep.

Tremors may also be associated with mycotoxins, some poisonous plants, several chemical poisons, and diffuse nonsuppurative encephalitis. The tremor is similar to that seen with cerebellar disease in most cases, and the diagnosis must depend on other signs and the history.

Myoclonus

The most common cause of myoclonus in domestic animals is associated with canine distemper. Synonyms include flexor spasm, canine chorea, and tremor. It is characterized by a repetitive contraction of a muscle or group of muscles at rates up to 60 per minute. It may occur in more than one muscle group in a dog, and different groups may be affected as the disease progresses. At any one time, the myoclonus is constant in the same groups of muscles. The myoclonus may persist during sleep. Any muscle group may be affected, but the condition is most frequent in the appendicular or masticatory muscles. The cause is unknown, but once established, the LMN and interneuron pool of the affected segment are sufficient for the movement. Transection of the spinal cord above and below the affected segment and sectioning of the dorsal root afferents does not abolish the movement. Ventral root section stops the myoclonus. Minimal histologic changes are seen in the affected segments. Distemper myoclonus may occur during the acute phase of the disease, but more frequently it occurs in the chronic phases. The myoclonus may persist for years after the animal recovers from the initial disease. Spontaneous remission is sometimes seen. Inherited myoclonus of cattle is caused by a deficit of glycine/strychnine receptors in the spinal cord.

Diseases

Tetanus and Tetany

Tetanus

Tetanus is caused by the toxin produced by the bacterium *Clostridium tetani*, a spore-bearing, anaerobic bacillus.[5] The spores are resistant to most sporicidal agents and can remain viable for years.[10] The organisms may be found in soil and are common in the feces of many species. Infection usually occurs through contamination of wounds. Deep wounds with poor oxygenation are most susceptible. The toxin is liberated, binds to gangliosides in nerves, and travels to the spinal cord by retrograde axonal transport. In the spinal cord, the toxin passes transsynaptically to inhibitory interneurons. It specifically blocks the release of the inhibitory neurotransmitters glycine and GABA.[5,6]

If the toxin ascends in a nerve of a limb, that limb will exhibit tetanus first, followed by the opposite limb, and eventually the entire body. If the toxin circulates in the blood, signs of tetanus start in the head. Prolapse of the nictitating membrane and contraction of the facial muscles and the muscles of mastication are seen prior to development of tetanus in the rest of the body.[10]

All domestic animals are susceptible to tetanus. The ruminants and dog are more resistant than the horse. Birds are naturally resistant.

The clinical signs of tetanus occur 5 to 10 days after infection and include increased muscle tone, usually in all the limbs and in the muscles of the head. In the early stages, the prolapsed nictitating membrane, contraction of the muscles of facial expression, and contraction of the muscles of mastication are characteristic. The lips are drawn in an exaggerated "grin," in erect-eared breeds the ears are drawn toward each other, and the jaws are tightly closed. Other early signs are a stiff gait and elevation of the tail. In the later stages the animal is recumbent, with extension of all four limbs and opisthotonos. Signs are enhanced by stimulation. Death may occur from respiratory paralysis. Autonomic effects may also be present. Bradycardia because of increased parasympathetic activity has been reported in the dog,[11] and increased sympathetic activity has been demonstrated experimentally and in human patients.[5]

The diagnosis is based on the characteristic clinical signs and evidence of infection. The source of infection is not always evident. Intra-abdominal infections, such as metritis, enteritis, and abscesses, may be a cause.

Treatment includes wound debridement and systemic administration of crystalline penicillin (20,000–50,000 IU/kg four times daily for dogs) and tetanus antitoxin (25–110 IU/kg intravenously [IV] for dogs, 10,000 IU for the horse). The benzodiazepines, such as diazepam or clonazepam, may be helpful by enhancing GABA inhibition. Nursing care must include a quiet environment, frequent turning if the animal is recumbent, and skin cleanliness. Oral intake may be impossible, so that parenteral fluids and nutrients may be needed. Nasogastric or pharyngostomy tubes may be used. Respiratory assistance may be required. Bloat must be watched for in ruminants and susceptible breeds of dogs. The prognosis is usually good for dogs and cats unless respiratory problems occur. Horses or cows that become recumbent have a poor prognosis.

Immunization with toxoid is recommended in horses. It is given to newborn foals, and boosters are given at least every few years. Toxoid is given any time there is injury, surgery, or before parturition.[12]

Metabolic Causes of Tetany

Hypocalcemia. Hypocalcemia results in tetany when serum calcium concentrations drop below 6 mg/dl. Calcium ion concentrations control neuronal membrane permeability; however, both protein-bound and ionized calcium are measured when serum calcium levels are quantitated. Thus, in hypoproteinemic conditions, low total serum calcium levels may be encountered without concomitant tetany. In dogs, cats, and horses, hypocalcemic tetany may result from hypoparathyroidism, postparturient eclampsia (rare in cats), terminal renal failure, protein-losing enteropathy, and severe alkalosis. Hypocalcemia in cows usually causes weakness, sometimes with a tremor.

Postparturient eclampsia (puerperal tetany) in the bitch usually occurs within 3 weeks after whelping. Small breed dogs with nervous temperaments are more prone to this disorder. The exact mechanism of postparturient hypocalcemia in the bitch is not known; however, calcium losses from fetal ossification and lactation combined with deficient osteoclastic activity or calcium absorption are probably responsible for the altered calcium homeostasis. Although some bitches may become hypoglycemic during puerperal tetany, lowered blood glucose values probably are not important in the production of tetany. Some authors believe that nervous dogs are predisposed to puerperal tetany because they hyperventilate during parturition, inducing a respiratory alkalosis. Alkalosis favors the protein binding of calcium, thus lowering the concentrations of ionized calcium. Since ionized calcium is biologically active, alkalosis would enhance the development of tetany.

The early clinical signs include nervousness, pacing, whining, and panting. Muscle spasm and ataxia are subsequent signs. These early manifestations usually progress to tonic-clonic tetanic spasms. The dogs are often febrile and, in severe cases, major motor seizures may be encountered.

The diagnosis of puerperal tetany is based on the clinical signs and low blood calcium concentrations. Upon presentation, a blood sample should be collected for calcium analysis. Five to 10 ml of 10% calcium gluconate should be given slowly IV while the heart rate and rhythm are monitored simultaneously. Two to 5 ml of 10% calcium gluconate diluted with equal volumes of normal saline can be given intramuscularly (IM) to prolong the calcium effect. Severely hyperthermic patients (body temperature greater than 105°F) should be cooled with ice packs or alcohol soaks. Animals that continue to have seizures or that remain excessively irritable or restless can be mildly sedated with diazepam or phenobarbital. For maintenance therapy, puppies should be separated from the bitch for 24 hours and supplemented with bitch's milk formula. Full nursing should be restricted for an additional 48 hours. Calcium lactate is given in oral dosages of 0.5 to 2.0 g/day.

Eclampsia of mares is rarely encountered except in draft horses. Most cases reportedly occur in lactating mares near the tenth day post parturition or 1 to 2 days after weaning. Factors that may predispose to eclampsia in mares include grazing on a lush pasture, strenuous work, and prolonged transport. Affected mares tend to sweat profusely, develop muscle spasticity of the limbs, and become ataxic. Rapid respiration, muscular fibrillation, and trismus are evident, but there is no protrusion of the membrana nictitans. The rectal temperature is normal or mildly elevated, and the pulse may be rapid and irregular. Swallowing may be impeded, and urination and defecation may cease. Within 24 hours, tetanic convulsions develop, followed by death within an additional 24 hours. The diagnosis is based on clinical signs and the presence of reduced serum calcium concentrations (4–6 mg/dl). Treatment with IV calcium solutions produces rapid, complete recovery.

Hypoparathyroidism results in decreased secretion of parathormone (PTH) with subsequent hypocalcemia and hyperphosphatemia. This condition has been recognized and studied most frequently in dogs, but also occurs in cats. Although the exact cause is unknown, the majority of dogs have histologic parathyroid changes indicative of a primary autoimmune disease (lymphocytic-plasmacytic cellular infiltration). A parathyroid deficiency also may occur following thyroid gland surgery. An acute form of the disease is characterized by a sudden onset of tetany or convulsions, or both. A chronic form of the disease is associated with recurrent depression, lethargy, anorexia, vomiting, intermittent facial and forelimb spasm, and latent tetany. Primary hypoparathyroidism is suspected in a dog with persistent hypocalcemia and hyperphosphatemia in the presence of normal renal function. Decreased concentrations of PTH in the presence of hypocalcemia substantiate the diagnosis; however, this test is not widely available for use in the dog.

Primary hypoparathyroidism is treated with drugs to overcome the PTH deficiency. Dihydrotachysterol, ergocalciferol (vitamin D_2) and calcitriol (1,25-dihydroxycholecalciferol) are the products frequently recommended. The clinician must individualize the dosage by following the serum calcium levels of each patient twice a week. Approximate initial dosages of these drugs are: dihydrotachysterol, 0.01 mg/kg/day; ergocalciferol, 1,000–2,000 U/kg/day; and calcitriol, 0.25 μg once a day. The clinician should monitor the serum calcium concentrations carefully in order to prevent hypercalcemia. The effect of vitamin D therapy may be delayed for 2 to 3 weeks. Calcium supplementation must be administered with caution, since its use with vitamin D increases the probability of hypercalcemic toxicity.

Hypomagnesemic Tetanies. These syndromes occur primarily in ruminants. Several hypomagnesemic conditions have been described, including grass tetany, wheat pasture poisoning, milk tetany of calves, and transport tetany. The basic pathophysiology of each is similar and probably is related to decreased dietary intake, reduced mobilization, or increased excretion of magnesium.

Grass tetany occurs in the lactating bovine that grazes in a lush pasture. It also occurs in the pregnant and lactating ewe and occasionally is seen in feeder cattle. Lush pastures are low in magnesium, and when magnesium requirements are increased, as in the case of the lactating bovine, clinical signs are likely to occur. Early signs include restlessness, extreme alertness, and muscular twitching. Animals may become excitable, belligerent, and even aggressive. Stimulation may induce severe signs of tetany, ataxia, and bellowing. Animals may become recumbent with opisthotonos and paddling movements. The diagnosis of grass tetany is supported by laboratory findings of hypomagnesmia (<1 mg/dl), hypocalcemia (<7 mg/dl), and high normal levels of potassium. Therapy should correct the immediate ionic imbalance and should supplement the dietary intake of magnesium. Magnesium lactate in a 3.3% solution (2.2 ml/kg), magnesium gluconate in a 15% solution (0.44 ml/kg), and magnesium sulfate in a 20% solution (0.44 ml/kg) can be given slowly IV or subcutaneously. Commercial combination solutions may also be used effectively. Magnesium oxide, 1 g/45 kg/day, should be force-fed or supplied in blocks containing protein supplements and molasses. Animals on high-risk pastures should be given magnesium oxide or chloride supplements.

Wheat pasture poisoning is very similar to grass tetany, except that it occurs in cattle and sheep that graze in a cereal grain pasture during its early growth. The diagnosis and the treatment are the same as those for grass tetany.

Milk tetany occurs in 2- to 4-month-old calves that are fed only milk. The signs may occur after episodes of diarrhea. The digestive disorders may decrease magnesium absorption, thus complicating the magnesium deficiency. The clinical signs include hyperesthesia, nervousness, recumbency, and seizures. Repeated attacks may occur. The diagnosis is based on the history, the clinical signs, and a serum magnesium concentration below 0.7 mg/dl. Calves respond to parenteral magnesium ionic therapy. Susceptible calves should be given magnesium oxide supplements, 1 g/day.

Transport tetany occurs following stressful events, such as transportation, vaccination, deworming, adverse weather, and marked dietary changes. It occurs in both cattle and sheep. A dietary reduction in calcium, magnesium, and potassium coupled with stress produces ionic imbalances that result in a wide range of clinical signs, from spastic to flaccid paralysis. The signs usually begin within 24 hours of the stress but may be delayed for 72 hours. Early manifestations include restlessness, anorexia, and excitement. These signs progress to muscular trembling, teeth grinding, ataxia, and recumbency. Opisthotonos, paddling, and coma may develop. Treatment consists of the parenteral administration of polyionic glucose solutions and attentive nursing care.

Renal Disease. The terminal stages of renal failure may cause tetany or seizures. Chronic renal disease may be associated with muscle wasting and weakness. Polyneuropathy and polymyopathy have been seen in human beings with chronic renal disease, especially those on hemodialysis, but are not well documented in animals. Alterations in electrolyte metabolism, especially the metabolism of calcium, may cause signs related to the nervous system, as already discussed.

Toxicoses

Strychnine. Strychnine is a rodenticide that is sometimes used in malicious poisonings of small animals. It produces tetanic spasms that are exacerbated by auditory or tactile stimuli. The animal is fully conscious. The signs may appear within 10 minutes to 2 hours after ingestion.[13] The clinical signs are strongly suggestive of the diagnosis. Tetanus is not as acute in onset. Hypocalcemia can be quickly ruled out by finding normal serum calcium concentrations in affected dogs. Other toxins cause signs other than tetany. Metaldehyde causes tetany that progresses rapidly to seizures. Organophosphates cause tremor, seizures, and autonomic signs. Chemical analysis of the stomach contents may confirm the diagnosis.

Treatment is directed at limiting absorption and controlling the tetany. Induction of vomiting or gastric lavage with activated charcoal is used to reduce the absorption. Tetany is controlled with pentobarbital sodium given IV to effect. Caution must be used to avoid overdosing. Endotracheal intubation and maintenance of respiration is mandatory. Inhalation anesthesia may be used to avoid large doses of barbiturates for prolonged periods. Diuresis is established with IV fluids. Acidification of the urine is recommended to enhance elimination, which should be completed in 24 to 48 hours.

Spasticity

Anomalous and Hereditary

Hereditary Myotonia. Myotonic myopathy, a condition of sustained contractions of the muscles, is an inherited disorder in dogs, goats, and horses. Table 11–2 lists the heredity and muscular changes in these animals. In the goat, the signs are noticed shortly after birth, while the signs in the dog are usually not recognized until 6 weeks to 3 months of age. This difference probably reflects the degree of mobility at these ages in the species affected. The horse has a much milder form that is usually not recognized until the animal is about 6 months of age.

The signs are a progressive stiffening of the gait with exercise. The muscles maintain contraction after a normal contraction is elicited. The limbs become stiff and abducted in a sawhorse posture. With time, the muscles become hypertrophied, especially in the proximal parts of the limbs and in the neck. Percussion of a muscle causes a prolonged contraction of that part of the muscle, with a resultant dimple or bulge. In long-haired animals, the dimple is easily seen on the tongue. Electromyography (EMG) is useful to detect the characteristic "myotonic" discharge—a high-frequency, waxing-waning series of potentials. It sounds like a dive bomber or a revving motorcycle engine. Similar potentials without the waxing-waning character are found with many other forms of myopathy, such as inflammatory myositis. Both forms may be found in acquired myotonias from increased adrenocortical hormones, whether acquired or iatrogenic.

Dogs and horses with myotonia may live a reasonable life. Cell membrane–stabilizing drugs have been used to provide some relief. Procainamide (500 mg given orally four times a day for dogs) has been recommended.[14]

TABLE 11–2 Myotonia

Species Breed	*Heredity*	*Dystrophic Changes*	*References*
Canine			
Chow chow	Autosomal recessive (?)	Minimal	63–69
Staffordshire terrier	Unknown	Minimal	67, 70
Rhodesian ridgeback	Unknown	Moderate	71
Cavalier King Charles spaniel	Unknown	Minimal	72
Great Dane	Unknown	Minimal	73
Golden retriever	Unknown	Marked	14, 16, 64
Irish terrier	X-linked autosomal recessive	Marked	16, 74
Caprine	Autosomal dominant or recessive	Minimal	75–77
Equine	Unknown	Unknown	78

Acquired Myotonia. Several forms of myopathy may have myotonic features. Inflammatory myopathy, whether immune mediated or caused by an infectious agent such as toxoplasmosis, may have myotonic discharges on the EMG and some increased contraction of the muscles. Endocrine myopathy, notably that caused by increased circulating corticosteroids, frequently has some myotonia associated with the degenerative changes. Hyperadrenocorticism (Cushing's syndrome) may be caused by adrenal tumors, pituitary tumors, or exogenous administration of corticosteroids. The myopathic changes occur late in the course of the syndrome, when polyuria, polydipsia, abdominal distention, and cutaneous changes are usually evident. A stiff gait or weakness on exercise may be recognized. Clinical signs generally improve dramatically with appropriate therapy for the hyperadrenocorticism. Myotonic discharges may persist for weeks to months, even with resolution of the other signs of Cushing's syndrome.

Spastic Paresis. Spastic paresis, also called Elso heel and spastic paralysis, occurs in young cattle of many breeds. Although it is thought to be heritable, the evidence is not clear.

Affected calves are recognized between the ages of 1 week and 12 months. The signs are usually bilateral, but one side is often worse. The pelvic limbs are straight, especially at the hock. The limb is advanced like a pendulum, and may be held caudally in extension. Some improvement is seen with walking, but it never becomes normal. Forceful attempts to flex the limb cause increased tone and clonic contractions of the extensors.[15] The pathogenesis appears to be an increase in the activity of the gamma efferent system. Section of the dorsal roots or blocking of the small gamma motor neurons reduces the clinical signs.[16] Lowered levels of homovanillic acid, the main metabolite of dopamine, were found in the cerebrospinal fluid (CSF) of affected calves, suggesting a primary defect in dopamine metabolism.[17] Surgical management by sectioning the tibial nerve or severance of all or part of the gastrocnemius and flexor tendons allows the cattle to reach market age.[15] A genetic basis is suspected.

Spastic Syndrome. Periodic spasticity, crampiness, stretches, or Standings disease are names given a syndrome affecting the extensor muscles of the lumbar region and pelvic limbs. The condition is similar to spastic paresis except that it occurs in older animals and is more episodic. The episodes of muscle spasms are induced by movement and are not seen at rest. It may occur in one limb or both, in which case the movements alternate from side to side. The affected limb is raised and extended caudally or forcefully flexed. The episodes increase in severity with time. One study of the nerves and muscles of an affected bull failed to reveal any significant changes.[18] Evidence for an autosomal dominant inheritance is reported.[12]

Shivering. A syndrome of spasms of the pelvic limbs, including flexion, abduction, and shaking when the limb is moved, has been called shivering. The tail may also exhibit tremors and be held elevated. The thigh muscles atrophy. The disorder is seen most often in draft horses. No lesion or treatment has been described.[16,19]

Stringhalt. Two forms of stringhalt are described. The gait is characterized by hyperflexion of one or both pelvic limbs during movement. Australian stringhalt occurs in epidemics and may involve the thoracic limbs. Degeneration is reported in the distal sciatic nerve. A toxic factor is postulated, especially for the epidemic form. Several plants have been investigated, but there is no clear cause known.[20] Many horses improve slowly over a time span of weeks to a year. Affected animals should be removed from access to toxic plants and rested. Tenectomy of the lateral digital extensor tendon may help in severe cases.[12]

Scotty Cramp. Scottish terriers are affected by an inherited disorder characterized by episodic hypertonus of the muscles. The syndrome is inherited as a recessive trait.[21,22] The clinical signs are similar to those described for myotonia. Episodes are precipitated by exercise, fear or excitement, and some drugs. The limbs gradually become stiff, the back is arched, and the animal becomes reluctant to move. The thoracic limbs initially tend to abduct, and the pelvic limbs often have both flexor and extensor hypertonus, resulting in a high-stepping, dysmetric gait. The animal becomes so stiff after a time that it falls down. Facial muscles may be involved. The severity is variable between dogs, some being only mildly affected, others incapacitated.

There are no gross or histologic lesions of the nervous system or muscles. The cause is believed to be an alteration in serotonin metabolism. The signs are made worse by the administration of agents that decrease serotonin levels in the central nervous system (CNS), such as methysergide (Sansert, Sandoz Pharmaceuticals). Drugs that increase serotonin levels, such as monoamine oxidase inhibitors, provide a beneficial effect. Methysergide can be used to help confirm the diagnosis. A dose of 0.3 mg/kg orally will increase the signs in most cases. A maximum dose of 0.6 mg/kg is recommended.[22] Diazepam is recommended at a dose of 0.5–1.5 mg/kg every 8 hours to reduce the clinical signs. Vitamin E, 125 IU/kg once a day, has been effective in reducing the frequency, but not the severity of episodes.

Muscle Spasms

Metabolic

Exertional Myopathy. Exertional myopathy may occur in any species but is most common in athletic animals after exercise. Racing or working horses and racing greyhounds are frequently affected. It is also seen in newly captured wild animals. Working horses tend to have the problem shortly after exercise following several days of rest.

The signs are stiffness and extension of the limbs, distress, and pain and swelling of the muscles. The pathogenesis is thought to be metabolic acidosis in the muscle, swelling, local ischemia, muscle cell necrosis, and myoglobinuria. The myoglobinuria may be severe enough to cause nephropathy. Renal failure may occur in severe cases resulting in death of the animal. Elevated serum levels of muscle enzymes (CPK, LDH, AST) aid in the diagnosis. Type II muscle fibers are affected to a greater extent, but not exclusively, in horses.[23]

Treatment entails administration of IV fluids to maintain renal function and bicarbonate to correct the acidosis, cooling the animal, and rest.[16,24] Dantrolene and phenytoin may help alleviate attacks, but they are still considered experimental.[12]

Tremor (Table 11–3)

Cerebellar Diseases

The primary cerebellar degenerations, anomalies, malformations, viral degenerations, toxic syndromes, idiopathic cerebellitis, and miscellaneous causes of cerebellar disease are discussed in Chapter 9. These diseases produce all of the signs of cerebellar disease, including tremor.

Idiopathic Cerebellitis. An acute onset of tremor is seen primarily in small, white, adult dogs. Maltese, poodles, and West Highland white terriers are affected most frequently, but the condition can occur in other breeds that are not white.[25] We have seen several in silver poodles, for example. The tremor worsens with movement, an intention tremor, and disappears at rest. Tremor of the eye is common. The disease is nonprogressive after the first 2 to 3 days.

TABLE 11–3 Tremor Syndromes

	Syndromes Categorized by Time of Disease Onset			
Species	**At or Within a Few Days of Birth**	**A Few Weeks/Months to Adult**	**Adult**	**Any Age**
Dogs	1. Inherited hypomyelination/dysmyelination	1. Inadequate glycogen stores 2. Glycogen storage disease	1. Metabolic diseases (Hypocalcemia, hypoglycemia, hypoadrenocorticism, hyperthyroidism) 2. Idiopathic tremor syndrome (white dogs)	1. Hexachlorophene toxicity
Pigs	1. Congenital hypomyelinogenesis (type A-I to A-V, B)	1. Encephalomyocarditis virus disease 2. Pseudorabies 3. Talfan/Teschen disease 4. Inadequate glycogen stores		1. Organic arsenical toxicity 2. Organic mercurial toxicity
Cattle	1. Shaker calf syndrome 2. Inherited congenital myoclonus 3. Maple syrup urine disease 4. Citrullinemia 5. Hereditary hypomyelinogenesis 6. Bovine viral diarrhea	1. Milk tetany 2. Polioencephalomalacia 3. Glycogen storage disease 4. White muscle disease	1. Metabolic diseases (Hypocalcemia, hypomagnesemia, hypoglycemia/ketosis)	1. Monensin toxicity 2. Urea toxicity 3. Organic mercurial toxicity 4. Hexachlorophene toxicity 5. Tremorogenic pasture grasses 6. Louping ill (rare)
Sheep and goats	1. Border disease (sheep) 2. Congenital swayback (goats)	1. Systemic neuraxial dystrophy (sheep) 2. Polioencephalomalacia 3. Glycogen storage disease (sheep) 4. White muscle disease (sheep)	1. Metabolic diseases—sheep (see cattle, above) 2. Visna (sheep) 3. Scrapie	1. Louping ill (sheep) 2. Tremorogenic pasture grasses 3. Urea toxicity (sheep) 4. Hexachlorophene toxicity
Horses		1. Shaker foal syndrome (botulism) 2. Inadequate glycogen stores 3. White muscle disease	1. Hyperkalemic periodic paralysis	1. Yellow star thistle poisoning 2. Tremorogenic pasture grasses
Cats		1. Glycogen storage disease	1. Hyperthyroidism	1. Hexachlorophene toxicity
All Species		1. Lysomal storage disease 2. Hepatic encephalopathy		1. End-stage liver failure 2. Poisonings—organophosphate/carbamate, metaldehyde, chlorinated hydrocarbons, strychnine, lead 3. Botulism

From Cuddon PA: Tremor syndromes. Prog Vet Neurol 1:285–299, 1990. Used by permission.

Spontaneous remission may occur. Other than the tremor and a slight degree of ataxia, the neurologic examination is normal. The tremor is worse than usually expected with cerebellar disease and the ataxia is less. The few dogs necropsied had mild nonsuppurative inflammation of the nervous system, not confined to the cerebellum.[16] Speculated causes include viral or immune-mediated inflammatory disease. The relation to the white coat color has led to hypotheses on the relation to tyrosine metabolism; however, as Parker points out, these are not albino animals.[26] Treatment is with immunosuppressive doses of corticosteroids, diazepam, or both. The corticosteroids should be given in decreasing doses for 8 to 12 weeks. Stopping therapy early may lead to relapse. Clinical improvement is expected in 2 to 3 days. The response to treatment is usually dramatic, but some dogs are less responsive. Relapses following recovery have been seen.

Demyelinating Diseases

The primary demyelinating diseases, such as globoid cell leukodystrophy, and those secondary to systemic diseases, such as canine distemper, frequently cause cerebellar signs, including tremor. These diseases are discussed in Chapter 16.

TABLE 11–4 Disorders of Abnormal Myelin Development

Species/Breed	Inherited	References
Canine		
Springer spaniel	Yes	27, 28, 79, 80
Chow chow	Probably	27, 28, 81–84
Samoyeds	Probably	27, 28, 85
Weimaraner	Probably	27, 28, 86–88
Bernese mountain dog	Probably	89
Lurcher	Unknown	27, 28, 90
Dalmatian	Unknown	91
Spaniel	Unknown	27
Australian silky terrier	Unknown	16
Porcine		
Type A-I	No, hog cholera virus	30–32
Type A-II	No, unknown virus	30–32
Type A-III Landrace	Yes	29, 33–35
Type A-IV saddleback	Yes	29, 31, 36, 37
Type A-V	No, toxic	30
Type B	Unknown	30
Ovine		
Border disease	No, virus (BVD?)	38, 39
Bovine		
Jersey	?	32, 40
Shorthorn	?	32, 41
Angus–shorthorn	?	32, 92
Hereford	?	32, 41, 53

Anomalous or Hereditary

Hypomyelination. Hypomyelination is a developmental disorder of normal myelin causing thinly myelinated and some nonmyelinated axons. Dysmyelination is similar, but with predominantly abnormal myelin.[27] Both terms have been used in describing these diseases. It is an inherited defect in some species and breeds, and also occurs secondary to *in utero* infection with several viral agents.[28] It is distinct from demyelinating diseases in which the myelin develops normally and is later destroyed by external agents (e.g., canine distemper) and from metabolic storage disease (e.g., globoid cell leukodystrophy). Table 11–4 lists the primary disorders of myelin development.

The clinical signs of these syndromes are usually noticed in the first few weeks of life. The signs are very similar to those of cerebellar disease (see Chap. 9), with ataxia, tremor, dysmetria, and pendular nystagmus being common in most animals. The primary difference is that most of the myelin disorders have a larger amplitude movement disorder in addition to the fine tremor. In fact, one of the original names for the condition in pigs was myoclonia congenita.[29] In the chow chow's that we have evaluated in our clinic, there is a large amplitude, repetitive, clonic movement in most affected dogs.

The diagnosis in dogs is based on the history, presenting signs, and lack of positive findings on any diagnostic test. Generally more than one pup in a litter is affected. It is difficult to distinguish these syndromes from other causes of cerebellar disease or demyelination. Most of the demyelinating diseases will not be apparent at such an early age.

Six different myelin disorders have been defined in pigs (see Table 11–4).[29–37] Only two of these—type A-III, which is sex-linked in Landrace, and type A-IV, which is inherited as an autosomal recessive trait in saddlebacks—are inherited. Affected pigs develop signs at 2 to 3 days of age. Myelin is abnormal in the saddlebacks, and oligodendrocytes are reduced in the Landrace. There is no treatment for the inherited forms.

Sheep with border disease have a hairy fleece that is characteristic and are often called hairy shakers.[38,39] Border disease is caused by a virus that is transmitted to the lamb in utero. Affected lambs are often stunted and may have skeletal deformities. Hereford calves have a rare degenerative disorder characterized by neurofilament accumulation in neurons. Tremor is a prominent sign hours after birth. Bovine diarrhea virus has been implicated in hypomyelination in other cattle.[12,32,40–42]

Many animals that are not severely affected improve with age, but assistance with feeding is usually necessary as they cannot nurse properly. In springer spaniels, the males do not show much improvement, but the carrier females are less severely affected and improve considerably with maturation. The chow chows and Weimaraners improve to near-normal behavior with maturity. Sheep and pigs may recover if assisted with nutrition. Cattle may also improve, but the degenerative disease in Herefords is progressive and fatal. There is no treatment.

Toxicoses

Mycotoxicoses. A mycotoxin, penitrem A, from cottage cheese caused tremors and seizures in a dog.[43] Mycotoxins associated with plants in large animals are discussed in the next section and listed in Chapter 16.

Poisonous Plants. Plant toxicoses causing tremors usually affect multiple animals in a group, are seasonal, and often occur late in the growth of the plants.[12] Food animals are affected more frequently than horses. Tremors are often associated with ataxia, dysmetria, and in some cases seizures.

Dallis grass and some other similar grasses are infested with *Claviceps paspali*, which produces a neurotoxin. Phalaris neurotoxicity is caused by alkaloids that interfere with serotonin release. Perennial ryegrass is infested with mycotoxins, while annual ryegrass has a toxin produced by a *Corynebacterium*.[25] See Table 16–25 for details.

Heavy Metal Poisoning. Lead is the most common heavy metal causing toxicosis in animals. GI and CNS signs dominate the clinical picture in most cases. Horses seem to be more resistant and generally have peripheral neuropathies and respiratory problems.[44] In cats and dogs, vomiting and diarrhea may be seen, especially in acute poisoning. Cattle may bloat and have diarrhea. CNS signs include seizures, blindness, abnormal behavior, and tremors.[13,45,46] Tremors are usually associated with chronic low-grade poisoning, and probably are caused by the demyelinating effects of lead. The acute cases often have laminar cerebrocortical necrosis accounting for the predominance of cerebral signs. Lead poisoning and other heavy metal toxicities, including diagnosis and management, are discussed in Chapter 16.

Hexachlorophene. Hexachlorophene, an ingredient in antiseptic soaps, may cause generalized tremors, especially in young animals. Oral administration of hexachlorophene in an attempt to reproduce the clinical syndrome caused vomiting and diarrhea, salivation, tachypnea, and depression.[47] Clinical cases of hexachlorophene toxicity have resulted from both topical and oral contact. Examples include puppies exposed from nursing mammary glands that were washed daily with hexachlorophene soap; a cat with a skin lesion near the mouth that was washed with undiluted hexachlorophene soap; and a dog that ingested a bar of hexachlorophene soap.[48–50] Lesions are primarily vacuolation of the white matter. Treatment is eliminating exposure and supportive care. Acute intoxication may be helped by osmotic diuresis.[48] Dogs often recover with time.

Organophosphates and Chlorinated Hydrocarbons. Organophosphate compounds may cause tremor in some cases of intoxication. The tremor usually precedes the more common findings of seizures and neuromuscular weakness. Chlorinated hydrocarbons often produce tremor as a major component of toxicity. Fine tremor or fasciculation of the muscles may be accompanied by seizures, tonic spasms, and autonomic manifestations. These toxicities are discussed in Chapter 16.

Myoclonus

Anomalous or Hereditary

Inherited Congenital Myoclonus. This syndrome is also described as neuraxial edema in the literature (Table 11–5). Healy et al. differentiated two syndromes found in Hereford and Polled Hereford cattle.[51] Congenital myoclonus occurs primarily in Polled Herefords and their crossbreeds. It is inherited as an autosomal recessive trait with onset prior to birth. There are no histologic lesions in these animals, but they have a deficit of glycine/strychnine receptors in the spinal cord.[52] The clinical syndrome is characterized by a stimulus-responsive myoclonic spasm. Many of the calves have traumatic lesions of the hip joints. The second disease was found in Polled Herefords and Herefords. Clinical signs developed after birth and consisted of dullness, opisthotonos, and recumbency. These animals had a characteristic status spongiosus of the nervous system. Ketone concentrations were high in the urine, with a distinct aroma of burnt sugar. Healy et al. compare this syndrome to

TABLE 11–5 Spongy Degenerations

Species/Breed	Signs	Age	Lesion	References
Canine				
Labrador retriever	Ataxia, extensor rigidity, tremor	4–6 mo.	Intramyelin, astrocytes	54, 55
Saluki	Seizures, behavioral change	3 mo.	Gray and white matter	56
Samoyed	Tremors	12 days	White matter	57
Silky terrier	Myoclonus of paravertebral muscles			57
Feline				
Egyptian Mau	Ataxia	7 wk	Intramyelin	58
Bovine				
Hereford, Polled Hereford	Recumbency, dullness, opisthotonus	1–3 days	Gray and white matter, maple syrup urine	42, 51
"Neuraxial Edema," Not Spongiform Degeneration				
Bovine				
Polled Hereford	Myoclonus	Birth	No lesion; deficiency of glycine, strychnine receptors	51, 52

maple syrup urine disease in man, one of several disorders of amino acid metabolism. The disease appears to be inherited as an autosomal recessive trait. The exact nature of the amino acid abnormality is not known. Neuraxial edema has also been reported in conjunction with hypomyelinogenesis in Hereford calves, but subsequent studies demonstrated that this was hypomyelinogenesis.[42,53]

Spongy Degeneration. A group of diseases characterized by intra- and extracellular vacuoles in either gray matter, white matter, or both produce a variety of signs including ataxia and tremor, spasticity, opisthotonos, and myoclonus. Table 11–5 lists the diseases described in dogs, cats, and cattle.[42,51,52,54–58] All of these syndromes occur in neonatal animals except the one described in Labrador retrievers. Congenital, infantile, and juvenile forms are described in humans.[55] Some of these diseases, such as maple syrup urine disease, are related to abnormal amino acid metabolism and can be managed in a limited way by controlling dietary intake of certain amino acids. All of these syndromes are rare.

Familial Reflex Myoclonus in Labrador Retrievers. A myoclonic syndrome of a group of Labrador retrievers has many characteristics of the congenital myoclonus in Hereford cattle.[59] The abnormality was recognized at 3 weeks of age. Clinical, laboratory, electrophysiologic, and tissue evaluations were done at 6 weeks of age. The pups were unable to rise without assistance. The extensor muscle tone was increased, but neurologic examination was normal otherwise. There was increased resistance to manipulation of the limbs or neck. Muscles were of normal size and there was no dimpling on percussion. The characteristic finding was increased muscle contraction with any tactile or auditory stimulus, or to voluntary activity. The muscle activity included all four limbs, opisthotonos, and contractures of the muscles of facial expression and the muscles of mastication. Laboratory values were normal. EMG showed large motor unit potentials (up to 5,000 μV), and a stereotyped set of three evoked compound muscle action potentials in response to a tactile stimulus. Normal dogs had no response to the same stimulus. Muscle biopsies were normal. Necropsy revealed mild esophageal dilation, but no other gross or histologic lesions. The authors suggest a similarity to the spastic mutant mouse that has a deficiency in glycine receptors.[59] We have examined one Labrador pup with a similar clinical presentation. No gross or histologic lesions were seen at necropsy.

Idiopathic

"Tic" in a Horse. A myoclonic twitch in the thoracic limb of a horse occurred following an unknown traumatic accident.[60] The limb was stiff and lame and had swelling and abrasions of the distal portions. A week following the injury a twitch developed in the triceps and latissimus dorsi muscles. The contractions were at a relatively constant rate of about 30 to 60 per minute. All tests were negative. A large number of drugs were tried, with no improvement. The twitch disappeared in 11 weeks.

Inflammation

Canine Distemper Myoclonus. The most common involuntary movement disorder recognized in domestic animals for many years occurs secondary to canine distemper. The syndrome was recognized and described as early as 1862.[61] It has been called chorea and the flexor spasm syndrome. Chorea is continual, irregular, rapid jerky movements of varying groups of muscles. Myoclonus is repetitive, rhythmic contractions of the same group of muscles.[3] The more appropriate term for the syndrome following distemper is myoclonus. Any group of muscles may be affected. Frequently it is confined to the flexor group in one limb, but myoclonus of combinations of muscle groups in more than one limb, facial muscles, or the muscles of mastication are also seen. The syndrome may occur before, during, or after the overt encephalitis typical of distemper. Most often it is a later developing sequela that may persist after all other clinical signs have resolved.[61] The myoclonus often persists during sleep and light anesthesia.

Experimental studies have demonstrated that the abnormality lies in the spinal cord or brain stem segment in intrinsic neural circuits.[62] Sectioning the spinal cord cranial and caudal to the segments containing the LMN to the affected muscle groups does not abolish the response, nor does sectioning the dorsal roots. Sectioning the ventral roots does eliminate it.[62] There is no effective pharmacologic treatment. Anticonvulsants have no benefit. Fortunately, the decreased incidence of canine distemper with modern vaccination programs makes this syndrome a relatively rare occurrence. Some individual animals seem to improve with time. If the myoclonus does not interfere with eating or locomotion, the dog can live with it.

CASE HISTORIES

Case History 11A

Signalment

Canine, Maltese, male, 4 years old.

History

Owner noticed shaking 3 days ago. She thought the dog was cold, but the shaking has persisted. The shaking abates when the dog sleeps, but is otherwise always present to some degree. The dog seems to feel good otherwise, and appetite and eliminations are normal.

Physical Examination

Normal except for a fine tremor.

Neurologic Examination

Normal except for the shaking, which is a fine tremor of the limbs, head, and trunk. The tremor is accentuated when the dog gets excited or starts to move, and tends to subside at rest. The gait is slightly ataxic and dysmetric. All postural reactions, spinal reflexes, cranial nerves, and sensation are normal.

Complete sections G and H before reviewing Case Summary.

G. Assessment (Anatomic diagnosis and estimation of prognosis)

H. Plan (Diagnostic)

Rule-outs	*Procedure*
1.	
2.	
3.	
4.	

Case History 11B

Signalment

Bovine, Holstein-Friesian, female, 9 months old.

History

A lameness developed in the right pelvic limb at 6 months of age and has gradually progressed.

Physical Examination

The animal is normal except for lameness in the right pelvic limb. The gait is hindered by inability to flex the limb. The stifle and hock are extended and do not flex at gait. The joints are normal on palpation.

Neurologic Examination

Normal except for the right pelvic limb. There is increased tone in the gastrocnemius muscle. The limb cannot be flexed. Sensation to the limb is normal.

Complete sections G and H before reviewing Case Summary.

G. Assessment (Anatomic diagnosis and estimation of prognosis)

H. Plan (Diagnostic)

Rule-outs	*Procedure*
1.	
2.	
3.	
4.	

Case History 11C

Signalment

Canine, chow chow, female, 3 months old.

History

The puppy had a lameness of several weeks' duration. The owners reported the puppy seemed to tire easily. She was one of five in a litter; the others are normal.

Physical Examination

All systems were normal, except the puppy was unusually well muscled.

Neurologic Examination

A. Observation
   1. Mental status: Alert.
   2. Posture: The limbs were abducted and the joints were straighter than normal.
   3. Gait: The pup had some difficulty getting up. The gait was stiff. The thoracic limbs were abducted and rotated medially. The pelvic limbs were dragged the first few steps, then were abducted. After a few steps the gait improved.

   The remainder of the neurologic examination was normal.

G. Assessment (Anatomic diagnosis and estimation of prognosis)

H. Plan (Diagnostic)

Rule-outs	*Procedure*
1.	
2.	
3.	
4.	

Assessment 11A

Anatomic diagnosis. The tremor is characteristic of a cerebellar intention tremor. However, the animal has minimal ataxia and severe tremor, which is not characteristic of most cerebellar diseases. A more generalized disorder should be considered. Because of the breed, idiopathic cerebellitis is a likely possibility.

Diagnostic plan. Two options are available, an aggressive approach, including CSF analysis, EEG, and possibly CT, or a trial on corticosteroids to rule out idiopathic cerebellitis. The owners chose to be aggressive. Hematology, serum chemistries, and urinalysis were normal. Skull radiographs were normal. CSF analysis disclosed a protein concentration of 20 mg/dl, a total WBC count of 9 cells, and a differential cell count of 95% lymphocytes and 5% monocytes.

The WBC count is slightly high (normal, <5 cells), but everything else is normal.

Therapeutic plan. A trial of corticosteroids, prednisolone (2 mg/kg twice daily), was given for 1 week. The clinical signs resolved. The dose was cut in half for one week, and then reduced to 0.5 mg/kg every other day for 2 weeks. Medication was stopped, and tremors recurred in 3 days. Alternate-day dosage was resumed, with remission of signs. Medication was stopped again after 3 weeks, with no recurrence of signs.

Case summary. The decision to pursue aggressive diagnostic procedures should be made by the owner. The possibility of exacerbating an infectious disease with corticosteroids must be considered when a therapeutic trial is considered. Idiopathic cerebellitis responds to treatment, but relapses are common.

Assessment 11B

Anatomic diagnosis. The lack of neurologic deficits other than increased tone in the gastrocnemius muscle is significant. Other diseases that must be considered are arthropathies, including infections and arthrogryposis, and upward fixation of the patella.

1. Spastic paresis: Local anesthetic block of the tibial nerve should relieve the lameness temporarily, as it did in this case. The other diseases would not be improved with this procedure.

Therapeutic plan. Tibial neuroectomy, either partial or total, provides relief of the signs. The primary branches supplying the gastrocnemius muscle were transected. These were identified by electrical stimulation during surgery.

Case summary. The calf had a relatively normal gait in 5 days. (Case from Yamada H, et al: A successful case of spastic paresis in a calf by partial tibial neurectomy. Jpn J Vet Sci 51:213–214, 1989.)

Assessment 11C

Anatomic diagnosis. The increased tone in all muscles of the limbs with no neurologic deficits suggests a muscle disease. Increased size of the musculature, some improvement after moving, and the breed should suggest congenital myotonia. Other possibilities include myositis, and other myopathies.

1. Muscle disease: Creatine phosphokinase (CK) was increased. Other laboratory values were normal. EMG disclosed prolonged insertion activity that increased and then decreased in amplitude and frequency. Percussion of muscles, including the tongue, caused prolonged contraction, producing a dimple. Nerve conduction velocities were normal. Muscle biopsies showed hypertrophy and a few atrophic fibers. These findings are consistent with myotonia.

Therapeutic plan. The pup was treated with procainamide, which partially relieved the signs. A trial with phenytoin resulted in no improvement.

Case summary. Congenital myotonia is an inherited disease in chow chows. Treatment relieves the signs to some degree, but a cure is not available. (Case from Amann JF, Tomlinson J, Hankison JK: Myotonia in a chow chow. J Am Vet Med Assoc 187:415–417, 1985.)

REFERENCES

1. Thach WT, Montgomery EB: Motor system. In Pearlman AL, Collins RC (eds): Neurological Pathophysiology. New York, Oxford University Press, 1984, pp 151–178.

2. Taylor EJ: Dorland's Illustrated Medical Dictionary. Philadelphia, WB Saunders, 1988.
3. Hallett M, Ravits J: Involuntary movements. In Asbury AK, McKhann GM, McDonald WI (eds): Diseases of the Nervous System. Philadelphia, Ardmore Medical Books, 1986, pp 452–460.
4. Liles SL, Davis GD: Athetoid and choreiform hyperkinesias produced by caudate lesions in the cat. Science 164:195–197, 1969.
5. Bleck T: Pharmacology of tetanus. Clin Neuropharmacol 9:103–120, 1986.
6. Luttgen PJ: An outline of neurotransmitters and neurotransmission: Part II. Function and dysfunction. J Am Anim Hosp Assoc 23:663–673, 1987.
7. Kornegay JN, Mayhew IG: Metabolic, toxic, and nutritional diseases of the nervous system. In Oliver JE, Hoerlein BF, Mayhew IG: Veterinary Neurology. Philadelphia, WB Saunders, 1987, pp 255–277.
8. Furman RE, Barchi RL: Pathophysiology of myotonia and periodic paralysis. In Asbury AK, McKhann GM, McDonald WI (eds): Diseases of the Nervous System. Philadelphia, Ardmore Medical Books, 1986, pp 208–226.
9. Roberts TDM: Neurophysiology of Postural Mechanisms. New York, Plenum Press, 1967.
10. Timoney JF, Gillespie JH, Scott FW, et al: Hagan and Bruner's Microbiology and Infectious Diseases of Domestic Animals. Ithaca, Comstock Publishing Associates, 1988.
11. Panciera DL, Baldwin CJ, Keene BW: Electrocardiographic abnormalities associated with tetanus in two dogs. J Am Vet Med Assoc 192:225–227, 1988.
12. Mayhew IG: Large Animal Neurology: A Handbook for Veterinary Clinicians. Philadelphia, Lea & Febiger, 1989.
13. Grauer GF, Hjelle JJ: Section 16. Toxicology. In Morgan RV (ed): Handbook of Small Animal Practice. New York, Churchill Livingstone, 1988, pp 1081–1128.
14. Duncan ID, Griffiths I: Neuromuscular diseases. In Kornegay JN (ed): Neurologic Disorders. New York, Churchill Livingstone, 1986.
15. Denniston JC, Shive RJ, Friedli U, et al: Spastic paresis syndrome in calves. J Am Vet Med Assoc 152:1138–1149, 1968.
16. de Lahunta A: Veterinary Neuroanatomy and Clinical Neurology, 2nd ed. Philadelphia, WB Saunders, 1983.
17. DeLey G, DeMoor A: Bovine spastic paralysis: Cerebrospinal fluid concentrations of homovanillic acid and 5-hydroxyindoleacetic acid in normal and spastic calves. Am J Vet Res 36:227–228, 1975.
18. Wells GAH, Hawkins SAC, O'Toole DT, et al: Spastic syndrome in a Holstein bull: A histologic study. Vet Pathol 24:345–353, 1987.
19. Palmer AC: Introduction to Animal Neurology, 2nd ed. Oxford, England, Blackwell Scientific Publishing, 1976.
20. Cahill JI, Goulden BE, Pearce HG: A review and some observations on stringhalt. NZ Vet J 33:101–104, 1985.
21. Meyers KM, Padgett GA, Dickson WM: The genetic basis of a kinetic disorder of Scottish terrier dogs. J Hered 61:189–192, 1970.
22. Clemmons RM, Peters RI, Meyers KM: Scotty cramp: A review of cause, characteristics, diagnosis and treatment. Comp Cont Educ Pract Vet 2:385–390, 1980.
23. McEwen S, Hulland T: Histochemical and morphometric evaluation of skeletal muscle from horses with exertional rhabdomyolysis (tying-up). Vet Pathol 23:400–410, 1986.
24. Braund KG: Diseases of peripheral nerves, cranial nerves, and muscle. In Oliver JE, Hoerlein BF, Mayhew IG: Veterinary Neurology. Philadelphia, WB Saunders, 1987, pp 353–392.
25. Cuddon PA: Tremor syndromes. Prog Vet Neurol 1:285–299, 1990.
26. Parker AJ: How do I treat? "Little white shakers." Prog Vet Neurol 2:151, 1991.
27. Duncan I: Abnormalities of myelination of the central nervous system associated with congenital tremor. J Vet Intern Med 1:10–23, 1987.
28. Duncan I: Congenital tremor and abnormalities of myelination. In: Proceedings of an ACVIM Forum, San Diego, 1987, pp 869–872.
29. Done J: The congenital tremor syndrome in pigs. Vet Ann 16:98–102, 1975.
30. Done JT, Bradley R: Nervous and muscular system. In Leman AD (ed): Diseases of Swine. Ames, Iowa, Iowa State University Press, 1985.
31. Emmerson JL, Delez AL: Cerebellar hypoplasia, hypomyelinogenesis and congenital tremors of pigs associated with prenatal hog cholera vaccination of sows. J Am Vet Med Assoc 147:47–54, 1965.
32. Braund KG: Degenerative and developmental diseases. In Oliver JE, Hoerlein BF, Mayhew IG (eds): Veterinary Neurology. Philadelphia, WB Saunders, 1987, pp 185–215.
33. Foulkes JA: Myelin and dysmyelination in domestic animals. Vet Bull 8:441–450, 1974.
34. Done JT: Congenital nervous diseases of pigs: A review. Lab Animal 2:207–217, 1968.
35. Done J, Woolley J, Upcott D, et al: Porcine congenital tremor type AII: Spinal cord morphometry. Br Vet J 142:145, 1986.
36. Harding JDJ, Done JT, Harbourne JF, et al: Congenital tremor type A III in pigs: An hereditary sex-linked cerebrospinal hypomyelinogenesis. Vet Rec 92:527–529, 1973.
37. Patterson DSP, Sweasey D, Brush PJ, et al: Neurochemistry of the spinal cord in British saddleback piglets affected with congenital tremor type A-IV, a second form of hereditary cerebrospinal hypomyelingenesis. J Neurochem 21:397–406, 1973.
38. Saperstein G, Leipold HW, Dennis SM: Congenital defects in sheep. J Am Vet Med Assoc 167:324–322, 1974.
39. Clarke GL, Osburn BI: Transmissible congenital demyelinating encephalopathy of lambs. Vet Pathol 15:68–82, 1978.
40. Saunders LZ, Sweet JD, Martin SM, et al: Hereditary congenital ataxia in Jersey calves. Cornell Vet 42:559–591, 1952.
41. Hulland TJ: Cerebellar ataxia in calves. Can J Comp Med 21:72–76, 1957.
42. Duffell S: Neuraxial oedema of Hereford calves with and without hypomyelinogenesis. Vet Rec 117:95–98, 1986.
43. Hocking AD: Intoxication by tremorgenic mycotoxin (pentrem A) in a dog. Aust Vet J 65:82–85, 1988.
44. Dollahite JW, Younger RL, Crookshank HR, et al: Chronic lead poisoning in horses. Am J Vet Res 39:961–964, 1978.
45. Zook BC, Carpenter JL, Leeds EB: Lead poisoning in dogs. J Am Vet Med Assoc 155:1329–1342, 1969.
46. Knecht CD, Crabtree J, Katherman A: Clinical, clinicopathologic, and electroencephalographic features of lead poisoning in dogs. J Am Vet Med Assoc 175:196–201, 1979.
47. Scott DW, Bolton GR, Lorenz MD: Hexachlorophene toxicosis in dogs. J Am Vet Med Assoc 162:947–949, 1973.
48. Thompson J, Senior D, Pinson D, et al: Neurotoxicosis associated with the use of hexachlorophene in a cat. J Am Vet Med Assoc 190:1311–1312, 1987.
49. Ward BC, Jones BD, Rubin GJ: Hexachlorophene toxicity in dogs. J Am Anim Hosp Assoc 9:167–169, 1973.
50. Bath ML: Hexachlorophene toxicity in dogs. J Small Anim Pract 19:241–244, 1978.
51. Healy P, Harper P, Dennis J: Diagnosis of neuraxial oedema in calves. Aust Vet J 63:95–96, 1986.

52. Gundlach AL, Dodd PR, Grabara CSG, et al: Deficit of spinal cord glycine/strychnine receptors in inherited myoclonus of poll hereford calves. Science 241:1807–1810, 1988.
53. Duffell SA, Harper PAW, Healy PJ, et al: Congenital hypomyelinogenesis of Hereford calves. Vet Rec 123:423–424, 1988.
54. O'Brien DP, Zachary JF: Clinical features of spongy degeneration of the central nervous system in two Labrador retriever littermates. J Am Vet Med Assoc 186:1207–1210, 1985.
55. Zachary JF, O'Brien DP: Spongy degeneration of the central nervous system in two canine littermates. Vet Pathol 22:561–571, 1985.
56. Luttgen PJ, Storts RW: Central nervous system status spongiosus. In: Proceedings of an ACVIM Forum, San Diego 1987, p 841.
57. Braund K: Clinical Syndromes in Veterinary Neurology. Baltimore, Williams & Wilkins, 1986.
58. Kelly DF, Gaskell CJ: Spongy degeneration of the central nervous system in kittens. Acta Neuropathol 35:151–158, 1976.
59. Fox JG, Averill DR, Hallett M, et al: Familial reflex myoclonus in Labrador retrievers. Am J Vet Res 45:2367–2370, 1984.
60. Beech J: Forelimb tic in a horse. J Am Vet Med Assoc 180:258–260, 1982.
61. Whittier JW: Flexor spasm syndrome in the carnivore. Am J Vet Res 17:720–732, 1956.
62. Breazile JE, Blaugh BS, Nail N: Experimental study of canine distemper myoclonus. Am J Vet Res 27:1375–1379, 1966.
63. Shores A, Redding RW, Braund KG, et al: Myotonia congenita in a chow chow pup. J Am Vet Med Assoc 188:532–533, 1986.
64. Braund KG: Identifying degenerative and developmental myopathies. Vet Med 81:713–718, 1986.
65. Shelton G, Cardinet H: Pathophysiologic basis of canine muscle disorders. J Vet Intern Med 1:36–44, 1987.
66. Farrow BRH: Canine myotonia. In: Proceedings of the Sixth Annual Veterinary Medical Forum, 1988, pp 64–66.
67. Nafe LA, Shires P: Myotonia in the dog. In: Proceedings of an ACVIM Forum, 1984, pp 191–192.
68. Jones BR, Anderson LJ, Barnes GRG, et al: Myotonia in related chow chow dogs. NZ Vet J 25:217–220, 1977.
69. Farrow BRH, Malik R: Hereditary myotonia in the chow chow. J Small Anim Pract 22:451–465, 1981.
70. Shires PK, Nafe LA, Hulse DA: Myotonia in a Staffordshire terrier. J Am Vet Med Assoc 183:229–232, 1983.
71. Simpson ST, Braund KG: Myotonic dystrophy-like disease in a dog. J Am Vet Med Assoc 186:495–498, 1985.
72. Wright JA, Smyth JBA, Brownlie SE, et al: A myopathy associated with muscle hypertonicity in the cavalier King Charles spaniel. J Comp Pathol 97:559–565, 1987.
73. Honhold N, Smith DA: Myotonia in the Great Dane. Vet Rec 119:162, 1986.
74. Wentink GH, van der Linde-Sipman JS, Meijer AEF, et al: Myopathy with a possible recessive X-linked inheritance in a litter of Irish terriers. Vet Pathol 9:328–349, 1972.
75. Bryant SH: Altered membrane potentials in myotonia. In Bolis L, Hoffman LA (eds): Membranes and Diseases. New York, Raven Press, 1976.
76. Bryant SH: Myotonia in the goat. Ann NY Acad Sci 317:314–325, 1979.
77. Atkinson JB, LeQuire VS: Myotonia congenita. Comp Pathol Bull 17:3–4, 1985.
78. Steinberg S, Bothelo S: Myotonia in a horse. Science 137:979, 1962.
79. Griffiths IR, Duncan ID, McCulloch M, et al: Shaking pups: A disorder of central myelination in the spaniel dog. Part 1. Clinical, genetic, and light microscopical observations. J Neurol Sci 50:423–433, 1981.
80. Farrow BRH: Tremor syndromes in dogs. In: Proceedings of the Sixth Annual Veterinary Medical Forum, Washington, DC, 1988, pp 57–60.
81. Vandevelde M, Braund K, Luttgen PJ, et al: Dysmyelination in chow chow dogs: Further studies in older dogs. Acta Neuropathol 55:81–87, 1981.
82. Vandevelde M, Braund KG, Walker T, et al: Dysmyelination of the central nervous system in the chow-chow dog. Acta Neuropathol 42:211–215, 1978.
83. Duncan I: Congenital tremor and abnormalities of myelination. In: Proceedings of the Fifth Annual Veterinary Medical Forum, San Diego, 1987, pp 869–873.
84. Farrow B: Generalized tremor syndrome. In Kirk RW (ed): Current Veterinary Therapy. IX. Philadelphia, WB Saunders, 1986.
85. Cummings J, Summers B, de Lahunta A, et al: Tremors in Samoyed pups with oligodendrocyte deficiencies and hypomyelination. Acta Neuropathol 71:267–277, 1986.
86. Kornegay J: Hypomyelination in weimaraner dogs. Acta Neuropathol 72:394–401, 1987.
87. Comont PSV, Palmer AC, Williams AE: Weakness associated with myelopathy in a weimaraner puppy. J Small Anim Pract 29:367–372, 1988.
88. Kornegay JN: Dysmyelinogenesis in dogs. In: Proceedings of the Third Annual Medical Forum, ACVIM, San Diego, 1985.
89. Palmer A, Blakemore W, Wallace M, et al: Recognition of 'trembler', a hypomyelination condition in the bernese mountain dog. Vet Rec 120:609–612, 1987.
90. Mayhew IG, Blakemore WF, Palmer AC, et al: Tremor syndromes and hypomyelination in Lurcher pups. J Small Anim Pract 25:551–559, 1984.
91. Greene CE, Vandevelde M, Hoff EJ: Congenital cerebrospinal hypomyelinogenesis in a pup. J Am Vet Med Assoc 171:534–536, 1977.
92. Young S: Hypomyelinogenesis congenita (cerebellar ataxia) in Angus–Shorthorn calves. Cornell Vet 52:84–93, 1962.

12

Blindness, Anisocoria, and Abnormal Eye Movements

Problems related to abnormalities of the eyes and the visual pathways are especially useful in the formulation of a neurologic diagnosis.[1] The retina and the optic nerve are the only sensory receptors and the only nerve that can be examined directly. The sensory and motor pathways of vision and eye movements traverse the brain from the orbit to the occipital region of the cerebral cortex and the medulla oblongata, so that diseases affecting the brain are likely to affect some portion of the visual system. The retina is often affected by systemic diseases.

Lesion Localization

The visual system will be considered in three parts: (1) vision, (2) pupillary light reflexes, and (3) eye movements. Combinations of abnormal signs should lead to an anatomic diagnosis.

Vision

The visual pathways are presented in Figures 12–1 and 12–2. Methods of testing vision were discussed in Chapter 1. Lesions of the lateral geniculate nucleus of the thalamus, the optic radiation (fiber tracts), or the occipital cortex cause a loss of sight without affecting pupillary reflexes (Table 12–1). Many of these lesions are unilateral, resulting in a loss of vision in the contralateral field. Bilateral lesions, such as may occur with encephalitis or hydrocephalus, cause complete blindness. Lesions of the retina, the optic nerve, the optic chiasm, or the optic tracts will cause blindness and pupillary abnormalities (see Fig. 12–1). Optic chiasm lesions almost always cause bilateral blindness. Retinal and optic nerve lesions are frequently bilateral (e.g., retinal atrophy, optic neuritis) but may be unilateral (e.g., trauma, neoplasia). Optic tract lesions causing clinical signs are rare.

The degree of decussation of optic nerve fibers at the optic chiasm varies in different species. As a rule, the more lateral the eyes are placed in the skull, the greater the degree of decussation. In primates, essentially all of the fibers from the nasal half of the retina cross, whereas all of the fibers from the temporal half of the retina remain ipsilateral. In carnivores, approximately one half of the fibers of the temporal retina cross, and all of the nasal retinal fibers cross. In most herbivores 80% or more of the fibers cross. Rabbits have almost all crossed fibers. Therefore, visual field testing may be of importance for lesion localization in dogs and cats, but each eye can be considered to have an independent pathway in other domestic animals.

Assessment of the visual field is difficult. The usual methods of the menace and visual placing reactions test the lateral field and the crossing fibers. Deficits in these responses that are central to the optic chiasm are usually on the contralateral side of the brain.

Caution must be exercised in the interpretation of visual deficits. Because the examiner must rely on motor or behavioral reactions, he or she should use several tests to confirm an

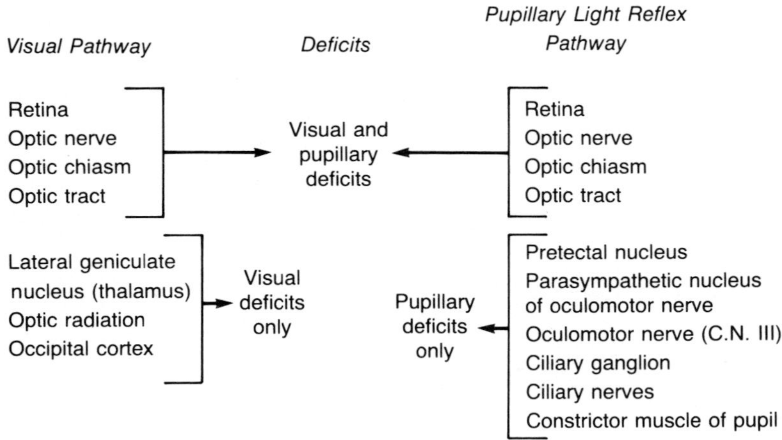

Figure 12–1 Deficits from lesions of the visual and pupillary light reflex pathways.

impression that the animal does not see. See Chapter 1 for details.

Pupillary Light Reflexes

The pathway for pupillary light reflexes is outlined and illustrated in Figures 12–1 to 12–3 and in Table 12–1. The methods of testing pupillary reflexes have been described in Chapter 1.

Lesions of cranial nerve (CN) III (the oculomotor nerve, including the ciliary ganglion and the short ciliary nerves) or of the constrictor muscle of the pupil cause loss of pupillary constriction in response to light on the affected side without affecting vision. Bilateral lesions are unusual except in lesions of the brain stem. Lesions of the pretectal nucleus or the parasympathetic nucleus of CN III cause loss of pupillary constriction. Usually both eyes are affected, because the nuclei are anatomically close together in the brain stem. Lesions of the retina, the optic nerve, or the optic chiasm cause loss of constriction of the pupil on the affected side in response to direct stimulation, but the pupil reacts to light shined in the opposite eye. Vision is impaired in the affected eye (see Table 12–1).

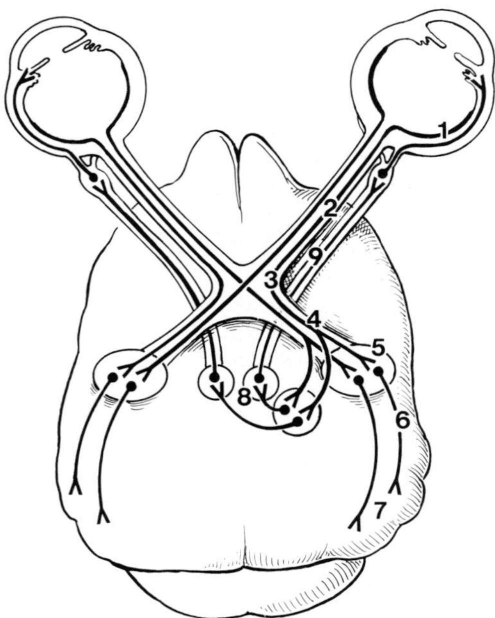

Figure 12–2 Pathways for vision and the pupillary light reflex pathway.

The sympathetic control of the dilator muscle of the pupil is illustrated in Figure 12–3. Sympathetic activation is produced by emotional reactions, such as fear and rage. The sympathetic nerves also innervate smooth muscle in the periorbital fascia and the eyelids, including the third eyelid in some species. Lesions of this pathway cause a constricted pupil (miosis), a slight retraction of the globe because of loss of tone in the periorbita (enophthalmos), a narrowing of the palpebral fissure (ptosis), and extrusion of the third eyelid.[2] Sweating of the ipsilateral face is seen in horses.[3] This cluster of signs is called Horner's syndrome. Horner's syndrome usually is not associated with visual deficits. Localization is dependent on associated clinical signs. For example, avulsion of the brachial plexus may cause a monoparesis and Horner's syndrome on the same side. T1–T3 spinal cord lesions cause upper motor neuron (UMN) signs in the pelvic limb, lower motor neuron (LMN) signs in the thoracic limb, and Horner's syndrome. Middle ear disease is frequently associated with Horner's syndrome in the dog because the sympathetic fibers pass through the tympanic bulla. Guttural pouch infections may cause Horner's syndrome in horses.

TABLE 12–1 Signs of Lesions in the Visual Pathways

Complete Lesion on Right Side	Vision		Resting Pupil		Pupillary Light Reflex	
	Right Eye	Left Eye	Right Eye	Left Eye	Light in Right Eye	Light in Left Eye
1. Retina or optic nerve	Absent	Normal	Slightly dilated	Normal	No response	Both constrict
2. Orbit (CN II, III)	Absent	Normal	Dilated	Normal	No response	Left constricts
3. Optic chiasm (bilateral)*	Absent	Absent	Dilated	Dilated	No response	No response
4. Optic tract	Normal	Absent†	Normal	Normal or slightly dilated	Both constrict	Both constrict
5. Lateral geniculate nucleus	Normal	Absent†	Normal	Normal	Both constrict	Both constrict
6. Optic radiation	Normal	Absent†	Normal	Normal	Both constrict	Both constrict
7. Occipital cortex	Normal	Absent†	Normal	Normal	Both constrict	Both constrict
8. Parasympathetic nucleus of CN III (bilateral)*	Normal	Normal	Dilated	Dilated	No response	No response
9. Oculomotor nerve	Normal	Normal	Dilated	Normal	Left constricts	Left constricts
10. Sympathetic nerve	Normal	Normal	Constricted	Normal	Both constrict	Both constrict

* Unilateral lesions of these structures are rare.
† Possibly loss of sight in left visual field with partial sparing of right visual field.

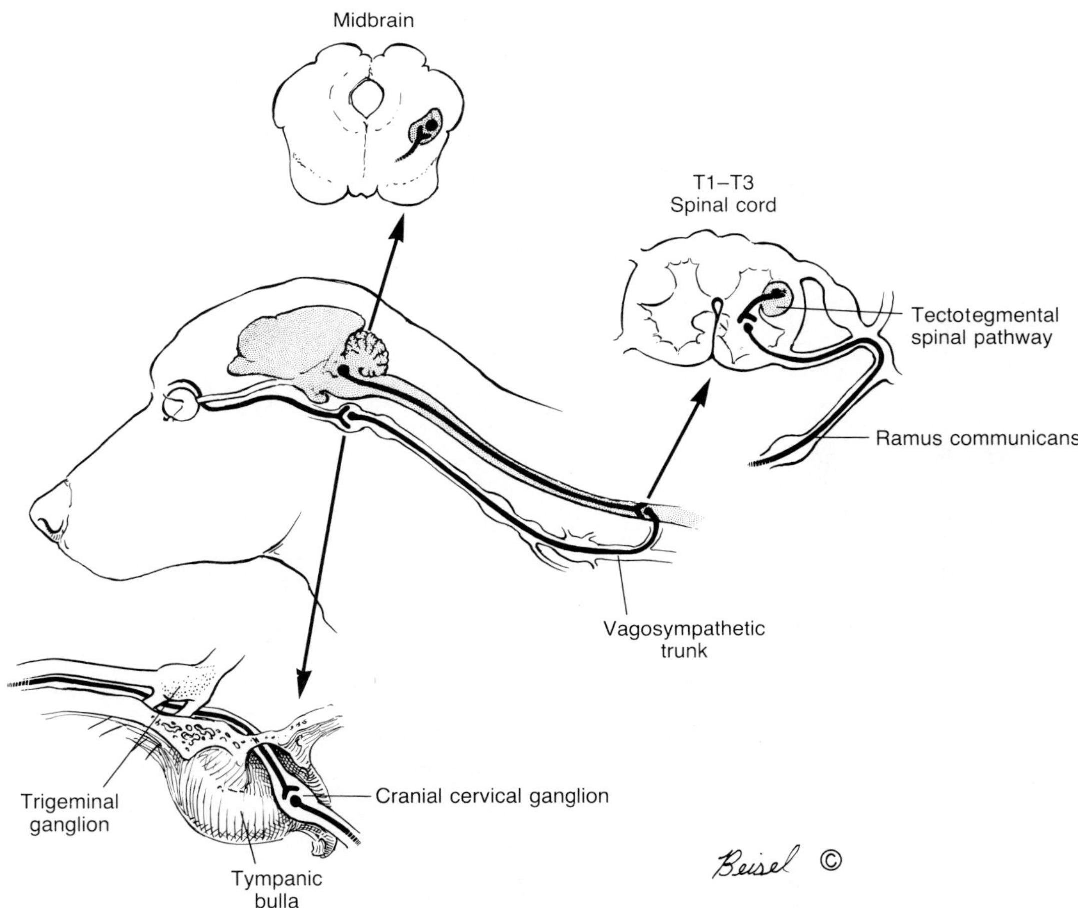

Figure 12–3 Pathway of sympathetic innervation of the eye. (From Greene CE, Oliver JE Jr: Neurologic examination. In Ettinger SE (ed): Textbook of Veterinary Internal Medicine, 2nd ed. Philadelphia, WB Saunders, 1982. Used by permission.)

Differentiation of pre- and postganglionic lesions can be determined in the first few weeks of Horner's syndrome. Instillation of 1% hydroxyamphetamine causes good dilation of a normal eye or one with a preganglionic lesion, but minimal dilation of an eye with a postganglionic lesion. Instillation of 10% phenylephrine causes minimal dilation of a normal eye or one with a presynaptic lesion, but good dilation of an eye with a postganglionic lesion.[1,2]

Eye Movements

The extraocular eye muscles are innervated by CN III (oculomotor), CN IV (trochlear), and CN VI (abducent) (Fig. 12–4). Eye movements are

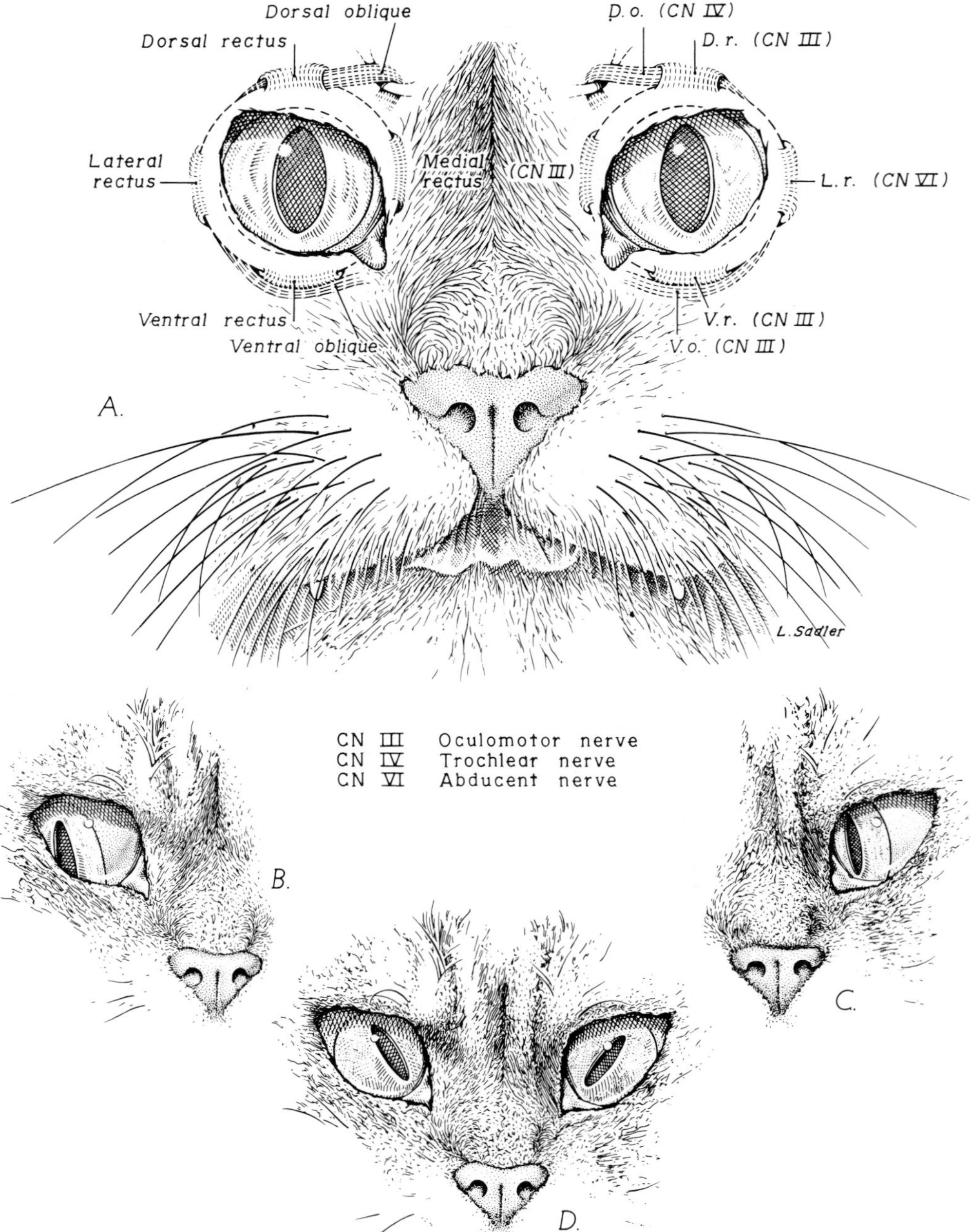

Figure 12–4 Functional anatomy of the extraocular muscles. *A*. Direction of strabismus following paralysis of the oculomotor (*B*), abducent (*C*), and trochlear (*D*) neurons. (From de Lahunta A: Veterinary Neuroanatomy and Clinical Neurology. Philadelphia, WB Saunders, 1977. Used by permission.)

controlled by UMNs from the cerebral cortex and through brain stem vestibular reflexes. The eye muscles normally act in a synergistic or antagonistic manner to provide coordinated conjugate movements. The testing of eye movements has been discussed in Chapter 1. Abnormalities of eye movements include paralysis of gaze in a direction related to a muscle or a group of muscles; strabismus, or deviation of the globe; loss of conjugate movements; and nystagmus.

When the globe is fixed, regardless of head position, a lesion of CN III, CN IV, or CN VI is suspected. Lesions of the trochlear nerve (CN IV) may cause a slight rotation of the globe, which is difficult to evaluate in animals that have a round pupil (see Fig. 12–4).[4] Lesions of CN III cause a ventrolateral strabismus, and lesions of CN VI cause a medial strabismus. Several weeks after an injury the globe may return to its normal midposition, but there is loss of movement dorsally, medially, and ventrally with a lesion of CN III and laterally with a lesion of CN VI (see Fig. 12—4). Positional strabismus (dysconjugate deviation of the eye in certain head positions) is characteristic of lesions of the vestibular system. Typically, the eye ipsilateral to the vestibular abnormality is ventral in the palpebral fissure when the nose is elevated. In this case, eye movements can be elicited in all directions by appropriate movements of the head, demonstrating that all extraocular muscles are functional (see Chap. 9). Both eyes tend to maintain a horizontal position in large animals; therefore they are ventrally placed when the head is elevated, although the affected side may be deviated relative to the normal side.

The function of the extraocular muscles has not been established in large animals. It is assumed that the movements and the physiologic deficits produced after lesions of the cranial nerves are similar to those that occur in other species.[5]

Conjugate eye movements require coordination of the three cranial nerves and their muscles. The pathway responsible for this coordination is the medial longitudinal fasciculus (MLF), which runs in the center of the brain stem from the vestibular nuclei to the nuclei of CN III, CN IV, and CN VI. Lesions of the MLF may cause dysconjugate movements or, more commonly, a lack of eye movements in response to moving the head (internuclear ophthalmoplegia). Lesions of the MLF are seen most commonly after an acute head injury that produces hemorrhage in the center of the brain stem (see Chap. 13). Ophthalmoplegia has also been reported from thyroid adenocarcinoma invading the cavernous sinus intracranially and affecting the three cranial nerves.[6]

Nystagmus is involuntary rhythmic movement of the eyes. Normal nystagmus may be visual in origin (for example, watching telephone poles go by from a moving car) or it may be vestibular in origin (for example, turning the head rapidly). The visual and vestibular types are called jerk nystagmus, because there is a slow phase to one side followed by a rapid recovery movement (jerk). The direction of the nystagmus is classified according to the fast component. Nystagmus also is categorized by the direction of the movement (horizontal, vertical, or rotatory) and according to whether it changes direction with varying head positions. Jerk nystagmus that is horizontal or rotatory and that does not change direction with varying head positions is indicative of peripheral vestibular disease. All other forms of jerk nystagmus are associated with central vestibular

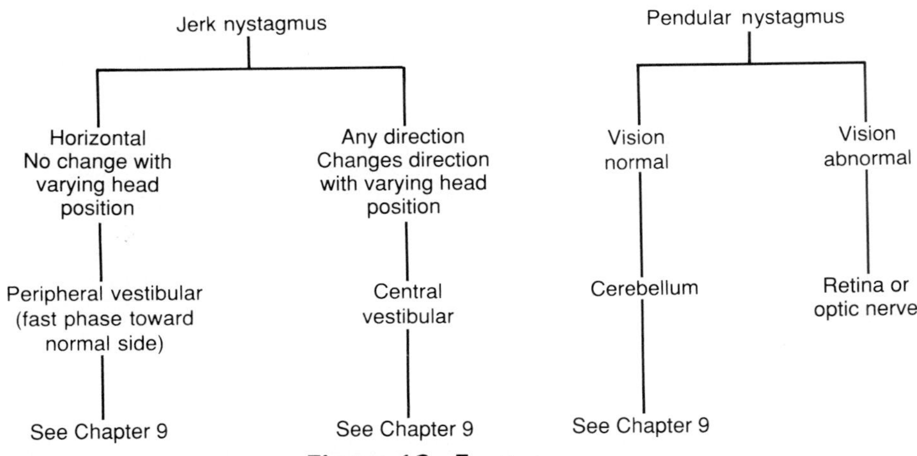

Figure 12–5 Nystagmus.

brain stem lesions (including lesions of the flocculonodular lobe of the cerebellum) (Fig. 12–5; see also Chap. 9).

A less frequently seen form, called pendular nystagmus, consists of small oscillations of the eye that do not have fast and slow components. Pendular nystagmus usually is seen with cerebellar disease and is most pronounced during fixation of the gaze. It may also be seen in animals with visual deficits.

Except for lesions of the globe and the orbit, most diseases affecting the visual system produce other clinical signs that are related to abnormal function of surrounding structures. For example, masses affecting the optic chiasm or the optic tracts usually affect hypothalamic function. Lesions of CN III, CN IV, or CN VI cause other brain stem signs. Lesions of the occipital cortex affect other cerebral functions. The combination of signs defines the location of the lesion.

Diseases

The most common diseases causing clinical signs of blindness, pupillary abnormalities, and ocular movement disorders are mentioned in Tables 12–2 through 12–4. Many diseases cause abnormality in more than one of these func-

TABLE 12–2 Etiology of Blindness*

Disease Category	*Nonprogressive*	*Acute Progressive*	*Chronic Progressive*
Degenerative			Storage diseases (R, C) (16) Retinal degenerations (R) Demyelinating diseases (O, C) (16)
Anomalous	Hypoplasia (O) Coloboma (O) Retinal dysplasia (R) Collie eye syndrome (R) Cerebral malformations (C) (13)		Hydrocephalus (C) (13)
Metabolic	Hyperthermia (C) (16) Hypoxia (C) (13)	Hypoglycemia (C) (13) Hepatic encephalopathy	Hypoglycemia (C) (13) Hepatic encephalopathy (C) (13)
Neoplastic (16)		Lymphosarcoma (R) Malignant melanoma (R)	1. Primary (16) a. Pituitary adenoma (O, X, C) b. Meningioma (O, X, C) c. Gliomas (O, X, C) d. Ependymoma (C) e. Choroid plexus papilloma (C) 2. Metastatic (R, O, X, C) 3. Lymphoreticular (R, O, X, C) 4. Skull origin (C)
Nutritional		Polioencephalomalacia thiamine—ruminants (O) (13)	Hypovitaminosis A (R, O) Taurine deficiency—cats (R)
Inflammatory (16)		Canine distemper (R, O, X, C) Feline coronavirus (R, O, X, C) Toxoplasmosis (R, C) Thromboembolic meningoencephalitis—bovine (R, C) Bovine virus diarrhea (R, O) Systemic mycoses (O, X, C) Bacterial infections (O, X, C)	Canine distemper (R, O, X, C) Feline coronavirus (R, O, X, C) Toxoplasmosis (R, C) Systemic mycoses (O, X, C) Bacterial infections (O, X, C) Granulomatous meningoencephalitis—dogs (O, X, C) Protothecosis (C) Immune mediated (O)
Toxic (16)		Lead and other heavy metals (C) Hexachlorophene (C)	Lead and other heavy metals (C) Hexachlorophene (C)
Traumatic (13)	Retinal detachment Retinal hemorrhage Edema (O, X, C) Hemorrhage (O, X, C)	Edema (O, X, C) Hemorrhage (O, X, C)	
Vascular (13)	Infarcts (R, C) Hemorrhages (R, O, X, C)		

* Abbreviations: R = retina, O = optic nerve, X = optic chiasm, C = optic tract and cerebral cortex. Numbers in parentheses refer to chapters in which entities are discussed.

TABLE 12–3 Etiology of Pupillary Abnormalities*

Disease Category	*Nonprogressive*	*Acute Progressive*	*Chronic Progressive*
Degenerative			Retinal degenerations (R)
Anomalous	Hypoplasia (O) Coloboma (O) Retinal dysplasia (R) Collie eye syndrome (R)		Hydrocephalus† (13)
Neoplastic			Any rostrotentorial tumor† (16)
Nutritional		Thiamine deficiency—dogs and cats (16)	
Idiopathic	Pupillotonia Anisocoria—cats (may be FeLV)	Feline dysautonomia (10)	
Inflammatory		Retrobulbar abscess Many infectious diseases (16) Middle ear infections (9)	
Toxic		Lead† (16)	
Traumatic (13)	Brain stem hemorrhage Brachial plexus lesions (6)	Hematoma†	Cerebral edema†

* Abbreviations: R = retina, O = optic nerve. Numbers in parentheses refer to chapters in which entities are discussed.
† Oculomotor signs secondary to tentorial herniation.

tions. The history and the physical and neurologic examinations should provide the clinician with a list of the most probable diseases to be considered. Most of the diseases presented in the figures are discussed in other chapters. Only those that are related primarily to the visual system are discussed here.

Degenerative Diseases

An abnormality of the intracellular enzyme systems causes an accumulation of the products of metabolism in the neurons. Affected neurons function abnormally and eventually die. This group of diseases is listed in Figures 12–2

TABLE 12–4 Etiology of Ocular Movement Disorders*

Disease Category	*Nonprogressive*	*Acute Progressive*	*Chronic Progressive*
Degenerative			Storage diseases (R, C) (16) Demyelinating diseases (O, C) (16)
Anomalous	Strabismus with optic pathway anomalies—cats		Hydrocephalus (C) (13)
Neoplastic			Any tumor affecting the brain stem, cerebellum, vestibular system, or CN III, IV, VI (16)
Nutritional		Thiamine deficiency—dogs and cats (16)	
Inflammatory		Any inflammatory disease affecting brain stem, cerebellum, vestibular system, or CN III, IV, or VI (9, 16)	
Toxic		Hexachlorophene (16)	
Traumatic (13)	Lesions of the brain stem, cerebellum, vestibular system, or CN III, IV, VI		
Vascular (13)	Lesions of the brain stem, cerebellum, vestibular system, or CN III, IV, VI		

* Numbers in parentheses refer to chapters in which entities are discussed.

through 12–4 as storage diseases (see Chap. 16). Because neurons are affected, the retina, the lateral geniculate nucleus, and the occipital cortex are the most obvious targets in the visual system. Cranial nerve nuclei usually are not affected until late in the disease. The diseases are hereditary, progressive, and invariably fatal. The formulation of an antemortem diagnosis is difficult except by assessment of the history, knowledge of the breed selectivity, and exclusion of other diagnoses. A brain biopsy can confirm a diagnosis. A biopsy of other tissues may provide a diagnosis in some of the systemic storage diseases.

Demyelinating diseases also are considered degenerative diseases; for example, one type, globoid cell leukodystrophy, is caused by an abnormal enzyme system similar to that of the neuronal storage diseases. The signs of cerebellar and spinal cord tract involvement (UMN signs, proprioception deficits) are characteristic of the clinical syndrome. Visual pathways (optic nerve, optic tract, optic radiation) may be affected. Demyelination also may occur secondary to inflammatory diseases, especially canine distemper. The visual pathways are often affected, but other signs predominate.

Primary retinal degenerations are common causes of blindness, especially in the dog. It is important to realize that some dogs with severe retinal degeneration and functional blindness may still have intact pupillary light reflexes. These degenerations are generally called progressive retinal atrophy with several variants, such as central progressive retinal atrophy. Numerous breeds of dogs and a few breeds of cats are affected. The affected breeds are listed in several textbooks of veterinary ophthalmology and in a comprehensive review by Whitley.[7–9]

Anomalies

Hydrocephalus, which may be the result of a congenital anomaly or may be secondary to mass lesions or inflammation, affects primarily the optic radiations and the occipital cortex through enlargement of the lateral ventricles. Hydrocephalus should always be considered in a blind animal that has intact pupillary light reflexes. A diagnosis of hydrocephalus requires computed tomography, ventricular tap, pneumoventriculography, or electroencephalography (see Chap. 13).

Primary retinal anomalies are relatively common in the dog but less frequent in other species. The anomalies include coloboma, optic nerve hypoplasia, the collie eye anomaly, and various forms of retinal dysplasia. As with the retinal degenerations, numerous breeds of dogs, a few breeds of cats, and large animals are affected. The types of anomaly and the breeds affected are listed in the references.[7–9] These diseases cause blindness and in some cases nystagmus and pupillary abnormalities.

Cats with visual pathway abnormalities, primarily Siamese and white cats, often have a medial strabismus and pendular nystagmus, but good vestibular eye movements. Pendular nystagmus is also seen in dairy cows. One survey of 2,932 cows in New York state reported an incidence of 0.51% in several breeds. It has also been reported as a familial problem in Ayrshire bulls.[10,11] Medial strabismus has been reported in several breeds of cattle, apparently as an inherited trait in some.[12]

Metabolic Diseases

A disease that alters the normal biochemical processes of the eye or the central nervous system (CNS) may produce signs of abnormal vision, although other signs usually are more apparent. Diabetes mellitus may cause vascular changes, including retinal hemorrhage. Cataracts are common and make retinal examination difficult.

Diseases that affect cortical function may produce blindness with intact pupillary light reflexes. Examples include hypoglycemia, hepatic encephalopathy, and uremia. Acute metabolic problems, such as hypoxia and hyperthermia, usually affect the cerebral cortex most severely. Cortical blindness frequently follows severe hypoxic episodes, such as cardiac arrest (see Chaps. 13 and 16).

Neoplasms

Visual pathway abnormalities are often helpful for localizing intracranial tumors. Primary tumors of the globe are apparent on a physical examination.[7]

Tumors of the pituitary gland may cause visual field deficits from compression of the optic chiasm; however, most pituitary tumors grow dorsally into the hypothalamus instead of spreading out rostrally and caudally. Visual signs therefore are seen very late in the development of the mass.[13]

A lymphosarcoma may infiltrate all portions of the globe. Involvement of the orbit may cause exophthalmos (especially in cattle). Compression of the optic nerves may cause papilledema or atrophy of the optic disk.

Reticulosis, which is considered either inflammatory or neoplastic by various authors, may infiltrate the optic nerves and cause atrophy or swelling of the optic disk, depending on the degree of involvement.

Neoplasia of the CNS is discussed in Chapter 16.

Nutritional Deficiencies

Animals that are fed normal commercial rations rarely have nutritional deficiencies severe enough to cause CNS abnormality. Hypovitaminosis A causes abnormal bone growth with stenosis of the optic foramen, which secondarily constricts the optic nerve, producing papilledema in the early stages, followed eventually by retinal degeneration. This syndrome is seen more commonly in calves than in companion animals.[14]

Feline central retinal degeneration (FCRD) can be produced by diets that are deficient in the amino acid taurine. Cats that are fed commercial dog food exclusively develop FCRD.[14]

Polioencephalomalacia of ruminants is characterized by cerebral necrosis and edema. Signs of cerebral dysfunction, including blindness, are seen. The pupillary light reflexes are usually normal, unless edema has caused tentorial herniation with compression of the oculomotor nerves. Extorsion of the globe, presumably from damage to the trochlear nucleus (CN IV), is seen in this syndrome. The disease is caused by an excess of thiaminase in the rumen, which produces an acute thiamine deficiency. Thiamine deficiency in small animals, primarily in cats, causes hemorrhages and malacia in the brain stem. Eye movements and pupillary reflexes may be affected (see Chap. 16).

Idiopathic

Several diseases are currently of unknown etiology and are included here.

Feline dysautonomia, also called the Key-Gaskell syndrome, is a diffuse disorder of the autonomic nervous system of unknown etiology.[15] It has been most frequently reported in Great Britain, but several cases have been recognized in other countries, including the United States.[16] A similar syndrome has also been reported in dogs.[17,18] One of the primary signs is dilation of the pupils without evidence of blindness. The nictitating membrane is frequently prolapsed. The other manifestations of this disease are discussed in Chapter 10.

Pupillotonia is a pupil that is slow to react to light, both on direct and consensual responses. It is thought to be immune system mediated. Primary abnormalities of the visual and oculomotor pathways must be excluded. Only one case has been reported.[19]

Inflammations

Systemic infectious diseases with CNS involvement frequently affect the visual system. Retinal lesions are common in canine distemper, feline infectious peritonitis, toxoplasmosis, rickettsial diseases, the systemic mycoses, and thromboembolic meningoencephalitis.[14,20–22] A fundic examination may help to confirm the diagnosis.

Optic neuropathy includes degenerative, compressive ischemic, and inflammatory conditions of the optic nerve. Optic neuritis is inflammation of the optic nerve. Sudden blindness may be noticed if both eyes are affected. Papilledema and vascular congestion are seen on a fundic examination if that portion of the nerve is affected. Atrophy of the disk is seen as the process resolves. The electroretinogram can differentiate primary retinal disease from optic nerve disease. Sudden acquired retinal degeneration (SARD) also causes acute blindness, and the fundus may appear normal. The ERG will be abnormal in SARD. Canine distemper, toxoplasmosis, and cryptococcosis are among the infectious diseases causing optic neuritis. Granulomatous meningoencephalitis (inflammatory reticulosis) frequently affects the optic nerve.[23] Many of the diseases causing optic neuropathy are not treatable and may lead to death; however, a number of cases are seen without evidence of systemic disease. Edema and inflammation may lead to loss of function of the nerve, regardless of the outcome of the primary disease. Early treatment therefore should include antiedema doses of corticosteroids. Other supportive or antibiotic therapy is given as indicated by the condition of the animal. The prognosis is guarded to poor. In one report of 12 dogs with optic neuropathy, 7 remained alive, and 5 of them were blind. The other 2 had partial vision.[24]

Vestibular disease, whether inflammatory or from other causes, will produce nystagmus.

Toxic Disorders

Heavy metal poisoning, especially lead poisoning, may produce cortical blindness. Toxins that affect the brain stem or cerebellum, such as hexachlorophene, may cause nystagmus (see Chap. 16).

Trauma

Any portion of the visual system may be affected by trauma. Assessing the function of the oculomotor nerve is of primary importance in evaluating patients with head injury. Brain swelling that leads to tentorial herniation compresses the oculomotor nerve at the tentorium cerebelli. One of the earliest signs of tentorial herniation is a fixed, dilated pupil ipsilateral to the herniation (if it is unilateral). A paralysis of the extraocular muscles that produces a ventrolateral strabismus follows the mydriasis. Hemorrhage in the brain stem also produces abnormal pupils. Hemorrhage above or below the oculomotor nucleus (midbrain) may destroy the UMN to the sympathetic pathway, producing small but responsive pupils. Midbrain hemorrhage may cause fixed, dilated pupils if the oculomotor nucleus is destroyed with the sympathetic pathway intact, but most cases have fixed, midposition pupils because both pathways are affected. Serial assessment of pupillary function together with mental status, motor function, and other cranial nerve signs is very important for the evaluation of patients with head trauma. Bilateral, fixed, dilated, or midposition pupils from the time of injury strongly suggests brain stem hemorrhage that is often irreversible, and progressive dilation of the pupils suggests a developing tentorial herniation that may be treatable (see Chap. 13).

Traumatic injuries of the eye can cause abnormal vision or pupillary responses.

Vascular

Cerebral infarction, primarily seen in the cat, may cause contralateral vision loss (see Chap. 13).

CASE HISTORIES

The case histories in this chapter emphasize localization of the lesion. Only the pertinent neuroophthalmologic findings will be given. Make your decision before reading the assessment.

Case History 12A

*Neurologic Examination**

Vision: Normal.

Pupillary light reflexes (PLR): The right pupil is dilated.

	Reaction	
Shine light	OS	OD
OS	+	−
OD	+	−

* *Key:* OS = left eye, OD = right eye.

Eye position and movement: Left eye is normal; fixed ventrolateral strabismus in right eye.

Case History 12B

Neurologic Examination

Vision: Normal in left eye; absent in right eye.

PLR: The right pupil is larger than the left.

	Reaction	
Shine light	OS	OD
OS	+	+
OD	−	−

Eye position and movement: Normal.

Case History 12C

Neurologic Examination

Vision: Absent in both eyes.

PLR: The pupil size is normal; the pupils are symmetric.

	Reaction	
Shine light	OS	OD
OS	+	+
OD	+	+

Eye position and movement: The vestibular eye movements are normal. No strabismus, but the animal does not follow moving objects.

Case History 12D

Neurologic Examination

Vision: Normal in both eyes.

PLR: The pupil size is normal; the pupils are symmetric.

	Reaction	
Shine light	OS	OD
OS	+	+
OD	+	+

Eye position and movement: Medial strabismus of the left eye. Dorsal and ventral movements can be elicited by moving the head. The right eye is normal.

Case History 12E

Neurologic Examination

Vision: Absent in both eyes.

PLR: The pupils are dilated bilaterally.

	Reaction	
Shine light	OS	OD
OS	−	−
OD	−	−

Eye position and movement: Normal eye position and normal vestibular eye movements, but the animal does not follow moving objects.

Case History 12F

Neurologic Examination

Vision: Normal in both eyes.
PLR: The pupil size is normal.

	Reaction	
Shine light	OS	OD
OS	+	+
OD	+	+

Eye position and movement: The eyes are in the normal midposition, but no vestibular eye movements can be elicited.

Assessment 12A

Right oculomotor nerve (CN III) lesion. The unilateral lesion suggests a lesion after the nerve leaves the brain stem, since the nuclei are only millimeters apart.

Assessment 12B

Right optic nerve or retinal lesion. A funduscopic examination is likely to differentiate between these two disorders. An electroretinogram may be necessary if there are no visible retinal lesions.

Assessment 12C

Bilateral occipital cortex or optic radiation lesions. This finding suggests a diffuse lesion, such as hydrocephalus, encephalitis, or increased intracranial pressure.

Assessment 12D

Left abducent nerve (CN VI) lesion. Isolated lesions of CN VI are rare. In a clinical case, other signs of brain stem disease would probably be present.

Assessment 12E

Optic chiasm, bilateral optic nerve, or bilateral retinal lesions. This situation is one in which two lesions (actually a diffuse disease) are more common than a single chiasmatic lesion. Retinopathies and optic neuropathies are seen more often than are primary lesions of the optic chiasm.

Assessment 12F

Medial longitudinal fasciculus (MLF) lesion. This lesion is in the tract connecting the vestibular nuclei to the nuclei of CN III, CN IV, and CN VI. Alternatively, there could be a lesion of CN III, CN IV, and CN VI bilaterally, but there should be pupillary abnormalities with oculomotor involvement. In either case, other signs probably would predominate. MLF lesions usually are associated with severe brain stem lesions (hemorrhage, tumor), and the animal is often comatose when these disorders are present.

REFERENCES

1. Neer TM: Horner's syndrome: Anatomy, diagnosis, and causes. Comp Cont Educ Pract Vet 6:740–747, 1984.
2. Van Den Broek A: Horner's syndrome in cats and dogs: A review. J Small Anim Pract 28:929–940, 1987.
3. Sweeney RW, Sweeney CR: Transient Horner's syndrome following intravenous injections in two horses. J Am Vet Med Assoc 185:802–803, 1984.
4. de Lahunta A: Veterinary Neuroanatomy and Clinical Neurology, 2nd ed. Philadelphia, WB Saunders, 1983.
5. Mayhew IG: Large Animal Neurology: A Handbook for Veterinary Clinicians. Philadelphia, Lea & Febiger, 1989.
6. Lewis GT, Blanchard GL, Trapp AL, et al: Ophthalmoplegia caused by thyroid adenocarcinoma invasion of the cavernous sinuses in the dog. J Am Anim Hosp Assoc 20:805–812, 1984.
7. Slatter D: Fundamentals of Veterinary Ophthalmology. Philadelphia, WB Saunders, 1981.
8. Whitley RD: Focusing on eye disorders among purebred dogs. Vet Med 83:50–63, 1988.
9. Barnett KC: Inherited eye disease in the dog and cat. J Small Anim Pract 29:462–475, 1988.
10. Nurmio P, Remes E, Talanti S, et al: Familial undulatory nystagmus in Ayrshire bulls in Finland. Nord Vet Med 34:130–132, 1982.
11. McConnon JM, White ME, Smith MC, et al: Pendular nystagmus in dairy cattle. J Am Vet Med Assoc 182:812–813, 1983.
12. Power EP: Bilateral convergent strabismus in two friesian cows. Ir Vet 41:357–358, 1987.
13. Davidson MG, Nasisse MP, Breitschwerdt EB, et al: Acute blindness associated with intracranial tumors in dogs and cats: Eight cases (1984–1989). J Am Vet Med Assoc 199:755–758, 1991.
14. Aguirre GD, Gross SL: Ocular manifestations of selected systemic diseases. Comp Cont Educ Pract Vet 2:144–153, 1980.
15. Edney A, Gaskell C, Sharp N: Feline dysautonomia—An emerging disease. J Small Anim Pract 28:333–416, 1987.
16. Guilford WG, O'Brien DP, Allert A, et al: Diagnosis of dysautonomia in a cat by autonomic nervous system function testing. J Am Vet Med Assoc 193:823–828, 1988.
17. Pollin M, Sullivan M: A canine dysautonomia resembling the Key-Gaskell syndrome. Vet Rec 118:402–403, 1986.
18. Presthus J, Bjerkas I: Canine dysautonomia in Norway. Vet Rec 120:463–464, 1987.
19. Gerding PA, Brightman AH, Brogdon J: Pupillotonia in a dog. J Am Vet Med Assoc 189:1477–1478, 1986.
20. Martin CL: Retinopathies of food animals. In Howard JL (ed): Current Veterinary Therapy: Food Animal Practice. Philadelphia, WB Saunders, 1981, pp 1067–1072.
21. Gelatt KN, Whitley RD, Samuelson DA, et al: Ocular manifestations of viral disease in small animals. Comp Cont Educ Pract Vet 7:968–978, 1985.
22. Ellett EW, Playter RF, Pierce KR: Retinal lesions associated with induced canine ehrlichiosis: A preliminary report. J Am Anim Hosp Assoc 9:214–218, 1973.
23. Nafe LA, Carter JD: Caninie optic neuritis. Comp Cont Educ Pract Vet 3:978–984, 1981.
24. Fischer CA, Jones GT: Optic neuritis in dogs. J Am Vet Med Assoc 160:68–79, 1972.

13

Stupor or Coma

Altered states of consciousness are always related to abnormal brain function. The nomenclature of these disorders is often confusing, because the terms extend beyond simple medical analysis and encompass psychology, philosophy, and other disciplines. Applying the terminology used in human medicine to animals is difficult because we must interpret behavior to assess mental status. For the purposes of the clinician, the following definitions are adequate:

Normal: The animal is alert, responsive to external stimuli, aware of its surroundings, and responds to commands as expected.

Depressed: The animal is lethargic and less responsive to its environment but still has the capability to respond in a normal manner. Most sick animals are depressed.

Disoriented, confused: Although the animal can respond to its environment, it may do so in an inappropriate manner.

Stuporous: The animal appears to be asleep when undisturbed but can be aroused by strong stimulation, especially pain. There is no clear boundary between lethargy and stupor.

Comatose: The animal is unconscious and does not respond to any stimulus except by reflex activity. For example, a strong toe pinch may elicit a flexion reflex or may increase extensor posturing but does not cause a behavioral reaction, such as crying, biting, or turning the head.

Vegetative: The animal lacks awareness of the environment but there is arousal. Brain stem function is present, but cortical responses are absent.[1]

Brain dead: The animal is in coma, is apneic, lacks all brain stem reflexes, and has electrocerebral silence. Currently in human medicine, electrocerebral silence includes all evoked responses as well as a flat electroencephalogram (EEG).

Confusion, stupor, and coma invariably are related to abnormal brain function.

Lesion Localization

Consciousness is maintained by sensory stimuli that act through the *ascending reticular activating system* (ARAS) on the cerebral cortex (Fig. 13–1). Decreasing levels of consciousness indicate abnormal function of the cerebral cortex or interference with cortical activation by the ARAS.

All sensory pathways have collateral input into the reticular formation of the pons and the midbrain. The reticular formation projects diffusely to the cerebral cortex, maintaining a background of activity through cholinergic synapses on cortical neurons. A balance is maintained between the ARAS and an adrenergic system that projects from nuclei in the midbrain and the diencephalon and that may be considered the sleep system.[2–4] Alterations in the balance of these two systems can produce signs ranging from hyperexcitability to coma. Narcolepsy, a syndrome of sleep attacks, will be discussed in Chapter 14.

Stupor and coma are caused by (1) diffuse, bilateral cerebral disease, (2) metabolic or toxic encephalopathies, (3) compression of the ros-

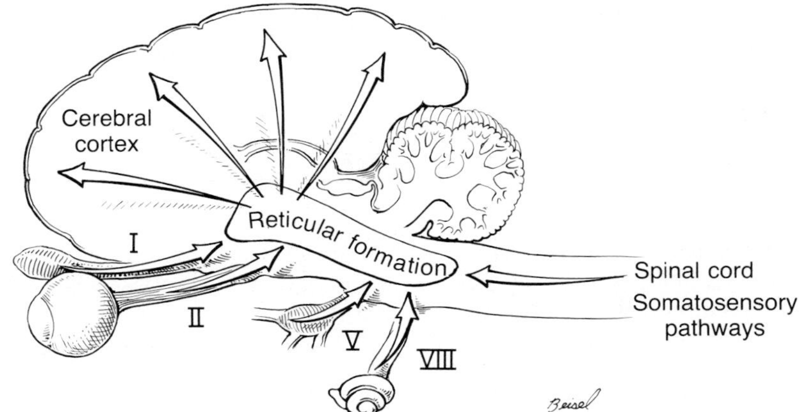

Figure 13–1 Reticular activating system (RAS). The reticular system of the brain stem receives input from most sensory systems. Diffuse projections from the RAS to the cerebral cortex maintain consciousness.

tral brain stem (midbrain, pons), or (4) destructive lesions of the rostral brain stem.

An anatomic diagnosis can be made on the basis of mental status, motor function, and neuro-ophthalmologic signs (vision, pupils, and eye movements—see Chap. 12 and Table 13–1). Alterations in the respiratory pattern may be correlated with levels of brain stem pathology, but they are less reliable than the other signs.

Diffuse cerebral disease usually does not produce localizing signs, although some inflammatory processes may be somewhat asymmetric. Voluntary motor activity and postural reactions are absent or severely depressed. Rhythmic walking movements, reflecting brain stem and spinal cord activity, may be elicited if the animal is suspended in a normal standing posture. Vision is absent, although the pupils are normal. Oculocephalic responses (vestibular eye movements) are normal, but the animal will not follow moving objects. Normal pupils and oculocephalic responses indicate an intact brain stem, whereas loss of vision and voluntary motor activity indicates an abnormal cerebral cortex. In the severest form, diffuse cerebral pathology will produce the chronic vegetative state where the animal has brain stem reflexes, but no behavioral reactions. Signs of meningeal irritation include pain on palpation of the head and the neck, rigidity of the neck muscles, and resistance to flexion of the neck. Meningeal irritation may be caused by infection, immune reactions, or the presence of blood in the subarachnoid space.

TABLE 13–1 Signs of Lesions Causing Stupor and Coma

Lesion	*Motor Function*	*Vision*	*Pupils*	*Eye Movements*
Severe diffuse cerebral cortex lesions	Tetraparesis (poorly coordinated walking movements); postural reactions absent	Absent	Normal	Normal, but no visual following
Metabolic or toxic encephalopathy	Tetraparesis without increased extensor tone; reflexes may be depressed	Absent	Usually normal, but may be altered in intoxication	Normal, but no visual following; absent in deep coma
Bilateral compression of rostral brain stem	Tetraparesis; increased tone in extensor muscles (decerebrate rigidity)	Absent in herniation, present in primary brain stem lesions	Dilated or midposition, unresponsive	Bilateral ventral lateral strabismus, poor vestibular eye movements
Unilateral compression of rostral brain stem	Hemiparesis or tetraparesis; increased extensor tone on affected side	Present – may be contralateral loss in herniation	Dilated, ipsilateral	Ipsilateral ventrolateral strabismus, poor vestibular eye movements
Destructive lesion, rostral brain stem	Tetraparesis; increased extensor tone (decerebrate rigidity)	Present – animal may not respond if comatose	Midposition unresponsive	No vestibular eye movements, may have bilateral ventrolateral strabismus

TABLE 13–2 Classification of Brain Swelling

Increased Vascular Volume	*Cellular Swelling*	*Interstitial Edema*
Arterial dilation Venous obstruction	Cytotoxic Metabolic storage	Vasogenic Osmotic Compressive Hydrocephalic

Metabolic or *toxic encephalopathies* usually depress higher (cortical) function early and affect brain stem functions later. They do not produce focal localizing signs. The signs are generally the same as those of diffuse cortical lesions but may have other components, depending on the cause. For example, barbiturates may cause depression of the spinal reflexes, organophosphate insecticides may cause muscle fasciculation and autonomic signs, and a number of toxins may cause seizures. Specific entities will be discussed in Chapter 16.

Compression of the brain stem may be caused by a mass (tumor, abscess) adjacent to the brain stem or by herniation of the cerebral cortex under the tentorium cerebelli, which secondarily compresses the brain stem.[5]

The skull forms an inelastic case around the brain. Any developing mass (tumor, abscess, hematoma), increase in the volume of the brain (cerebral edema), or deformation of the skull must displace cerebrospinal fluid (CSF), blood, or nervous tissue. An increase in brain bulk may come from changes in any of the three compartments, i.e., *vascular, cellular,* and *extracellular* (Table 13–2).[6] In addition, many disease processes cause increased brain volume by multiple mechanisms. For example, trauma may cause vasogenic edema, venous obstruction, and an osmotic edema. Tumors may cause vasogenic, compressive, and hydrocephalic changes. There is approximately 7 ml of CSF in the average dog. Blood volume is maintained nearly constant up to pressures equaling arterial pressure. Increased pressure causes displacement of the cerebral hemispheres caudally under the tentorium cerebelli, resulting in compression of the brain stem (Figs. 13–2 and 13–3). Unilateral masses produce a herniation on the same side, whereas cerebral edema usually causes a bilateral herniation.

If the pressure continues to rise, or if the mass starts in the caudotentorial compartment, the cerebellum may herniate through the foramen magnum, compressing the medulla oblongata. The respiratory pathways are blocked, resulting in death.

The signs of brain stem compression from

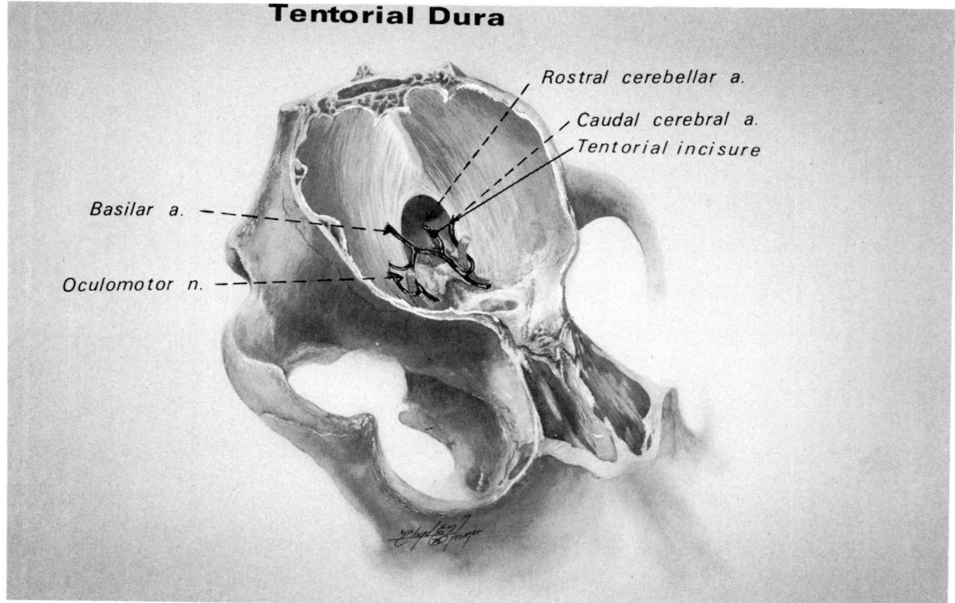

Figure 13–2 Increased pressure rostral to the tentorium cerebelli causes herniation of the cerebral cortex under the tentorium, resulting in compression of the brain stem.

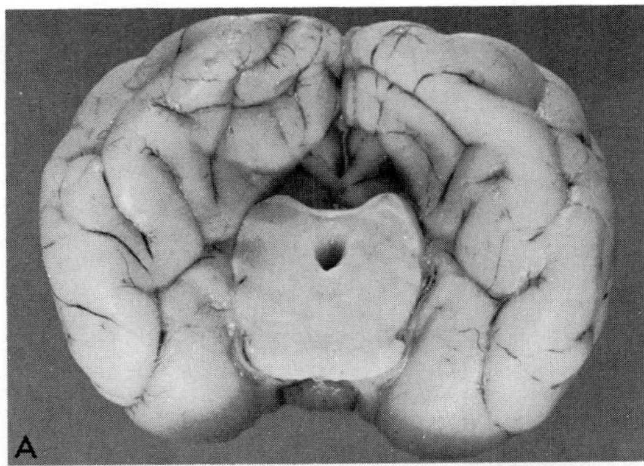

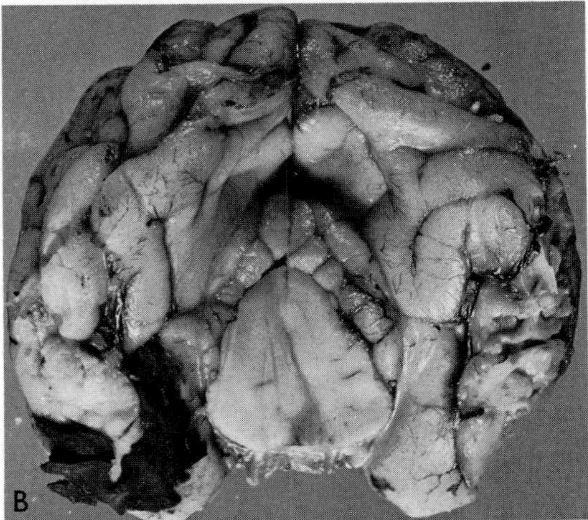

Figure 13–3 Caudal view of the brain, transected at the midbrain. *A*. Normal brain. Note the open mesencephalic aqueduct. *B*. Severe cerebral edema has caused herniation of the cerebrum under the tentorium cerebelli, resulting in compression and distortion of the brain stem. The mesencephalic aqueduct is closed, causing further increases in intracranial pressure. (From Oliver JE Jr: Neurologic emergencies in small animals. Vet Clin North Am 2:341–357, 1972. Used by permission.)

tentorial herniation are outlined in Tables 13–3 and 13–4. Masses that compress the brain stem usually cause similar signs, although the animal's mental status is not altered as severely, because the cerebral cortex is not directly affected. The involvement of CN III is particularly important to the clinician, because it is one of the earliest detectable signs of herniation. In some cases, pupillary dilation may be preceded by a slight pupillary constriction. Either of these signs indicates impending deterioration of the patient, and treatment must be instituted quickly.

Destructive lesions of the brain stem are most frequently parenchymal hemorrhages following head injury. Neoplasia and inflammation also may produce a destructive lesion. Table 13–5 lists the signs of a focal lesion at various levels of the brain stem.

Diseases

The causes of stupor and coma are classified in Table 13–6 according to the presence or absence of focal, lateralizing, or meningeal signs and the onset and the progression of the signs.

Focal or Lateralizing Signs

Acute Progressive

Trauma. Head injuries in domestic animals are most often the result of motor vehicle accidents. Most of the available information relates to dogs, but other species respond similarly to injuries of the brain.[7]

The terms that are commonly used in describing head injury are defined in Table 13–7.

TABLE 13–3 Signs Characteristic of Progressive Bilateral Tentorial Herniation

Level	*Consciousness*	*Pupils*	*Eye Movements*	*Motor Function*	*Autonomic Responses*
Cerebral	Apathy	Small but reactive	Normal	Hemiparesis	Normal to irregular responses
Late diencephalic	Stupor	Small but reactive	Normal	Hemiparesis to tetraparesis	Cheyne-Stokes respiration
Midbrain	Coma	Dilated bilaterally	Poor vestibular eye movements	Decerebrate rigidity	Hyperventilation
Pons	Coma	Midposition unresponsive	Vestibular eye movements absent	Tetraparesis; decreased muscle tone	Rapid, shallow respiration
Medulla oblongata	Coma	Midposition, dilated terminally	Absent	Tetraparesis; decreased muscle tone	Irregular to apnea, pulse slowing

Modified with permission from Oliver JE Jr: Neurologic emergencies in small animals. Vet Clin North Am 2:341–357, 1972.

TABLE 13–4 Signs Characteristic of Progressive Unilateral Tentorial Herniation

Level	*Consciousness*	*Pupils*	*Eye Movements*	*Motor Function*	*Autonomic Responses*
CN III	Normal to stupor	Ipsilateral dilation	Normal to slight lateral strabismus	Normal to hemiparesis	Normal
Early midbrain	Stupor	Ipsilateral to bilateral dilation	Ipsilateral ventrolateral strabismus	Hemiparesis, ipsi- or contralateral	Normal
Late midbrain	Coma	Dilated bilaterally to fixed midposition	Ventrolateral strabismus to fixed midposition	Decerebrate rigidity	Hyperventilation
Pons	Coma	Midposition, unresponsive	Vestibular eye movements absent	Tetraparesis; decreased muscle tone	Rapid, shallow respiration
Medulla oblongata	Coma	Midposition, dilated terminally	Absent	Tetraparesis; decreased muscle tone	Irregular to apnea; pulse slowing

Modified with permission from Oliver JE Jr: Neurologic emergencies in small animals. Vet Clin North Am 2:341–357, 1972.

The clinical differentiation of concussion from contusion is not clear and has no significance for clinical management. Cerebral edema can be assumed to exist in any patient with neurologic signs following head injury. The most common types of intracranial hemorrhage are subarachnoid and intramedullary. Surgical treatment is of no benefit in either case.

Differentiation of the signs of diffuse cerebral and focal brain stem lesions from the signs of tentorial herniation was discussed earlier and is summarized in Table 13–8.

Shores has modified coma scales used in assessing human patients for use in animals (Table 13–9).[8,9] The patient's status in each of three categories—motor activity, brain stem reflexes, and level of consciousness—is assessed. Total scores of 3 to 8 indicate a grave prognosis, scores of 9 to 14 indicate a poor to guarded prognosis, and scores of 15 to 18 indicate a good prognosis. The scale has not been evaluated on large numbers of patients to assess its reliability, but it emphasizes the importance of these clinical parameters. Serial evaluations are important to determine if there is improvement.

The treatment of head injury cannot be separated from management of the whole patient. Multiple-system injuries are common in animals that have been hit by cars. The owner may be instructed by telephone to establish a patent airway by extending the animal's head and pulling the tongue forward if the animal is unconscious. The animal should be carried on a piece of plywood or some similar rigid support to avoid displacement of the vertebral column.[10]

The priorities for management on presentation of the animal to the veterinary clinic are (1) maintenance of adequate ventilation by endotracheal catheter or tracheostomy if necessary and (2) treatment of shock (Table 13–10). An

TABLE 13–5 Signs Characteristic of Focal Brain Stem Hemorrhage At One Level*

Level	*Consciousness*	*Pupils*	*Eye Movements*	*Motor Function*	*Autonomic Responses*
Diencephalon	Apathy to stupor	Small but reactive	Normal	Hemiparesis to tetraparesis	Normal to Cheyne-Stokes respiration
Midbrain	Stupor to coma	Dilated bilaterally or midposition, unresponsive	Bilateral ventrolateral strabismus	Decerebrate rigidity	Hyperventilation (variable)
Pons	Coma	Midposition, unresponsive	Vestibular eye movements absent	Decerebrate tetraparesis, or decreased muscle tone	Rapid, shallow respiration; loss of micturition reflex
Medulla oblongata	Coma	Midposition, dilated terminally	Absent	Tetraparesis; decreased muscle tone	Irregular to apnea, pulse slowing

Modified with permission from Oliver JE Jr: Neurologic emergencies in small animals. Vet Clin North Am 2:341–357, 1972.

* Assuming a large intramedullary hemorrhage confined primarily to one level. The most frequent is in the caudal midbrain and the pons following acute head injury. Asymmetric or smaller lesions will produce less severe signs.

TABLE 13–6 Etiology of Stupor and Coma*

Condition	Acute Nonprogressive	Acute Progressive	Chronic Progressive
Focal or Lateralizing Signs			
Neoplastic (16)		Metastatic	Primary Gliomas Meningiomas
Traumatic (13)	*Parenchymal hemorrhage*	Epidural, subdural hematoma Intracarotid injections (large animals)	Subdural hematoma
Vascular (13)	Hemorrhage, infarction		
No Focal or Lateralizing Signs, But Evidence of Meningeal Irritation			
Inflammatory (16)		*Meningitis* *Meningoencephalitis*	
Traumatic (13)	Subarachnoid hemorrhage		
No Focal, Lateralizing, or Meningeal Signs			
Degenerative (16)			Storage diseases
Anomalous	Malformation of brain Lissencephaly Hydranencephaly Otocephaly		*Hydrocephalus*
Metabolic (16)		*Hypoglycemia* *Hepatic encephalopathy* Uremic encephalopathy Diabetic coma Hypothyroid coma Heat stroke Hypoxia	
Nutritional (16)		*Thiamine deficiency* (polioencephalomalacia)	
Idiopathic (14)		Epilepsy (postictal) Narcolepsy	*Neonatal maladjustment syndrome*
Inflammatory (16)		Encephalitis (many)	Encephalitis
Toxic (16)		Heavy metals Barbiturates and other drugs Carbon monoxide	Water intoxication Various plants Enterotoxemia
Traumatic (13)		*Cerebral edema*	

* *Italics* indicate most common diseases clinically. Numbers in parentheses refer to chapters in which conditions are discussed.

TABLE 13–7 Terminology of Head Injury

Concussion: Transient loss of consciousness without structural pathology.

Contusion: Pathologic alterations in the brain, including edema, petechial hemorrhage, disruption of nerve fibers, and so forth.

Coup and Contrecoup: Injuries at the point of impact (coup) and at the opposite pole of the brain (contrecoup).

Cerebral Edema: An increase in intracellular (gray matter) and extracellular (white matter) fluid, present in most head injuries.

Hemorrhage:

Epidural: Bleeding between the dura and the calvaria. It usually is caused by a skull fracture with laceration of a meningeal artery. Relatively rare in animals.

Subdural: Bleeding between the dura and the arachnoid. It usually is caused by disruption of the bridging veins, so it develops slowly. Relatively rare in animals.

Subarachnoid: Bleeding into the subarachnoid space. It usually is caused by disruption of the veins or the arteries of the arachnoid. Relatively common in animals.

Intramedullary (intracerebral): Bleeding into the tissue of the brain. It usually is caused by disruption of the intramedullary vessels. Relatively common in animals.

Skull Fractures:

Linear: Fractures of the calvaria that are not displaced.

Depressed: Fractures of the calvaria that encroach on the brain.

Compound (open): Fractures of the calvaria that have a laceration of the skin.

TABLE 13–8 Comparison of Acute Brain Stem Hemorrhage with Tentorial Herniation Following Head Injury

Feature Compared	*Brain Stem Hemorrhage*	*Tentorial Herniation*
Onset	Early	Delayed
Course	Usually static	Progressive
Mental status	Coma, stupor if small lesion	Depressed, progressing to coma
Pupils	Fixed midposition, may be dilated if small lesion	Miosis, progressing to unilateral or bilateral dilation; fixed midposition late
Eye movements	Absent	Normal, progressing to fixed
Motor function	Decerebrate posturing	Normal or hemiparesis, progressing to decerebrate posture
Respiration	Hyperventilation or cluster breathing	Normal or Cheyne-Stokes

TABLE 13–9 Small Animal Coma Scale*

Neurologic Function Assessed	*Score*
Motor Activity	
Normal gait, normal spinal reflexes	6
Hemiparesis, tetraparesis, or decerebrate activity	5
Recumbent, intermittent extensor rigidity	4
Recumbent, constant extensor rigidity	3
Recumbent, constant extensor rigidity with opisthotonus	2
Recumbent, hypotonia of muscles, depressed or absent spinal reflexes	1
Brain Stem Reflexes	
Normal pupillary light reflexes and oculocephalic reflexes	6
Slow pupillary light reflexes and normal to reduced oculocephalic reflexes	5
Bilateral, unresponsive miosis with normal to reduced oculocephalic reflexes	4
Pinpoint pupils with reduced to absent oculocephalic reflexes	3
Unilateral, unresponsive mydriasis with reduced to absent oculocephalic reflexes	2
Bilateral, unresponsive mydriasis with reduced to absent oculocephalic reflexes	1
Level of Consciousness	
Occasional periods of alertness and responsive to environment	6
Depression or delirium, capable of responding to environment but response may be inappropriate	5
Stupor, responsive to visual stimuli	4
Stupor, responsive to auditory stimuli	3
Stupor, responsive only to repeated noxious stimuli	2
Coma, unresponsive to repeated noxious stimuli	1
Assessment	
Good prognosis	15–18
Guarded prognosis	9–14
Grave prognosis	3–8

Modified with permission from Shores A: Craniocerebral trauma. In Kirk RW (ed): Current Veterinary Therapy X. Philadelphia, WB Saunders, 1989.

* Neurologic function is assessed for each of the three categories and a grade of 1 to 6 is assigned according to the descriptions for each grade. The total score is the sum of the three category scores.

TABLE 13–10 Management of Intracranial Injury

Emergency Management: Treat shock, maintain airway, stop bleeding, provide cardiopulmonary resuscitation
Evaluate: History, physical examination, neurologic examination

Assessment:*	Level and Type of Injury			
	Cerebral Nonprogressive	Cerebral Progressive	Brain stem Progressive	Brain stem Nonprogressive
Coma scale score:	15–18	9–14	3–8	3–8
Management:	Corticosteroids, monitor	Corticosteroids, mannitol, DMSO,† monitor	CT, skull radiography, corticosteroids mannitol, DMSO, surgical decompression	Corticosteroids, mannitol, DMSO, monitor
Prognosis:	Usually good	Guarded	Poor unless reverses	Poor

* For assessment see Tables 13–1 through 13–5. Progressive signs will frequently follow the pattern from left to right in the table.
† DMSO is not licensed for systemic use, but is frequently recommended for large animals.

intravenous (IV) catheter should be established and lactated Ringer's solution administered to maintain a route for other medications. IV corticosteroids usually are given for shock and are beneficial in reducing or preventing traumatic cerebral edema. The efficacy of corticosteroids in trauma-induced edema has been questioned, but several studies have provided objective evidence of reduced intracranial pressure with high doses.[11] Several studies of spinal cord trauma also indicate efficacy.[11,12] Because spinal cord and brain tissue respond to injury in a similar manner, we assume that similar methods would be effective in brain injury. The two key factors appear to be adequate dose and early administration. The soluble steroids are essential in early therapy. Methylprednisolone is given at a dose of 30 mg/kg IV, followed by 5 mg/kg/hr in an IV drip. The treatment must be given as early as possible, preferably within the first hour after injury. Within 6 hours of injury there is neuronal and axonal loss that is irreversible. A recent study indicated that patients with spinal cord injury had less recovery of function than with placebo treatment when the first dose was administered more than 8 hours after injury.[12] Mannitol (0.25–1 g/kg) should be given IV if the patient is comatose but not if the patient is hypovolemic.[13]

The extent of the injury must be determined quickly. Cardiopulmonary function, internal hemorrhage, and fractures of the limbs or the spinal column should be evaluated.[7] The nervous system should then be evaluated as has been described previously. Evaluations of the level of consciousness, pupillary function and eye movements, dysfunction of other cranial nerves, and motor function are adequate for the assessment of the level and the extent of the damage to the central nervous system (CNS).

After the patient is stabilized, frequent monitoring of the severity of signs is imperative. The coma scale is useful for comparison between examinations. Radiography should be performed on the patient with minimal deficits (alert or depressed) in order to detect skull fractures, and the animal should be observed closely for 24 to 48 hours for progressive signs. Depressed skull fractures in conscious patients are elevated surgically when the animal is stable. Animals with linear fractures do not need surgery unless progressive signs indicate continuing intracranial hemorrhage. Open fractures are debrided and closed as early as possible.

Stuporous or comatose patients require more critical assessment and care and have a poorer prognosis. Brain stem hemorrhage usually can be differentiated from tentorial herniation from the time course of the neurologic signs (see Fig. 13–4 and Table 13–8). Intramedullary brain stem hemorrhage, which usually occurs in the midbrain or the pons, produces coma immediately after the trauma, and there is little or no improvement in this case (Fig. 13–5). Tentorial herniation may develop from cerebral edema (usually bilateral) or from rostrotentorial hemorrhage (epidural, subdural). The progression of signs is usually characteristic (see Tables 13–3 and 13–4). Animals with brain stem hemorrhage rarely recover, and those that do usually have severe neurologic deficits. Tentorial herniation must be managed early in order for the treatment to be successful. Severe tentorial herniation with compression and distortion of the brain stem produces secondary brain hemorrhages that are irreversible. In addi-

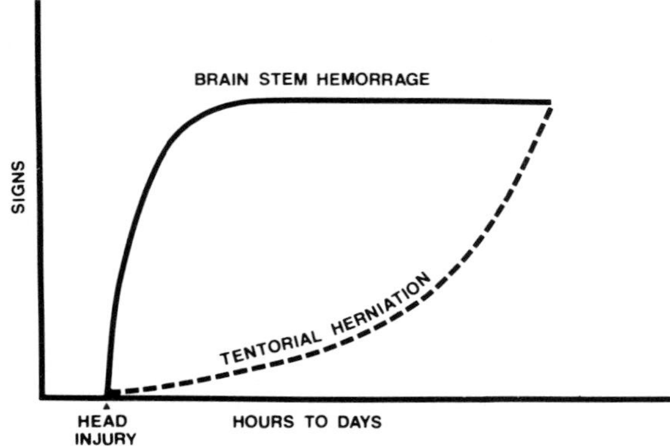

Figure 13–4 Sign-time graph of head injury. Tentorial herniation and brain stem hemorrhage may be differentiated by the clinical course. (From Oliver JE Jr: Neurologic emergencies in small animals. Vet Clin North Am 2:341–357, 1972. Used by permission.)

tion, increased pressure transmitted to the caudotentorial compartment produces cerebellar herniation through the foramen magnum, causing death by interference with the medullary respiratory centers (Fig. 13–6).

Brain stem hemorrhage is treated as was outlined previously: with the administration of corticosteroids and mannitol, maintenance of ventilation, and provision of nursing care. The initial management of tentorial herniation involves the same procedures. If the signs do not improve or if progression is observed in the first few hours, craniotomy for evacuation of the hematoma and relief of intracranial pressure is indicated.[14]

The management of the comatose patient must include maintaining hydration and nutrition; regulating body temperature; providing

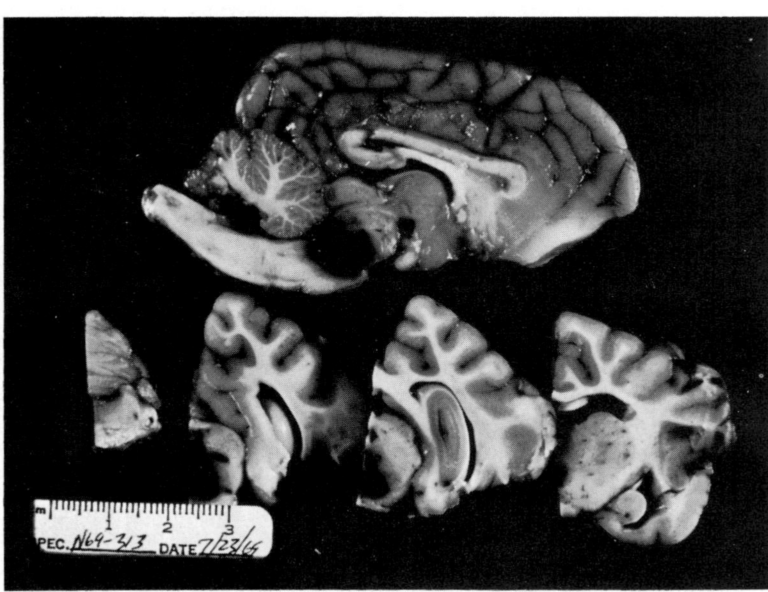

Figure 13–5 Brain stem hemorrhage in a boxer dog that was hit by a car. The hemorrhage extends from the caudal midbrain into the middle of the pons. The sulci and the gyri of the cortex are prominent, indicating minimal brain swelling. There is no evidence of tentorial herniation. (Compare the brain stem section second from the right with that in Fig. 13–3.) (From Oliver JE Jr: Neurologic examination. VM/SAC 67:654–659, 1972. Used by permission.)

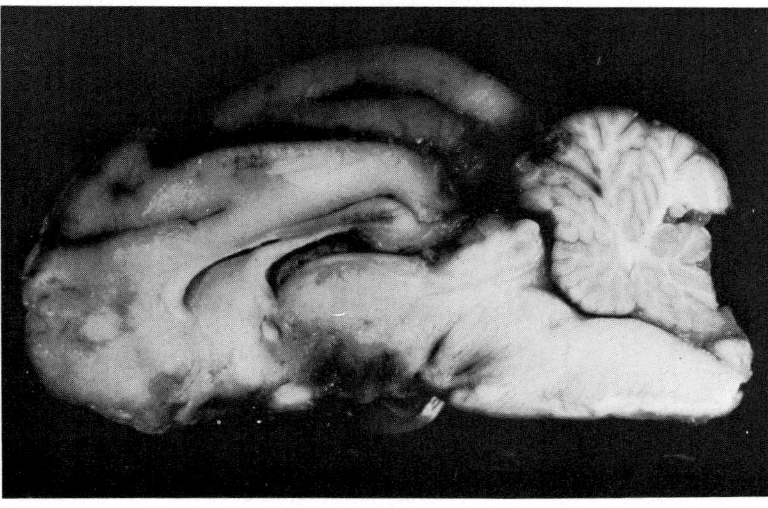

Figure 13–6 Brain of a cat with head trauma. There is tentorial herniation with compression of the rostral cerebellum and foramen magnum herniation with compression of the caudal cerebellum and the brain stem. (Courtesy of Joe N. Kornegay, D.V.M.)

adequate ventilation (including hyperventilation in the early stages); preventing decubital ulcers by frequent turning, meticulous cleaning of the skin, and cushioning with sponge rubber or fleece pads; and maintaining urinary and fecal elimination.

Management of the comatose patient can be time-consuming and expensive but is rewarding when successful.

Acute Nonprogressive

Vascular Diseases. *Vascular diseases* include occlusions causing infarctions and disruption of vessels causing hemorrhage.[15] Primary vascular changes, such as arteriosclerosis, are rare in animals.[16,17] Atherosclerosis can be produced with atherogenic diets and may be more common in animals with hypothyroidism.[18] Most vascular lesions are caused by emboli from sepsis or neoplasia. Fibrocartilaginous emboli from degenerating disks cause infarction in the spinal cord (see Chap. 7). The causes of vascular diseases are listed in Table 13–11.

A *stroke*, or a *cerebrovascular accident* (CVA), is an acute onset of neurologic deficit from spontaneous intracranial hemorrhage or occlusion of an intracranial blood vessel by a thrombus or an embolus. *Cerebral vasospasm* is a temporary constriction of an intracranial artery, causing transient ischemia. A vasospasm is difficult to document clinically. Transient loss of consciousness (syncope) is usually caused by a cardiac arrhythmia, not by a vasospasm (see Chap. 14).

TABLE 13–11 Etiology of Vascular Disease in the Brain*

Hemorrhage
Trauma
Infectious disease (rickettsial, septicemia, infectious canine hepatitis) (16)
Toxins (warfarin) (16)
Neoplasia (16)
Disseminated intravascular coagulopathy
Idiopathic thrombocytopenic purpura
Intracarotid injections (equine)
Neonatal maladjustment syndrome (foals)
Vascular anomalies
Infarction
Septic emboli (endocarditis, septicemia, thromboembolic meningoencephalitis) (16)
Neoplasia (metastases) (16)
Parasites (*Dirofilaria*) (16)
Idiopathic feline cerebral infarction
Vasospasm, vascular insufficiency, heart failure
Emboli secondary to surgery (air, fat, clot)

* Numbers in parentheses refer to chapters in which the conditions are discussed.

Hemorrhage in the brain is usually caused by trauma. All other causes of hemorrhage combined have a much lower incidence than does trauma. Small hemorrhages (petechiae) are seen on examination of the brain with inflammation as the primary problem, but other changes predominate.[19] The exception are those infections, such as Rocky Mountain spotted fever, that cause thrombocytopenia and vasculitis.[20] Hemorrhage producing stroke syndromes probably is seen most often in neoplasms that have compromised an artery (Fig. 13–7). Systemic coagulation disorders, such as disseminated intravascular coagulopathy (DIC) or idiopathic thrombocytopenic purpura (ITP), usually are recognized by systemic signs.[21]

An infarction is usually caused by septic emboli, frequently in association with endocarditis (Fig. 13–8). Cardiomyopathy should be considered in small animals with suspected cerebral infarctions. Thromboembolic meningoencephalitis (TEME) is an acute disease of cattle that is characterized by infarcts produced by septic emboli. Disseminated coagulopathy subsequently may develop. The disease is caused by *Hemophilus somnus* and usually is seen in feedlot cattle. Cerebral signs predominate, but brain stem infarctions may produce focal signs (see Chapter 16). Metastatic neoplasia or parasites, including the microfilaria of *Dirofilaria immitis*, are less common causes of vascular occlusion.[22,23] Air, fat, or blood clots may be introduced into the circulation during surgical procedures. Air emboli are of particular concern during vascular surgery of the head and the neck.

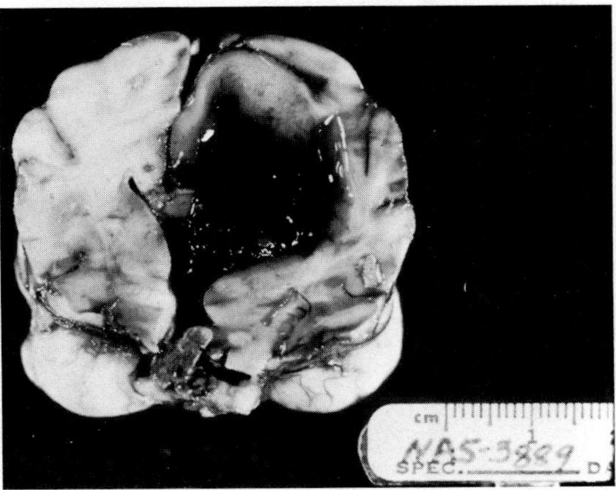

Figure 13–7 Massive hemorrhage in an oligodendrioglioma in a Samoyed. There were no clinical signs prior to an acute episode related to the hemorrhage.

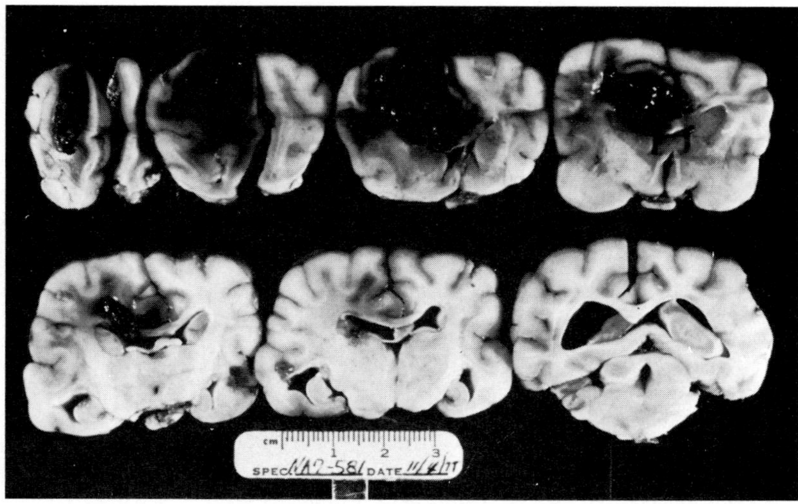

Figure 13–8 Hemorrhagic infarct in a dog with endocarditis. There is a cingulate herniation across the midline.

Idiopathic feline cerebral infarction has been described as a distinct syndrome. The etiology of the infarction has not been established, although vasculitis and thrombosis have been reported as causes.[24,25] There is no breed, sex, or age predilection. It has not been correlated with feline cardiomyopathy, although an association with this disorder should be considered in the differential diagnosis. The lesions are often confined to the distribution of the middle cerebral artery (Fig. 13–9). The rostral and caudal cerebral arteries are affected less often, possibly because they anastomose with each other, offering a source of collateral circulation, except in their terminal branches (Fig 13–10).[26]

Clinical signs of hemorrhage and infarction depend on the location and the extent of the involvement. In all cases of vascular occlusion or hemorrhage, a sudden onset with little or no progression is characteristic. Depending on the state of oxygenation and other factors, neuronal death begins in 3 to 10 minutes. Because most vascular lesions are unilateral, clinical signs are frequently more severe or are confined entirely to one side. Diffuse cerebral or rostral brain stem lesions may cause loss of consciousness that may persist (coma) or may be transient. Hemiparesis is frequent, and behavioral changes may be present.

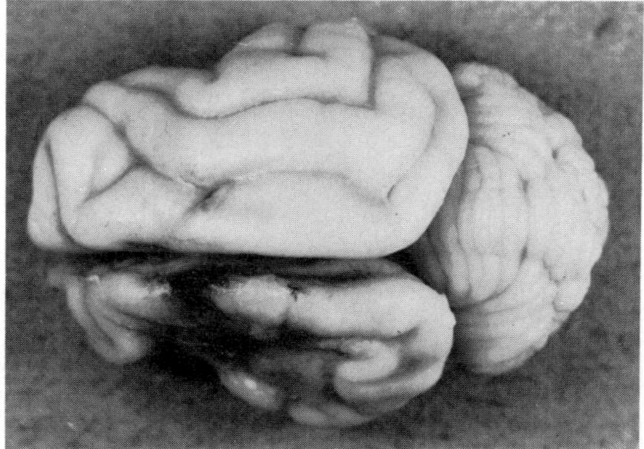

Figure 13–9 Infarction of the left cerebral hemisphere of a cat.

The management of the unconscious patient is discussed in the section on trauma in this chapter. Less severe lesions are usually not life-threatening; however, the amount of residual damage may depend on the adequacy of therapy. Although there is still some question of their efficacy, corticosteroids should be given in antiedema doses (30 mg/kg of methylprednisolone sodium succinate) in order to control edema.[27] Adequate ventilation must be assured if respiration is compromised. Anticoagulants generally are not used unless a clotting problem is known (DIC). If the source of the problem, such as bacterial endocarditis, can be identified, specific antibiotic therapy is instituted.

Most animals that are diagnosed clinically as likely to have CVAs recover. Unless the lesion is large or involves the brain stem, neurologic function is adequate for survival. An idiopathic feline cerebral infarction is characterized by massive cortical damage that causes seizures or behavioral disorders, which often are unacceptable in a pet.

Chronic Progressive

Neoplasia. Neoplasms of the brain may cause stupor and coma, depending on the location, the rate of growth, the development of ce-

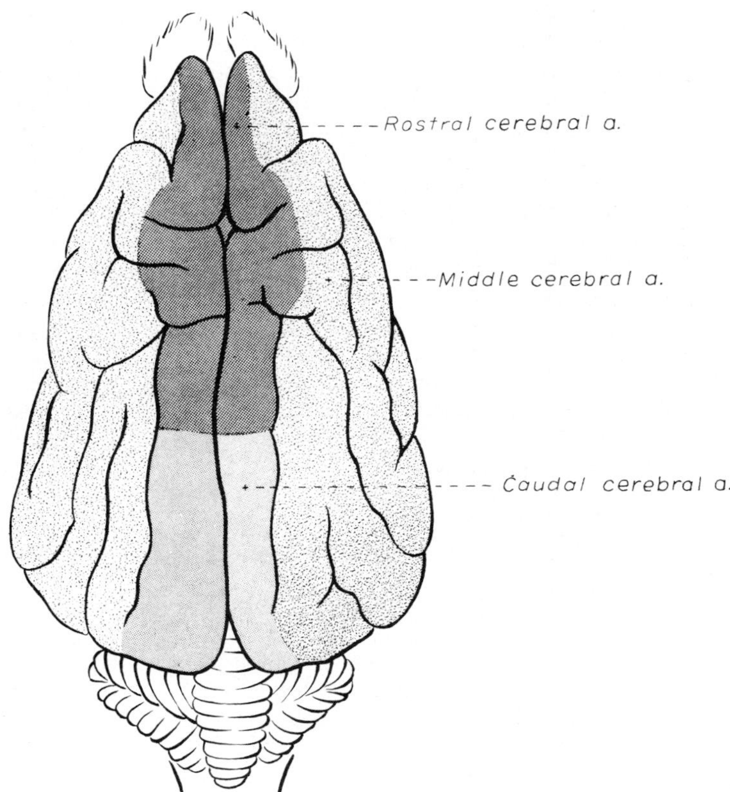

Figure 13–10 Areas of the brain supplied by the cerebral arteries. (From Evans HE, Christensen GC: Miller's Anatomy of the Dog, 2nd ed. Philadelphia, WB Saunders, 1979. Used by permission.)

rebral edema, and alterations in circulation. A sudden onset of stupor or coma has been seen in cases of acute hemorrhage into a cerebral brain tumor. The signs were attributed to an acute increase in intracranial pressure (see Fig. 13–7). Neoplasia will be discussed in Chapter 16.

No Focal or Lateralizing Signs, But Evidence of Meningeal Irritation

Acute Progressive

Inflammation. Inflammatory diseases of the CNS may affect both the nervous tissue and the meninges, although one of these entities may be more severely involved than the other. Stupor or coma is the result of a direct effect on neurons, cerebral edema, increased intracranial pressure from hydrocephalus, hypoxia from vasculitis, or systemic metabolic abnormalities.

Viral agents tend to have a greater effect on the nervous tissue, with only minimal involvement of the meninges. Vasculitis is common with viral or rickettsial infection. Bacterial and fungal agents produce a greater meningeal reaction. The formulation of a diagnosis usually requires an analysis of CSF (see Chap. 4).

The management of patients with stupor or coma secondary to inflammatory disease includes treatment of the primary disease, if possible, and management of the increased intracranial pressure. Cerebral edema should be treated with corticosteroids only if the animal is stuporous or worse. Depression of the immune system is a serious side effect of corticosteroids in a patient with infectious disease; however, the consequence of not treating the increased intracranial pressure is worse, namely, death of the animal. (See Chapter 16 for a complete discussion of inflammatory diseases and Chapter 5 for a discussion of treatment protocols.)

No Focal or Lateralizing Signs

Acute Progressive

Inflammation. Many of the viral encephalitides cause depression, stupor, or coma. They will be discussed in Chapter 16.

Metabolic Diseases. Nervous tissue depends on a continuous supply of glucose and oxygen for normal function. It is protected from toxic substances by the blood-brain barrier. Alterations in brain metabolism can cause severe clinical signs ranging from depression to coma and from tremors to seizures. The most common metabolic problems causing stupor or coma are listed in Table 13–6. Hypoglycemia will be discussed in Chapter 14. Hepatic encephalopathy, uremic encephalopathy, and diabetic coma are discussed in Chapter 16.

Heat stroke is an acute failure of the heat-regulating mechanisms of the body, which results in a body temperature that exceeds 40° C (105° F).[28,29] High ambient temperature, high humidity, and poor ventilation are the inciting factors. Brachycephalic breeds of dogs are especially susceptible. A long-haired coat, obesity, and a high fever may also predispose to heat stroke.

The primary mechanism for dissipation of heat in dogs and cats is panting. The air flow is unidirectional—in through the nose and out through the mouth.[30] The large surface area of the nasal turbinates promotes heat exchange. Prolonged panting causes a respiratory alkalosis that later is modified by a metabolic acidosis, presumably from increased muscular activity. If hyperthermia continues, two major complications are seen, either of which can cause death. Cerebral edema and DIC occur frequently, although the precise cause is not known. Although all of the CNS is involved, the neurons of the cerebral cortex and the cerebellum seem to be most susceptible to permanent damage.[31,32] The diagnosis of heat stroke is based on the clinical signs and the elevation of the body temperature.

The three major objectives of treatment are to reduce body temperature, prevent cerebral edema, and manage DIC if it develops. A corticosteroid should be given IV in an antiedema dose. The clinician lowers the body temperature by immersing the animal in cold or iced water. The rectal temperature should be monitored continuously by thermistor or at 10-minute intervals. To prevent hypothermia, cooling is stopped when the rectal temperature reaches 39.5° C (103° F). Ice water enemas may be used in refractory cases, but they prevent accurate monitoring of body temperature unless an esophageal thermistor is available. If shivering interferes with the cooling process, a tranquilizer (acetylpromazine, 0.1 mg/kg) may be given.

If the animal shows evidence of cerebral edema, and especially if signs of tentorial herniation are present (see Table 13–3), mannitol (0.25–1 g/kg) should be administered IV. If serious blood loss or DIC is a complication, mannitol should not be given.

Fluids should be given IV if hemoconcentration or peripheral circulatory failure is present. Overhydration must be avoided. Ringer's solution is the fluid of choice unless specific replacement therapy can be determined by serum electrolyte determination.

Hemorrhagic diarrhea, petechiae, or excessive bleeding from venipuncture sites signifies the onset of DIC. IV heparin (50–150 IU/kg) therapy should be instituted immediately. Coagulation studies can confirm the presence of DIC.[21,29]

The patient should be monitored carefully for at least 24 hours after normothermia is achieved so that recurrences can be avoided. The prognosis for patients with heat stroke is relatively good if they are treated early, before signs of cerebral edema or DIC develop.

Hypoxia is an inadequate supply of oxygen for normal brain function. Arterial oxygen tension levels below 50 mm Hg are detrimental to brain function. Increased levels of carbon dioxide have a profound effect on cerebral blood flow. Since there are no oxygen reserves in the brain, merely a few minutes of hypoxia can cause irreversible damage. More than 10 minutes of hypoxia produces neuronal death. The cerebral cortex is most susceptible to hypoxic damage, and the lower brain stem is most resistant.

The most frequent causes of hypoxia in animals are anesthesia, cardiopulmonary failure, suffocation, paralysis of respiration, carbon monoxide poisoning, and cyanide poisoning.

Despite the almost universal use of inhalation anesthesia with controlled ventilation, complications of anesthesia are common. Cardiac arrhythmias, overdose of the anesthetic agent, improper intubation, and faulty apparatus are but a few of the problems encountered. Meticulous attention to detail in the administration and the monitoring of anesthesia is essential.

Heart, lung, and peripheral circulatory failure rival anesthesia as the most common cause of hypoxia. Heart and lung disease may cause a mild to severe hypoxemia. If the condition does not cause unconsciousness, the danger of cerebral damage is low. Shock may cause profound cerebral hypoxia and irreversible damage to the brain. A primary concern in the management of shock is the maintenance of adequate ventilation. The management of the various forms of cardiopulmonary failure is beyond the scope of this text.[21]

Suffocation is a less frequent problem in animals. Examples of causes are aspiration of vomitus (especially in injured or anesthetized animals), aspiration of foreign bodies, and drowning.

Paralysis of respiration may occur with lesions of the CNS between the medullary respiratory centers and the origin of the phrenic nerve at C5–C7 (sometimes C4). The lesion may affect the respiratory center directly, or it may interrupt the descending pathway in the cervical spinal cord and produce the same effect: apnea. Lesions in the lower cervical (C7) or the upper thoracic region may block the pathway to the intercostal innervation, but the intact phrenic pathway will allow diaphragmatic ("abdominal") breathing to occur. The most common cause of this lesion is trauma. If the damage to the CNS is irreversible, life can be maintained only by use of a respirator. Generalized lower motor neuron (LMN) disease also may cause respiratory paralysis through its effect on both the intercostal nerves and the phrenic nerve (see Chap. 8).

Carbon monoxide poisoning is seen occasionally in animals that have been transported in a car trunk. Carbon monoxide combines with hemoglobin, preventing the formation of oxyhemoglobin. The animal typically has bright red mucous membranes and rapid, shallow respiration. Transfusion of fresh (not stored) whole blood and administration of oxygen may be effective if hypoxia has not persisted for too long.

Cyanide poisoning is rare, except in ruminants that eat plants containing hydrocyanic acid (cherry trees, sorghum grasses, and others). Cyanide interferes with the cellular utilization of oxygen through blockage of the cytochrome system.[33] Treatment is with sodium nitrite and sodium thiosulfate.

Nutritional Diseases. Thiamine deficiency may cause stupor or coma, especially in ruminants. Polioencephalomalacia, a symmetric laminar necrosis of the cerebral cortex, is seen in cattle, sheep, and goats. Increased intracranial pressure is common. Thiamine deficiency will be discussed in Chapter 16.

Chronic Progressive

Toxic Disorders. A large number of toxic agents may produce stupor and coma, especially in the terminal stages (see Chap. 16). An overdose of certain drugs, including barbiturates, tranquilizers, or narcotics, may produce stupor or coma as a primary effect.[33] The drugs may have been given deliberately or may have been ingested accidentally. Historical information may be clear ("he ate my bottle of pills") or misleading ("we never have anything like that around"). A comparison of the signs of coma caused by drugs with those of coma caused by structural changes in the brain is provided in Table 13–1. Spinal reflexes and respiration are depressed more severely by sedative drugs than by most structural lesions, whereas pupillary responses are less affected.

Most patients that have overdosed on CNS depressants can be saved with proper management. If the animal is not in coma, attentive nursing is usually all that is necessary. Gastric lavage and use of activated charcoal is useful if the drug was ingested recently. The maintenance of adequate respiration is the most important consideration for patients in coma. Controlled respiration through an endotracheal catheter is essential. Diuresis is promoted by the IV administration of glucose or mannitol. Urine output must be monitored through an indwelling urethral catheter. The excretion of many agents (e.g., barbiturates) is dependent on the rate of urine formation. Hydration and acid-base balance must be maintained. Periodic evaluation of serum electrolytes and blood gases is of great benefit in the management of persistent coma. The combination of diuresis and controlled ventilation can lead to serious changes in a short time. Stimulant drugs have been used in the past but appear to be of little benefit, since they do not affect the rate of metabolism or excretion of most drugs.

Degenerative Diseases. *Storage diseases*, inherited degenerative diseases with accumulation of metabolic products in neurons, may cause depression or stupor. The animal may be in a coma terminally. Other signs, such as ataxia or seizures, are more common in the early stages of the disease (see Chap. 16).

Anomalies. *Hydrocephalus* is an enlargement of the cerebral ventricular system secondary to an increased amount of CSF. Excessive CSF may be the result of obstruction to flow (noncommunicating or obstructive hydrocephalus), poor absorption, or increased production (communicating hydrocephalus). Hydrocephalus may be seen in any species.

Most of the CSF is produced by the choroid plexus in the lateral, third, and fourth ventricles, but a substantial portion travels through the ependyma lining the ventricles and the subarachnoid space around the brain and the spinal cord. CSF flows from the lateral ventricles through the interventricular foramina to the third ventricle. It continues caudally through the mesencephalic aqueduct to the fourth ventricle and into the subarachnoid space through the lateral apertures of the fourth ventricle. In the subarachnoid space, most of the fluid moves around the brain stem into the rostrotentorial compartment. Most of the absorption occurs through the arachnoid villi in the dorsal sagittal sinus (Fig. 13–11).

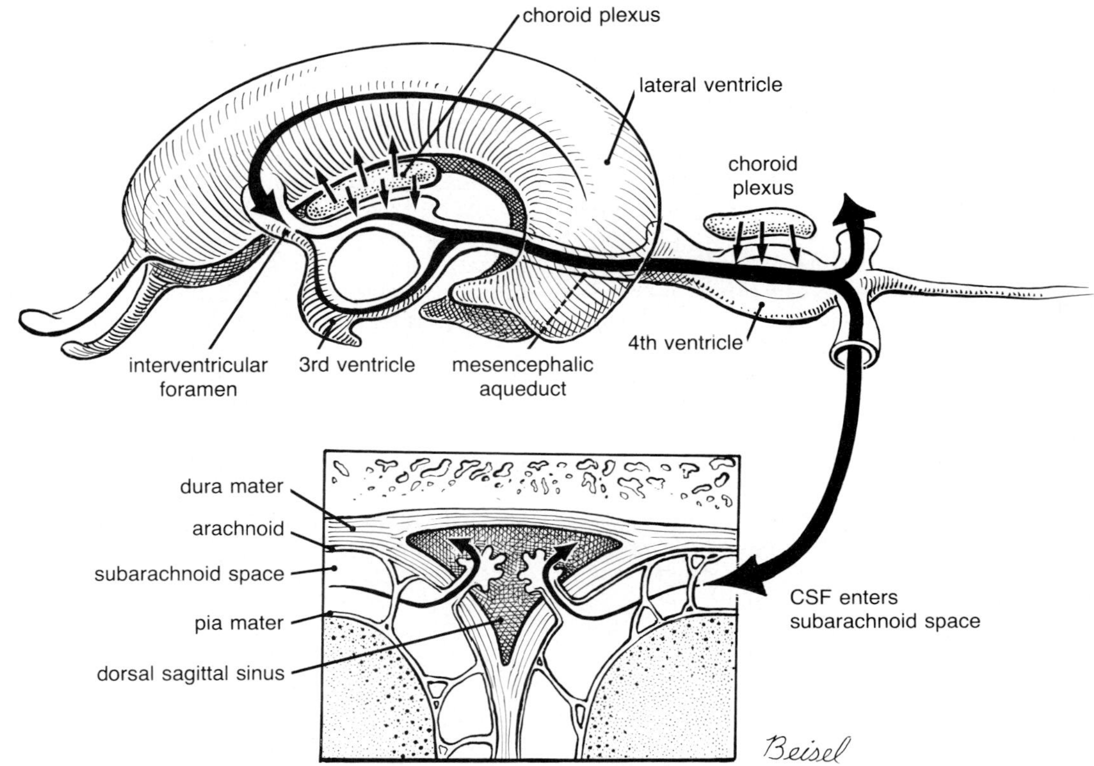

Figure 13–11 Cerebrospinal fluid is produced in all areas of the central nervous system. The bulk of the fluid flows from the lateral ventricles to the third ventricle to the mesencephalic aqueduct and continues from the fourth ventricle to the lateral apertures and then to the subarachnoid space, where it is absorbed.

Overproduction of CSF by a choroid plexus papilloma is rare. Communicating hydrocephalus from decreased absorption of CSF is usually the result of inflammation of the meninges. Inflammation is usually caused by infectious diseases, such as canine distemper, but may be secondary to subarachnoid hemorrhage or to the presence of foreign materials, such as radiographic contrast materials injected in the subarachnoid space.[34] Obstruction of the flow of CSF occurs most commonly at the mesencephalic aqueduct. Malformations of the aqueduct range from complete absence to stenosis. Obstruction of the aqueduct also can be secondary to inflammation or compression by a mass. For example, brain stem tumors that cause obstruction of the aqueduct produce hydrocephalus.[35,36]

Most cases of hydrocephalus that are seen in veterinary practice are congenital. The disorder may be caused by environmental or genetic factors. Hereditary hydrocephalus has been reported in Hereford cattle.[37] There have not been enough studies of the pathology of congenital hydrocephalus in the dog to determine the primary defect. Some patients have stenosis or atresia of the mesencephalic aqueduct, but others do not. Multiple branching of the aqueduct, called "forking," has been reported in both dogs and human beings.[36,38] A statistically significant correlation between small body size and hydrocephalus has been demonstrated in dogs (Table 13–12).[39]

Ventricular enlargement without clinical signs is a common finding in some toy breeds, especially Chihuahuas. A kennel of Chihuahuas was studied by Redding.[40] Subclinical hydrocephalus was common. Behavioral changes could be correlated with abnormal EEGs in

TABLE 13–12 Breeds of Dogs at Increased Risk for Hydrocephalus

Maltese	Toy poodle
Yorkshire terrier	Cairn terrier
English bulldog	Boston terrier
Chihuahua	Pug
Lhasa apso	Pekingese
Pomeranian	

Data from Selby LA, Hayes HM, Becker SV: Episootiologic features of canine hydrocephalus. Am J Vet Res 40:411–414, 1979.

many instances. A selective breeding program in which the EEG was used to screen breeding animals reduced the incidence of hydrocephalus. Redding concluded that the dogs had a compensated hydrocephalus (a balance between production and absorption of CSF) that could be decompensated by relatively mild changes, such as trauma or infection. These observations correlate with our clinical impression. Redding also observed a high incidence of enlargement of the foramen magnum (occipital dysplasia—see Chap. 9) in these dogs. Whether this abnormality is related to the cause of hydrocephalus or whether it is secondary to increased pressure is still debatable. The clinical signs are related to (1) the age at onset, (2) the degree of imbalance between production and absorption of CSF, and (3) the location of the defect (communicating or noncommunicating).

Simpson[38] studied a series of hydrocephalic Maltese dogs. Less than 20% had seizures, with most seizures occurring during the first year of life. Behavioral problems were the most frequent complaint. Learned responses, such as house training, were difficult or impossible to achieve in 75% of the dogs.

Congenital hydrocephalus is usually recognized in the very young animal. The increase in intracranial volume occurs before the sutures of the skull have closed, allowing for enlargement of the calvaria. The enlargement of the head, the open sutures and fontanelles, and the poor development of the animal may be recognized shortly after birth. Affected dogs are usually presented to the veterinarian when they are between 2 and 3 months of age. Palpation of the skull may reveal the open sutures and fontanelles. In compensated hydrocephalus the fontanelle may be open, but there is no tension as the brain is palpated. Active hydrocephalus with increased pressure often causes a bulging of the soft tissue through the fontanelle, and palpation reveals the increased tension. The head is enlarged. The prominent frontal areas encroach on the orbits, causing a ventrolateral deviation of the eyes (Fig. 13–12). Oculomotor

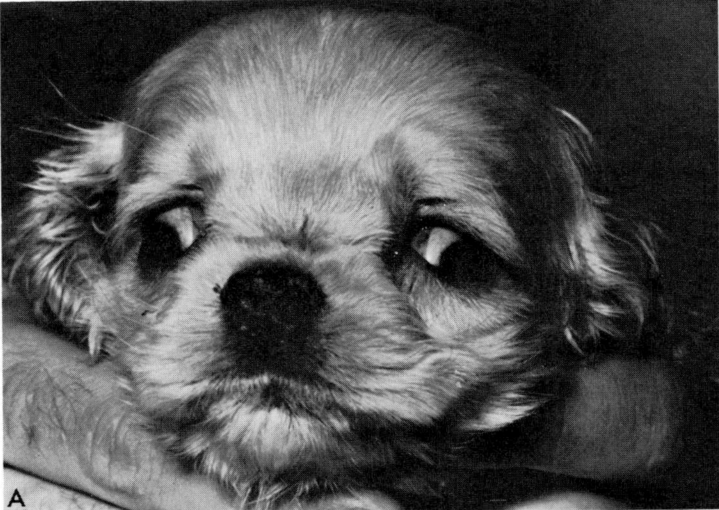

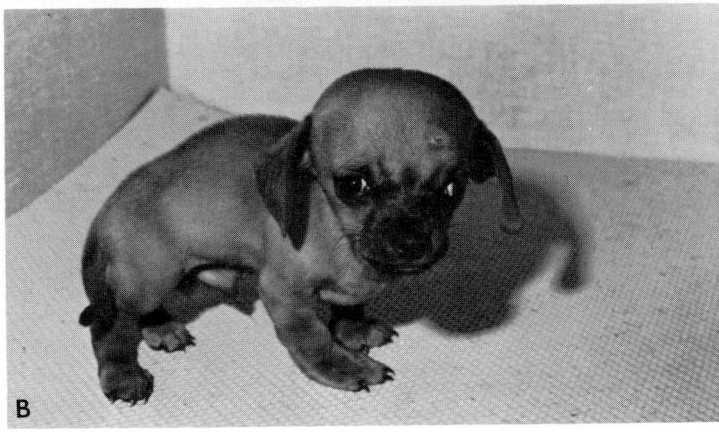

Figure 13–12 Cocker spaniel (*A*) and dachshund (*B*) puppies with hydrocephalus. The large, rounded head and the ventrolateral deviation of the eyes are characteristic.

nerve function (pupils and eye movements—see Chap. 12) is usually normal, indicating that the eye deviation is mechanical, not neurologic, in origin. The widening of the skull is detected by palpation of the parietal area where the space between the skull and the zygomatic arch is narrowed. Head pain may be evident in some animals when the skull is palpated.

Young animals with hydrocephalus usually are smaller and less developed than their littermates. They are often depressed, have episodic behavioral changes (such as aggression or confusion), and frequently have seizures (see Chap. 14). Their mental development is retarded, so they do not learn as readily as their littermates. Visual deficits with normal pupillary responses are common because of damage to the optic radiation and the occipital cortex (see Chap. 12). Motor function may range from almost normal gait to severe tetraparesis. Papilledema may be seen on fundic examination in a small percentage of cases.

Hydrocephalus in the adult animal is more difficult to recognize. The skull is normal because the sutures have fused prior to the increase in pressure. The clinical signs develop more rapidly and are more severe, but they are dependent on the relative balance of production and absorption of CSF. Seizures are a frequent sign in the early stages. Depression, which may progress to stupor or coma, is common. Since hydrocephalus in the adult is usually secondary to inflammation or a mass, signs of the primary problem may predominate early in the course of the disease. Complete obstruction of the CSF causes a rapidly progressive hydrocephalus, which may cause tentorial herniation, cerebellar herniation, or both.

The diagnosis of hydrocephalus in the young animal is relatively certain if the characteristic signs are present. Although the clinical signs of severe hydrocephalus are typical, less severe involvement may produce a more subtle picture. Behavioral changes or seizures may be the only complaint. In these cases, ancillary studies are necessary to confirm the diagnosis.

EEG is the first test used in our clinic, because it is noninvasive and the recordings are usually diagnostic (Fig. 13–13). High-voltage, slow wave activity (25–200 μV, 1–6 Hz) that is hypersynchronous (similar in all leads) may be seen both in dogs that are awake and in those that are anesthetized. A fast component (10–12 Hz) often is superimposed on the slow waves. In severe hydrocephalus, in which the large slow waves (1–4 Hz) predominate, the EEG is sufficient for diagnosis. Earlier forms, in which faster activity is more prominent, may be confused with inflammatory disease. Adult dogs may have faster activity also.[38] Since many veterinary practices do not have EEG capabilities, the diagnosis must be confirmed by other procedures.

Two procedures, computed tomography (CT) and ultrasonography (US) through the open fontanelles, are the most accurate and least invasive methods of diagnosis (Fig. 13–14).[38]

If CT and US are not available, radiographs of the skull may demonstrate changes that are compatible with hydrocephalus. If expense is a consideration, radiographs are not essential, and the diagnosis can be confirmed by ventricular tap. Skull radiographs can confirm open suture lines and fontanelles. Increased intracranial pressure for an extended period causes thinning of the skull with loss of the normal

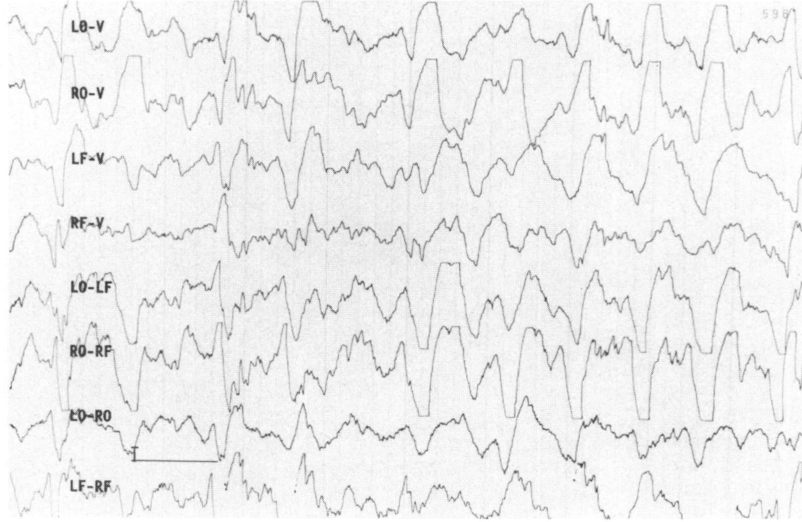

Figure 13–13 Electroencephalogram of a hydrocephalic dog. The recording is characterized by low-frequency, high-voltage activity that is synchronized, generalized, and symmetric. *L* = left, *R* = right, *O* = occipital, *F* = frontal, *V* = vertex. Calibration markers: horizontal bar = 1 sec; vertical bar = 50 μV.

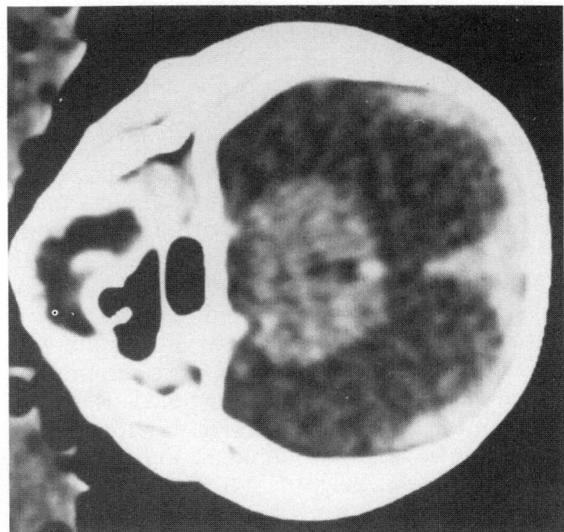

Figure 13–14 CT scan of a hydrocephalic Chihuahua dog, female, 10 months old, with a history of seizures, progressive dementia, and postural reaction deficits. The ventricles are the dark areas occupying most of the cranial vault.

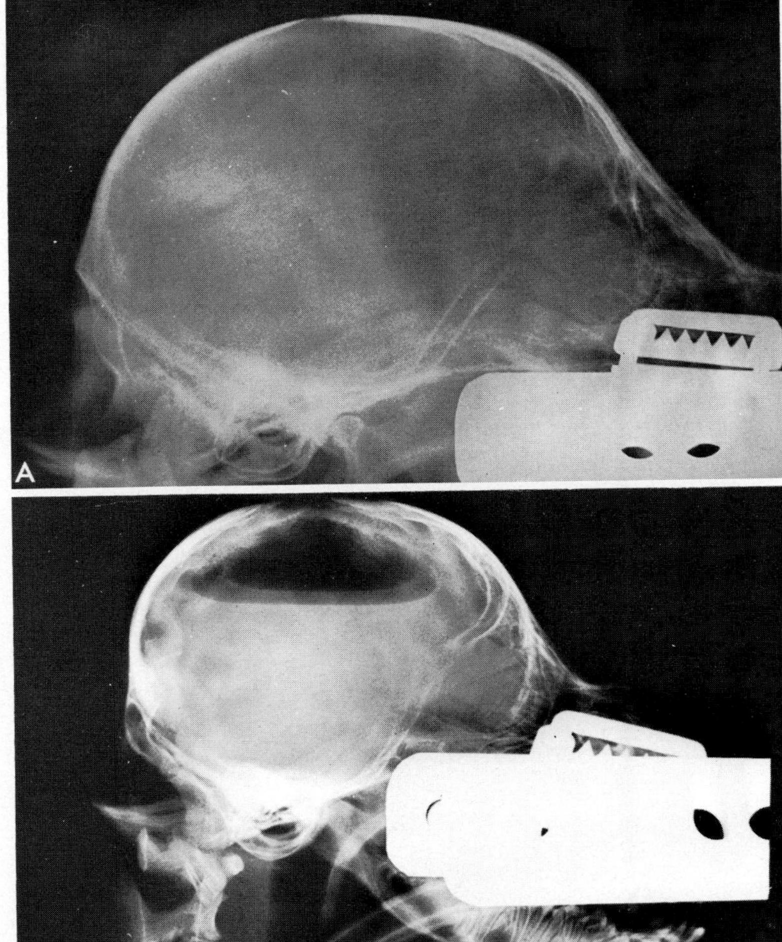

Figure 13–15 *A.* Radiograph of a hydrocephalic dog. Notice the "ground-glass" appearance of the calvaria, caused by loss of the digital impressions from chronic increased pressure. The fontanelle is open on the dorsum of the skull, and the osseous tentorium is absent. *B.* Pneumoventriculogram of a dog with hydrocephalus.

digitate impressions on the inner surface of the calvaria. The cranium has a "ground-glass" appearance (Fig. 13–15A). Rostral displacement and thinning of the wing of the sphenoid bone and loss of the osseous tentorium cerebelli also may be seen.

The diagnosis can be confirmed in severe cases by a ventricular tap under general anesthesia. A spinal needle is inserted directly into the ventricle. The depth that is necessary to obtain fluid provides an estimate of the thickness of the cerebral cortex. Normal animals have a lateral ventricle that is only a few millimeters thick. Careful needle placement is required to obtain fluid. Severe hydrocephalus causes thinning of the cerebral cortex (Fig. 13–16), so that fluid may be obtained within 0.5 to 1.0 cm of the inner surface of the skull. If it is necessary to go deeper than 1.0 to 1.5 cm to obtain fluid, pneumoventriculography is performed to confirm the ventricular enlargement. The distances given are primarily for toy-breed dogs or cats; those for larger animals of any species may vary somewhat. Fluid never should be aspirated with a syringe, because the cerebral cortex may collapse, causing a subdural hematoma (Fig. 13–17). Fluid may be allowed to escape under its own pressure, providing some therapeutic benefit in addition to establishing the diagnosis. Analysis of the CSF may be useful for formulating an etiologic diagnosis (see Chap. 4). In a potentially hydrocephalic animal with an open fontanelle, there is less risk in obtaining the CSF for analysis from the ventricle than from the cerebellomedullary cistern.

If the results of the ventricular tap are not diagnostic, pneumoventriculography is performed (see Fig. 13–15B). Positive contrast ventriculography may be necessary to determine whether the hydrocephalus is communicating or noncommunicating. Because therapy generally will be the same in either case, the increased risks involved in the use of positive contrast material usually are not justified.

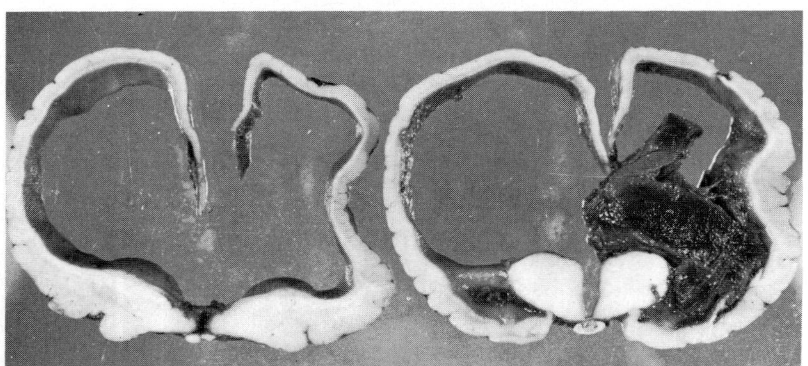

Figure 13–16 Severe hydrocephalus in a Chihuahua. Notice the thinning of the cerebral cortex. There is an intraventricular hematoma.

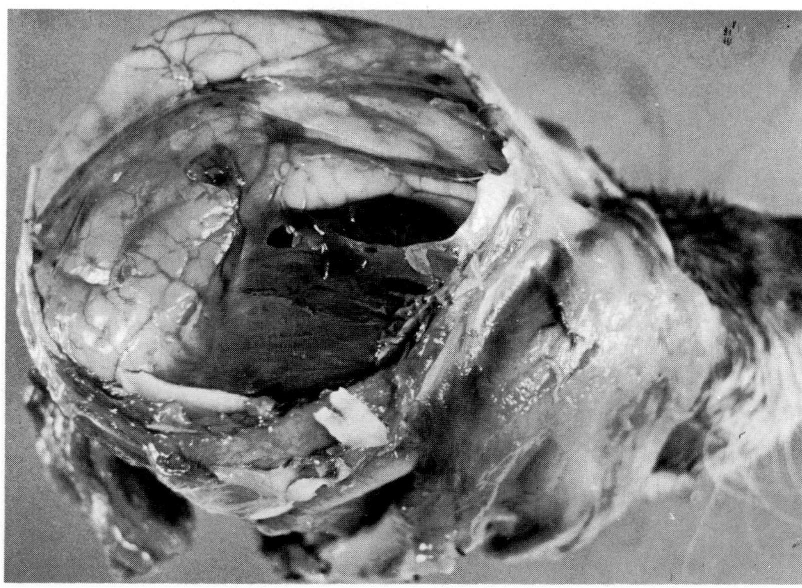

Figure 13–17 A dog with hydrocephalus and a large subdural hematoma that resulted when too much fluid was aspirated from the lateral ventricle. (From Oliver JE Jr, Knecht CD: Diseases of the brain. In Ettinger SJ: Textbook of Veterinary Internal Medicine, 1st ed. Philadelphia, WB Saunders, 1975. Used by permission.)

In summary, CT or US are the best diagnostic tests that are not invasive. If either is available, the other tests are not necessary. Ventricular tap may be needed for therapeutic benefit in acute cases, and is the safest method for obtaining CSF if it is needed to substantiate an etiologic diagnosis.

The treatment of hydrocephalus depends on the cause of the disorder and the status of the animal. Acquired hydrocephalus in the adult animal requires resolution of the inciting factor. Neoplasia will be discussed in Chapter 16. An inflammatory disease may cause permanent reduction of absorptive capacity, and the hydrocephalus must be managed separately. Hydrocephalic patients usually fit into one of the following categories: (1) acute with rapidly progressing signs in a previously normal animal or one that previously has been static, (2) chronic progressive deterioration, or (3) static signs that may be mild to severe.

Acute progressive signs indicate a poor prognosis and the need for vigorous treatment. A ventricular tap should be done, and fluid should be allowed to flow under its own pressure with the animal in sternal recumbency and the head elevated slightly above the shoulders. Fluid should not be aspirated. An osmotic diuretic (mannitol, 1 g/kg) should be given slowly by IV drip to reduce cerebral edema. A corticosteroid (methylprednisolone, 30 mg/kg IV) should be given to reduce CSF production and edema. The dosage of mannitol should be repeated twice at 6-hour intervals. Corticosteroids may be continued as in trauma (5 mg/kg/hr IV). If the animal is stable, the glucocorticoid can be given in anti-inflammatory doses. Anticonvulsants should be used if needed. If the animal survives and the neurologic status permits, the same long-term treatment should be provided as for chronic progressive cases.

Animals with chronic progressive hydrocephalus, as indicated by the history and serial neurologic examinations, may be treated medically or surgically. Progression should be stopped, and some clinical improvement should be seen as a result of treatment. The owner must be made aware, however, that the animal will not be totally normal. If the neurologic status is too poor for the animal to function as a pet, then treatment should not be continued. Medical treatment usually is tried first.[38] Dexamethasone, 0.25 mg/5 kg b.i.d., or prednisone, 0.25–0.5 mg/kg b.i.d., should be given orally. Clinical improvement is expected within 3 days. If improvement is seen, the dosage should be reduced by half after 1 week. After another week, glucocorticoids are given once every other day. If signs are stable, medication may be discontinued and repeated only as signs develop. Many animals stabilize in remission and only occasionally require medication. Others may require continuous medication, in which case signs of Cushing's disease may appear. The objective of medical treatment is to provide remission of signs with the least possible amount of medication. Low-dose, alternate-day therapy can be used for extended periods without problems.

Surgical treatment is reserved for those cases that cannot be stabilized medically. Surgical treatment entails placement of a drainage tube from the lateral ventricle through a one-way valve to the right atrium or the peritoneal cavity. The major disadvantages of surgery are the expense and the postoperative complications. The complications include the necessity of replacing the tubing as the animal grows, occlusion of the tubes by fibrous tissue or clots, and sepsis. The shunts can be very effective and have functioned well in some dogs for up to 8 years.[14]

Other anomalies of the brain may cause alterations in mental status (see Table 13–5). Some are so grossly abnormal that they are not usually compatible with life, such as hydranencephaly and otocephaly. Others are more typically characterized by seizures and will be discussed in Chapter 14.

CASE HISTORIES

The cases in this chapter have the common sign of alteration in mental status. After reading the history and the results of the examination, the student should make a problem list, localize the lesion, list the rule-outs and formulate a plan for the diagnosis of each, and make a prognosis. Then read the assessment section and the results of the diagnostic procedures.

Case History 13A

Signalment

Canine, boxer, female, 6 months old.

History

The dog was hit by a car 6 hours before presentation. She was unconscious after being hit and has not regained consciousness.

Physical Examination

The dog is unconscious and in lateral recumbency. The temperature is 100.6° F, the pulse is 75, and the respirations are 25 and shallow. The color of the membranes is good, and the capillary refill time is rapid. There is a small abrasion on the muzzle on the left side. There are no palpable fractures or luxations. Heart and lung sounds are normal.

Neurologic Examination

The dog is unconscious and does not respond to painful stimuli, except for the withdrawal reflexes. All four limbs are in rigid extension. When the dog is forced to flex the limbs, there is considerable resistance to a point, and then they collapse. The postural reactions are absent. When the animal is moved into an erect position, the head and the neck arch dorsally. The myotatic reflexes cannot be evaluated because of the rigid extension of the limbs. Strong stimuli cause an increase in extension followed by a brief partial flexion that reverts to extension almost immediately. Tests for vision are negative. The pupils are small, symmetric, and slightly reactive. In a darkened room, they dilate only slightly (about 2 to 3 mm). Vestibular eye movements are absent. The globes are in the center of the palpebral fissure. The palpebral reflex is present but weak. There is no evidence of conscious perception of pain from a pinch of the face or a stimulation of the nasal mucosa. The gag reflex is present. The tongue retracts symmetrically, but there are no licking movements.

Case History 13B

Signalment

Canine, Samoyed, male, 4 years old.

History

The dog has hip dysplasia, but there were no other significant medical problems. At 8:00 A.M. the dog started walking aimlessly, bumping into walls and doors. Within one-half hour the rear limbs began to abduct, and the dog fell. When the owner picked him up, he growled. At 9:00 A.M. the dog was seen by the referring veterinarian, who reported the following:

Mental status: The dog is depressed.

Posture and gait: The dog is unable to walk and falls to the right side.

Postural reactions: Very poor to absent in the right front and the right rear limbs; normal in the left front and the left rear limbs.

Spinal reflexes: Normal.

Cranial nerves: The menace reaction is poor bilaterally; otherwise, the reactions are normal.

The dog was brought to our clinic at 6:00 P.M., 10 hours after the onset of the signs.

Neurologic Examination

The dog is in coma. The temperature is 105° F. There is minimal increase in extensor tonus of the limbs. The postural reactions are absent. The spinal reflexes are normal. The menace reaction is absent. The pupils are widely dilated and unresponsive to light. The eyes are deviated ventrolaterally and do not respond to head movements. The palpebral reflex is present, but there is no behavioral response to a pinch of the face or a touch of the nasal mucosa. There is a weak gag reflex and good retraction of the tongue.

Case History 13C

Signalment

Canine, Chihuahua, male, 3 months old.

History

Lack of coordination and intermittent depression began at age 2 months. The dog has had no known illness, and his vaccinations have been given on schedule.

Physical Examination

The head is dome-shaped with a large, open fontanelle. The only other abnormalities appear on the neurologic examination.

Neurologic Examination

The dog is depressed and does not seem to have a normal awareness of his environment. Loud noises produce a startle reaction, but the response is not oriented toward the sound. The dog can walk but is reluctant to do so. Once he starts walking, he progresses to a wall and then stands with his head against the wall. Some dysmetria and a mild ataxia are present. The postural reactions are depressed in all four limbs, and worse in the pelvic limbs than in the thoracic limbs. The spinal reflexes are normal. There is no menace reaction, and the dog does not appear to be able to see. The visual placing reaction is absent, although the tactile placing reaction is present but slow. The pupillary reflexes are normal. The eyes appear deviated ventrolaterally, although vestibular eye movements are present in all directions. Other cranial nerves are normal. Sensation is intact, although reactions to painful stimuli are slow and poorly directed.

Assessment 13A

The dog is in coma and exhibits decerebrate rigidity. Decerebrate rigidity is caused by loss of the voluntary upper motor neuron (UMN) pathways with retention of the reticulospinal and vestibulospinal pathways, which are facilitatory to the extensor motor neurons. The loss of postural reactions confirms the absence of voluntary UMN pathways. The arching of the head and the neck is opisthotonos. The spinal reflexes are difficult to assess when the limbs are in extensor rigidity, but it is apparent that the extensor neurons are intact. The visual tests will be negative in an unconscious animal, since we depend on behavioral responses for our assessment. The pupillary reactions indicate that the oculomotor nerve is intact bilaterally. The small size of the pupil suggests loss of sympathetic input or irritation of the oculomotor nerve.

The symmetry suggests that it is loss of sympathetic tone. The absent eye movements indicate paralysis of CN III, CN IV, and CN VI, or a lesion of the medial longitudinal fasciculus (MLF) connecting those nuclei with the vestibular nucleus. Because the parasympathetic component of CN III is functional, a lesion of the MLF is more likely. Other cranial nerves appear relatively normal, considering the level of consciousness.

Localization: Brain stem, caudal to CN III (midbrain), rostral to CN VII (rostral medulla), including the midline MLF and a large portion of the reticular activating system (coma). Therefore, it probably is a large intramedullary lesion of the pons.

Rule-outs: Trauma is known. An acute onset of coma without improvement for 6 hours suggests brain stem hemorrhage rather than tentorial herniation. The clinical signs are consistent with this hypothesis. Tentorial herniation usually affects CN III early. The signs indicate a lesion of the pons rather than the midbrain, which is compressed by tentorial herniation. There are no simple diagnostic tests to confirm intramedullary hemorrhage of the brain stem. The alternatives are to treat and observe for change or to use other tests to rule out epidural or subdural hemorrhage absolutely. Radiographs would demonstrate a skull fracture, but this finding probably would not alter the plan.

Skull radiographs were taken, and it was found that a linear fracture extended across the floor of the cranial vault—a basilar fracture. Basilar fractures have been associated with severe brain lesions in the cases we have seen.

Prognosis: Poor.

Plan: Treat medically (corticosteroids, mannitol, IV fluids, nursing care) and observe for 48 hours.

Results: The dog's neurologic status did not change in 48 hours. The owners requested euthanasia. The brain is shown in Figure 13–5.

Assessment 13B

Localization: The lesion involves the brain stem. Dilated pupils (CN III) and coma (reticular activating system) indicate that there is midbrain involvement. CN V and CN VII are intact (palpebral reflex), indicating that the pons and the medulla (also CN IX, CN X, CN XII) are intact. The progression of signs from the cerebrum (pacing, blindness, postural reaction deficits) to the midbrain suggests tentorial herniation. The early signs were unilateral, indicating a left cerebral lesion with rapid progression to bilateral tentorial herniation.

Rule-outs: The sudden onset of severe signs usually indicates trauma or vascular lesions. The dog was in the house and had not been out since the night before, making trauma unlikely. Severe cerebral vascular lesions in dogs are unusual, but this hypothesis seems most likely. Vascular lesions may be associated with other pathologies, such as parasites or neoplasia.

Rule out (1) vascular lesion and (2) trauma.

Plan: Spontaneous epidural or subdural hemorrhages have not been reported in dogs. Parenchymal hemorrhages are not likely to be helped by surgery. These factors, plus the severity of the signs, made the prognosis very poor. The only useful diagnostic test is CT, but it was not available. The animal was given intensive medical treatment (mannitol, corticosteroids, fluids) and was monitored carefully until the next day. The temperature cycled frequently, varying from 101° to 107° F. There was no change in the neurologic status after 18 hours, and the owner requested euthanasia.

Necropsy: The dog had an oligodendroglioma of the left cerebrum with a massive hemorrhage (see Fig. 13–7).

Assessment 13C

The primary problems are depression, loss of vision, and postural reaction deficits with a reasonably normal gait. All of these conditions are compatible with lesions above the brain stem. Postural reaction deficits without significant gait deficits usually are caused by cerebral or diencephalic lesions. Loss of vision with intact pupillary light reflexes indicates that the pathways from the eye to the midbrain and CN III are intact, but there is bilateral damage to the lateral geniculate nucleus, the optic radiations, or the cerebral cortex. Intact vestibular eye movements indicate that the brain stem pathways (MLF) and CN III, CN IV, and CN VI are intact. The deviation of the eyes must have another cause. Depression is not localizing but is compatible with diffuse cerebral or diencephalic disease.

Localization: Cerebrum or diencephalon, diffuse.

Rule-outs: The problems are slowly progressive, with an onset at an early age. Inflammatory disease would have to be considered. The inherited degenerative diseases also may cause a syndrome such as this one, but none of these disorders has been reported in the Chihuahua. Hydrocephalus is commonly seen in this breed. The signs are usually cortical in origin. Blindness is frequent. The dog has a dome-shaped head with an open fontanelle, which is typical of congenital hydrocephalus. Many Chihuahuas have these skull changes without enlarged ventricles, however. The deviation of the eyes is seen in hydrocephalics because of the malformation of the bones of the orbit (see Fig. 13–12). Hydrocephalus would have to be our first choice until the presence of another condition is proved.

Rule-outs: (1) hydrocephalus, (2) inflammation, and (3) degenerative disease.

Plan: Skull radiographs will not reveal much more than we already can see and feel (shape and open fontanelle). An EEG may be useful but probably will not be absolutely diagnostic because the dog is immature, and we can expect high-voltage slow waves in a normal 3-month-old dog. The best diagnostic test is CT, but it was not available. The next most direct diagnostic test for hydrocephalus is a ventricular tap with a pneumoventriculogram if the tap is not diagnostic. The tap can be made through the lateral margin of the open fontanelle. If fluid is obtained with the needle inserted less than 2 cm, then the ventricles are enlarged. If there is doubt, 2 ml of air can be injected and a radiograph made to confirm the size of the ventricles. The CSF that is obtained can be analyzed. A cisternal tap is contraindicated, because it may cause cerebral herniation if hydrocephalus is present. Degenerative diseases cannot be diagnosed except by biopsy or necropsy in most cases.

Prognosis: Guarded.

Plan:

1. Rule out hydrocephalus: Ventricular tap, CSF analysis, pneumoventriculogram.
2. Rule out inflammation: CSF analysis.
3. Rule out degenerative diseases: Exclusion.

Results: Under general anesthesia, a ventricular tap was performed. Fluid was obtained with the needle only 1 cm below the scalp. The owners refused treatment for the dog, and he was destroyed.

Many dogs with this degree of abnormality will improve with treatment; however, vision may be permanently lost. If vision is present, the prognosis is much better.

Also review Case History E in Chapters 1, 2, and 4.

REFERENCES

1. Cartlidge NEF: States of altered consciousness. In Swash M, Kennard C: Scientific Basis of Clinical Neurology. Edinburgh, Churchill Livingstone, 1985.
2. Hendricks JC, Morrison AR: Normal and abnormal sleep in mammals. J Am Vet Med Assoc 178:121–126, 1981.
3. Siegel J, Tomaszewski K, Nienhuis R: Behavioral states in the chronic medullary and midpontine cat. EEG Clin Neurophysiol 63:274–288, 1986.
4. Kaitin KI, Kilduff TS, Dement WC: Evidence for excessive sleepiness in canine narcoleptics. EEG Clin Neurophysiol 65:447–454, 1986.
5. Kornegay JN, Oliver JE Jr, Gorgacz EJ: Clinicopathologic features of brain herniation in animals. J Am Vet Med Assoc 182:1111–1116, 1983.
6. Milhorat TH: Cerebrospinal Fluid and the Brain Edemas. New York, Neuroscience Society of New York, 1987.
7. Griffiths IR: Central nervous system trauma. In Oliver JE, Hoerlien BF, Mayhew IG: Veterinary Neurology. Philadelphia, WB Saunders, 1987, pp 303–320.
8. Shores A: Development of a coma scale for dogs: Prognostic value in cranio-cerebral trauma. In: Proceedings of the Sixth Annual Veterinary Medical Forum, Washington, DC, 1988, pp 251–253.
9. Shores A: Craniocerebral trauma. In Kirk RW (ed): Current Veterinary Therapy X. Philadelphia, WB Saunders, 1989, pp 847–853.
10. Oliver JE: Neurologic emergencies in small animals. Vet Clin North Am 2:341–357, 1972.
11. Bracken MB, Shepard MJ, Collins WF, et al: A randomized, controlled trial of methylprednisolone or naloxone in the treatment of acute spinal-cord injury. N Engl J Med 322:1405–1411, 1990.
12. Bracken MB, Shepard MJ, Collins WF, et al: Methylprednisolone or naloxone treatment after acute spinal cord injury: 1-year follow-up data. J Neurosurg 76:23–31, 1992.
13. Parker AJ: Blood pressure changes and lethality of mannitol infusion in dogs. Am J Vet Res 34:1523–1528, 1973.
14. Oliver J, Hoerlein B: Cranial Surgery. In Oliver JE, Hoerlein BF, Mayhew IG (eds): Veterinary Neurology. Philadelphia, WB Saunders, 1987, pp 470–492.
15. Joseph RJ, Greenlee PG, Carillo JM, et al: Canine cerebrovascular disease: Clinical and pathologic findings in 17 cases. J Am Anim Hosp Assoc 24:569–576, 1988.
16. Fankhauser R, Luginbuhl H, McGrath JT: Cerebrovascular disease in various animal species. Ann NY Acad Sci 127:817–860, 1965.
17. Detweiler DK, Ratcliffe HL, Luginbuhl H: The significance of naturally ocurring coronary and cerebral arterial disease in animals. Ann NY Acad Sci 127:868–881, 1968.
18. Zachary J, Patterson J, Rusley M: Neurologic manifestations of cerebrovascular atherosclerosis associated with primary hypothyroidism in a dog. J Am Vet Med Assoc 186:499–503, 1985.
19. Braund KG, Brewer BD, Mayhew IG: Inflammatory, infectious, immune, parasitic, and vascular diseases. In Oliver JE, Hoerlein BF, and Mayhew IG (eds): Veterinary Neurology. Philadelphia, WB Saunders, 1987, pp 216–254.
20. Greene CE: Rocky Mountain spotted fever and ehrlichiosis. In Kirk RW (ed): Current Veterinary Therapy IX. Philadelphia, WB Saunders, 1986, pp 1080–1084.
21. Morgan RV: Handbook of Small Animal Practice. New York, Churchill Livingstone, 1988.
22. Patton CS, Garner FM: Cerebral infarction by heartworms (*Dirofilaria immitis*) in a dog. J Am Vet Med Assoc 5:600–605, 1970.
23. Segedy AK, Hayden DW: Cerebral vascular accident caused by *Dirofilaria immitis* in a dog. J Am Anim Hosp Assoc 14:752–756, 1978.
24. Bernstein N, Fiske R: Feline ischemic encephalopathy in a cat. J Am Anim Hosp Assoc 22:205–206, 1985.
25. de Lahunta A: Feline ischemic encephalopathy: A cerebral infarction syndrome. In Kirk RW (ed): Current Veterinary Therapy VI. Philadelphia, WB Saunders, 1977, pp 905–907.
26. Rasmessen TB: Experimental ligation of the cerebral arteries of the dog. Thesis, University of Minnesota, St Paul, MN, 1938.
27. Wimalaratna HSK, Capildeo R: Management of stroke: The place of steroids. In Capildeo R (ed): Steroids in Diseases of the Central Nervous System. New York, John Wiley & Sons, 1989, pp 275–290.
28. Kornegay JN, and Mayhew IG: Metabolic, toxic, and nutritional diseases of the nervous system. In Oliver JE, Hoerlein BF, Mayhew IG: Veterinary Neurology. Philadelphia, WB Saunders, 1987, pp 255–277.
29. Schall WD: Heat stroke. In Kirk RW (ed): Current Veterinary Therapy VII. Philadelphia, WB Saunders, 1980.
30. Schmidt-Nielsen K, Bretz WL, Taylor CR: Panting in dogs: Unidirectional air flow over evaporative surfaces. Science 169:1102–1104, 1970.
31. Mehta AC, Baker RN: Persistent neurological deficits in heat stroke. Neurology 20:336–340, 1970.
32. Krum SH, Osborne CA: Heat stroke in the dog: A polysystemic disorder. J Am Vet Med Assoc 170:531–535, 1977.
33. Osweiler GD, Carson TL, Buck WB, et al: Clinical and Diagnostic Veterinary Toxicology, 3rd ed. Dubuque, IA, Kendall/Hunt Publishing Co, 1985.
34. Braund KG: Degenerative and developmental diseases. In Oliver JE, Hoerlein BF, Mayhew IG (eds): Veterinary Neurology. Philadelphia, WB Saunders, 1987, pp 185–215.

35. Cox NR, Shores A, McCoy CP, et al: Obstructive hydrocephalus due to neoplasia in a Rottweiler puppy. J Am Anim Hosp Assoc 26:335–338, 1990.
36. Russell DS: Observations on the pathology of hydrocephalus. Medical Research Council Special Report No. 265. London, Her Majesty's Stationery Office, 1949.
37. Axthelm MK, Leipold HW, Phillips RM: Congenital internal hydrocephalus in polled Hereford cattle. Vet Med Small Anim Clin 76:567–570, 1981.
38. Simpson ST: Hydrocephalus. In Kirk RW (ed): Current Veterinary Therapy X. Philadelphia, WB Saunders, 1989, pp 842–846.
39. Selby L, Hayes H, Becker S: Epizootiologic features of canine hydrocephalus. Am J Vet Res 40:411–413, 1979.
40. Hoerlein BF: Canine Neurology: Diagnosis and Treatment, 3rd ed. Philadelphia, WB Saunders, 1978.

14

Seizures and Narcolepsy

Epilepsy is a disorder of the brain that is characterized by recurring seizures. *Seizures, fits,* and *convulsions* are synonymous terms used to describe the manifestations of abnormal brain function that are characterized by paroxysmal stereotyped alterations in behavior. The term convulsion is reserved for seizures with a generalized motor component. Narcolepsy is a disorder of the brain that is marked by sudden recurring attacks of sleep. Narcolepsy will be discussed at the end of this chapter. Syncope is transient loss of consciousness caused by ischemia of the brain. The most common cause in animals is cardiac arrhythmia. The history is usually indicative of syncope rather than seizures, but when in doubt careful auscultation of the heart and an electrocardiogram (ECG) may disclose the problem.

A seizure has several components. The actual seizure is called the *ictus*. Prior to the seizure (preictally), there may be a period of altered behavior, called the *aura*. People with seizures report varying sensation, apprehension, and so forth during the aura. Animals may hide, appear nervous, or seek out their owners at this time. The ictus usually lasts for 1 to 2 minutes, but there is considerable variation. Following the seizure (the postictal phase), the animal may return to normal in seconds to minutes or may be restless, lethargic, confused, disoriented, or blind for minutes to hours. The aura and the postictal phase do not have any relationship to the severity or the cause of the seizures.

The behavioral changes of seizures are composed of one or more of the following involuntary phenomena: (1) loss or derangement of consciousness or memory (amnesia), (2) alteration of muscle tone or movement, (3) alteration of sensation, including hallucinations of special senses (e.g., visual, auditory, olfactory), (4) disturbances of the autonomic nervous system (e.g., salivation, urination, defecation), and (5) other psychic manifestations, abnormal thought processes, or moods (recognized as behavioral changes, e.g., fear, rage).[1]

It should be noted that one or more of the aforementioned changes are present in a seizure. For example, loss of consciousness is usually associated with a generalized motor seizure but may not be a part of a seizure with behavioral manifestations. Behavioral or psychic changes are not necessarily seizure disorders; however, if the changes are paroxysmal, seizures are strongly considered.

Seizures may occur in any animal, but they have been reported more frequently in the dog.

Pathophysiology

Seizures are always a sign of abnormal brain function. The dysfunction may be from a primary lesion in the brain or may be secondary to a metabolic abnormality (e.g., hypoglycemia, toxicity).

There are two main categories of seizures: those in which the seizure discharge originates in a circumscribed area of the brain, and those in which the discharge appears to involve the two cerebral hemispheres bilaterally and synchronously from the start. Most of the information on seizure genesis is taken from models of focal seizures.

Two components are recognized as the basis for focal seizure disorders: the seizure focus and the spread of the abnormal activity to other areas of the brain. The paroxysmal alterations in behavior are associated with synchronous excessive discharge in large aggregates of neurons—the seizure focus.[2] If the activity of the seizure focus spreads to other parts of the brain, a generalized cerebral dysrhythmia results, which produces the behavioral change that is recognized as a seizure (Fig. 14–1).

Seizure foci apparently are present in many individuals who do not have seizures. Some populations of neurons in the brain (e.g., the hippocampus) are much more likely to develop seizure activity than others. The seizure focus has been studied extensively in a variety of experimental models and in naturally occurring epilepsy. Neurons in seizure foci are characterized by large-amplitude, prolonged membrane depolarizations with associated high-frequency bursts of spikes, the paroxysmal depolarizing shift. These changes cause paroxysmal interictal spikes in the electroencephalogram (EEG).[3,4] The number of epileptic neurons correlates with the frequency of seizures.

Generalized seizures may also develop simultaneously in many areas of the brain. The two forms of generalized seizures are tonic/clonic convulsions and absence attacks. The latter are rarely recognized in animals. Much of the research on generalized seizures has been done in the cat generalized penicillin model. Large doses of parenteral penicillin cause generalized spike-wave discharges on the EEG and behavioral unresponsiveness like absence attacks.[2] The cause of the diffuse cortical hyperexcitability is still not clear. Reduction of dendrite inhibition or potentiation of excitation mediated by glutamate and aspartate are suggested mechanisms.[2] Alteration of γ-aminobutyric acid (GABA) inhibition is likely involved in the transition to generalized convulsions.

Seizures can be generated in any individual by pharmacologic, metabolic, or electrical changes; however, the threshold for stimulation varies widely. Normal individuals may require potent convulsant drugs (e.g., pentylenetetrazol) or electrical shock to exceed the threshold. A lower seizure threshold may allow production of convulsions by conditions such as fever, photic stimulation, or minor alterations in body chemistry (e.g., hypoglycemia, hypocalcemia, hyperventilation). Finally, some individuals have seizures with no apparent stimulus. The range from normal individuals to those who have spontaneous fits is a continuum without sharply defined boundaries. The threshold for seizures may be an inherited trait.

Recent studies indicate that the expression of individual seizures is different from the development of a lasting seizure-prone state.[5] Antagonists to N-methyl-D-aspartate (NMDA) prevented the progressive development of seizures, but did not block previously induced seizure activity.

Classification

The classification of seizures based on clinical signs is useful from a descriptive standpoint and may also be helpful in localization (Table 14–1).[6]

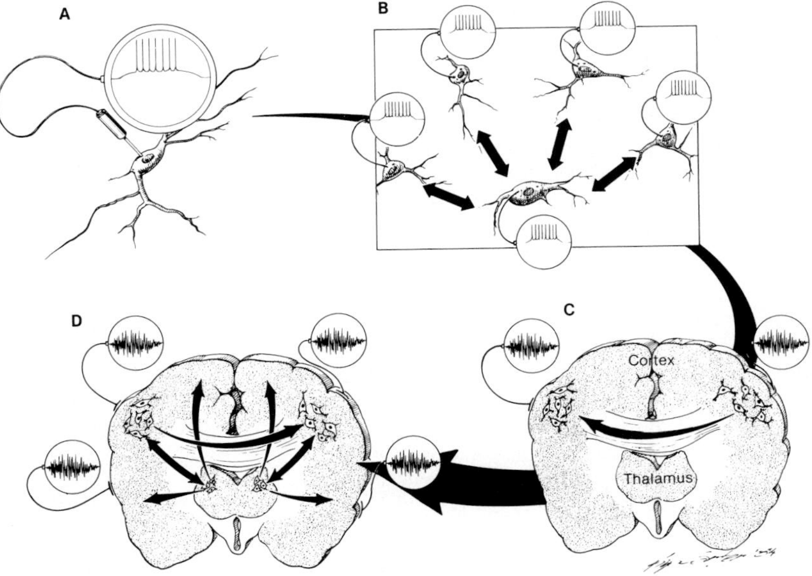

Figure 14–1 Spread of seizure activity from a focal area to the entire cerebrum. *A*. Paroxysmal depolarization shift in a neuron. *B*. Spread of activity to surrounding neurons. *C*. Propogation of seizure activity to other cortical areas by axonal conduction. *D*. Generalization of seizure activity through the diencephalon. (From Oliver JE, Hoerlein BF, Mayhew IG (eds): Veterinary Neurology. Philadelphia, WB Saunders, 1987. Used by permission.)

TABLE 14–1 Classification of Seizures: Clinical Signs

Clinical Manifestation	*EEG*	*Etiology*	*Anatomic Location*
Generalized Seizures, Bilateral Symmetric Seizures, or Seizures Without Local Onset			
Primary generalized, tonic/clonic (grand mal, major motor)	Generalized dysrhythmia from onset, symmetric, often normal interictal unless they are activated or have organic or toxic origin	1. Genetic predisposition 2. Diffuse or multiple organic lesions 3. Toxic or metabolic	1. Unlocalized, multifocal 2. Diencephalic
Absences with or without motor phenomena (petit mal) — rare or rarely recognized in animals	Generalized 3-per-second spike-and-wave dysrhythmia, symmetric (human)	Usually genetic predisposition (human)	1. Unlocalized, multifocal 2. Diencephalic
Partial Seizures or Seizures Beginning Locally			
Partial motor (may generalize to tonic/clonic seizure) — signs depend on site of discharge	Focal dysrhythmia (spikes, slow waves), may generalize secondarily	Acquired organic lesion (see Tables 14–2 and 14–3)	Focal cortical or subcortical
Psychomotor (may generalize or appear as complex behavioral change — running, fear, aggression)	Dysrhythmia related to temporal lobe (unproven in animals)	Acquired organic lesion (see Tables 14–2 and 14–3)	Limbic system (hippocampus, temporal or pyriform lobe)

Modified with permission from Oliver JE Jr: Seizure disorders in companion animals. Comp Cont Ed Pract Vet 2:77–86, 1980.

Gastaut has proposed that generalized seizures be called *primary generalized epilepsy* if no etiology can be ascertained and *secondary generalized epilepsy* if any organic cause can be found.[7] Primary generalized epilepsy includes essential epilepsy, true epilepsy, idiopathic epilepsy, genetic epilepsy, and centrencephalic epilepsy. Partial or focal seizures are usually acquired, thus ruling out primary generalized epilepsy.[8]

Generalized Seizures

Tonic/clonic seizures (grand mal, major motor) are the most frequently recognized convulsions in animals. The seizure frequently is preceded by an aura. The animal falls and becomes unconscious, the limbs are extended rigidly, opisthotonos usually is seen, and respiration stops (apnea). The tonic phase is usually brief (10 to 30 seconds) and is rapidly followed by clonic limb movements in the form of running or paddling activity. Chewing movements of the mouth are common. Visceral activity may start in the tonic or clonic phase of the ictus and may include pupillary dilation, salivation, urination, defecation, and piloerection. The clonic phase may alternate with tonic activity. The ictus usually lasts 1 to 2 minutes. The postictal phase may be a few minutes of rest followed by normal activity or may include confusion, disorientation, restlessness and pacing, and blindness lasting for minutes to hours.

Careful questioning of the owner is required to determine if the episode described is actually a seizure. Owners frequently confuse syncope or acute vestibular syndromes with seizures. If the event is repetitive and has the same appearance each time, then it is likely a seizure. Next, the clinician needs to know if the seizure starts as generalized, symmetric activity or if it has a focal component. The aura should not be confused with focal seizure activity. Any indication of focal motor activity preceding the generalized seizure, such as chewing, forced turning of the head, or clonic jerks of muscle groups, indicates a focal component, even if it generalizes secondarily.

Absences, or *petit mal seizures*, either are very uncommon in animals or, more likely, are uncommonly recognized. They are characterized by a brief (a matter of seconds) loss of contact with the environment, but without motor activity. Variations seen in human beings include minor motor components, such as facial twitching, loss of postural tone, and autonomic activity. Redding has reported one dog with absence attacks and characteristic EEG changes (4-Hz spike-wave complexes).[9] Unless these attacks are frequent or the owner is very observant, they are usually not recognized. Primary generalized seizures cannot be localized anatomically. Whether the seizure focus is single or multiple, the generalized signs preclude localization.

Partial Seizures

Partial motor seizures (focal motor, jacksonian) reflect the activity of a local seizure focus in an area producing motor activity. Movements are restricted to one part of the body, such as the face or one limb. Partial seizures frequently spread, resulting in a generalized convulsion. The focal component of the seizure onset is the key differential feature. Since partial seizures are invariably acquired, primary generalized epilepsy is not considered in the differential diagnosis. The true jacksonian seizure (which includes a focal onset followed by a slow progression of motor activity to adjacent structures, ultimately terminating in a generalized motor seizure) is rare in animals. The motor area of the cerebral cortex of domestic animals is small, allowing seizure activity to generalize rapidly. Patients with partial motor seizures are more likely to have focal EEG abnormalities in interictal periods than are those with generalized seizures. Partial sensory and autonomic seizures are not commonly recognized. Psychomotor seizures may have a predominance of autonomic signs.[1,7,8,10] Animals that have repetitive episodes of "fly-biting" may be having focal sensory seizures in the visual cortex; however, psychomotor seizures with a sensory component are the generally accepted explanation.[11]

Partial motor seizures are presumed to arise from a seizure focus near a primary motor area, usually the frontal cortex. In animals, partial motor seizures are indicative of a pathology in the contralateral cerebral hemisphere (e.g., a left thoracic limb seizure indicates a right cerebral cortex lesion).

Psychomotor seizures (partial seizures with complex symptomatology, behavioral seizures, emotional disorders) are paroxysmal episodes of abnormal behavior.[10–12] Examples include hysteria, rage, autonomic reactions (such as salivation), and hallucinations (such as "fly-biting"). Visceral activity such as diarrhea, vomiting, and abdominal discomfort may correlate with lesions of the limbic system.[10]

Differentiating psychomotor seizures from functional behavioral changes may be difficult. Psychomotor seizures usually will be preceded by an aura and followed by a postictal phase. The ictus is stereotyped and repetitive. Autonomic components of the ictus are common.

Psychomotor seizures indicate an abnormality in the limbic system. The most frequent locations are probably the hippocampus, the amygdala, and the temporal cortex. These areas commonly are involved in inflammatory diseases, such as canine distemper and rabies, and are damaged in tentorial herniation of any cause (see Chaps. 13 and 16).

Diseases

Seizures may be caused by any process that alters normal neuronal function. As with all neurologic diseases, the differential diagnosis is formulated in broad categories. The most likely diseases within each category then are considered. Tables 14–2 and 14–3 outline the major categories of diseases that are likely to produce seizures.

Idiopathic (Genetic)

Primary generalized epilepsy (idiopathic) has no demonstrable pathologic cause and may be inherited. Although it may occur in a number of species,[13] the most comprehensive studies have been those of human beings and dogs.[13–21]

In animals, primary generalized epilepsy usually occurs in the form of generalized tonic/clonic seizures. Absence attacks are common in human beings but are apparently rare in dogs.[19] Breeds of dogs that are known to have a genetic basis for epilepsy are listed in Table 14–4. Also listed are those breeds reported to have a high incidence of seizure disorders but for which genetic studies have not been documented. Whether these breeds have genetic epilepsy has not been proved. A study at the University of Pennsylvania found no evidence of an increased incidence of epilepsy in any breed. The incidence of seizures in all breeds closely matched the frequency of admission to the hospital for all problems.[22] The diagnosis of primary generalized epilepsy does not prove inheritance. Only careful breeding studies can prove a genetic trait.

An inherited epilepsy also has been reported in Brown Swiss and Swedish Red cattle.[23] A hereditary syndrome characterized by recurrent seizures and the gradual development of cerebellar ataxia occurs in purebred and crossbred Aberdeen Angus cattle. The seizures start in young calves but decline in frequency in those that survive to approximately 15 months of age. Most cattle are clinically normal by 2 years of age. Pathologic changes have been found in the Purkinje cells of the cerebellum.[24]

The first seizure in a dog with primary generalized epilepsy usually occurs between the ages of 6 months and 5 years.[1] Early onset of seizures in puppies from breeding of two epileptic Labrador retrievers has been described.[25] Three puppies of a litter of ten had seizures beginning at 8 to 9 weeks of age. Eventually five of eight surviving pups had seizures. In a large beagle colony, 29 dogs had their first seizure at a mean age of 30 months (range, 11 to 70 months).[15]

TABLE 14–2 Causes of Seizure Disorders of Dogs and Cats*

Classification	***Most Frequent Causes***	***Diagnostic Tests***
Degenerative (16)	Storage diseases	Breed, biopsy
Anomalies (13)	Hydrocephalus	PE, CT, EEG, ventriculography
	Lissencephaly	Breed, PE, EEG
Idiopathic (14)	Genetic Unknown	Breed, age, history Absence of other causes
Inflammation (16)	Viral: canine distemper, rabies, FIP Bacterial: any type Mycotic: cryptococcosis Protozoal: toxoplasmosis, neosporosis Granulomatous meningoencephalitis Immune meningoencephalitis Aberrant parasites	History, PE, CSF analysis, titers
Metabolic (16)	Electrolyte: hypocalcemia Carbohydrate: hypoglycemia Renal failure Hepatic failure, portocaval shunt Hypothyroidism (?)	PE and laboratory values
Neoplastic (16)	Primary: gliomas, meningiomas Metastatic	NE, CT
Nutritional (16)	Thiamine	History, response to treatment
Toxic (16)	Heavy metal: lead	History, blood lead levels
	Organophosphates	History, NE, cholinesterase levels
	Chlorinated hydrocarbons	History, NE
	Strychnine	History, NE
	Tetanus	History, NE
	Many others	
Traumatic (14)	Acute: immediately after head injury	History, PE, NE
	Chronic: weeks to years after head injury	History, EEG
Vascular	Infarctions (13)	History, NE, CT
	Arrhythmias	Auscultation, ECG

Modified from Oliver JE Jr: Seizure disorders in companion animals. Comp Cont Ed Pract Vet 2:77–86, 1980.

* Numbers in parentheses refer to chapters in which disease classes are discussed. PE = physical examination, CT = computed tomography, CSF = cerebrospinal fluid, EEG = electroencephalography, FIP = feline infectious peritonitis, NE = neurologic examination, PE = physical examination.

Many dogs with abnormal EEGs did not have seizures by 6 years of age but may have been at risk for future seizures. An incidence of 1% to 2% is reported from two university teaching hospitals.[26,27]

The clinician can make a diagnosis of primary generalized seizures only by excluding other causes. There are no positive diagnostic findings that will substantiate the diagnosis. The breed, the age, and the history may be highly suggestive, especially if there is a familial history of seizures (Tables 14–4 through 14–6). EEG abnormalities are not consistent.

Degenerative

Deficiencies in specific enzymes cause abnormal cellular metabolism with the accumulation of metabolic products within the neurons. These storage diseases may produce seizures as one part of the clinical syndrome (see Chap. 16).

Developmental

Disorders in this group may or may not be inherited but are distinguished from primary generalized epilepsy (genetic) by involving demonstrable pathologic changes in the brain. Hydrocephalus is the most common developmental disorder causing seizures (see Chap. 13). Other developmental defects that may produce convulsions are lissencephaly and porencephaly (see Tables 14–5 and 14–6).

Lissencephaly is a congenital absence of the convolutions of the cerebral cortex.[28,29] It has been reported in Lhasa apso dogs, wire-haired

TABLE 14–3 Causes of Seizure Disorders of Large Animals*

Classification	Most Frequent Causes	Diagnostic Tests
Degenerative (16)	Storage diseases (bovine, ovine)	Breed, biopsy
Anomalies (13)	Hydrocephalus Hydranencephaly	PE, CT, EEG
Idiopathic	Genetic (bovine) Unknown	Breed, age, history Absence of other causes
Inflammation (16)	Viral: infectious bovine rhinotracheitis, pseudorabies (bovine, porcine), rabies (all), thromboembolic meningoencephalitis (bovine), hog cholera, viral encephalomyelitis (equine) Bacterial: any type Aberrant parasites (all)	History, species, PE, CSF analysis, titers
Metabolic (16)	Electrolyte: hypocalcemia, hypomagnesemia, water intoxication (porcine) Carbohydrate: hypoglycemia, ketosis, pregnancy toxemia (ovine) Renal failure Hepatic failure	PE and laboratory values
Neoplastic (16)	Primary: gliomas, meningiomas Metastatic	NE, CSF, CT
Nutritional (16)	Thiamine (ruminants)	History, response to treatment
Toxic (16)	Heavy metal: lead, arsenic	History, blood lead levels
	Organophosphates	History, NE, cholinesterase levels
	Chlorinated hydrocarbons	History, NE
	Strychnine	History, NE
	Tetanus	History, NE
Traumatic (14)	Acute: immediately after head injury	History, PE, NE
Vascular	Infarction (13) Arrhythmias	History, NE Auscultation, ECG

* Numbers in parentheses refer to chapters in which disease classes are discussed. PE = physical examination, CT = computed tomagraphy, CSF = cerebrospinal fluid, EEG = electroencephalography, NE = neurologic examination, PE = physical examination.

TABLE 14–4 Breeds with Primary Generalized Epilepsy

Genetic Factor Proved or Highly Suspected
Beagle[15,19]
Dachshund[26]
German shepherd (Alsatian)[13]
Horak's laboratory dogs[19]
Keeshond[18]
Tervuren (Belgian) shepherd[14]
Aberdeen Angus cattle[24]
Brown Swiss cattle[62]
Swedish Red cattle[23]
High Incidence of Seizure Disorders[1,8,19,32,63]
Arabian foals
Boxer
Cocker spaniel
Collie
Golden retriever
Irish setter
Labrador retriever
Miniature schnauzer
Poodle
Saint Bernard
Siberian huskies
Wire-haired terrier

TABLE 14–5 Common Causes of Seizures at Different Ages

Age/Disease Class	Cause
<1 yr	
Degenerative	Storage diseases
Developmental	Hydrocephalus
Toxic	Heavy metals—lead, organophosphates, chlorinated hydrocarbons
Infectious	Canine distemper, encephalitis, other infectious diseases
Metabolic	Hypoglycemia—transient; enzyme deficiency; portacaval shunt; hepatic encephalopathy
Nutritional	Thiamine, parasitism
Traumatic	Acute
1–3 yr	
Genetic	Primary generalized epilepsy (may start at approximately 6 mo.) Others as above
>4 yr	
Metabolic	Hypoglycemia—secondary to beta-cell tumor; cardiovascular—arrhythmia, thromboembolism; hypocalcemia—hypoparathyroidism; hepatic encephalopathy—cirrhosis
Neoplastic	Primary or metastatic brain tumor

Modified with permission from Oliver JE Jr: Seizure disorders in companion animals. Comp Cont Ed Pract Vet 2:77–86, 1980.

TABLE 14–6 Causes of Seizures by Breed Predisposition

Breed	Cause
Alsatian (German shepherd)	Genetic
Beagle	Genetic
Belgian (Tervuren) shepherd	Genetic
Boston terrier	Hydrocephalus, neoplasia
Boxer	Neoplasia
Cairn terrier	Globoid cell leukodystrophy
Chihuahua	Hydrocephalus
English setter	Lipodystrophy
German shepherd (Alsatian)	Genetic
German short-haired pointer	Lipodystrophy
Irish setter	Genetic (suspected)
Keeshond	Genetic
Lhaso apso	Lissencephaly
Maltese	Portacaval shunts
Miniature pinscher	Hydrocephalus
Miniature schnauzer	Hyperlipoproteinemia, portacaval shunts
Pekingese	Hydrocephalus
Poodle, miniature and standard	Idiopathic
Poodle, toy	Hydrocephalus
Saint Bernard	Idiopathic
West Highland white terrier	Globoid cell leukodystrophy
Yorkshire terrier	Hydrocephalus, portacaval shunts

Modified with permission from Oliver JE Jr: Seizure disorders in companion animals. Comp Cont Ed Pract Vet 2:77–86, 1980.

fox terriers, Irish setters, and in one cat. Affected animals may have behavioral, visual, and slight proprioceptive deficits in addition to seizures.

Porencephaly is a cystic malformation of the cerebrum that usually communicates with the ventricle or the subarachnoid space. It may be congenital or acquired (degenerative).

Infectious

Any infectious disease has the potential to cause seizures if it invades the central nervous system (CNS). The most prevalent diseases are listed in Tables 14–2 and 14–3. Canine distemper virus is probably the most common cause of seizures in dogs. Seizures may appear without any noticeable clinical illness or may occur long after a clinical illness has been resolved. The diagnosis may require EEG.[30] Infectious diseases are discussed in Chapter 16.

Metabolic

Failure of one of the major organs or of the endocrine glands may produce alterations in electrolytes or glucose or the accumulation of toxic products, which results in seizures (see Tables 14–2, 14–3, and 14–5).[30] Some animals have a lower seizure threshold, and relatively minor alterations may cause seizures in these instances. The major metabolic disorders are discussed in Chapter 16.

Neoplastic

Intracranial neoplasia, either primary or metastatic, may cause seizures. The seizure activity is caused by an abnormality in neurons adjacent to the neoplasm that are compressed or distorted or that have an insufficient blood supply. Brain tumors are not electrically active.

Seizures may be the first sign of brain tumor. A neurologic deficit may not be apparent until weeks to months after the onset of seizures, especially if the mass is in the cerebral cortex. Older animals with a sudden onset of seizures should be considered to have a tumor until proven otherwise. Computed tomography (CT) is the diagnostic procedure of choice. Neoplasia is discussed in Chapter 16.

Nutritional

Seizures may be the terminal manifestation of a number of nutritional disorders. The B-complex vitamins are most frequently incriminated. Thiamine deficiency causes polioencephalomalacia in ruminants. Similar lesions are seen in dogs and cats with thiamine deficiency, except that the lesions are predominantly in the brain stem nuclei.

Animals that are fed most commercial rations do not develop thiamine deficiencies. Dogs that are fed only cooked meat develop paraparesis that progresses to convulsions. Early treatment with thiamine reverses the clinical progression of the disease. Thiamine deficiency in cats has been attributed to fish-based cat foods that contain thiaminase. Supplementation with thiamine eliminates the problem. Cats typically have a seizure syndrome that is characterized by ventroflexion of the head, ataxia, behavior changes, dilated pupils, and eventually coma. Since thiamine toxicity is unlikely, it is best to give thiamine to all cats with seizures. A dose of 50 to 100 mg is given intravenously (IV) the first day; thereafter, daily intramuscular (IM) injections are given until a response is obtained or another diagnosis is established.[1]

Toxic

Many toxins affect the CNS, and most can cause seizures. The diagnosis usually depends on the history, the identification of the toxic substance from analysis of body tissues or intestinal contents, and the animal's response to treatment.

Lead poisoning is a frequent intoxication in animals. Other clinical signs may include depression, tremor, and ataxia, which sometimes is associated with gastrointestinal signs. Seizures are often psychomotor. Peripheral blood changes may include nucleated erythrocytes (RBCs) and basophilic stippling of RBCs without anemia. The changes in the RBCs are transient and may not be present in chronic lead poisoning. Blood lead determination is diagnostic. Calcium ethylenediamine tetraacetic acid (CaEDTA) is used in treatment.[31]

Strychnine causes a tonic seizure that is exacerbated by stimulation. The animal remains conscious unless respiration stops. Strychnine blocks inhibitory interneurons in the spinal cord, causing a release of motor neuron activity.

Organophosphate and chlorinated hydrocarbon insecticides are a common cause of seizures. Toxic disorders are discussed in Chapter 16.

Traumatic

Seizures may be seen immediately after acute head trauma as the result of direct neuronal injury. Posttraumatic seizures may occur many weeks to several years after a head injury. Posttraumatic epilepsy may be focal or generalized, depending on the location of the brain lesion. The focus develops secondary to a scar in the brain at the site of the initial injury. The focal abnormality may be recognized on EEG. The diagnosis is based on the correlation of historical information with the development of seizures and the elimination of other causes. The treatment is directed at controlling the seizures.[6]

Plans for Diagnosis and Management of Seizure Disorders

Most animals with seizures present with a similar history—episodic convulsions. Therefore, a protocol for diagnosis and management that includes a defined data base is useful.[6,32]

Data Base

The recommended data base is formulated at two levels to rule out the two major groups of problems causing seizures: (1) extracranial abnormalities, such as metabolic, toxic, and nutritional problems; and (2) intracranial diseases, such as encephalitis, brain tumors, anomalies, degenerative diseases, and traumatic injuries. Idiopathic or primary generalized epilepsy is assumed from the history, signalment, and exclusion of other causes. (Table 14–7). The minimum data base can be obtained at any veterinary clinic with an access to clinical pathology services. The specific serum chemistry analyses can be modified to fit those available in an automated service. The only expense other than the initial examination is the cost of laboratory studies. The risk to the patient is minimal.

The minimum data base screens for primary neurologic disease (neurologic examination) and metabolic or systemic disorders (physical examination, laboratory examination).

TABLE 14–7 Data Base for Seizure Disorders*

Minimum Data Base
- Patient profile
  - Species, breed, age, sex
- History
  - Immunizations: kind, dates, by whom
  - Environment
  - Age at onset
  - Frequency, course
  - Description of seizure: general or partial; duration; aura; postictus; time of day; relation to exercise, food, sleep, or stimuli
  - Previous or present illness or injury
  - Behavioral changes
- Physical examination
  - Complete examination of systems, including specifically:
    - Musculoskeletal: size, shape of skull, evidence of trauma, atrophy of any muscles
    - Cardiovascular: color of mucous membranes, evidence of arrhythmias, murmurs
    - Funduscopic examination
- Neurologic examination
  - Complete examination. Note time of last seizure. If it was within 24–48 hours and neurologic examination is abnormal, repeat in 24 hours.
- Clinical pathology
  - CBC
  - Urinalysis
  - BUN, ALT, ALP, calcium, fasting blood glucose levels (GGT, SDH in large animals)
  - Others as indicated (e.g., blood lead level, Coggins test)

Complete Data Base
- Computed tomography or magnetic resonance imaging
- CSF analysis: cell count, total and differential; protein levels; pressure
- Skull radiographs: ventrodorsal, lateral, frontal
- EEG

* Abbreviations: CBC = complete blood cell count, BUN = serum urea nitrogen, ALT = serum alanine transaminase, ALP = alkaline phosphatase, GGT = γ-glutamyltransferase, SDH = sorbitol dehydrogenase.

The more complete data base includes cerebrospinal fluid (CSF) analysis, skull radiography, CT, and EEG (see Table 14–7). CSF analysis and radiography can be performed at most clinics, but EEG usually is not available except at referral centers. CT is available to many veterinarians through local hospitals or mobile units. CT should be the first test if a brain tumor is suspected. These tests are performed when the minimum data base indicates the presence of neurologic disease or if the seizures have not been controlled with medication. These procedures are not recommended as a part of the minimum data base because of the low yield in animals with normal findings, the increased risk because anesthesia is required, and the increased cost to the client.

CT and magnetic resonance (MR) imaging have largely replaced the various contrast-enhanced imaging procedures for evaluating structural alterations in the brain. Arteriography and ventriculography are no longer used because of the risk and poor diagnostic results. Ventriculography may be used in the diagnosis of hydrocephalus, but it is being replaced by ultrasound.[33]

Plan for Management

A minimum data base should be completed for every patient having more than one seizure. Patients having only one isolated seizure should be given thorough physical and neurologic examinations. If no abnormalities are found, the owners should be advised to watch for further seizures.

Information from the minimum data base yields one of three findings: (1) a definitive diagnosis, (2) a possible cause of the seizures that requires further tests to confirm, or (3) no suggestion of the cause (Fig. 14–2).

Seizures occur episodically; therefore, the veterinarian frequently must evaluate an animal without ever seeing a convulsion. The history must be taken carefully and must include a complete description of the seizures and their frequency, duration, and severity. The first goal

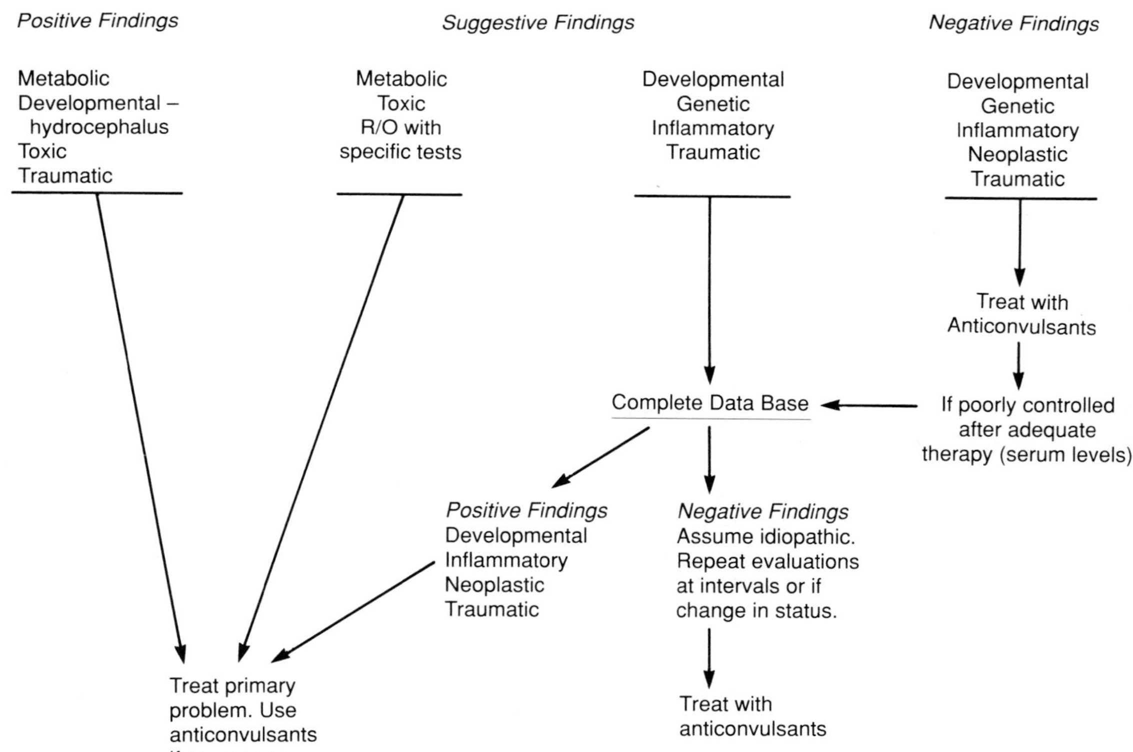

Figure 14–2 Plan for the diagnosis and management of seizures. R/O = rule out. Positive findings confirm the diagnosis, negative findings eliminate the diagnosis. (Modified from Oliver JE Jr: Protocol for diagnosis of seizure disorders in companion animals. J Am Vet Med Assoc 172:824, 1978. Used by permission.)

is to determine that the animal is having convulsions. For example, transient vestibular dysfunction and drug reactions may resemble seizures. The most frequent problem to be confused with seizures is syncope (transient loss of consciousness). Syncope is caused by a loss of the blood supply to the brain or hypoglycemia. Cardiac arrhythmia is the most common cause. Acute vestibular episodes may also be mistaken for seizures. Vestibular disease usually causes other deficits such as a head tilt or ataxia.

The history also provides information related to the onset and the progression of the disease (see Fig. 14–2). Seizures, by definition, are acute in onset; however, the owner may be able to recognize a chronic progression of signs, with seizures being only one component. The diagnostic tests that are most likely to be useful in each disease are listed in Tables 14–2 and 14–3. The minimum data base will rule out most metabolic diseases. Other diseases may or may not be suggested by the minimum data base.

Positive findings include evidence of a metabolic or toxic disease, or an abnormal neurologic examination indicating central nervous system (CNS) disease. Suggestive findings include some indication of metabolic abnormality that may require further tests. For example, serum albumin and urea nitrogen levels may be low, suggesting liver disease. If there are no positive or suggestive findings in the minimum data base, the animal should be treated with anticonvulsants.

Failure to control the seizures after adequate therapy (see Plans for Treatment) warrants a complete data base to rule out neurologic disease. Any change in neurologic signs also indicates a complete evaluation. A dog or cat with onset of seizures after the age of 5 years most likely has an acquired disease. Brain tumors must be high on the list of rule-outs in all such cases even when there are no neurologic signs. The safest and most accurate method of diagnosis is CT or MR imaging. Therefore, we recommend a scan for all of these animals as the first test. If it is negative, CSF analysis, EEG, and survey radiography may be done (Table 14–7).

Some breeds have primary generalized epilepsy that is difficult to control. The most common examples are German shepherds, Saint Bernards, and Irish setters.[1,8] Negative findings on the complete data base for an animal that has been poorly controlled with adequate anticonvulsant medication suggest a poor prognosis. The treatment may be altered by changing the dosage or the drugs, combining drugs, or changing the schedule of administration. Periodic reevaluation may reveal a progressive disease that was missed originally.

Plans for Treatment

Successful treatment depends more on client education and cooperation than any other single factor. Treatment failures are usually the result of (1) a progressive disease, (2) refractory epilepsy, or (3) inadequate client education or poor client compliance. A progressive disease is identified by repeated examinations. Refractory epilepsy is expected in the breeds that have been listed previously. Client education is a variable that the clinician can control.

The client should understand that successful treatment may be manifested by (1) a reduction in the frequency of seizures, (2) a decreased duration of seizures, or (3) a reduction in the severity of seizures. Although complete elimination of seizures is certainly a goal, it is not a realistic expectation for most animals.

The client should be given the following basic rules for treating epileptic animals:

1. Do not judge the efficacy of the medication for at least 2 weeks. Give the medication a chance.
2. Do not change or discontinue the medication suddenly. Status epilepticus may follow.
3. Phenothiazine tranquilizers are *contraindicated* in epileptics.
4. Allow for changes in the animal's environment (e.g., give more medication when increased excitement is expected).
5. Medication may be required for life. Do not decrease dosages rapidly or too soon after seizure control is achieved.
6. No single drug or combination works in all cases. Adjustments in the dosage, the schedule, or the combination of drugs probably will be required. Finding the right combination usually occurs by trial and error.

We usually do not recommend treatment for animals that have had only one seizure. It is useful to know the frequency and severity of the seizures in order to assess the response to treatment. We usually do not treat animals while we are establishing a diagnosis, unless the seizures are frequent and severe (more than one per day).

We do recommend treating seizures if they are recurrent or intense, and especially if they tend to cluster (several in one day). Owners should be advised that each time a seizure discharge spreads, it increases the probability that it will spread again.

The final decision on treatment must be made by the client. In essence, if the client feels that the seizures are more of a problem than is giving the medication, then treatment is in order.

The ideal anticonvulsant should suppress seizures completely without side effects or toxicity. Unfortunately, such a drug is not known. Phenobarbital is the initial drug of choice for treating seizures in dogs and cats.[34–37] Phenobarbital is effective, inexpensive, and convenient for administration. The usual starting dosage is 2.5 mg/kg given orally twice daily. Most dogs will require at least 5 mg/kg to achieve therapeutic blood levels, but absorption and excretion vary considerably between individuals. The lower dosage is used if seizures are infrequent and occur as single episodes. Higher dosages are recommended if seizures are frequent or tend to cluster. The dosage is adjusted according to results and side effects. Sedation may occur, but usually disappears in the first week. Polyphagia, polydipsia, and polyuria may be seen in some patients. Hepatotoxicity is seen in a small number of cases, but it is less frequent than with most other anticonvulsants.[38] If seizures are not controlled or if side effects persist, serum levels of phenobarbital are measured. Blood samples for analysis are obtained just before medication is given since one wants to measure the lowest concentration in the serum. The usual therapeutic range is 15–45 μg/ml.[34–36] Many dogs need levels near the high end to achieve control. Dosages as high as 10–20 mg/kg/day may be needed in some dogs to maintain therapeutic blood levels. The response to treatment is more important than the blood level, but monitoring serum levels of phenobarbital may help determine the cause of inadequate seizure control. Monitoring for evidence of hepatotoxicity or other side effects is of minimal value in most cases. Routine blood counts and serum chemistries are usually recommended at 6-month intervals. However, a recent report on monitoring of human epileptics indicates that there is little benefit, except in high-risk patients.[39] High-risk groups include those with known or presumed biochemical disorders, a history of adverse drug reactions, or neurodegenerative disease.

If phenobarbital is not effective, primidone may be tried. A portion of the primidone molecule is metabolized to phenobarbital, and the remainder is phenylethylmalonamide (PEMA). Phenobarbital is the primary component found in the serum and is assumed to be the primary active agent.[34,37,40] Primidone at a dosage of 50 mg/kg/day produces effective blood levels of phenobarbital (>10 μg/ml). Although primidone and PEMA concentrations are much lower, they may have an additive effect.[40] The efficacy of primidone in patients with seizures has been demonstrated clinically for years. However, several studies indicate that it has little or no advantage over phenobarbital, and hepatotoxicity is more frequent.[34,41] Side effects include depression, polydipsia, polyphagia, and hepatic necrosis. The side effects may be dramatic, but they are usually transient. The usual dosage is 50 mg/kg/day, divided into three doses. One half to twice this dosage may be used, depending on the individual animal's response. Larger animals should be started on a lower dose until tolerance is induced. Primidone is not approved for use in food animals or horses, because the dosage and the anticonvulsive effects are unknown.

Animals that cannot be controlled with adequate levels of phenobarbital may be tried on combination therapy. Phenobarbital is continued while other drugs are added to the regimen. Guidelines for use of the few alternative drugs available are not clearly documented by controlled trials in most cases. These drugs are not approved for use in animals, so owner consent should be obtained.

Currently, the first choice for alternate therapy is potassium bromide (KBR).[42,43] KBR was the principal anticonvulsant for humans in the late 1800s until phenobarbital was introduced in the early 1900s. The therapeutic range is not far from the level that produces toxic side effects such as skin eruptions, sedation, and weakness. These problems have been rarely seen in animals, despite the increased use of KBR in recent years. The dosage of KBR is 40 mg/kg once a day.[42,43] Chemical grade KBR can be used in capsules or dissolved in sucrose or water (250 mg/ml), which is mixed with food. KBR is slow to reach steady state and has a long half-life (Table 14–8). Increased chloride in the diet increases the rate of renal excretion of bromide.[44] Two to three weeks are required to reach therapeutic levels. Steady state is reached in about 4 months. KBR combined with phenobarbital has controlled seizures in dogs refractory to phenobarbital alone.[43]

Phenytoin is probably the most widely used anticonvulsant in human beings. Its use in animals is limited because of studies showing marked species differences in the metabolism of the drug. The pharmacokinetics vary, depending on the route of administration, pretreatment, and treatment with other drugs. The action of the drug also varies among individuals, even of the same breed.[40] The approximate

TABLE 14–8 Anticonvulsant Drugs for Dogs and Cats

Drug	*Dosage (mg/kg)*	*Serum Concentration (μg/ml)*	*Half-Life (hr ± SE)*	*Time to Steady State (days)*
Phenobarbital	1.5–5 q12h	15–45	70 ± 16	10–18
Potassium bromide	20–60 q24h or divided	1,000–1,500	25 days	4 mo.
Diazepam (cats)	0.5–1 q12h	200–500 ng/ml	1.5–2	
Clonazepam	0.02–0.5 q12h	0.02–0.08	1.4 ± 0.3	
Valproic acid	60 q8h	40–100	1.7 ± 0.4	6–10
Primidone	10–15 q8h (dog)	5–15 (human)	9–12	6–8
Metabolites				
PEMA		4–20 (human)	10–16	
Phenobarbital (see above)		15–45	70 ± 16	10–18
Not recommended				
Phenytoin	35 q8h	10	4.4 ± 0.78	0.5–1
Carbamazepine		5–12 (human)	1.1–1.9	4–12 hr

plasma half-life of phenytoin is 22 to 28 hours in human beings, 3 to 4 hours in dogs, and 24 to 108 hours in cats. In addition, blood concentrations of phenytoin in the dog do not reach therapeutic levels (10 μg/ml, based on human clinical and canine research data) at the dosages prescribed for human beings.[40,45] Laboratory studies indicate that at least 35 mg/kg t.i.d. is needed to reach therapeutic levels in the dog.[45] In another study, therapeutic levels were achieved with 3–5 mg/lb t.i.d., but the reported concentrations were only 1.5–3.0 μg/ml.[46] The variability in serum levels and the short half-life make phenytoin of little benefit in most dogs.

Mephobarbital is longer-acting than phenobarbital and is given once daily. Its efficacy is essentially the same as that of phenobarbital because it is metabolized into two molecules of phenobarbital. It offers a once-a-day medication schedule at a greater expense.

TABLE 14–9 Protocol for Anticonvulsant Medication

Dogs
Phenobarbital, 2.5–5 mg/kg b.i.d. Reduce dosage after 1 week if sedation is a problem. Measure serum levels after 2 weeks to establish a baseline standard. Increase dosage to maintain control as needed and measure serum levels 2 weeks after changes in dosage.

If seizures are not controlled, add potassium bromide (KBR) in a dosage of 40 mg/kg once a day in addition to the phenobarbital. Serum levels of KBR (1000–1500 μg/ml) may be reached in about 4 months. If seizures are frequent or severe, clonazepam (0.5 mg/kg b.i.d.) may be used during the time KBR is reaching therapeutic levels.

See text for other alternatives

Cats
Phenobarbital as above.

Diazepam, 0.5–1 mg/kg b.i.d. or t.i.d. (may be combined with phenobarbital).

Horses and Food Animals
Phenobarbital as above.

Phenytoin, 20 mg/kg b.i.d., for horses only (not approved or tested).

Diazepam is used in the treatment of status epilepticus and may be administered in conjunction with other drugs in the treatment of epilepsy. The duration of action is short in the dog, requiring t.i.d. or q.i.d. administration. In the cat, dosages of 0.5–2.0 mg/kg t.i.d. are effective.[34,43] Phenobarbital and diazepam are the only anticonvulsants recommended for cats (Table 14–9).

Clonazepam, a longer acting benzodiazepine, is effective for short-term control of refractory seizures. The beneficial effect seems to last for only a few months. Some hepatotoxicity has been a problem in dogs on clonazepam for longer than a few months. Currently, we use it during the time that KBR is reaching therapeutic effect (1–3 months), then stop it. The dosage is 0.5 mg/kg twice daily.

Sodium valproate in combination with phenobarbital has been useful in a limited number of cases. The half-life is short, and therapeutic levels are difficult to achieve. There is some evidence that brain levels may be higher and that other metabolites may have some effect. It may be tried in combination with phenobarbital at a dose of 60 mg/kg.[35,47]

Paramethadione and related drugs of that group are primarily used for absence seizures in humans. Paramethadione is reported to be effective in tonic/clonic seizures at a dosage of 10–60 mg/kg/day.[48]

Progestational agents have been beneficial in some cases, especially for patients with psychomotor-type seizures.

A protocol for the treatment of seizures is outlined in Table 14–9.

TABLE 14–10 Protocol for Treatment of Status Epilepticus

1. Stop the seizure. Administer diazepam, 10–50 mg in 10-mg boluses IV. Diazepam usually gives at least temporary remission, allowing time for succeeding steps. Clonazepam may also be used in a dosage of 0.05–0.2 mg/kg for a longer duration of action. If seizures are not controlled, administer phenobarbital sodium (2–4 mg/kg IV at 30-minute intervals). If neither is effective, administer sodium pentobarbital to effect (estimated dosage, 10–15 mg/kg). Pentobarbital must be given cautiously, because diazepam and phenobarbital may potentiate its effect. Ultra-short-acting barbiturates should not be used because they may potentiate seizure activity.
2. When the seizures have stopped, ensure ventilation of the patient. An endotracheal tube should be placed if the patient is unconscious.
3. Place an IV catheter, draw blood for hematology and chemistry analyses, and start a drip with lactated Ringer's solution. Measure blood glucose levels as soon as possible.
4. Give 50% dextrose IV (2–3 ml for toy breeds, 50 ml for giant breeds). If the seizures are not violent or if there are interictal quiet periods, you may perform steps 3 and 4 first. Hypoglycemia is the one cause of status that can be treated directly.
5. Ruminants and cats should be given thiamine IV in 0.5–1-g doses, repeated several times in 24–48 hours.
6. If you suspect hypocalcemia, give an IV calcium preparation. Monitor the heart rate.
7. Once the seizures are under control, evaluate the animal to try to determine the cause of the seizures. If a cause can be found (e.g., toxicity), it should be treated specifically.
8. Monitor the body temperature. If it reaches 105° F, cool the animal with ice to a temperature of 103° F. Maintain the temperature in a normal range.
9. Continue to control the seizures. IV or IM phenobarbital should be given until oral medication can be used. The normal movements of anesthetic recovery should not be mistaken for seizures.

Status epilepticus is the condition of rapidly recurring convulsions without complete recovery between seizures. This is a serious emergency that can result in death of the patient. Causes of status epilepticus include (1) toxicities or metabolic abnormalities, (2) withdrawal of anticonvulsant medication, (3) ineffective anticonvulsant medication, and (4) progressive brain disease. A protocol for the treatment of status epilepticus is presented in Table 14–10.

Narcolepsy

Narcolepsy is a brain disorder characterized by recurring sudden attacks of sleep.[49] Cataplexy (loss of muscle tone) commonly accompanies the attacks. Two other components that have been described in human beings—sleep paralysis and hallucinations—are difficult to verify in animals because of the subjective nature of the conditions.[50]

Dogs with narcolepsy typically have episodes in which they suddenly fall asleep, often while excited or during emotional stimulation. Eating is the most common precipitating factor in reported cases. The dog will start to eat and suddenly will fall to the ground asleep. Noise, shaking, or other stimuli will arouse the animal, and often it will resume eating, only to fall asleep again. Continual stimulation, such as petting or shaking, may prevent the attack. The episodes often are repeated many times a day.[49–52] Narcolepsy also has been reported in ponies, horses, and a Brahman bull.[50,53,54]

Normal sleep is characterized on the EEG by a change from low-voltage, fast-wave activity in the animal that is awake to high-voltage, slow-wave activity in the animal that is asleep. Rapid eye movement (REM) sleep develops after approximately 90 minutes of slow-wave sleep and may recur intermittently thereafter. REM sleep is associated with dreaming and is characterized by eye movements, occasional facial movements, and desynchronized low-voltage, fast-wave activity of the EEG.[55]

The sleep attacks of narcolepsy are the same as REM sleep with no intervening slow-wave sleep. Partial attacks and cataplectic episodes may occur without EEG changes.[51]

Narcolepsy has been seen in human beings following CNS infection or trauma, and an immune mechanism is suspected in some cases.[50] A biochemical alteration of the neuronal membrane is presumed. Studies in dogs with narcolepsy have demonstrated some biochemical abnormalities.[56–59] There are increased numbers of dopamine and muscarinic receptors, but no change in benzodiazepine receptors. The reticular activating system of the rostral brain stem presumably is associated with sleep and the more caudal portions of the reticular formation in the pons with cataplexy.

A genetic basis for narcolepsy in some breeds is suspected. An autosomal recessive inheritance has been demonstrated in Doberman pinschers and Labrador retrievers.[60] Numerous other breeds of dogs have been diagnosed as narcoleptics, but breeding studies have not been done, or have been inconclusive.

A diagnosis usually can be made by observation of the characteristic signs if cataplexy is a prominent part of the syndrome. In the absence of cataplexy, the problem probably will not be recognized by the owner. The EEG is the only available diagnostic test. Sleep beginning with

REM sleep is characteristic. Polygraphic recording of the EMG, eye movements, and EEG simultaneously for extended periods is the most definitive test.[60] Anticholinergic compounds increase the frequency and duration of cataplectic attacks in narcoleptic animals, but have no effect on normal animals.[60] A dose of physostigmine salicylate (0.025–0.1 mg/kg IV) produces cataplectic attacks in susceptible animals.

Treatment with stimulants is partially effective. Dextroamphetamine (5–10 mg t.i.d.) and methylphenidate (Ritalin, 5–10 mg b.i.d. or t.i.d.) have stopped the sleep attacks but have produced undesirable behavioral changes in some cases.[49,60] Excessive somnolence is not a significant problem for most dogs; therefore, managing the cataplectic episodes is of more importance. Imipramine at a dosage of 0.5–1.0 mg/kg t.i.d. is more effective in preventing cataplexy.[60] A combination of methylphenidate and imipramine is recommended to control sleep attacks and cataplexy. The medication should be given at a level to reduce attacks but not completely eliminate them, because that may require dangerously high dosages. Giving the medication intermittently also reduces the development of tolerance. Protriptyline at a dosage of 10 mg once a day was effective in controlling hypersomnia in a dog.[61] This dog did not have cataplexy.

Combining amphetamines and imipramine is potentially dangerous, because amphetamines cause a release of catacholamines and imipramine blocks their reuptake. Hypertensive episodes can result.

A balanced regimen of therapy must be developed for each individual to attain a relatively normal sleep-wakefulness cycle.

CASE HISTORIES

Seizures are a common neurologic problem in dogs. Most patients with seizures do not have other neurologic deficits. The following case histories demonstrate the approach to management. Localizing signs of brain disease are not present in these cases, because they are discussed in other chapters. After reading the history and the preliminary laboratory data, the student should develop a plan for further diagnosis or treatment of each case. Then read our assessment.

Case History 14A

Signalment

Canine, miniature poodle, male, 18 months old.

History

The dog has received all vaccinations on schedule and has had no major medical problems. The first seizure occurred 2 months ago. The second seizure was observed last night at approximately 6:00 P.M.

The owner describes the seizure as follows: The dog seemed somewhat apprehensive for approximately 30 minutes, seeking attention from the owner. Suddenly he fell down, extended all four limbs, and arched the head and the neck. After approximately 30 seconds he started making running movements of the limbs with some chewing movements of the mouth. There was some salivation, and the dog urinated. The owner tried to hold and rub the dog, and the movements stopped after approximately 1 minute. In about 2 or 3 minutes, the dog was able to get up. He seemed a little disoriented for a few minutes, and then he seemed normal.

Other than during the two seizures, the dog has appeared to be healthy. He is fed a variety of commercial dog foods twice daily. Water consumption and urination are thought to be normal.

Physical and Neurologic Examinations

No abnormalities are found.

Laboratory Examination

The complete blood cell (CBC) count and the chemistry profile (see Table 14–7) are normal.

Case History 14B

Signalment

Canine, cairn terrier, male, 6 years old.

History

The dog has had no serious illnesses and has had booster vaccinations annually. Ten weeks ago the dog had a generalized motor seizure that lasted approximately 5 minutes. The dog seemed blind and confused for approximately 4 hours afterward. Two weeks ago the dog had a second seizure. Since that time he has not acted "right." His appetite is diminished, he does not play in the way that he did, and he has urinated and defecated in the house several times, which he had not done for years. Last night he had another seizure that lasted over 5 minutes. Today he is very depressed.

Physical Examination

No abnormalities are found other than depression.

Neurologic Examination

The dog can be coaxed to walk, but he prefers to lie down. The gait is good, with a suggestion of slight symmetric dysmetria. The limbs seem to be lifted a bit high and to be put down with increased force. There is no ataxia, however. The postural reactions also seem slightly dysmetric. The spinal reflexes are normal, as are the cranial nerves, although the menace reaction seems a little sluggish. This response is considered within normal limits when the depression is taken into account.

Case History 14C

Signalment

Canine, German shepherd, female, 4 years old.

History

All vaccinations, including annual boosters, have been given. There have been no major illnesses. Generalized motor seizures started 18 months ago. The first few were 2 to 3 months apart, but recently they have been 2 to 3 weeks apart. Several recent seizures were prolonged (approaching status epilepticus) and were controlled with general anesthesia. Several anticonvulsants, including phenobarbital, phenytoin, and primidone, in dosages that appear to be adequate, have been used in the last year, with no apparent control of the fits. The seizures have occurred at various times of day, including at night, when the dog is asleep. Laboratory evaluations performed on several occasions by the referring veterinarian have not revealed any abnormalities. The owner feels that neither he nor the dog can continue to tolerate these seizures.

Physical and Neurologic Examinations

No abnormalities are found.

Laboratory Examination

No abnormalities are found.

Case History 14D

Signalment

Feline, domestic short hair, female, 14 months old.

History

The cat took up residence at the owner's home 6 months ago. She was vaccinated for the usual feline diseases, including rabies, at that time. She has not been ill except for seizures, which started 6 weeks ago. The first seizure, which occurred in the evening, was described as a brief period during which the cat suddenly looked "glassy-eyed," stiffened all four limbs, and arched the neck. The seizure lasted less than a minute. The second and third seizures were similar and occurred approximately 1 week apart. In the last 3 weeks, the cat has had at least two seizures per week. The last two were generalized motor seizures. The most recent seizure was described as starting like the first one. The cat then twisted to the right, urinated, and began paddling, first with the right limb and then with all four limbs. The seizure lasted approximately 2 minutes, and the cat acted dazed and depressed for approximately 2 hours.

Physical Examination

No abnormalities are found.

Neurologic Examination

The only abnormality is a slight anisocoria, with the left pupil slightly smaller than the right. Both pupils are reactive to light, although the right seems slightly slower to react than the left. The iris and the fundus appear normal.

Case History 14E

Signalment

Canine, dachshund, male, 6 months old.

History

The dog suddenly became lethargic and exhibited a staggering gait. The owners believe that the onset of signs occurred shortly after he was seen eating some unknown substance in the front yard. Observation of the dog for several days revealed the following pattern of behavior: The dog suddenly collapses to the ground while walking. He appears to be asleep for a few seconds and then awakens, gets up, and behaves normally. While eating, the dog collapses with food in his mouth, wakes up in less than a minute, and continues eating. This pattern might be repeated every 2 to 3 minutes during a meal. The dog can be aroused from sleep easily by noise or touch. No other abnormalities are observed. The dog had not been ill previously and has had all vaccinations.

Physical and Neurologic Examinations

Other than the behavior just described, no abnormalities are found.

Laboratory Examination

All tests, including an ECG, are normal.

Assessment 14A

The seizures are generalized tonic/clonic (grand mal, major motor—see Table 14–1). To the owner's knowledge, they have occurred twice. The seizures are single and are of short duration. There is no history of illnesses or injuries, and the physical, neurologic, and laboratory examinations are normal. Although a genetic basis for epilepsy has not been demonstrated in miniature poodles, it is suspected because of the relatively frequent occurrence of seizures in this breed without specific cause.

There is nothing in the data base to justify further diagnostic tests at this time. We would recommend prophylactic medication in order to determine if the seizures can be prevented. If the owner feels that giving medication is a serious problem, we would suggest observing the animal closely for further seizures and then starting medication if another seizure occurs. The owner should be warned that the dog probably will have more seizures and that medication is the preferred alternative. The medication of choice is phenobarbital.

Assessment 14B

A 6-year-old dog with a sudden onset of seizures probably has an acquired brain problem. The disorder appears to be progressive. The depression suggests brain abnormalities, which may be primary or secondary to metabolic or toxic abnormalities. Dysmetria, especially when it is subtle and occurs in a terrier, may or may not be significant. It could indicate a diffuse abnormality with cerebellar involvement. A laboratory profile is indicated.

Laboratory examination.

CBC	
Packed cell volume	37%
Hemoglobin	14.5 g/dl
WBCs	10,950
Neutrophils	7,400
Lymphocytes	2,400
Monocytes	450
Eosinophils	700
Nucleated RBCs	3 per high-power field
Some polychromasia	
Serum plasma protein	6.5 g/dl
Albumin	3.3 g/dl
Serum urea nitrogen	14 mg/dl
Alkaline phosphatase	80 IU/L
ALT	30 IU/L
Calcium	9.9 mg/dl
Glucose	95 mg/dl
Urinalysis	Normal

There is no evidence of systemic infectious disease (normal WBCs and differential). Severe liver disease is unlikely (normal ALT and alkaline phosphatase, serum albumin, and serum urea nitrogen levels). Calcium and glucose levels are normal. The only unusual findings are nucleated RBCs and polychromasia with a normal packed cell volume and hematocrit (no anemia). This finding is suggestive of lead poisoning. A sample of whole blood was submitted, and 65 μg of lead per 100 ml was reported. These results are diagnostic of lead poisoning. Chelation therapy with calcium EDTA was successful. The source of the lead was not found for several weeks, until the owners discovered a thoroughly chewed bowling trophy under a bed.

Assessment 14C

The history is typical of a form of epilepsy, presumably genetic, that is seen in German shepherd dogs and a few other large breeds. The seizures begin in early adult life and are severe. They often are multiple and are refractory to anticonvulsant therapy. It would be worthwhile to perform EEG and CSF analysis in order to rule out inflammatory disease, but the results of these tests probably will be normal. An EEG may reveal some nonspecific abnormality, such as diffuse spike discharge. If phenobarbital is ineffective, as in this case, potassium bromide in combination with phenobarbital is the best alternative. The prognosis for significant control is poor, but some dogs can be managed effectively.

Assessment 14D

Seizures in cats usually are caused by organic disease. Unfortunately, most of the causes are diseases with a poor prognosis. The progression from a partial motor seizure to generalized seizures also suggests primary brain disease. Anisocoria frequently is seen in cats that have had positive tests for feline leukemia virus (FeLV). The signs also may be associated with feline infectious peritonitis (FIP—usually the "dry" form). Meningiomas also may cause seizures without other signs in the early stages. The age of the cat is more suggestive of viral diseases than of neoplasia.

Localization: cerebral or diencephalic; rule-outs: (1) FIP, (2) FeLV, and (3) meningioma.

Plan. Laboratory examination, titers for FeLV and FIP, CSF analysis, EEG. The significant findings are:

WBCs: 16,800
- 6,700 segmented neutrophils
- 2,500 bands
- 6,000 lymphocytes
- 800 eosinophils

Serum protein 9.0 g/dl
Albumin 3.0
Globulin 6.0
CSF:

Protein	110 mg/dl
Cells (total)	240/cu mm
Neutrophils	130/cu mm
Lymphocytes	110/cu mm

EEG: generalized high-voltage slow waves with spikes randomly superimposed
FeLV: Positive
FIP titer: Positive at 1:1600

All of the findings are characteristic of FIP. If costs are a factor, the laboratory examination (serum protein) and FeLV and FIP tests are adequate for diagnosis. Treatment of the CNS form of FIP has been uniformly unsuccessful. Many of these cats will have either uveitis or retinal lesions, or both, and a strong presumptive diagnosis can be made from the clinical examination alone.

Assessment 14E

The behavior of this dog is typical of narcolepsy-cataplexy. The EEG is useful for documenting the changes. Clinical management requires long-term therapy, because the disease is not reversible. A brief trial with therapy at home was unsatisfactory for this client, and euthanasia was performed.

REFERENCES

1. Oliver JE Jr: Seizure disorders and narcolepsy. In Oliver JE, Hoerlein BF, Mayhew IG: Veterinary Neurology. Philadelphia, WB Saunders, 1987, pp 285–302.
2. Gloor P, Fariello RG: Generalized epilepsy: Some of its cellular mechanisms differ from those of focal epilepsy. Trends Neurosci 11:63–68, 1988.

3. Russo ME: The pathophysiology of epilepsy. Cornell Vet 71:221–247, 1981.
4. Bleck TP, Klawans HL: Convulsive disorders: Mechanisms of epilepsy and anticonvulsant action. Clin Neuropharmacol 13:121–128, 1990.
5. Stasheff SF, Anderson WW, Clark S, et al: NMDA antagonists differentiate epileptogenesis from seizure expression in an in vitro model. Science 245:648–651, 1989.
6. Oliver JE Jr: Seizure disorders in companion animals. Comp Cont Educ Pract Vet 2:77–85, 1980.
7. Gastaut H: Clinical and electroencephalographic classification of epileptic seizures. Suppl Epilepsia 10:512–513, 1969.
8. Holliday TA: Seizure disorders. Vet Clin North Am 10:3–29, 1980.
9. Redding RW: Electroencephalography. In Oliver JE, Hoerlein BF, Mayhew IG: Veterinary Neurology. Philadelphia, WB Saunders, 1987, pp 111–144.
10. Breitschwerdt EB, Breazile JE, Broadhurst JJ: Clinical and electroencephalographic findings associated with ten cases of suspected limbic epilepsy in the dog. J Am Anim Hosp Assoc 15:27–50, 1979.
11. Crowell-Davis SL, Lappin M, Oliver JE: Stimulus-responsive psychomotor epilepsy in a Doberman pinscher. J Am Anim Hosp Assoc 25:57–60, 1989.
12. Gastaut H, Toga M, Naquet R: Clinical, electrographical and anatomical study of epilepsy induced in dogs by the ingestion of agenized proteins. In Baldwin M, Bailey P (eds): Temporal Lobe Epilepsy. Springfield, Ill, Charles C Thomas, 1958, pp 268–295.
13. Falco MJ, Barker J, Wallace ME: The genetics of epilepsy in the British Alsatian. J Small Anim Pract 15:685–692, 1974.
14. Van der Velden A: Fits in Tervuren shepherd dogs: A presumed hereditary trait. J Small Anim Pract 9:63–70, 1968.
15. Biefelt SW, Redman HC, Broadhurst JJ: Sire and sex-related differences in rates of epileptiform seizures in a purebred beagle dog colony. Am J Vet Res 32:2039–2048, 1971.
16. Hegreberg GA, Padget GA: Inherited progressive epilepsy of the dog with comparisons to Lafora's disease of man. Fed Proc 35:1202–1205, 1976.
17. Tomchick T: Familial Lafora's disease in the beagle dog. Fed Proc 32:8–21, 1973.
18. Wallace ME: Keeshonds: A genetic study of epilepsy and EEG readings. J Small Anim Pract 16:1–10, 1975.
19. Holliday TA: Epilepsy in animals. In Frey H-H and Janz D (eds): Handbook of Experimental Pharmacology. Vol 74. Berlin, Springer-Verlag, 1985, pp 55–76.
20. Cunningham JG, Farnbach GC: Inheritance and idiopathic canine epilepsy. J Am Anim Hosp Assoc 24:421–424, 1988.
21. Borden J, Manuelidis L: Movement of the X chromosome in epilepsy. Science 242:1687–1691, 1988.
22. Farnbach GC: Seizures in the dog: Part I. Basis, classification, and predilection. Comp Cont Educ Pract Vet 6:569–576, 1984.
23. Chrisman CL: Epilepsy and seizures. In Howard JL (ed): Current Veterinary Therapy: Food Animal Practice. Philadelphia, WB Saunders, 1981, pp 1082–1083.
24. Barlow R: Morphogenesis of cerebellar lesions in bovine familial convulsions and ataxia. Vet Pathol 18:151–162, 1981.
25. Gerard VA, Conarck CN: Identifying the cause of an early onset of seizures in puppies with epileptic parents. Vet Med 86:1060–1061, 1991.
26. Holliday TA, Cunningham JG, Gutnick MJ: Comparative clinical and electroencephalographic studies of canine epilepsy. Epilepsia 11:281–292, 1971.
27. Bunch SE: Anticonvulsant drug therapy in companion animals. In Kirk RW (ed): Current Veterinary Therapy VIII. Philadelphia, WB Saunders, 1983, pp 746–754.
28. Braund KG: Degenerative and developmental diseases. In Oliver JE, Hoerlein BF, Mayhew IG: Veterinary Neurology. Philadelphia, WB Saunders, 1987, pp 185–215.
29. Greene CE, Vandevelde M, Braund K: Lissencephaly in two Lhasa Apso dogs. J Am Vet Med Assoc 169:405–410, 1976.
30. Oliver JE, Hoerlein BF, Mayhew IG: Veterinary Neurology. Philadelphia, WB Saunders, 1987.
31. Kornegay JN, Mayhew IG: Metabolic, toxic, and nutritional diseases of the nervous system. In Oliver JE, Hoerlein BF, Mayhew IG: Veterinary Neurology. Philadelphia, WB Saunders, 1987, pp 255–277.
32. Oliver JE Jr: Protocol for the diagnosis of seizure disorders in companion animals. J Am Vet Med Assoc 172: 822–824, 1978.
33. Hudson JA, Simpson ST, Buxton DF, et al: Ultrasonographic diagnosis of canine hydrocephalus. J Vet Radiol 31:50–58, 1990.
34. Schwartz-Porsche D, Loscher W, Frey HH: Therapeutic efficacy of phenobarbital and primidone in canine epilepsy: A comparison. J Vet Pharmacol Therap 8:113–119, 1985.
35. Lane SB, Bunch SE: Medical management of recurrent seizures in dogs and cats. J Vet Intern Med 4:26–39, 1990.
36. Farnbach GC: Serum concentrations and efficacy of phenytoin, phenobarbital, and primidone in canine epilepsy. J Am Vet Med Assoc 184:1117–1120, 1984.
37. Frey H-H: Use of anticonvulsants in small animals. Vet Rec 118:484–486, 1986.
38. Dayrell-Hart B, Steinberg SA, VanWinkle TJ, et al: Hepatotoxicity of phenobarbital in dogs: 18 cases (1985–1989). J Am Vet Med Assoc 199:1060–1066, 1991.
39. Pellock JM, Willmore LJ: A rational guide to routine blood monitoring in patients receiving antiepileptic drugs. Neurology 41:961–964, 1991.
40. Frey H-H, Loscher W: Pharmacokinetics of anti-epileptic drugs in the dog: A review. J Vet Pharmacol Ther 8:219–233, 1985.
41. Farnbach GC: Efficacy of primidone in dogs with seizures unresponsive to phenobarbital. J Am Vet Med Assoc 185:867–868, 1984.
42. Schwartz-Porsche D, Boenigk HE, Lorenz JH: Bromidtherapie bei den Epilepsien des Hunds: Erste Erfahrungen. Kurzreferate, Regionale Arbeitstagung Nord DVG–Fachgruppe. Kleintierkrankheiten. Timmendorfer Strand, 1987.
43. Schwartz-Porsche D: Epidemiological, clinical, and pharmacokinetic studies in spontaneously epileptic dogs and cats. In: Proceedings of an ACVIM forum, Washington, DC, 1986, vol 11, pp 61–63.
44. Sisson A, LeCouteur RA: Potassium bromide as an adjunct to phenobarbital for the management of uncontrolled seizures in the dog. Prog Vet Neurol 1:114–115, 1990.
45. Sanders JE, Yeary RA: Serum concentrations of orally administered diphenylhydantoin in dogs. J Am Vet Med Assoc 172:153–156, 1978.
46. Pasten LJ: Diphenylhydantoin in the canine: Clinical aspects and determination of therapeutic blood levels. J Am Anim Hosp Assoc 13:247–254, 1977.
47. Nafe LA, Parker A, Kay WJ: Sodium valproate: A preliminary clinical trial in epileptic dogs. J Am Anim Hosp Assoc 17:131–133, 1981.
48. Parker AJ: A preliminary report on a new anti-epileptic medication for dogs. J Am Anim Hosp Assoc 11:437–438, 1975.
49. Knecht CD, Oliver JE, Redding R, et al: Narcolepsy in a dog and a cat. J Am Vet Med Assoc 162:1052–1053, 1973.

50. Richardson JW, Fredrickson P, Lin S: Narcolepsy update. Mayo Clin Proc 65:991–998, 1990.
51. Mitler MM, Soave O, Dement WC: Narcolepsy in seven dogs. J Am Vet Med Assoc 168:1036–1038, 1976.
52. Katherman AE: A comparative review of canine and human narcolepsy. Comp Cont Educ Pract Vet 2:818–822, 1980.
53. Sweeney CR, Hendricks JC, Beech J, et al: Narcolepsy in a horse. J Am Vet Med Assoc 183:126–128, 1983.
54. Strain GM, Olcott BM, Archer RM, et al: Narcolepsy in a Brahman bull. J Am Vet Med Assoc 185:538–541, 1984.
55. Wauquier A, Verheyen JL, Van Den Broeck WAE, et al: Visual and computer-based analysis of 24 H sleep-waking patterns in the dog. EEG Clin Neurophysiol 46:33–48, 1979.
56. Mitler MM, Dement WC, Guilleminault C, et al: Canine Narcolepsy. In Rose FC, Behan PO (eds): Animal Models of Neurological Disease. Kent, Great Britain, Putman Medical Ltd, 1980, pp 226–238.
57. Delashaw JB Jr, Foutz AS, Guilleminault C, et al: Cholinergic mechanisms and cataplexy in dogs. Exp Neurol 66:745–757, 1979.
58. Bowersox S, Kilduff K, Zeller-DeAmicis L, et al: Brain dopamine receptor levels elevated in canine narcolepsy. Brain Res 402:44–48, 1987.
59. Fruhstorfer B, Mignot E, Bowersox S, et al: Canine narcolepsy is associated with an elevated number of α_2-receptors in the locus coeruleus. Brain Res 500:209–214, 1989.
60. Baker TL, Mitler MM, Foutz AS, et al: Diagnosis and treatment of narcolepsy in animals. In Kirk RW (ed): Current Veterinary Therapy VIII. Philadelphia, WB Saunders, 1983, pp 755–759.
61. Shores A, Redding R: Narcoleptic hypersomnia syndrome responsive to protriptyline in a labrador retriever. J Am Anim Hosp Assoc 23:455–458, 1987.
62. Atkeson FW, Ibsen HL, Eldridge E: Inheritance of an epileptic type character in Brown Swiss cattle. J Hered 34:45, 1944.
63. Croft P: Fits in the dog. Vet Rec 88:118–120, 1971.

15

Pain

Animals do feel pain, yet this has been a point of argument for many years. For a review of the entire spectrum of animal pain the "Colloquium on recognition and alleviation of animal pain and distress"[1] and the text *Animal Pain*[2] are recommended.

In this chapter the pathophysiology of pain, some of the diseases with pain as the primary clinical sign, and the symptomatic treatment of pain will be reviewed.

Definitions of the terms related to the description of pain are essential for communication. Kitchell has provided an excellent working definition: "*Pain* in animals is an aversive sensory and emotional experience (a perception), which elicits protective motor actions, results in learned avoidance, and may modify species-specific traits of behavior, including social behavior."[3] Pain is a perception and is not a quantifiable entity. It is also incorrect to refer to painful stimuli or pain receptors, pathways, or nerve fibers. All of these are more accurately called *noxious* (noxious means injurious). Thus, there are noxious stimuli, nociceptors, nociceptive pathways, and so on.

Other terms frequently used or misused include the following.

Hyperesthesia denotes an increased sensitivity to stimulation. It has often been used to designate an unpleasant response to a nonnoxious stimulus.[3] We use the term as more generic than the others because of the difficulty in truly knowing if the animal perceives pain or not. Throughout this book, we use the term hyperesthesia to mean a behavioral reaction of the animal indicating that the stimulus was unpleasant, when we consider the stimulus to be nonnoxious. The most common usage is in describing an animal's response to palpation that does not evoke a reaction in some locations, but causes an aversive reaction in other areas.

Hyperpathia denotes an unpleasant painful response to a noxious stimulus, especially if repeated, and is characterized by delay, overreaction, and aftersensation.[3] This term has been used frequently in veterinary medicine, but is far more specific than just a "painful response." It would be difficult if not impossible to know that an animal actually has the sensations associated with hyperpathia.

Allodynia is pain resulting from a nonnoxious stimulus to normal skin. Because we are often assessing "painful" responses from structures other than skin, this term is not used often.

Lesion Localization

Pathophysiology of Pain

Nociception, the neural response to a noxious stimulus, has a specific set of complex pathways. Activation of these pathways leads to the sensation of pain.[3,4] The nociceptive pathway includes peripheral nociceptors, nerve fibers in peripheral nerves, spinal cord and brain stem relays, spinal cord and brain pathways, and central processing areas in the brain stem, thalamus, and cerebral cortex.

Nociceptors are specific receptors that respond to a variety of stimuli. They include mechanosensitive, thermosensitive, and polymodal (those responding to more than one kind of stimulus) receptors. Nociceptors are usually silent unless stimulated and require more intense stimuli than many other receptors. They respond to stimuli in proportion to the intensity of the stimulus. The nociceptors of the skin have been studied in most detail, but it is clear that nociception occurs from many structures. The nociceptors are generally "free nerve endings," although the endings are never completely free of surrounding structure.[4,5] The nerve fibers associated with nociception are either A-delta, which are small myelinated axons, or C-polymodal, which are nonmyelinated. Excitation of cutaneous A-delta receptors causes a "pricking pain" in humans, while excitation of C-polymodal receptors causes a "burning pain."[6] Release of certain chemicals (acetylcholine, histamine, bradykinin) excites nociceptors, but it is not likely that these chemicals are necessary for all nociception.

Nociceptive afferent fibers generally enter the spinal cord through the dorsal root. The afferent fibers synapse on relay neurons in the dorsal horn of the spinal cord that send axons cranially. There are also segmental connections for reflexes, for example the flexion reflex. Many of the dorsal horn neurons have synapses from nociceptors in muscle, joint, and other structures. This convergence of nociceptive pathways in the spinal cord may be one of the mechanisms of referred pain.[6]

The nociceptive spinal cord pathways include spinothalamic, spinoreticular, spinomesencephalic, spinocervical tracts, and the dorsal column postsynaptic system. The relative significance and location of these tracts vary between species. For example, a major part of the spinothalamic tract is in the dorsal lateral funiculus in cats, as compared to the ventrolateral funiculus in primates.[4,7] The spinoreticular and spinomesencephalic tracts probably have less discriminative capacity than the spinothalamic tracts. The domestic animals have multisynaptic, bilateral nociceptive pathways, probably in the propriospinal system, that are resistant to destruction. The spinal tracts relay in the thalamus before reaching the cerebral cortex.

Nociception from the head is carried in branches of the trigeminal (V), facial (VII), glossopharyngeal (IX), and vagus (X) nerves. Fibers synapse in the nucleus caudalis of the trigeminal nerve, then follow routes to the cerebrum similar to the spinal pathways.

Mechanisms of Pain

Nociceptive stimulation causes two kinds of reactions. Superficial pain is discriminative, allowing precise localization of the stimulus. Deep pain is motivational, causing the animal to exhibit a change in behavior. Both superficial and deep pain are used clinically to localize lesions. Deep pain is also used as an important test for prognosis in spinal cord lesions. In gen-

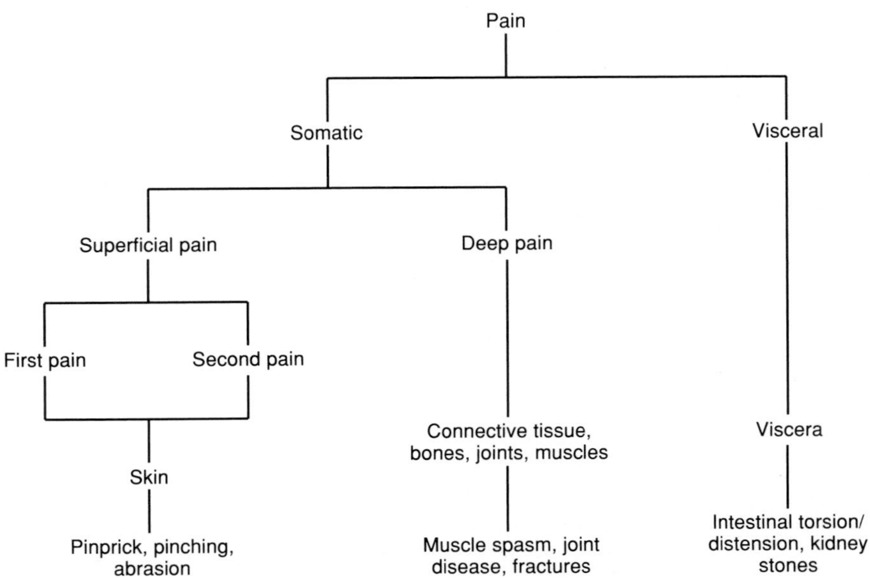

Figure 15–1 Qualities of pain.

eral, superficial pain comes from the more superficial structures, while deep pain comes from receptors in muscle, joints, and bone (Fig. 15–1).[8]

Examination

The methods for evaluating an animal's ability to perceive pain were discussed in Chapter 1.

Recognition of the signs of pain in animals is important for diagnosis and appropriate, humane care. The perception of pain is apparently similar in most mammalian species, but the relative reaction to pain varies considerably even in the same species. Many animals give little outward indication that they are in pain, when we recognize that the physical abnormality must be painful. For example, a dog with a fracture of a limb often shows little outward signs of pain and suffering, but we know it must be in considerable pain.

Animals with severe pain show one or more of the following changes:

- Decreased activity
- Depressed mentation
- Change in normal attitude (i.e., aggression, withdrawal)
- Gait abnormality—lameness, stilted, stiff limbs, reluctance to go up or down stairs, reluctance to jump
- Chewing, biting, or licking of a painful area
- Autonomic signs, such as salivation, pupillary dilation, or sweating (in the horse)

Localization of painful areas is accomplished by a combination of observation, palpation, and manipulation. After observing for the changes listed above, the clinician systematically palpates the animal. It is usually best to start caudally and work cranially to localize pain. Generally, nervous system disease will cause decreased sensation caudal to the lesion, increased sensation at the location of the problem, and normal sensation cranial to the lesion. This is especially true of spinal cord lesions. Palpating from caudal to cranial goes from decreased sensation through the painful area to normal sensation, maximizing the ability of the examiner to recognize the abnormal area. If abnormality is identified, the palpation can be done in reverse direction to help narrow the location.

Palpation of the vertebral column can be done by pressing on the spinous processes or squeezing the articular or transverse processes, depending on the size of the animal and examiner. Placing the other hand on the abdomen of small animals while palpating detects increased tension in the muscles as painful areas are approached. Pressing on the ribs may also be helpful in recognizing thoracic vertebral pain, such as that seen in diskospondylitis. Careful palpation can distinguish vertebral from abdominal pain. A few animals will be in so much pain that localization is impossible. Sedation often allows a more accurate examination.

Manipulation of the limbs is used to identify joint pain. The vertebral column can also be manipulated to elicit pain if palpation is unsuccessful. Flexion, extension, and turning of the head and neck often elicits pain in problems affecting the cervical vertebrae. Extension of the lumbosacral region causes pain in animals with degenerative lumbosacral disease.

Palpation of the head, temporal muscles, and mandible, and opening the mouth are important in assessing cranial structures.

Diseases

The diseases that frequently cause pain are listed in Table 15–1. Most of these are discussed in other chapters, as indicated in the table. The only neurologic disease that frequently causes pain without other clinical signs is meningitis.

Meningitis

Inflammation of the meninges, or *meningitis*, may be caused by many infectious agents, including bacterial, viral, fungal, protozoal, and rickettsial organisms.[9] A complete list is in the tables in Chapter 16. In addition, autoimmune diseases can cause meningitis, and there are some diseases of unknown origin, including granulomatous meningoencephalomyelitis (GME),[10] a meningitis characterized by an eosinophilic CSF,[11] and a suppurative, noninfectious meningitis.[12,13] A vasculitis and meningitis seen in dogs, primarily beagles, has been called the "canine pain syndrome."[14] Bacterial infections are probably more common in large animals than in pets. They are most common in neonatal foals, calves, and lambs. *Staphylococcus* spp. are most frequent in dogs in our clinic. Bacterial infections occur by hematogenous spread from infections in other parts of the body, by direct extension from adjacent structures, such as the sinuses, eyes, or ears, and from direct trauma, including surgery and CSF collection. The organisms spread through the CSF to both spinal and intracranial meninges. Vasculitis is common, especially in rickettsial infections and immune-mediated disease.[9,14]

TABLE 15–1 Etiology of Pain*

Localization/ Class	*Acute Nonprogressive*	*Acute Progressive*	*Chronic Progressive*
Multifocal or Diffuse			
Inflammatory		Meningitis Myositis (8) Neuritis (8)	
Localized			
Degenerative		Disk (type I) (7)	Disk (type II) (7) Spondylosis (7) Lumbosacral stenosis (7) Cervical vertebral spondylopathy (8)
Anomalous		Atlantoaxial instability (8) Hydrocephalus (13)	
Neoplastic (16)			Vertebral Extradural Intradural-extramedullary
Inflammation (7)		Diskospondylitis Osteomyelitis Abscess	
Trauma (7)	Fractures Luxations		
Vascular	Ischemic myopathy (7)		Immune vasculitis

* Numbers in parentheses refer to chapters in which entities are discussed.

Regardless of the cause of meningitis, the potential for the inflammatory process to extend to the nervous tissue is always present. The resulting encephalitis, myelitis, or encephalomyelitis causes other clinical signs, such as seizures, paresis, ataxia, or altered mental status, reflecting the location and extent of the inflammation. Cranial and spinal nerves may be affected. Communicating hydrocephalus may develop because of reduced absorption of CSF in the subarachnoid space and through the venous sinuses. Occlusion of the CSF pathways may also cause obstructive hydrocephalus.

Animals with meningitis are frequently ill. The onset is usually acute and signs are progressive. They may be lethargic and reluctant to eat. Many animals, especially dogs, have cervical rigidity with generalized pain that seems worse in the cervical region. Palpation of the vertebral column and head usually causes the animal to splint the muscles and appear uncomfortable, as contrasted with palpation of limb musculature. However, small animals may appear to be painful everywhere. They frequently walk as if they did not want to jar their body, as if "walking on egg shells." A fever may be present.

The diagnosis is supported by finding increased white blood cells (WBCs) in the CSF. Bacterial infections generally have a WBC count of 500 to 1,000 cells, with a predominance of neutrophils. Rickettsial infections have variable numbers and mixed populations of cells. Ehrlichiosis is more likely to have mononuclear cells predominating, while Rocky Mountain spotted fever may have more neutrophils.[9,15] Fungal infections have very high WBC counts with a mixed population of cells, sometimes including many eosinophils. Antibiotic or corticosteroid therapy may reduce the numbers of WBCs, especially neutrophils. Organisms may be seen on appropriately stained sediment or on electron microscopy. Cryptococcal organisms are best seen with an India ink preparation. Culture and sensitivity testing in all suspected cases is an important diagnostic aid. The results are most likely to be rewarding when there is a neutrophilic pleocytosis. The protein content of the CSF is elevated in meningitis and highest in bacterial and fungal infections (usually >100 mg/dl).

Antibiotic treatment of bacterial and rickettsial infections is discussed in Chapter 5. Treatment of other infections is outlined in Chapter 16.

Treatment

Relief of pain in animals was often ignored in the past. Greater awareness of the signs associated with pain has resulted in more aggressive management.[16,17] Pain management in human beings includes three categories of therapy—

pharmacologic, physical, and psychological.[18] Pharmacologic and physical methods are used commonly in animals, but psychological methods are rarely used.

Pharmacologic Management. Analgesic agents include narcotics, anti-inflammatory agents, anesthetics, and psychotropic drugs (Tables 15–2 through 15–7). Anesthetic agents will not be discussed. Species variability is important in selecting agents to control pain.[19] For example, the cat, horse, and ruminant may become hyperexcitable with doses of morphine that pro-

TABLE 15–2 Analgesic Agents for Dogs

Analgesic	*Dosage (mg/kg), Route*	*Duration of Action (hr)*	*Comments and Side Effects*
Opioids			
Morphine	0.1–2.0 IM, SC	3–6	Vomiting, defecation, poor temperature control
Oxymorphone	0.05–0.22 IV, IM, SC	2–6	Auditory hypersensitivity
Meperidine	2–6 IM, SC	1–2	
Codeine	1–2 PO	6	Oral therapy combined with acetaminophen or aspirin
Pentazocine	0.1–4 IM	2–4	
Butorphanol	0.2–0.4 IV, IM, SC	2–6	Minimal side effects
Buprenorphine	0.01–0.02 IV, IM, SC	6–12	
Nonsteroidal Anti-inflammatory Drugs			
Aspirin	10–20 PO	2–4	Combine with codeine, give every 8–12 hr
Acetaminophen	10–20 PO	2–4	Combine with codeine, give every 8–12 hr
Flunixin	0.5–2.2 IM, IV	6–8	Caution with repeated doses
Phenylbutazone	10 PO 22 IV	6–8	Maximum of 800 mg/day
Other Analgesic Agents			
Xylazine	0.05–0.2 IV, IM	1–3	Best when combined with opioid

TABLE 15–3 Analgesic Agents for Cats

Analgesic	*Dosage (mg/kg), Route*	*Duration of Action (hr)*	*Comments and Side Effects*
Opioids			
Morphine	0.1 IM, SC	3–6	Excitement with higher doses
Oxymorphone	0.05–0.22 IV, IM, SC	2–6	Excitement with higher doses, auditory hypersensitivity
Meperidine	2–10 IM, SC	1–2	
Pentazocine	0.75–3 IM, SC, IV	2–4	Higher doses have been used
Butorphanol	0.2–0.4 IV, IM, SC	2–6	Minimal side effects
Buprenorphine	0.005–0.01 IM, SC	6–12	
Nonsteroidal Anti-inflammatory Drugs			
Aspirin	10 PO	48	Caution with repetitive doses
Other Analgesic Agents			
Ketamine	2–4 IV, IM	0.5	Dissociative anesthetic
Xylazine	0.05–0.2 IV, IM	0.5	Best combined with other agents

TABLE 15–4 Analgesic Agents for Horses

Analgesic	Dosage (mg/kg), Route	Frequency of Administration (hr)	Comments and Side Effects
Opioids			
Morphine	0.2–0.3 IM, IV, SC	4–7	Best after giving xylazine; excitement with higher doses
Meperidine	2–4 IM, IV	0.5–1	Excitement, hypotension (IV)
Pentazocine	0.33–0.66 IM, SC, IV	1	
Butorphanol	0.1–0.2 IM	2–4	Excitement with higher doses
Fentanyl	0.1 IV, IM, SC	2	Pacing
Methadone	0.25 IM, IV	6	
Nonsteroidal Anti-inflammatory Drugs			
Aspirin	30–50 PO	12	
Dipyrone	5–10 g (total dose) SC, IM, IV	8–24	
Flunixin	1.1 IM, IV, PO	24	Repeat for colic-induced pain, no more than 5 days
Phenylbutazone	4–8 PO 3–6 IV	24 (PO) 12 (IV)	Maximum dose, 8.8 mg/kg/day
Naproxen	10 PO	12	
Meclofenamic acid	2.2 PO	24	Lower dose if used more than 5–7 days
Other Analgesic Agents			
Xylazine	1.1 IV 2.2 IM	0.5	Best combined with other agents

TABLE 15–5 Analgesic Agents for Cattle

Analgesic	Dosage (mg/kg), Route	Duration of Action (hr)	Comments and Side Effects
Opioids			
Meperidine	3.3–4.4 IM, SC	1–2	Regulatory concern
Nonsteroidal Anti-inflammatory Drugs			
Aspirin	50–100 PO	12	
Phenylbutazone	10–20 PO	24	
Other Analgesic Agents			
Xylazine	0.1–0.2 IM	Once	Brahman sensitive, not approved for use (FDA)

TABLE 15–6 Analgesic Agents for Sheep and Goats

Analgesic	Dosage (mg/kg), Route	Frequency of Administration (hr)	Comments and Side Effects
Opioids			
Meperidine	1–3 IM	12	
Pentazocine	3.0 IM	4	
Buprenorphine	0.005–0.2 IM	12	
Other Analgesic Agents			
Sodium salicylate	1–4 g (total dose), IV	24	
Xylazine	0.05–0.2 IM	Once	Combinations used

TABLE 15–7 Analgesic Agents for Swine

Analgesic	Dosage (mg/kg), Route	Frequency of Administration (hr)
Opioids		
Meperidine	2.0 IM	4
Pentazocine	3.0 IM	4
Buprenorphine	0.005–0.01 IM	12
Nonsteroidal Anti-inflammatory Drugs		
Sodium salicylate	1–4 g (total dose), IV	24
Aspirin	10 PO	6

duce sedation in the dog. These effects may be prevented by combining the narcotic with other agents, such as the phenothiazine tranquilizers or xylazine.

Narcotics are the most effective analgesics, providing relief in most cases regardless of the cause of the pain. Their effect is primarily in the central nervous system, and cause depression of behavior and respiration. Opioid narcotics are controlled drugs. They are frequently used for postoperative and trauma-induced pain. Newer synthetic agents with both agonist and antagonist opioid effects include butorphanol and buprenorphine.[17,20–22] These agents are not controlled, provide moderate analgesic effects, and have less depressive effects.

Anti-inflammatory drugs are most effective in pain associated with inflammation. The nonsteroidal anti-inflammatory drugs (NSAIDs) are widely used, and their action is potentiated by combination with the opioids.[21] A combination of codeine and acetaminophen or aspirin is frequently used for spinal pain associated with disk disease or surgery. NSAIDs are primarily peripherally acting agents that reduce the interaction of humoral substances (e.g., kinins, substance P, histamine, eicosanoids) with pain receptors. These agents have the potential for causing a variety of side effects, especially gastrointestinal hemorrhage. There is considerable species variability in their effectiveness and the severity of side effects.[20,21]

Xylazine is the most common α_2-agonist currently in use, but detomidine for horses, and medetomidine for dogs and cats, have become available recently.[14,20] Xylazine produces mild analgesia in small animals, moderate visceral (but not limb) analgesia in horses, and nearly anesthetic effects in ruminants.

Other psychotropic drugs include tranquilizers and ketamine. The tranquilizers, including phenothiazine derivatives, benzodiazepines, and butyrophenones, are primarily useful in reducing anxiety associated with pain. They may potentiate the effects of other analgesic agents but should not be used alone in the treatment of pain. Ketamine is a dissociative anesthetic and is not generally used for the management of pain.

Physical Therapy. A variety of therapeutic techniques are useful in reducing swelling, pain, and discomfort from injury. Commonly available methods are applications of heat or cold, passive exercise, hydrotherapy, and massage. Electrical stimulation is being used in humans with success, but there is little information available on its use in veterinary medicine.

Psychological Therapy. The use of biofeedback, operant conditioning, hypnosis, and meditation is a component of chronic pain therapy in humans. These techniques are probably not applicable to animals.

Acupuncture. Acupuncture is still controversial, although there is substantial evidence for the benefits of its use in treating pain. If used with pain relief as the goal, and not as a substitute for correction of the cause of pain, then it is appropriate.[23–25]

REFERENCES

1. Colloquium on recognition and alleviation of animal pain and distress. J Am Vet Med Assoc 191:1184–1298, 1987.
2. Short CE, Poznak AV: Animal Pain. New York, Churchill Livingstone, 1992.
3. Kitchell R: Problems in defining pain and peripheral mechanisms of pain. J Am Vet Med Assoc 191:1195–1199, 1987.
4. Willis WD, Coggeshall RE: Sensory mechanisms of the spinal cord. New York, Plenum Press, 1991.
5. Kruger L, Rodin BE: Peripheral mechanisms involved in pain. In Kitchell RL, Erickson HH, Carstens E, Davis LE (eds): Animal Pain Perception and Alleviation. Bethesda, Md, American Physiological Society, 1983, pp 1–26.
6. Willis WD Jr: The Pain System: The Neural Basis of Nociceptive Transmission in the Mammalian Nervous System. Basel, S Karger, 1985.
7. Willis W, Chung J: Central mechanisms of pain. J Am Vet Med Assoc 191:1200–1202, 1987.

8. Schmidt RF: Fundamentals of Sensory Physiology. Berlin, Springer-Verlag, 1986.
9. Meric SM: Canine meningitis: A changing emphasis. J Vet Intern Med 2:26–35, 1988.
10. Cook JR Jr: Granulomatous meningoencephalomyelitis. Vet Med Rep 1:321–327, 1989.
11. Smith-Maxie LL, Parent JP, Rand J, et al: Cerebrospinal fluid analysis and clinical outcome of eight dogs with eosinophilic meningoencephalomyelitis. J Vet Intern Med 3:167–174, 1989.
12. Russo E, Lees G, Hall C: Corticosteroid-responsive aseptic suppurative meningitis in three dogs. Southwest Vet 35:197–201, 1983.
13. Meric S, Perman V, Hardy R: Corticosteroid-responsive meningitis in ten dogs. J Am Anim Hosp Assoc 21:677–684, 1985.
14. Burns JC, Felsburg PJ, Wilson H, et al: Canine pain syndrome is a model for the study of Kawaski disease. Perspect Biol Med 35:68–73, 1991.
15. Greene CE: Update on neurologic and serologic findings on RMSF in dogs. In: Proceedings of an ACVIM Forum, San Diego, 1987, pp 691–692.
16. Tranquilli WJ, Raffe MR: Understanding pain and analgesic therapy in pets. Vet Med 841:680–686, 1989.
17. Potthoff A, Carithers RW: Pain and analgesia in dogs and cats. Comp Cont Educ Pract Vet 11:887–897, 1989.
18. Maciewicz R, Mucke L: Pain. In Johnson RT (ed): Current Therapy in Neurologic Disease. Philadelphia, BC Decker, 1987, pp 43–48.
19. Benson G, Thurmon J: Species difference as a consideration in alleviation of animal pain and distress. J Am Vet Med Assoc 191:1227–1230, 1987.
20. Tranquilli WJ, Fikes L, Raffe MR: Selecting the right analgesics: Indications and dosage requirements. Vet Med 84:692–697, 1989.
21. Jenkins W: Pharmacologic aspects of analgesic drugs in animals: An overview. J Am Vet Med Assoc 191:1231–1240, 1987.
22. Raffe MR, Tranquilli WJ: Classifying commonly used analgesic agents. Vet Med 84:687–690, 1989.
23. Latshaw W: Current theories of pain perception related to acupuncture. J Am Anim Hosp Assoc 11:449–450, 1975.
24. Vincent C, Richardson P: The evaluation of therapeutic acupuncture: Concepts and methods. Pain 24:1–13, 1986.
25. Martin B, Klide A: Use of acupuncture for the treatment of chronic back pain in horses: Stimulation of acupuncture points with saline solution injections. J Am Vet Med Assoc 190:1177–1180, 1987.

16

Systemic or Multifocal Signs

The first step in the management of a neurologic problem is localization of the disease process to a single anatomic site. Localization has been emphasized throughout this book; however, a group of diseases that produce more than one lesion or that affect most of the central nervous system (CNS) simultaneously has not yet been discussed. These disorders are categorized as multifocal, systemic, or diffuse diseases. Some of them initially may appear as focal diseases but progress to affect other structures.

Lesion Localization

The key to the recognition of these diseases is a neurologic examination that indicates the involvement of two or more parts of the nervous system that are not closely related anatomically. The most obvious example is an abnormality in both the brain and the spinal cord. All of the possible combinations of signs of diffuse or multifocal diseases are too extensive to list, but Table 16–1 outlines some of the more common ones. Any time that the neurologic examination does not strongly indicate a single lesion, this group of diseases becomes more likely.

Diseases

The major disease categories producing systemic or multifocal signs are degenerative, metabolic, neoplastic, nutritional, inflammatory, and toxic disorders. Some of these diseases may be chiefly focal in the individual animal, such as primary CNS neoplasms, but they are capable of affecting any part of the nervous system and therefore are included in this section. Diseases that are primarily skeletal in origin will be mentioned but not discussed. All of these diseases are progressive. The acute or chronic onset and the rate of progression may be of some help in establishing the diagnosis (Table 16–2).

Degenerative Diseases

New primary degenerative diseases of the CNS continue to be recognized. These diseases are usually inherited and are relatively rare, but are important to specific breeds. They are also important because they often serve as excellent models of similar human diseases. Anyone recognizing one of these diseases should contact a neurologist or one of the authors of the papers listed in the references.

Three groups of diseases will be discussed: (1) storage diseases, (2) abiotrophies, and (3) degenerations of unknown cause. Primary vascular disease has been discussed in Chapter 7 (spinal cord) and Chapter 13 (brain).

Storage Diseases

A large group of diseases are characterized pathologically by the accumulation of metabolic products in cells (Table 16–3). A genetically based deficiency of an enzyme causes an

TABLE 16–1 Examples of Systemic or Multifocal Signs

LMN signs: More than one location, may include cranial nerves, e.g., diffuse LMN diseases, polyneuropathy (see Chap. 9)
Brain and spinal cord signs: Examples – pelvic limb paresis and seizures
Systemic disease and CNS signs: Examples – fever, anorexia, ataxia or seizures
Generalized pain: Example – meningitis
Cerebral cortex and brain stem: Examples – seizures and cranial nerve deficits, blindness, severe gait deficits
Bilateral cerebral cortex: Examples – blindness with normal pupils (may be seen with brain swelling, hydrocephalus) (see Chap. 13)
Cerebellum and paresis: Examples – head tremor, ataxia, severe gait deficits, paresis
Ascending paralysis: Example – pelvic limb paresis progressing to tetraparesis (focal cervical spinal cord lesion must be ruled out)

accumulation of the product in neurons, glia, or other cells. The effect of the disease may be caused by the accumulation of the product or may be a direct result of the metabolic disturbance.[1] The clinical signs and the progression of the disease are dependent on the pathologic process, so many of the conditions are similar. Two groups are commonly recognized: neuronal storage diseases, in which the product accumulates in neurons, and leukodystrophies, in which there is a progressive destruction of myelin.[2]

The storage diseases are rare. Most have been recognized in dogs or cats. Animals are usually normal at birth, but fail to grow normally. Most of the diseases that have been studied have a recessive mode of inheritance, so only a portion of the litter is affected. Inbreeding is common in most of the animals studied. Onset of clinical signs is usually in the first few months of life (see Table 16–3). All of the disorders are slowly progressive and lead to the death of the animal.[3] There is no treatment known for any of them; however, they are important diseases because (1) they are genetic disorders and can be eliminated by selective breeding; (2) they may be confused with conditions of nongenetic origin, such as viral diseases; and (3) they are important models for diseases of human beings. Colonies of animals with many of these diseases have been established at research institutions.

Abiotrophies and Other Degenerative Diseases

The normal neuron is not capable of dividing and reproducing itself but has the capacity to survive for the life of the animal. An abnormality of the metabolic pathways leads to early death of the neuron. This process is termed *abiotrophy*.[4] The classification proposed by de Lahunta is used in Table 16–4.[4] The degeneration is characterized as primarily motor neuronal, multisystemic, cerebellar, or peripheral. The multisystem disorders are further characterized as to the primary site of the degenerative process—cell body, cell process, myelin, and so forth.

Most of these diseases are seen in young animals, with the exception of degenerative myelopathy of German shepherd dogs (see Chap. 7 and Table 16–4). Clinical signs relate to the primary site affected. The motor neuron degenerations produce generalized lower motor neuron (LMN) signs (see Chap. 8), myelin disorders cause ataxia that progresses to paresis, and cerebellar degenerations cause ataxia, dysmetria, and tremor (see Chap. 9). The progression is generally slow (months) but unrelenting.

TABLE 16–2 Etiology of Systemic Diseases*

Classification	*Acute Progressive*	*Chronic Progressive*
Degenerative		Storage disease Abiotrophy
Metabolic	*Hepatic encephalopathy* *Hypoglycemia* Endocrine disease Renal disease	*Hepatic encephalopathy* Endocrine disease
Neoplastic	Metastatic	*Primary* Metastatic
Nutritional		Hypovitaminosis Hypervitaminosis
Inflammatory	Infectious	Infection – usually viral
Toxic	Most toxins	*Heavy metals* Other toxins, low dosages

* *Italics* indicate most common diseases seen clinically.

TABLE 16–3 Storage Diseases

Disease	Enzyme Deficit (Storage Product)	Signalment	Clinical Signs/ Diagnosis	Human Disease	References
Gangliosidosis GM_1					
Type 1	β-Galactosidase (ganglioside)	Beagle cross (3 mo.), Portuguese water dogs (5 mo.); domestic cats (2–3 mo.); Friesian cattle (CNS – 1 mo.)	Tremor, incoordination, spastic paraplegia, impaired vision; enzyme assay WBC, skin fibroblast cultures, biopsy of lymph node or cerebellum	Norman-Landing disease	77–80
Type 2	β-Galactosidase (ganglioside)	Siamese, Korat, and domestic cats (2–3 mo.); Suffolk sheep (4 mo.)	Same as Type 1	Derry's disease	81
Gangliosidosis GM_2					
Type 1	Hexosaminidase A (ganglioside)	German short-haired pointer dogs (6–9 mo.), Japanese spaniel (18 mo.)	Ataxia, incoordination, impaired vision, dementia; enzyme assay, WBC, biopsy of cerebrum	Tay-Sachs disease	82, 83
Type 2	Hexosaminidase A, B (ganglioside)	Domestic cats (2 mo.)	Same as cats with GM_1 gangliosidosis	Sandhoff's disease	84, 85
Type 3	Hexosaminidase A (ganglioside)	Mixed-breed dog (1.5 yr); Yorkshire swine (CNS – 3 mo.)	Ataxia, incoordination, tremor, hypermetria	Bernheimer-Seitelberger disease	86
Glucocerebrosidosis	β-Glucosidase (glucocerebroside)	Sydney silky dog (6–8 mo.)	Ataxia, incoordination, hypermetria; enzyme assay WBC, skin fibroblast cultures, biopsy of lymph node, liver, bone marrow, cerebellum	Gaucher's disease	87
Sphingomyelinosis	Sphingomyelinase (sphingomyelin)	Siamese, Balinese, domestic cats (2–4 mo.); poodle dogs (2–4 mo.)	Ataxia, incoordination, tremor, hypermetria, polyneuropathy; enzyme assay WBC, bone marrow, skin fibroblast cultures, biopsy of bone marrow, cerebellum	Niemann-Pick disease	88–91
Globoid cell leukodystrophy	β-Galactosidase (galactocerebrosidase)	Cairn terrier, West Highland (2–5 mo.); beagle, bluetick hound (4 mo.); miniature poodle (2 yr); basset hound (1.5–2 yr); Pomeranian (1.5 yr); domestic cat (5–6 wk); polled Dorset sheep (4–18 mo.)	Ataxia, incoordination, tremor, progressive paraparesis, hypermetria, impaired vision; CSF macrophages with myelin; enzyme assay WBC	Krabbe's disease	92–99

Metachromatic leukodystrophy	Arysulfatase (sulfatide)	Domestic cat (2 wk)	Progressive motor dysfunction, seizures, opisthotonos		100, 101
Mucopolysaccharidosis	Arylsulfatase B (mucopolysaccharide)	Siamese, domestic cat (4–7 mo.)	Progressive paraparesis	Maroteaux-Lamy disease	102–104
	α_1-Iduronidase (mucopolysaccharide)	Domestic cat (10 mo.); Plott hound (3–6 mo.), mixed dog (4–6 mo.)	Progressive paraparesis	Hurler's syndrome	103, 105–107
Glycoproteinosis	(? Glycoprotein)	Beagle, basset hound, poodle dogs (5 mo–9 yr)	Depression, progressive seizures; biopsy of lymph nodes, liver, cerebellum	Lafora's disease	3, 108, 109
Mannosidosis	α-Mannosidase (mannoside)	Domestic (7 mo.), Persian cat (8 wk); Angus, Murray grey cattle, Galloway calves (birth)	Ataxia, incoordination, tremor, and aggression (calves); assay of urine oligosaccharide	Mannosidosis	110–114
	β-Mannosidase (mannoside)	Nubian goats (birth–1 yr)	Ataxia, recumbency	β-Mannosidosis	115, 116
Glycogenosis	α-Glucosidase	Lapland dogs (1.5 yr), English springer spaniel (11 yr); domestic, Norwegian forest cats (5 mo.); Corriedale sheep (6 mo.); shorthorn, Brahman cattle (3–9 mo.)	Incoordination, exercise intolerance	Pompe's disease	117–125
Fucosidosis	α_1-Fucosidase	Springer spaniel dogs (2 yr)	Incoordination, behavioral changes, dysphonia, dysphagia, seizures; enzyme assay WBC		126–128
Ceroid lipofuscinosis	Unknown abnormality	English setter (1 yr), dachshund (3.5–7 yr), cocker spaniel (1.5 yr), Chihuahua, Saluki (2 yr), Tibetan terrier (3 yr), Australian cattle dog (14 mo.), border collie (18–22 mo.), blue-heeler (12 mo.), mixed dog (4 mo.); Siamese, domestic cats (2–7 yr); South Hampshire sheep (6–18 mo.); Rambouillet sheep (9–12 mo.), Devon cattle (14 mo.); Nubian goat (10 mo.)	Personality change, visual impairment, ataxia, incoordination, jaw champing, seizures; biopsy of lymph nodes, cerebellum	Batten's disease, ceroid lipofuscinosis	129–143

Modified with permission from Oliver JE, Hoerlein BF, Mayhew IG: Veterinary Neurology. Philadelphia, WB Saunders, 1987, Table 6–1.

TABLE 16–4 Abiotrophies and Degenerative Diseases of Unknown Cause

Anatomic Location	*Signalment*	*Clinical Signs*	*References*
Motor neuron	Swedish Lapland (5–7 wk), St. Bernard × Great Dane × bloodhound cross (8–14 wk), Brittany spaniel (6 wk, 6 mo., 1 yr), Rottweiler (1–4 wk), English pointer (5 mo.), German shepherd dogs (2 wk)	LMN degeneration with resulting paralysis and atrophy of muscles of trunk and limbs	4, 144–149
Multisystem			
Cell body	Cocker spaniel (1 yr), Cairn terrier (2.5–5 mo.); Angora goat (1 wk–4 mo.)	Cerebellar ataxia, spastic paresis	150–153
Cell processes	Smooth fox terrier (2.5–4 mo.), Jack Russell terrier dogs (2.5–4 mo.)	Degeneration of superficial tracts of lateral funiculi; cerebellar ataxia, dysmetria, spasticity; rapid early progression, then progresses slowly	4, 154
	Bull mastiff dog (6–9 wk)	Hydrocephalus also present; visual abnormality, cerebellar ataxia, primarily in pelvic limbs; head tremor, abnormal nystagmus, behavioral change	155
	German shepherd dogs (4–5 yr), Siberian huskies, sporadically in other dog breeds	Spinal cord affected; progressive pelvic limb ataxia and paresis	156–159
	Simmental (5–8 mo.), Limousin × (4 mo.) cattle	Multifocal encephalopathy, progressive ataxia, behavioral change; progresses to recumbency and death by 12 mo.	4, 55
	Brown Swiss cattle (5–8 mo.)	Progressive pelvic limb paresis and ataxia, thoracic limbs affected late	160–161
	Appaloosa, Morgan, Przewalskii, and other horses; Grant zebra (before 7–14 mo.)	Slowly progressive ataxia and paresis of all four limbs; some cases related to vitamin E deficiency	49, 50, 55
Myelin	Rottweiler dog (1.5–3.5 yr)	Ataxia, dysmetria, tetraparesis	162
	Labrador retriever dog (4–6 mo.)	Extensor rigidity and opisthotonos, progressive cerebellar ataxia	163
	Dalmatian dog (3–6 mo.)	Progressive visual deficiency and locomotor abnormality	4
	Saluki (3 mo.)	Seizures, behavioral change	164
	Afghan hound (3–13 mo.)	Pelvic limb ataxia and paresis, progressing to paraplegia in 7–10 days; Varying degrees of thoracic limb involvement later	165
	Egyptian Mau cat (7 wk)	Ataxia, seizures	166
	Charolais cattle (6–36 mo.)	Slowly progressive pelvic limb paresis and ataxia	3, 55
	Murray Grey cattle (birth–12 mo.)	Spastic pelvic limb paresis and ataxia	3, 55
	Polled Hereford cattle (1–3 d)	Dull, recumbent, opisthotonos	167

Neuraxonal dystrophy	Collie sheepdogs (2–4 mo.), Rottweiler 1–2 yr), Chihuahua dogs (7 wk)	Progressive cerebellar ataxia, tremor	168–171
	German shepherd dog (15 mo.)	Progressive pelvic limb paresis and ataxia	172–173
	Boxer dog (1–7 mo.)	Spastic pelvic limb paresis, late tetraparesis	174, 175
	Siamese cat (5 wk)	Progressive cerebellar ataxia	176
	Suffolk (1.5–5 mo.), Merino (1–4 yr), Coopworth (1–6 mo.) sheep	Progressive paresis and ataxia	177
	Morgan horse (6–12 mo.)	Spastic pelvic limb paresis and ataxia	178, 179
Neurofilaments	Collie dog (3 wk)	Paresis of limbs	180
	Domestic cats (3 wk)	Progressive paresis of all four limbs	181
	Yorkshire pig (5 wk)	Progressive paresis	182
	Grant zebra (2 wk)	Progressive tetraparesis	4
	Hereford cattle (birth)	Progressive spastic paraplegia	183
Cerebellum			
Autosomal recessive	Kerry blue terrier (8–16 wk), Gordon setter (6–30 mo.), rough-coated collie (4–12 wk)	Progressive cerebellar ataxia, dysmetria, tremor	184–190
Multiple litters	Airedale, Bernese mountain, Finnish harrier, Brittany spaniel, Border collie, beagle, Samoyed, Clumber spaniel, Akita, Bern running dogs	Progressive cerebellar ataxia, dysmetria, tremor	3, 4, 190–192
Single dog or litter	Miniature poodle, fox terrier, cairn terrier, cocker spaniel, Labrador retriever, golden retriever, Great Dane, Schnauzer × beagle, mixed-breed dogs	Progressive cerebellar ataxia, dysmetria, tremor	3, 4, 193
Cats	Domestic cats	Progressive cerebellar ataxia	190
Cattle	Aberdeen Angus, Ayrshire, Charolais, Hereford, Holstein, Shorthorn	Progressive cerebellar ataxia	3, 194–197
Horses	Arabian, Gotland pony, Oldberg	Progressive cerebellar ataxia	55
Sheep	Corriedale, Merino, Welsh mountain, Border Leicester	Progressive cerebellar ataxia	3, 4, 55, 198, 199
Swine	Yorkshire, saddleback	Progressive cerebellar ataxia	3, 55, 200
Astrocytes	Labrador retriever, Scottish terrier, Alpine sheep	Progressive spasticity and ataxia	4, 201
Schwann cells	Tibetan mastiff dog (7–12 wk)	Pelvic limb paresis	202, 203
Nociceptive neurons	English pointer, European short-haired pointer (11–12 wk)	Mutilation of digits, analgesia of distal extremity	204, 205
Sensory neuropathy	Long-haired dachshunds	Ataxia, urinary incontinence, proprioceptive deficits, decreased nociception	206
Distal neuropathy	Doberman pinscher dog (3 yr)	Pelvic limb gait and stance abnormality.	207

Like the storage diseases, the abiotrophies are rare, usually inherited, and eventually fatal. The course of the disease is usually longer than that of the storage diseases.

Differential Diagnosis of Degenerative Diseases

Many of these diseases have a similar clinical history and course. The findings on a neurologic examination may indicate a predominance of cerebral, cerebellar, or spinal cord signs. These findings and the age and breed of the animal should suggest a small number of possibilities (see Tables 16–3 and 16–4). In the early stages, neuronal diseases often can be differentiated from demyelinating diseases. Neuronal diseases (storage disease, abiotrophy) are more likely to have cerebral or LMN signs. Demyelinating diseases are more likely to have ascending ataxia and paresis of an upper motor neuron (UMN) type, often with tremors of the limbs. Proprioceptive positioning is commonly affected in demyelinating diseases but is rarely involved in the early stages of neuronal disease.

The degenerative diseases also must be differentiated from inflammatory, neoplastic, and toxic disorders. Specific diagnostic tests are available for most of these conditions and will be discussed later in this chapter.

Metabolic Disorders

Normal nervous system function depends on a closely regulated environment. Conversely, the homeostasis of the body is coordinated by the nervous system through the neuroendocrine, autonomic, and somatic systems. Disorders altering homeostasis often have profound effects on the nervous system.

Liver Diseases

Hepatic encephalopathy is a complex metabolic disorder resulting from abnormal liver function.

Pathogenesis. Hepatic encephalopathy has been reported in three types of liver disease: (1) severe parenchymal liver damage, either acute or chronic (cirrhosis, neoplasia, toxicosis), (2) anomalous portal venous circulation (rare in large animals), and (3) congenital urea cycle enzyme deficiencies (rare).[5] Parenchymal liver diseases other than cirrhosis (fatty infiltration, chronic active hepatitis, and so forth) usually do not cause hepatic encephalopathy except in the terminal stages of the disease. Pyrrolizidine alkaloids in certain plants, such as *Senecio* spp. and *Crotalaria* spp., cause parenchymal liver damage and hepatic encephalopathy in herbivores.

Parenchymal disease severely reduces the capacity of the liver to perform its normal metabolic functions. Portosystemic venous shunts divert a significant portion of the portal blood past the liver into the vena cava. Potentially toxic substances that normally are absorbed from the gastrointestinal (GI) tract and detoxified in the liver enter the systemic circulation. Urea cycle enzyme deficiencies prevent the metabolism of ammonia to urea.

The metabolic changes that cause the clinical syndrome of hepatic encephalopathy are a result of failure of the liver to (1) remove toxic products of gut metabolism, and (2) synthesize factors necessary for normal brain function.[5] Cerebral toxins include increased circulating ammonia, short-chain fatty acids, and degradation products of amino acids, including mercaptans, skatoles, and indoles. Altered amino acid and neurotransmitter concentrations in the brain also are found. Ammonia is probably the most important toxic substance, although the level of ammonia in the blood does not necessarily correlate with the severity of the CNS disturbance.[6]

Clinical Signs. Most animals with liver disease severe enough to produce hepatic encephalopathy also have other clinical signs such as GI disturbances, anorexia, weight loss, stunted growth, ascites, and polyuria-polydipsia.

The neurologic signs are frequently worse after feeding, especially if high-protein food is given. The release of nitrogenous materials into the portal circulation exacerbates the signs. Depression that may progress to stupor and coma is the most common neurologic sign. Other signs of cerebral involvement, such as behavior change, continuous pacing and head pressing, blindness, and seizures, also are common. Frequently the clinical picture is that of a waxing and waning diffuse cerebral abnormality. The postural reactions and reflexes are only minimally involved, except when the animal is nearly comatose. The cranial nerves are not markedly affected, except that vision may be impaired. Ptyalism is frequent, especially in cats.

A variety of factors may precipitate the neurologic signs of hepatic encephalopathy in an animal with marginal liver function (Table 16–5). Any source of protein in the digestive tract is a common cause. Hemorrhage in the GI tract, constipation, or increased fatty acids also may precipitate a crisis. Alterations in fluids, electrolytes, or pH may increase the blood and tissue ammonia levels. Decreased renal function reduces elimination of ammonia and other me-

TABLE 16–5 Management of Hepatic Encephalopathy (HE)

Factors That Exacerbate HE	*Management of HE*
Increased dietary protein and fatty acids	Low-protein, low-fat diet
Bacterial production of ammonia in large bowel	Diet, antibiotics
Constipation leading to bacterial production of ammonia in large bowel	Diet, laxatives, enemas in acute problems, lactulose
Gastrointestinal hemorrhage	Monitoring and treatment of ulcers, bleeding disorders, hookworms, whipworms
Hypokalemia, hypovolemia, alkalosis—aggravated by diuretics	Monitoring and correction of fluid and electrolyte imbalance, use of potassium-sparing diuretics with caution or not at all
Transfusion of stored blood	Use of fresh blood (only if essential)
Sedatives, narcotics, anesthetics	Use of depressant drugs with extreme caution (in lowest possible dosages), monitoring carefully
Infections, fevers	Monitoring and vigorous treatment

tabolites. Fever and infection cause increased tissue catabolism and increased nitrogen release. Stored blood for transfusions may have an excess of ammonia. Depressant drugs directly affect the brain and frequently are metabolized in the liver. The first evidence of hepatic dysfunction often has been poor recovery from anesthesia. Diuretics used to treat ascites may cause hepatic encephalopathy through their effect on potassium, renal output of ammonia, and alkalosis.

Diagnosis. A variety of clinicopathologic abnormalities may be present, depending on the cause. Microcytosis with normochromic erythrocytes, ammonium biurate crystals in the urine, lowered cholesterol, and lowered blood glucose levels may be seen in portacaval shunts. Frequently the serum albumin and serum urea nitrogen levels are low. Parenchymal disease frequently causes elevations in liver enzymes, such as serum alanine aminotransferase (ALT), aspartate aminotransferase (AST), and alkaline phosphatase (AP), but levels of these enzymes usually are not elevated significantly in shunts.[7] Hepatic dysfunction may be confirmed with tests such as the ammonia tolerance test, or serum bile acids measured after a 12-hour fast and 2 hours after a meal.[8] Hepatic ultrasonography (US) is a sensitive indicator of liver size, and the definitive diagnosis of a shunt requires US or contrast-enhanced radiography. Parenchymal disease requires a biopsy for confirmation.

Management. The successful medical management of hepatic encephalopathy depends on the cause of the liver disorder and the degree of liver malfunction. Animals with marginal liver function may be managed by reducing the sources of nitrogenous products in the GI tract (see Table 16–5). A high-carbohydrate, low-fat, low-protein diet with a high biologic value is indicated. If dietary management alone is inadequate, then oral, nonabsorbable antibiotics (such as neomycin) may be used to reduce the bacterial flora that split urea. Mild laxatives or lactulose (a nonabsorbable disaccharide) may be helpful.[9,10]

Acute crises of hepatic encephalopathy require more vigorous treatment. Protein sources must be removed completely. Enemas and laxatives are used to remove all nitrogenous material from the GI tract. Sedative drugs, methionine, and diuretics are discontinued. Sources of GI hemorrhage are corrected if they are present. Dehydration, hypokalemia, and alkalosis are managed with intravenous (IV) fluid therapy. Renal output must be maintained in order to eliminate nitrogenous products. Oxygen therapy may be necessary, especially in cases of coma. The prognosis for herbivores with hepatic encephalopathy from pyrrolizidine toxicity is poor.

Specific treatment of the cause is instituted if possible. Unfortunately, most chronic liver diseases and the urea cycle enzyme deficiency cannot be treated specifically. Portosystemic shunts may be corrected surgically if there is adequate portal circulation to the liver. Partial occlusion of the shunt may be effective. For details of the management of hepatic encephalopathy, the reader should consult the references.[6,11,12]

Renal Diseases

The terminal stages of renal failure may cause tetany or seizures. Chronic renal disease may be associated with muscle wasting and weakness. Polyneuropathy and polymyopathy have been seen in human beings with chronic renal disease, especially those on hemodialysis, but these have not been documented in animals. Alterations in electrolyte metabolism, especially calcium and potassium electrolyte metabolism, may cause signs that are related to the nervous system (discussed later in this chapter).

Endocrine Disorders

Endocrine disorders that affect electrolyte, calcium, magnesium, phosphorus, and glucose homeostasis may produce neurologic signs in affected animals. In addition, hormonal excess or deficiency may affect the function of nerves or muscle directly. Also, pituitary lesions may cause signs of hormonal and brain dysfunction if the disease extends into the hypothalamus. In this section, specific endocrine and metabolic diseases that produce prominent neurologic signs of weakness will be discussed. Those that cause involuntary movements, tremor, tetany, and spasticity are discussed in Chapter 11. Readers should seek other textbooks for in-depth descriptions of each disorder.

Generalized Weakness. Many endocrine and metabolic diseases result in generalized weakness because they affect neuromuscular functions. In certain conditions, clinical signs improve with rest and are exacerbated by exercise. The term *episodic weakness* has been applied to this condition (see Chap. 8). In this section, endocrine and metabolic diseases that produce episodic or generalized weakness are discussed.

HYPOCALCEMIA Parturient paresis, or milk fever, is a hypocalcemic metabolic disorder that occurs in mature dairy cows, sows, sheep, and, rarely, horses, usually within 48 hours of parturition. The affected cows are usually more than 5 years old, and the incidence is increased in heavy milk producers and in the Jersey breed. Many dairy cows are marginally hypocalcemic at parturition, and any factor that decreases the metabolic adjustment to this hypocalcemia may cause paresis. Such factors include milk yield versus calcium mobilization from bone and gut, calcium to phosphorus ratios in the diet, anorexia and decreased intestinal motility, and dietary pH.

The onset of parturient paresis is characterized by hypersensitivity and a stiff gait, followed by progressive muscular weakness, recumbency, depression, and coma. Stage 1 is often missed and is characterized by apprehension, anorexia, ataxia, and limb stiffness. Stage 2 is marked by recumbency and depression. The head is usually turned to the flank, and there may be an S-shaped curvature of the neck. Other signs include dilated pupils, decreased pupillary light reflexes, reduced anal reflex, decreased defecation and urination, no ruminal motility, protrusion of the tongue, and frequent straining. Stage 3 occurs in approximately 20% of cases and is characterized by lateral recumbency; severe depression or coma; subnormal temperature; a weak, irregular heart rate; and slow, irregular, shallow respirations. The pupils are dilated and unresponsive to light. Bloating may occur. Changes in serum ions include hypocalcemia, hypophosphatemia, and hypomagnesemia. With prolonged anorexia, serum sodium and potassium levels may decrease. IV calcium salts (Ca^{++}, 1 g/45 kg body weight) are usually effective. Calcium borogluconate is commonly used; a 25% solution contains 10.4 g of calcium per 500 ml. Milk fever can be prevented in susceptible cows or herds by the administration of vitamin D or its analogues or by manipulating the prepartum dietary calcium and phosphorus levels.

Hypocalcemic syndromes are well documented in dogs and cats. In both species, primary hypoparathyroidism is a documented cause of chronic hypocalcemia. In the cat, hypoparathyroidism is sometimes caused by surgical resection of the parathyroid glands which inadvertently occurs during surgical thyroidectomy for the treatment of hyperthyroidism. Hypocalcemia may be associated with chronic renal disease in dogs and cats. It is the major biochemical abnormality in dogs with eclampsia.

When the ionized calcium concentration of the serum falls below 6–7 mg/dl, the clinical signs of hypocalcemia are likely to occur. Tetanic muscle contractions are the most common clinical signs, but some dogs may develop muscle weakness early in the disease. Hypocalcemia is suspected when the total serum calcium concentration is less than 9.0 mg/dl and the serum albumin concentration is normal. Total serum ionized calcium concentrations are confirmatory. Once the diagnosis of hypocalcemia is confirmed, the underlying cause should be identified. The diagnosis of both eclampsia and iatrogenic hypoparathyroidism is usually obvious from the history and physical findings. Primary hypoparathyroidism may be confirmed through parathormone (PTH) assays conducted at specialized laboratories.[13]

Animals experiencing seizure should be given 10% calcium gluconate solution IV at a dosage of 0.5–1.5 ml/kg. The dosage should be slowly infused over a 10- to 20-minute period and the heart rate and Q-T interval should be closely monitored. The calcium dose can be repeated every 6 to 8 hours as a bolus injection.

Oral maintenance therapy is instituted when the total serum calcium concentration is consistently less than 6.5 mg/dl. Calcium gluconate or calcium lactate is administered orally in doses of 1–4 g for dogs and 0.5–1.0 g for cats. In parathyroid deficiency, vitamin D therapy is required. Dihydrotachysterol is a synthetic vitamin D that is active in the absence of PTH. The loading dose is 0.03 mg/kg/day orally for 3 to 4 days. The maintenance dose is 0.01–0.02 mg/kg/day. Each patient should be closely monitored, since hypercalcemia may be a complication of vitamin D therapy, especially when supplemental calcium salts are administered.[14]

KETONEMIC SYNDROMES These diseases occur primarily in ruminants and are characterized by hypoglycemia and the accumulation of ketones in body fluids. Conditions that have been recognized include bovine ketosis (acetonemia) and pregnancy toxemia of cattle, sheep, and goats. Unlike most monogastric animals, ruminants produce most of their glucose supplies from the gluconeogenesis of volatile fatty acids (acetic, propionic, and butyric acids). Nearly 50% of the glucose in the cow is normally derived from dietary propionic acid that is converted to glucose in the gluconeogenic pathway. Reduction of propionic acid production in the rumen can result in hypoglycemia and the subsequent mobilization of free fatty acids and glycerol from fat stores. The liver has a limited ability to utilize these fatty acids because the levels of oxaloacetate are low. Acetyl coenzyme A therefore is not incorporated into the tricarboxylic acid cycle and is converted into the ketone bodies acetoacetate and β-hydroxybutyrate. When the production of ketones by the liver exceeds peripheral utilization, pathologic ketosis results.

Both ketosis and primary hypoglycemia are involved in the development of the clinical signs. The most common signs include depression, partial to complete anorexia, weight loss, and decreased milk production. The neurologic signs that are present in some cows include ataxia, apparent blindness, salivation, tooth grinding, excessive licking, muscle twitching, head pressing, and hyperesthesia. Cows may charge blindly if they are disturbed. The diagnosis of bovine ketosis is based on the presence of elevated ketone levels in blood and milk with concomitant hypoglycemia. The smell of ketones may be perceived on the breath and in the urine. The immediate therapy is an IV injection of glucose, followed by oral administration of 125 to 250 g of propylene glycol twice a day. Glucocorticoids are also beneficial in cows that are not septic. Cows with severe nervous signs can be treated with 2 to 8 g of chloral hydrate orally twice a day for 3 to 5 days.

Pregnancy toxemia is a condition that is closely related pathophysiologically to bovine ketosis. It occurs in ewes during the last 6 weeks of pregnancy, when there is a large demand for glucose by developing fetuses. Pregnancy toxemia occurs in pastured or housed beef cows during the last 2 months of pregnancy. Overweight cows or those bearing twin calves are especially susceptible. In ewes and cows, the basic etiology is nutrition insufficient to maintain normal blood glucose concentrations when fetal glucose demands are high. Hypoglycemia precipitates the ketosis, as has been described earlier in this section. In sheep, clinical signs may develop in a flock and may extend for several weeks. Ewes become depressed and develop weakness, ataxia, and loss of muscle tone. Terminally, recumbency and coma develop. Neuromuscular disturbances include fine muscle tremors of the ears and the lips. In some cases, seizures may develop. "Stargazing" postures and grinding of the teeth are common. The neurologic signs in cattle include depression, excitability, and ataxia. The diagnosis of pregnancy toxemia is based on the history, the clinical signs, and the presence of ketosis and hypoglycemia. In sheep, flock treatment consists of increasing the availability of glucose precursors in the diet or drenching affected ewes twice daily with 200 ml of a warm 50% glycerol solution. The anabolic steroid trienbolone acetate also is beneficial in 30-mg doses intramuscularly (IM). Induction of parturition or fetal removal by cesarean section also may be needed to reduce the metabolic drain on the ewe. Cattle are treated by the method described for bovine ketosis. Pregnancy toxemia can be prevented by ensuring adequate nutrition during pregnancy.

DIABETES MELLITUS Diabetes mellitus may result in neurologic signs from at least four mechanisms. Insulin deficiency results in failure of glucose transport into muscle and adipose tissue. An early sign of diabetes may be exercise intolerance and weakness. If severe insulin deficiency occurs, ketonemia develops from a marked increase in lipolysis and serum fatty acids. The ensuing metabolic acidosis results in depressed cerebral function that culminates in coma and death. In the nontreated ketoacidotic dog or cat, hyperkalemia may be a serious complication that depresses neuromuscular and cardiovascular function. With therapy and correction of the acidosis, potassium ions reenter cells, and hypokalemia may be a complication that fosters muscle weakness and depression.

In some animals, the hyperglycemia may be severe, even though acidosis is absent. This syndrome is called *hyperosmolar nonketotic coma*. Clinical signs result from the hyperosmolar effects on the cerebral cortex. On rare occasions, diabetic patients may develop neuropathies with associated LMN signs in affected muscles.

The comatose diabetic animal is a difficult therapeutic challenge. The clinician must exercise great care in performing insulin, acid-base, electrolyte, and fluid therapy. Interested readers should consult other texts for an in-depth discussion of the diagnosis and management of the diabetic patient.

HYPOTHYROIDISM Deficiencies of thyroxine result in a marked decrease in cerebration and basal metabolic rate. Severely hypothyroid dogs may become very depressed or may appear dull and unresponsive. Coma may result in severe cases.[15,16] A very low-voltage electroencephalogram (EEG) usually is seen. The cerebral signs improve dramatically following replacement thyroid medication. Polyneuropathies have been recognized in dogs without the usual signs of hypothyroidism. Syndromes include laryngeal paralysis, vestibular and auditory dysfunction, and various peripheral nerve and cranial nerve palsies. The fact that the animal has a polyneuropathy rather than a single problem may require electromyography (EMG) or other electrodiagnostic tests. Thyroid stimulating hormone testing is necessary to confirm a diagnosis. Many of these animals respond well with thyroid supplementation, but it may take weeks to months for nerve function to recover.[17]

HYPERADRENOCORTICISM Hyperactivity of the adrenal cortex may result in generalized muscle weakness from the catabolic effects of glucocorticoids, which are secreted excessively in this disease. In addition, some dogs with this condition develop muscle degeneration that is known as *steroid-induced myopathy*. This syndrome has been described in Chapter 8.

Bilateral adrenal cortical hyperplasia is a common cause of canine hyperadrenocorticism. This condition may develop as a consequence of adrenocorticotropic hormone (ACTH)–producing pituitary tumors. Occasionally these pituitary tumors grow large enough to produce neurologic signs, including depression, confusion, seizures, and a variety of autonomic nervous system abnormalities. Neurologic signs rarely occur unless the tumor invades the hypothalamus.

Episodic Weakness. In Chapter 8, the problem of episodic weakness was introduced and the primary neuromuscular causes of this problem were discussed. In this section, the endocrinologic and metabolic causes of episodic weakness are described briefly.

HYPERCALCEMIA An increased concentration of serum calcium may result in neuromuscular, cardiovascular, and renal dysfunction. When the level of calcium in body fluids rises above normal, excitable cell membranes are depressed. Reflex activities of the CNS become sluggish, and muscles also become sluggish and weak. Hypercalcemia also will decrease the Q-T interval of the heart and will decrease myocardial function. Hypercalcemia impairs the renal concentrating ability. In prolonged hypercalcemia, mineralization of soft tissue may occur. The syndrome of hypercalcemic nephropathy is well documented in animals and culminates in chronic renal failure. In the dog, calcium levels above 12.5 mg/dl result in hypercalcemic signs. In some cases, muscle weakness is markedly worse during exercise and improves with rest.

Several causes of hypercalcemia exist, including primary hyperparathyroidism, pseudohyperparathyroidism, vitamin D intoxication, and iatrogenic calcium therapy. Primary hyperparathyroidism results from autonomously functioning parathyroid adenomas. These tumors secrete PTH in the face of increasing serum calcium concentrations. Certain nonendocrine tumors, such as lymphosarcomas, secrete substances with PTH-like activity that results in hypercalcemia. This syndrome is called pseudohyperparathyroidism. An excessive intake of vitamin D promotes increased absorption of calcium and may produce hypercalcemia.

The symptomatic therapy of hypercalcemia includes diuresis with fluids and furosemide. Corticosteroids also are beneficial, because they promote the renal excretion of calcium.

HYPERKALEMIA Increased serum concentrations of potassium decrease the activity of excitable membranes, especially cardiac muscle. An excessive extracellular concentration of potassium causes cardiac flaccidity and decreases the conduction of cardiac impulses through the atrioventricular (AV) node. Thus, heart rate and cardiac output may be severely depressed. In addition, the contraction of skeletal muscle also may be somewhat depressed. Hyperkalemia therefore manifests itself as generalized weakness that becomes worse with exercise.

Hyperkalemia may occur secondary to severe acidosis; however, the usual cause is adrenal insufficiency. Adrenal insufficiency may result in aldosterone deficiency, which produces hyperkalemia and hyponatremia. Typical signs include depression, anorexia, vomiting, diarrhea, weakness, bradycardia, and decreased cardiac output. The disease responds well to fluid and replacement adrenocortical hormone therapy.

Hyperkalemic periodic paralysis, an episodic syndrome of muscular weakness and fasciculations, occurs in Quarter Horses.[18] It is associated with a marked hyperkalemia without major acid-base imbalance or high serum activity of enzymes derived from muscle. The episodes occur spontaneously or can be induced by administration of potassium chloride orally. EMG changes include fibrillation potentials, positive sharp waves, and complex repetitive discharges. Histologic changes in muscle are minimal, but may include vacuolation of type 2b fibers or mild degenerative changes. Marked hyperkalemia is present during episodes. Intravenous administration of calcium, glucose, or bicarbonate results in recovery. Administration of acetazolamide, 2.2 mg/kg orally every 8 to 12 hours, prevents the episodes. Decreasing the potassium content of the feed may also be effective. This can be done by feeding oat hay, grain two to three times daily, and providing free access to salt.[18]

HYPOKALEMIA Decreased serum concentrations of potassium decrease the activity of skeletal muscle because the membranes are hyperpolarized. Muscle weakness and even paralysis may occur. The primary causes of hypokalemia include diuretic therapy, vomiting, diarrhea, alkalosis, and excessive mineralocorticoid therapy for adrenal insufficiency. Most patients respond well to potassium supplementation.

HYPOGLYCEMIA Hypoglycemia causes altered CNS function similar to that which occurs with hypoxia. The blood glucose concentration is of prime importance for normal neuronal metabolism, because glucose oxidation is the primary energy source. There are no glycogen stores in the CNS. Glucose enters nervous tissue by diffusion rather than by insulin facilitation. The severity of the CNS signs is related more to the rate of decrease than to the actual concentration of glucose. Sudden drops in glucose levels are more likely to cause seizures, whereas slowly developing hypoglycemia may cause weakness, paraparesis, behavioral changes, or severe depression.

Hypoglycemia in young animals may be secondary to malnutrition, parasitism, stress, or a GI abnormality. Puppies frequently present as extremely depressed or comatose. The blood glucose level is usually very low (<30 mg/100 ml). A blood sample should be obtained for glucose determination, and IV glucose should be administered immediately (2–4 ml of 20% glucose per kg). If seizures are present, diazepam should be administered if there is no immediate response to the glucose (see the section on the treatment of status epilepticus in Chap. 14). Continued signs of stupor or coma indicate brain swelling and are treated with corticosteroids and mannitol (see Chap. 13). Dietary regulation, including tube feeding if necessary, must be established in order for normoglycemia to be maintained.

Glycogen storage diseases also have been reported in puppies. Persistent recurrent hypoglycemia, hepatomegaly, acidosis, and ketosis suggest a glycogen storage disease. It is necessary to perform a biopsy in order to make a definitive diagnosis. The management of these cases is frequently unsuccessful.

Adult-onset hypoglycemia usually is caused by a functional tumor of the pancreatic beta cells (insulinoma). The excessive insulin produces an increased transfer of blood glucose into the nonneuronal cellular compartments, resulting in hypoglycemia and abnormal CNS metabolism. Although insulinomas are relatively rare, increasing awareness has resulted in more frequent diagnosis in recent years. Most of the tumors in dogs are carcinomas and have metastasized to the liver and other sites by the time a definitive diagnosis is made. Other neoplasms may induce hypoglycemia as well.[18]

Seizures are more frequently related to exercise, fasting (or, conversely, eating), and excitement. Other signs, such as weakness, muscle tremor, disorientation, and behavioral changes, are more common. The signs are episodic until irreversible neuronal damage occurs.

Hypoglycemia may mimic the other causes of seizures. Blood glucose concentrations after a 12-hour fast are usually below normal (<60 mg/100 ml). Longer fasts (24 to 48 hours) may be necessary in some cases, but animals should be monitored closely during this time. Plasma insulin levels are more specific for making a diagnosis. Values above 54 μg/ml in a fasting dog are considered abnormal (immunoreactive insulin test, or IRI). Serum IRI concentrations are near zero when plasma glucose concentrations are less than or equal to 30 mg/dl. The amended insulin-glucose ratio (AIGR) has been found to be the simplest and most sensitive indication of functional beta cell carcinoma, although abnormal AIGR results have been obtained in dogs with hypoglycemia caused by sepsis or tumors other than beta cell tumors. The AIGR is obtained by the application of the following ratio:

$$\frac{\text{Serum insulin } (\mu U/ml \times 100)}{\text{Plasma glucose } (mg/dl) - 30}$$

Normal values are less than 30 μU/mg glucose. The glucagon tolerance test may be used as an alternative procedure but carries a greater risk of profound hypoglycemia during the test.[19]

The management of patients in coma and status epilepticus was discussed in Chapters 13 and 14, respectively. Surgical removal of the tumor is indicated when the patient's condition has stabilized. The reported incidence of malignancy ranges from 56% to 82%; therefore, the prognosis is poor even with successful removal of the pancreatic focus. Animals with hyperinsulinism should be fed several small meals each day. Diets high in simple sugars should be avoided. Glucocorticoids, such as prednisolone, given at a dosage of 0.25–0.50 mg/kg/day, will help normalize the blood glucose concentration because of their anti-insulin effects. Diazoxide is the drug of choice for the medical management of hyperinsulinism (beta cell carcinoma) because it increases blood glucose concentrations through several mechanisms. The initial dose is 10 mg/kg divided twice a day orally. The dose may be gradually increased, but should not exceed 60 mg/kg/day.[14,19]

Neoplasms

Neoplasia affecting the nervous system is classified in three groups (Table 16–6). *Primary tumors* arise from cells that normally are found in the cranial vault, in the vertebral canal, or in the peripheral nerves. *Secondary tumors* metastasize from a primary tumor to the nervous system. *Tumors of surrounding structures* such as the skull or the vertebrae may be considered a form of secondary tumors. The peripheral nerves also may be invaded or compressed by tumors of other structures.

TABLE 16–6 Classification of Neoplasia of the Nervous System

Tumor Type	*Predilection Site*	*Species (Breed)*	*Incidence*
Primary Tumors			
Tumors of nerve cells			
Ganglioneuroma	Variable (cerebellum, cranial nerve roots, eye, cervical region)	Dogs, pigs, horses, cattle	Rare
Tumors of neuroepithelium			
Ependymoma	Ependymal surfaces	Dogs, cats, horses, cattle	Uncommon
Blastoma (neuroepithelioma)	Meninges to thoracolumbar spinal cord	Dogs	Uncommon
Plexus papilloma	Fourth ventricle	Dogs, horses, cattle	Common (dogs)
Tumors of glia			
Astrocytoma	Piriform area, convexity of cerebral hemispheres, thalamus, hypothalamus	Dogs (brachycephalic), cats, cattle	Common (dogs)
Oligodendroglioma	Cerebral hemispheres	Dogs (brachycephalic)	Common (dogs)
Glioblastoma	As for astrocytoma	Dogs (brachycephalic), cattle, pigs	Uncommon
Medulloblastoma	Cerebellum	Dogs, cats, pigs, calves	Common (dogs)
Gliomas, unclassified	Periventricular areas, especially subependymal plate	Dogs (brachycephalic), cattle, horses, sheep, pigs	Common (dogs)
Tumors of peripheral nerves and nerve sheaths			
Neurinoma (schwannoma)	Peripheral nerves	Dogs, cattle	Uncommon
Neurofibroma	Peripheral nerves	Dogs, cattle, horses, pigs, sheep	Common (dogs, cattle)
Neurofibrosarcoma	Peripheral nerves	Dogs, cats, horses	Common (dogs, cattle)
Tumors of the meninges, vessels, and other mesodermal structures			
Meningiomas	Falx cerebri	Dogs (dolichocephalic), cats, horses, cattle, sheep	Common (dogs, cats)
Angioblastoma	Variable (cerebral hemispheres, choroid plexus, medulla, spinal cord)	Dogs, horses, pigs	Rare

TABLE 16–6 Classification of Neoplasia of the Nervous System *Continued*

Tumor Type	*Predilection Site*	*Species (Breed)*	*Incidence*
Sarcoma	Variable (meninges, brain, spinal cord)	Dogs, cats, horses, cattle, sheep	Common (dogs, cats)
Focal granulomatous meningo-encephalo-myelitis (reticulosis)	Cerebral hemispheres, brain stem	Dogs, cats, horses, cattle	Common (dogs)
Tumors of the pineal and pituitary glands and of the cranio-pharyngeal duct			
Pinealoma	Pineal body	Dogs, horses, cattle	Rare
Pituitary adenoma	Pituitary gland	Dogs (brachycephalic), cats, horses, cattle, sheep	Common (dogs, horses)
Craniopharyngioma (germ cell tumors)	Hypophyseal-infundibular areas	Dogs	Rare
Tumors of heterotopic tissues (mal-formation tumors)			
Epidermoid, dermoid, teratoma	Variable (fourth ventricle and cere-bellopontine angle for epi-dermoid)	Dogs, horses, cattle, sheep	Rare
Secondary Tumors			
Metastatic tumors			
Mammary gland adenocarcinoma, pulmonary carcinoma, chemo-dectoma, prostatic carcinoma, hemangiosarcoma, fibrosar-coma, malignant melanoma, salivary gland adenocarcinoma	Variable	Dogs, cats, cattle, horses, sheep	Common
Lymphosarcoma	Spinal cord	Cats, cattle, dogs	Common (cattle, cats)
Primary Tumors from Surrounding Tissues			
Osteoma, osteosarcoma, chon-droma, chondrosarcoma, he-mangioma, hemangiosarcoma, fibrosarcoma, calcifying apo-neurotic fibromatosis, epider-moid cyst, lipoma	Variable (brain, spinal cord)	Dogs, cats, horses, cattle, pigs	Common (dogs, cats)

Modified with permission from Oliver JE, Hoerlein BF, Mayhew IG: Veterinary Neurology. Philadelphia, WB Saunders, 1987, p 279.

Pathogenesis

Tumors affect the function of the nervous system by (1) destruction of nervous tissue, (2) compression of surrounding structures, (3) interference with circulation and the development of cerebral edema, and (4) disturbance of cerebrospinal fluid (CSF) circulation. Secondary effects may include herniation of the cerebrum under the tentorium cerebelli or herniation of the cerebellum into the foramen magnum (see Chap. 13).

Primary tumors usually grow slowly, producing a clinical syndrome of chronic progression. If the mass obstructs or erodes a vessel, the resulting infarction or hemorrhage may produce an acute onset of a severe neurologic deficit (see Fig. 13–7). Secondary tumors, especially those that are highly malignant, also may have a more acute progression. Edema of surrounding tissues is frequent with neoplasia of the CNS. Brain tumors frequently produce signs of increased intracranial pressure. The progression may be more rapid if there is obstruction of CSF flow with secondary hydrocephalus.

Incidence

The frequency of occurrence of tumors affecting the nervous system of animals is not known. Brain tumors are estimated to occur at a rate of 14.5 per 100,000 dogs.[20] A complete evaluation of the nervous system usually is not performed except at referral institutions, which precludes an accurate estimate of the incidence of CNS neoplasia in the general population of any species. Primary tumors of the CNS are infrequently reported in food animals and horses. The relative frequencies of the types of tumors and the relative risks of some breeds of dogs have been established (Table 16–7).

Brain tumors, primarily gliomas, are found more frequently in boxers, Boston terriers, and

TABLE 16–7 Frequency of Neuroectodermal Brain Tumor Types in Dogs[20]

Cell Type	Number
Astrocytoma	92
Oligodendroglioma	99
Glioblastoma	40
Choroid plexus papilloma	42
Medulloblastoma	20
Ependymoma	19
Gliomatosis	4
Pinealoma	1
Unclassified glioma	24

TABLE 16–8 Common Sites and Signs of Brain Tumors

Site	Signs
Cerebrum	
Frontal lobe	Seizures, abnormal behavior, contralateral postural reactions
Occipital lobe	Seizures, contralateral visual field deficit
Temporal lobe	Seizures, abnormal behavior
Pituitary–hypothalamus	Behavioral, autonomic and endocrine signs: polyuria, polydipsia, changes in eating, sleeping, and behavior patterns, and so forth; later visual deficits
Brain stem	Gait and postural reaction deficits, cranial nerve signs
Cerebellopontine angle	CN V, CN VII, and CN VIII signs, hemiparesis

English bulldogs than in other breeds. The incidence of meningiomas is slightly higher in German shepherds, collies, poodles, and cats, and meningiomas are now thought to be the most common brain tumor of small animals.[21–23] Plexus papillomas are found most frequently in nonbrachycephalic breeds.[22] Neoplastic reticulosis is seen in all breeds. Spinal cord tumors have not been reported as often as brain tumors, but secondary tumors, either from vertebral involvement or metastases, are seen most frequently.[24] Horses and cattle are at slightly greater risk for peripheral nerve tumors.[24]

In general, the risk of neoplasia increases with age.[25] In one study, the risk for glial tumors in dogs peaked at 10 to 14 years of age, the risk for meningeal tumors peaked at seven to nine years, and the risk for peripheral nerve tumors peaked at two to three and seven to nine years. Younger dogs may have epidermoid-dermoid cysts, medulloblastomas, and teratomas. A unique tumor, currently called thoracolumbar spinal cord blastoma, occurs in large breed dogs of young age. It invariably occurs intradurally between T10 and L3.[26,27]

Clinical Signs

The signs of CNS tumors depend on the location of the mass (Table 16–8). In contrast to the other diseases discussed in this chapter, signs of focal abnormality are expected with CNS neoplasia. Metastatic disease and the diffuse neoplastic disorders (reticulosis, lymphosarcoma) are the exceptions. Although there is some evidence that the different types of tumors have sites of predilection, the number of reported cases is too low for predictions to be made with confidence.

Cerebral tumors can become relatively large (greater than 1 cm in diameter) before clinical signs are recognized. However, many animals with brain tumors may have vague signs, such as behavioral changes, for up to a year before showing overt neurologic signs.[23] Seizures may be the first sign of a cerebral tumor. An examination performed at the time of the first seizure may not reveal any neurologic deficits. Medical control of the seizures may be effective at first, but as the tumor expands, seizures usually become more frequent despite the use of anticonvulsant medication. Progression to include other clinical signs usually is recognized over a period of a few months.

In addition to signs related to the location of the lesion (see Table 16–8), signs related to the generalized increase in intracranial pressure frequently are present. Depression and dullness are common, and the animal often appears to have a headache. Papilledema may be seen in some animals.[28]

Many gliomas arise in the deeper structures of the cerebrum, possibly from the cells of the subependymal plate.[29] Involvement of the basal nuclei and the diencephalon is common (Fig. 16–1).

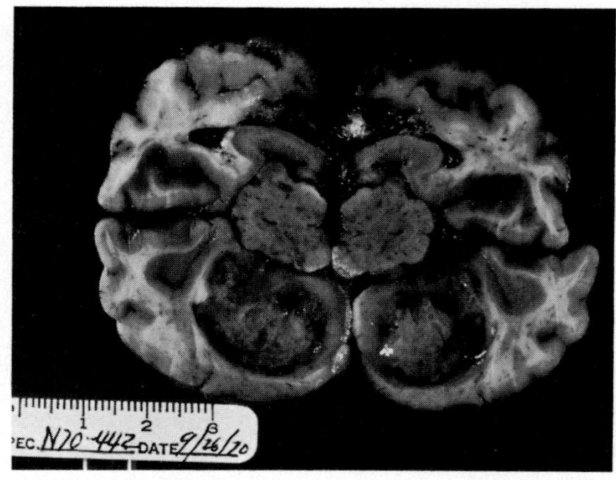

Figure 16–1 Grade IV astrocytoma in a boxer dog. Note compression of the brain stem.

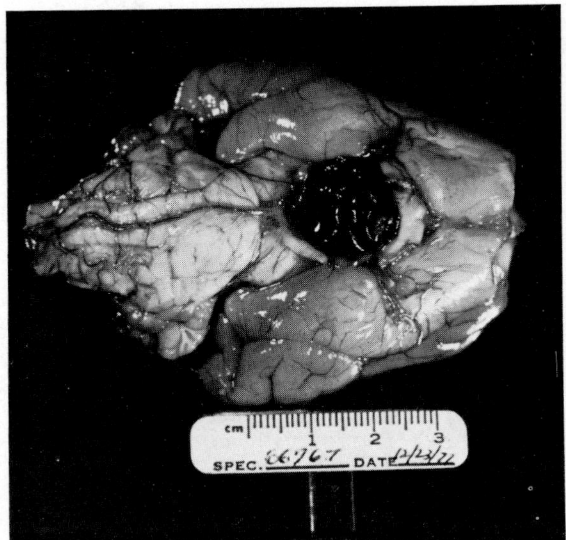

Figure 16–2 A pituitary tumor in a Labrador retriever with visual and postural reaction deficits and Horner's syndrome.

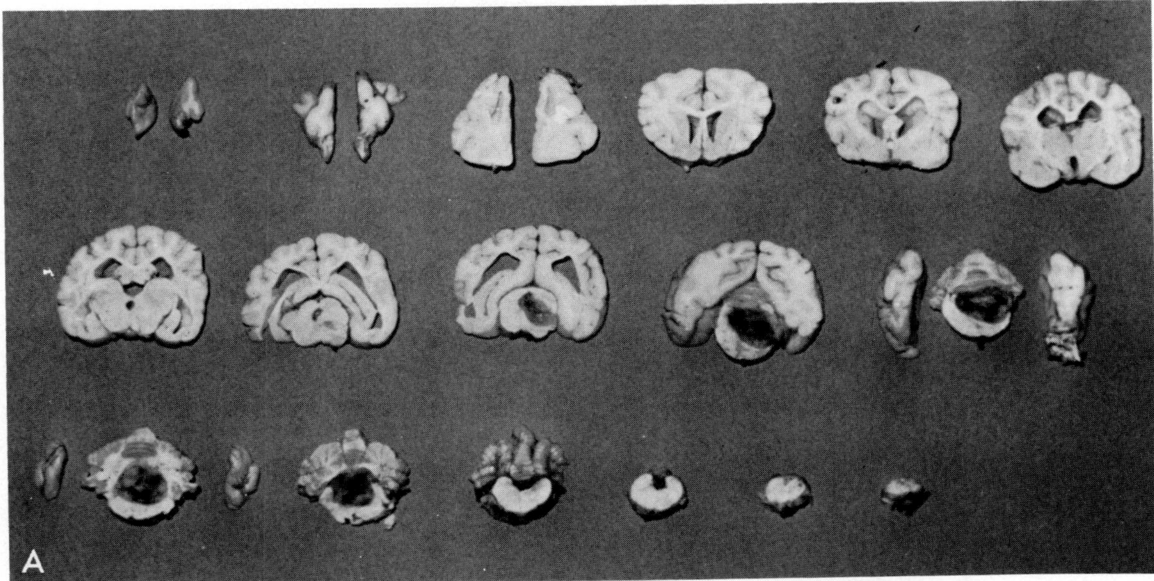

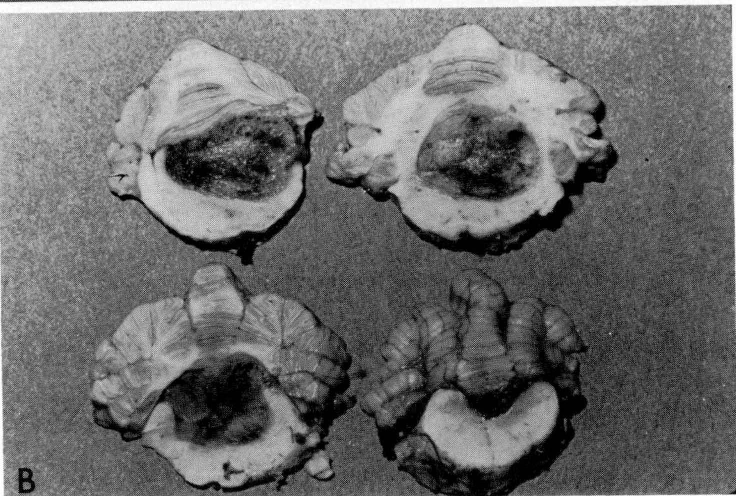

Figure 16–3 *A* and *B*. Oligodendroglioma in the brain stem, extending from the midbrain to the rostral medulla. The dog had a left facial paralysis, a right hemiparesis, and a forced gaze deviation to the right. This case is an exception to the usual rule of ipsilateral paresis with brain stem lesions, possibly related to the central location of the mass.

Pituitary tumors in animals tend to expand dorsally into the hypothalamus, producing seizures and changes in metabolic and endocrine function in the early stages. These tumors can become quite large before cranial nerve signs or motor signs are observed (Fig. 16–2). Blindness from compression of the optic nerves is not frequent but may occur.[30]

Brain stem tumors are characterized by gait deficits and cranial nerve signs (Fig. 16–3). Behavioral changes and seizures are usually absent in tumors of the brain stem and the cerebellum until the mass affects the reticular activating system or alters intracranial pressure by obstructing CSF circulation.

Spinal cord tumors usually produce signs of a segmental myelopathy. Extramedullary tumors often cause unilateral signs until late in their growth. The unilateral signs are in direct contrast to the usual bilateral signs seen with most other spinal cord compressive lesions (e.g., disk, vertebral luxation). Intramedullary lesions are more likely to produce bilateral signs. Intramedullary tumors rarely cause pain, whereas extramedullary tumors, especially extradural masses, usually do (Table 16–9).[25]

Peripheral nerve tumors other than neurofibromas of the nerve roots have been reported infrequently. Neoplasia must be considered in any mononeuropathy without evidence of trauma (see Chap. 6). Secondary tumors, especially lymphosarcomas, may invade or compress peripheral nerves.

Diagnosis

Brain Tumors. Until localizing signs develop, the diagnosis of a brain tumor may be extremely difficult to make. The primary groups of diseases that must be ruled out are outlined in Table 16–10. The more common degenerative diseases can be excluded on the basis of age at onset; however, tumors occasionally are seen in young animals. The other diseases, except for inflammation and vascular lesions, may be excluded when focal signs develop. Most inflammatory diseases, with the exception of brain abscesses and granulomatous meningoencephalomyelitis, are multifocal or diffuse in distribution; however, they may produce focal signs early in the course of the disease. Hemorrhages and infarcts are usually acute in onset and nonprogressive.

The most useful diagnostic test available today is computed tomography (CT) or magnetic resonance (MR) imaging (Figs. 16–4 and 16–5).[31] Both techniques are expensive and are not always available in general practice. However, many veterinarians can have them done at local hospitals or imaging centers, and many veterinary referral institutions have the service. In most suspected cases of brain tumor, CT should be performed as the first test after metabolic problems have been ruled out. All other tests are poor in comparison, and some have considerable risk for the patient.

CSF analysis may be helpful in the diagnosis

TABLE 16–9 Characteristics of Spinal Cord Tumors

	Tumor Location		
Characteristics	Extradural	Intradural-Extramedullary	Intramedullary
Frequency	50%	35%	15%
Tumor types	Bone tumors Metastatic tumors Lymphosarcoma	Neurofibromas Meningiomas Blastomas	Gliomas Ependymomas
Rate of growth	Rapid	Slow	Usually slow
Clinical signs			
Pain	Early severe	Early, variable	Unusual, late
Paresis	Early, rapidly progressive, usually bilateral	Late, slowly progressive, may be unilateral	Late, rapidly progressive, usually bilateral
Sensation	Usually intact until late	Usually intact until late	Usually intact until late
Course	Acute onset, rapid progression	Very slow progression	Insidious onset, rapid progression
Diagnosis			
CSF	Increased protein, normal cells	Increased protein, normal cells	Increased protein, normal cells, may be xanthochromia
Radiography	Skeletal lesions	Possibly large intervertebral foramen (neurofibroma)	Possible widened vertebral canal
Myelography	Extradural compression	Variable, may be cupping of dye column	Widened spinal cord, attenuated dye column

Modified with permission from Prata RG: Diagnosis of spinal cord tumors in the dog. Vet Clin North Am 7:165–185, 1977.

TABLE 16–10 Differential Diagnosis of Brain Tumors*

Characteristic	*Brain Tumor*	*Degenerative Disease*	*Metabolic Disease*	*Inflammatory Disease*	*Toxic Disease*	*Vascular Disease*
Age	Adult to old	Young	Any	Any	Any	Any
Progression	Slow	Slow	Variable, often waxing and waning	Usually fast	Slow (heavy metal)	Acute onset, not progressive
Focal signs	Yes	No	No	May be, especially abscess	No	Yes
CSF	Increased protein, variable cells	Increased protein (variable), normal cells	Normal	Increased protein, increased cells	Increased protein, normal cells (heavy metal)	Increased protein, normal cells, may be xanthochromic
EEG	May be focal (cortical) or diffuse HVSW	Diffuse abnormality	Diffuse abnormality	Diffuse abnormality	Diffuse abnormality	May be focal abnormality
CT, MR	Positive	Negative	Negative	Negative, except abscess	Negative	Positive, infarct or hemorrhage

* Abbreviations: HVSW = high-voltage slow waves, CT = computed tomography, MR = magnetic resonance imaging.

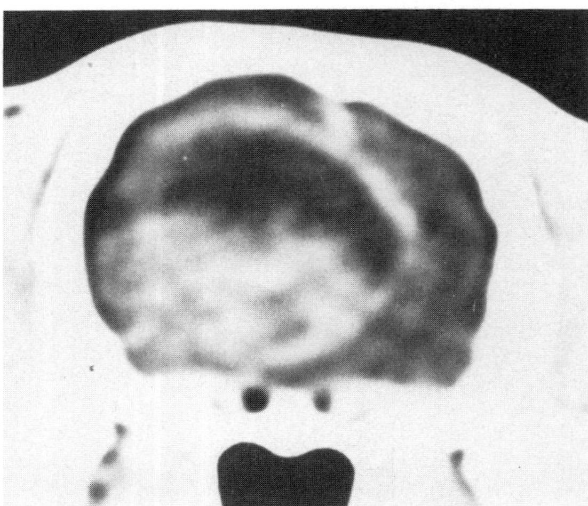

Figure 16–4 CT brain scan of a domestic cat, 10 months old, with a history of seizures for 5 months. The cat became acutely worse 5 days before the scan, with severe depression, proprioceptive deficits of the right limbs, and decreased menace reactions on the right. There is a massive lesion (3 cm in diameter) occupying most of the forebrain on the left side. The ventral portion and dorsal rim enhances with contrast material. The falx cerebri is displaced to the right. The histologic diagnosis was malignant ependymoma.

of neoplasia, but it provides limited information at best, and poses a significant risk for the patient at worst. Tumors generally cause an increase in pressure and protein content with no increase in cells. However, recent studies have shown that there is often an increase in cells in dogs with brain tumors.[32] In a series of 77 dogs, almost 10% were normal, and almost half of the dogs with tumors had increased white blood cell (WBC) counts in the CSF, some predominantly neutrophils. The risks of a CSF tap must be carefully weighed against the benefits. If there is increased intracranial pressure, the chances of causing a herniation of the brain are very high (see Chap. 4). We have seen cerebellar herniations following CSF taps in animals with no clinical evidence of increased pressure. We also have seen cases in which the patients were strongly suspected of having a tumor but proved to have bacterial infections (abscess and meningitis) and subsequently were cured with medical therapy. Ultimately, the decision must be made with the owner fully informed of the risks. If CT is negative, then the CSF analysis should be done.

EEG may aid in the diagnosis of cortical tumors by showing focal abnormality. Increased intracranial pressure may cause generalized high-voltage slow waves. Lateralization may be demonstrated in a small portion of the cases. Again, if CT is negative, an EEG is indicated.

Radiographic procedures other than CT or MR imaging are rarely used now. These include arteriography and radioisotope brain scans for cerebral lesions, and sinus venography and positive contrast thecography for lesions on the floor of the skull. If neoplasia is suspected early, thoracic and abdominal radiographs may help identify primary malignancy that may have metastasized to the brain.

Spinal Cord Tumors. The localization of spinal

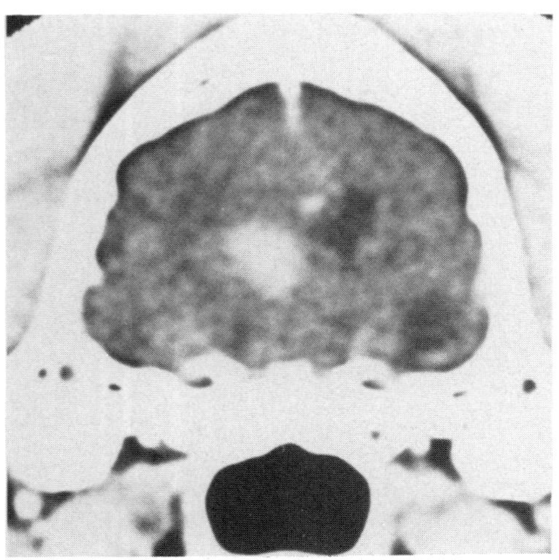

A

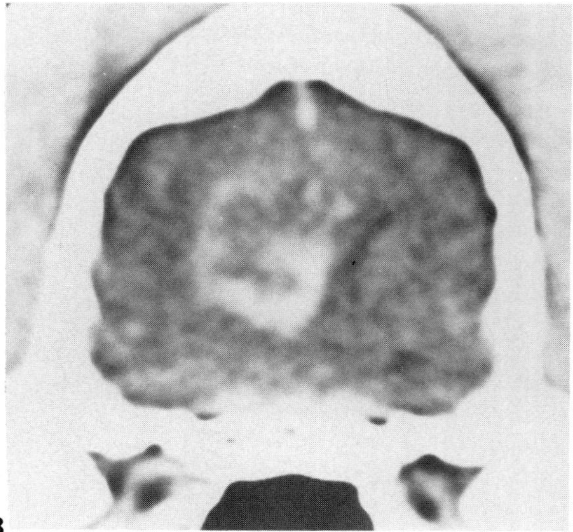

B

Figure 16–5 CT brain scans of a Labrador retriever, female, 9 years old, with a history of seizures for 1 week. Following the first seizure, the dog circled to the left and had postural reaction deficits on the right side. The right lateral ventricle is enlarged (*A*), the falx cerebri is displaced to the right side, and the mass in the left cerebrum has a ring of contrast enhancement (*B*). The mass was identified as a primary histiocytic lymphoma.

cord tumors can be accurate if LMN signs or pain are present. The differential diagnosis of spinal cord tumors is outlined in Table 16–11. Degenerative myelopathy, which occurs primarily in German shepherd dogs, is the only condition that is never painful. Myelitis initially may appear to be a focal disease, but progression to other parts of the spinal cord is the rule. These diseases cannot be differentiated on the basis of clinical evaluation alone.

Radiography is the most useful diagnostic procedure for confirmation of a diagnosis.[33] Vertebral changes may be seen in primary bone tumors, metastatic tumors, and some primary tumors of nervous tissue (see Fig. 7–10). Tumors of the spinal nerve may cause an enlarged intervertebral foramen (see Fig. 7–12). Slowly expanding tumors in the spinal canal may erode the lamina and the body of the vertebra, giving the appearance of a slightly enlarged vertebral canal (see Fig. 7–13). Myelography is necessary to confirm these findings, to demonstrate lesions that do not cause vertebral change, and to define the extent of the mass (Fig. 16–6; see also Fig. 4–2).[34]

CSF analysis is of limited benefit. Inflammation can be ruled out if there is no increase in cells. The other diseases usually cause an increase in protein levels with normal cell counts.

Peripheral Nerve Tumors. Peripheral nerve tumors that do not affect the spinal cord are difficult to diagnose. Any mononeuropathy without evidence of trauma is likely to be caused by a tumor. Peripheral nerve tumors are usually painful, especially if they can be palpated.[35–37]

Electrophysiologic testing is useful for establishing which nerve (or nerves) is involved.[38] A final diagnosis must be made by surgical removal and histopathologic examination.

Management

Brain Tumors. The objectives of therapy for a brain tumor are eradication of the tumor and control of secondary tumor effects such as edema.[23] Corticosteroids are often effective in

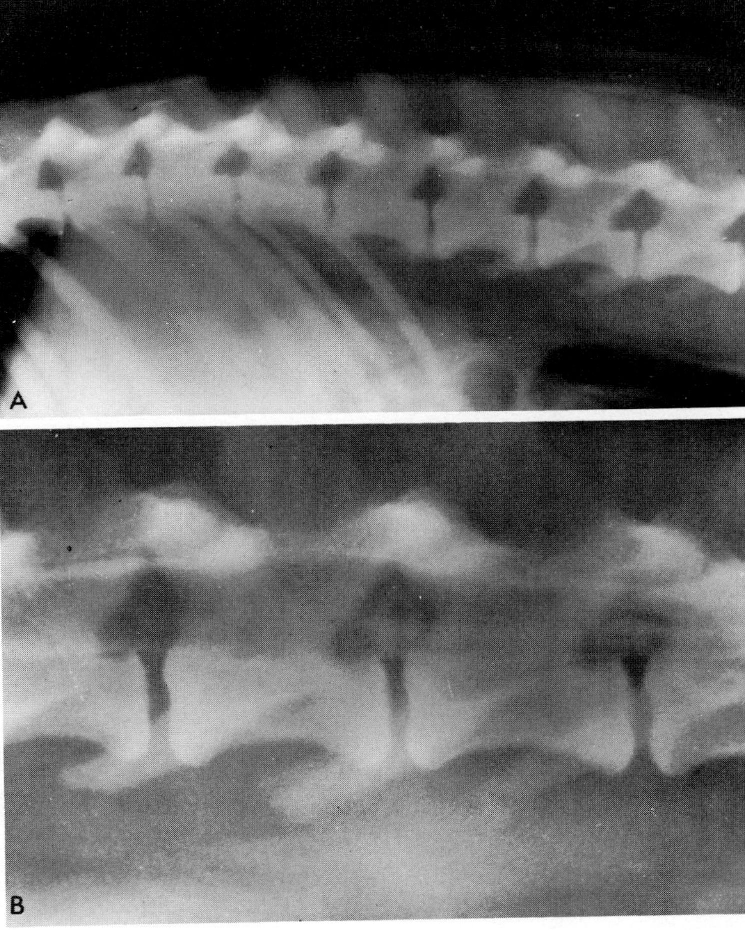

Figure 16–6. *A* Enlarged vertebral canal at L4. The canal is normally larger in this area because of the lumbosacral intumescence. *B*. Myelogram demonstrating an intramedullary mass. Note thinning of the dye column. There was an astrocytoma in the spinal cord.

TABLE 16–11 Differential Diagnosis of Spinal Cord Tumors

			Inflammation		
Characteristic	***Spinal Cord Tumor***	***Degenerative Myelopathy***	Meningitis and Myelitis	Diskospondylitis	***Type II Disk***
Age	Adult to old	>5 yr	Any	Any	>6 yr
Progression	Usually slow	Slow	Variable	Variable	Slow
Focal signs	Yes, unless metastatic; may be painful	T3–L3, not painful	Sometimes early, later progresses to other areas; frequently painful	Yes, may be multifocal; usually painful	Yes, may be painful
Radiography					
Survey	Sometimes vertebral changes	Normal, frequently have spondylosis because of age and breeds	Normal	Characteristic, osteomyelitis	May be normal, frequently have spondylosis because of age and breed
Myelography	Defines extent: extradural, intradural, intramedullary	Normal	Normal	May demonstrate extradural compression	Extradural compression at disk space
CSF	Increased protein, normal cells	Increased protein (variable), normal cells	Increased protein, increased cells	Variable, may be normal	Increased protein (variable), normal cells

reducing peritumoral edema. The growth of some types of tumors may also be reduced with corticosteroids. Improvement may be significant and may last for weeks to months. Acute episodes may be treated with IV methylprednisolone (30 mg/kg) or dexamethasone (2 mg/kg), while long-term treatment is usually with oral prednisolone (0.5 mg/kg every 48 hours). The oral dose is increased gradually until there is improvement, then adjusted to the smallest effective dosage.[39,40] Anticonvulsant therapy may also be needed. Eventually the growth of the tumor will cause severe clinical signs, often acutely after a period of relative normalcy.[25]

Four methods of treatment are available for eradication or reduction of the tumor mass: surgery, chemotherapy, radiation therapy, and immunotherapy. Only surgery and radiation therapy have been used in many animals, although the use of chemotherapy is increasing.

Surgery is usually the first consideration. The criteria for possible success include (1) a solitary noninvasive tumor, (2) a tumor that is on or near the surface of the cerebral hemisphere, (3) a neurologic status that is compatible with life, (4) accurate localization, (5) careful and complete surgical resection, and (6) intensive postoperative care. Meningiomas are most likely to meet the first two requirements. Newer techniques such as laser surgery, microsurgery, and intraoperative US are likely to enhance the chance of success.[25]

Radiation therapy has been used with moderate success and is being used more following surgical resection. It is effective in treating most kinds of tumors, both primary and secondary, including metastases, pituitary tumors, and skull tumors. Lymphoma and granulomatous meningoencephalomyelitis may also be sensitive to radiation.[23,41]

Few data are available regarding the medical treatment of brain tumors in animals. Corticosteroids may provide some improvement in clinical signs for a limited time, primarily by reducing cerebral edema, but may reduce tumor bulk and slow the growth as well. Specific chemotherapeutic agents that achieve adequate penetration of the brain include carmustine (BCNU), lomustine, and semustine. Cook has reported some success in a variety of tumor types for up to a year.[39] Other therapeutic agents are being tried, but no significant numbers have been reported as yet.

Immunotherapy, consisting of stimulating and culturing the patient's lymphocytes and returning them to the tumor bed during surgery, is a new therapeutic approach.[42] Limited trials suggest that this may be an effective treatment modality.

Although some improvement in outcome of treatment is being reported as protocols are refined, published studies are not encouraging. One review of 86 brain tumors is illustrative.[43] Median survival time was 1 month (range, 1 day to 42.4 months). The median survival time of those with no treatment ($N = 7$) was 0.2 months. In animals that underwent surgery alone it was 0.9 months, and in animals treated with cobalt 60 radiation therapy (some with hyperthermia or surgery in addition) it was 4.9 months. Animals with a solitary tumor had a better prognosis than those with multiple tumors. As protocols improve with experience, these results should also improve. However, owners should be aware of the limitations of therapy.

Spinal Cord Tumors. Surgical removal of spinal cord tumors is the treatment of choice. Extradural tumors would seem to be the most favorable for surgical removal. Unfortunately, extradural tumors are usually metastatic, with metastases also present elsewhere, or they are primary bone tumors. Resection of a vertebral tumor is likely to produce an unstable spine. Intradural-extramedullary tumors, which are usually meningiomas or nerve sheath tumors, are more likely to be resectable. An early diagnosis is critical. Intramedullary tumors, usually gliomas, ependymomas, or metastases, are frequently invasive and are not amenable to resection without destruction of the spinal cord. Microsurgical techniques should improve the prognosis for spinal cord tumors significantly.

Peripheral Nerve Tumors. Complete resection of primary peripheral nerve tumors can be readily accomplished with good results. The primary limiting factor is the functional significance of the affected nerve (see Chap. 6). Resection with anastomosis of the nerve is possible if the tumor is not too large.[25,35] Amputation of the limb with resection of the tumor is the alternative.

Nutritional Disorders

Nervous system disorders caused by nutritional deficiencies or excesses are uncommon in companion animals, but more common in food animals. Severe malnutrition can cause a variety of abnormalities that are related to multiple deficiencies. Vitamin deficiencies and excesses are the most common nutritional abnormalities seen in practice.

Hypovitaminosis

Vitamin A. Deficiencies in vitamin A may produce night blindness. Hypovitaminosis A in young animals may cause excessive thickening of the skull and the vertebrae with secondary compression of nervous tissue (especially of the cranial nerves as they pass through the foramina). Poor absorption of CSF may result in communicating hydrocephalus.[44] Hypovitaminosis A is rare or rarely recognized in companion animals but has been reported in food animals.[45–47] Blindness in cattle with vitamin A deficiency is caused by several pathologic mechanisms.[48] Papilledema occurs in adult animals secondary to increased CSF pressure, which is secondary to poor absorption. Photoreceptor abnormalities are also seen, especially affecting the rods, which leads to night blindness. In growing calves similar changes occur, but, in addition, the optic nerve is compressed by narrowing of the optic canals, resulting in ischemia and direct interference with the nerve.

***Vitamin* E.** A noninflammatory myopathy may be produced by vitamin E deficiency. Although myopathies are seen fairly often, vitamin E deficiencies are rare in companion animals. Calves and sheep have a myopathy associated with a deficiency in vitamin E and selenium. Swine may die suddenly because of the degeneration of cardiac muscle. An association of vitamin E deficiency with degenerative myelopathy in horses has been proposed (see Chap. 8).[49,50]

***Vitamin* B *Complex*.** Deficiencies in all of the B vitamins can cause pathologic changes in both the central and the peripheral nervous systems. Thiamine deficiency has been reported in dogs and cats, and ruminants.[45,51–54] The syndrome in dogs progresses from anorexia to pelvic limb paresis, tetraparesis, seizures, and coma in approximately 1 week.[54] Malacia and hemorrhage were found in multiple sites in the brain and the spinal cord, with the most severe lesions in the brain stem. Animals that were treated with thiamine recovered. A peripheral neuropathy with LMN paralysis also has been seen.[51] Cats with a thiamine deficiency often have a characteristic ventral flexion of the head and the neck, sometimes causing the chin to touch the sternum. Ataxia and seizures also may be present. The lesions are similar to those that occur in dogs.[45] The deficiency that was observed in dogs was produced by a diet consisting entirely of cooked meat or a specific thiamine-deficient diet.[54] Cat foods with fish as the primary ingredient contain thiaminase, which has been reported to cause the thiamine deficiency in cats.[45]

Treatment should be instituted immediately for any animal that is suspected of having thiamine deficiency. A dosage of 50 to 100 mg should be given IV and should be repeated IM daily until a response is obtained or another diagnosis is established.

Polioencephalomalacia (symmetric necrosis of the cerebral cortex) is caused by a thiamine deficiency in ruminants. The deficiency is the result of an increased breakdown of thiamine in the rumen by thiaminase-secreting bacteria. Usually the animals have been moved from a marginal pasture to a lush pasture, are in a feed lot, or have had some similar change in feeding patterns. Animals less than 2 years of age are most commonly affected.[53]

Clinical signs are primarily cerebral in origin and include depression, pacing, head pressing, blindness, ataxia, odontoprisis, opisthotonos, and seizures. A dorsomedial strabismus that has been attributed to trochlear nerve (CN IV) paralysis has been described. Increased intracranial pressure is common and may lead to tentorial herniation.

A symmetric laminar cortical necrosis is the most prominent pathologic finding. Edema of the brain with flattening of the gyri and herniations, and cerebral or cerebellar herniations may be present. Autofluorescence of the cut surface of the cerebral cortex under ultraviolet light is usually present.

Measurement of transketolase, the thiamine-dependent coenzyme, is helpful for making a diagnosis. The condition should be treated with thiamine, 250 to 1,000 mg IV or IM for 3 to 5 days. Steroids should be given if CNS signs are severe. Severely affected animals may have permanent cortical damage.[55]

Niacin and riboflavin deficiencies are less common, but since animals with thiamine deficiency also may have deficiencies in these vitamins, multiple B-complex preparations are indicated. The diet should be corrected in order to prevent recurrences.

Hypervitaminosis

***Vitamin* A.** Increased levels of vitamin A have been reported in cats with diets predominantly of liver. A hypertrophic bone formation on the vertebrae causes an ankylosing spondylosis, primarily of the cervical vertebrae but in some cases extending to the lumbar region. The clinical signs primarily relate to the rigidity of the vertebral column. Nerve compression occurs in severely affected cats. Alterations in the diet stop the progression of the spondylosis but do not significantly reduce the spondylosis that is present. Anti-inflammatory and analgesic drugs have been recommended, but they must be used with caution, especially in the cat.[45]

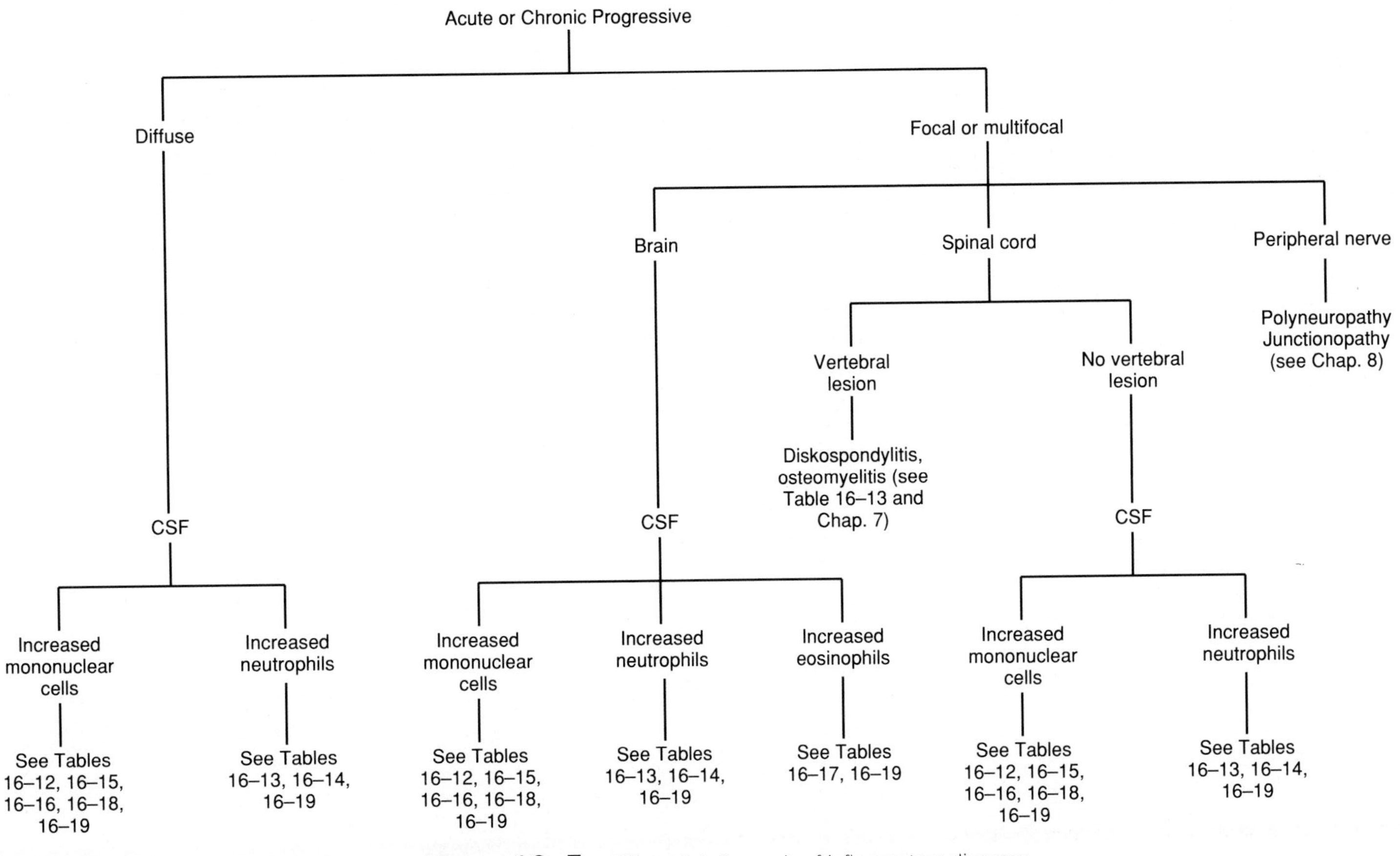

Figure 16–7 Differential diagnosis of inflammatory diseases.

Inflammatory Diseases

The inflammatory diseases of the nervous system are caused by infectious or parasitic organisms or immune reactions. Canine distemper, feline infectious peritonitis, equine protozoal myeloencephalitis, and bacterial infections, including thromboembolic meningoencephalitis and listeriosis, are common causes of disease. Some of the fungal diseases are common in endemic areas. Most of the other diseases are relatively uncommon, although granulomatous meningoencephalomyelitis in dogs is being recognized with increasing frequency. Inflammatory diseases are discussed in many textbooks.[56–61] The differential diagnosis is outlined in Figure 16–7 and will be discussed in the next section. The more common inflammatory diseases are outlined in Tables 16–12 to 16–19.

Diagnosis

Most of the inflammatory diseases are characterized by an acute onset. All of the inflammatory diseases are progressive. A diffuse or multifocal distribution is characteristic of most of the diseases in this group. The minimum data base (see Chap. 1) may provide evidence of systemic infection (such as alterations in WBC), although many primary CNS diseases do not produce a systemic response. Therefore, positive findings in laboratory data are useful, but negative findings do not rule out infectious disease. Focal deficits should be investigated according to the location of the lesion (see Chaps. 6–15).

CSF analysis is the single most useful test for establishing the diagnosis of inflammatory disease (see Chap. 4). Increases in CSF protein concentrations vary from low (50–100 mg/dl) in chronic viral diseases to very high (300+ mg/dl) in bacterial and fungal infections. Characteristic cell changes are: increased mononuclear cells (in viral diseases), increased neutrophils (in bacterial diseases), increased numbers of both mononuclear cells and neutrophils (in mycotic and protozoal diseases and feline infectious peritonitis), and increased numbers of mononuclear cells, neutrophils, and some eosinophils (in parasitic and immune-mediated diseases). However, with the increased use of newer cytologic methods, it is clear that these guidelines are only general tendencies. For example, chronic bacterial infections may have a mononuclear cell response, especially increases in macrophages, while some viral diseases are accompanied by significant numbers of neutrophils in the CSF. The presence of neutrophils in the CSF is not necessarily abnormal. The only cell that seems to be consistently abnormal is the macrophage. Clinical suspicion of an infection is an adequate indication for bacterial and fungal cultures and bacterial sensitivity tests. Anti-canine distemper virus antibody, if elevated in the CSF, is evidence of active infection of the nervous system. It is not elevated in vaccinated dogs or those with systemic distemper without CNS disease.[57]

Toxic Disorders

Toxicities are common in both small and large animals. Many toxic materials produce signs of CNS disorder (many of which are biochemical changes and potentially reversible), whereas others produce structural damage. The more common toxicants are listed in Table 16–20. Toxicologic disorders, including those caused by poisonous plants, are discussed in detail in several books.[45,62,63]

Diagnosis

A history of exposure to a toxic agent is the most important factor in establishing the diagnosis in cases of poisoning. CNS signs of intoxication include (1) seizures; (2) depression or coma; (3) tremors, ataxia, and paresis; and (4) LMN signs. Animals that present with any of these four signs must be considered as possible poisoning victims until proved otherwise. The primary groups of diseases that are likely to be confused with toxicosis are metabolic disorders and inflammatory diseases.

When an animal presents with signs suggestive of poisoning, the owner must be questioned carefully in an attempt to find a possible source. Animals that present in status epilepticus must be treated immediately, and the history must be obtained later (see Chap. 14). Direct questions regarding agents that are capable of producing the signs must be asked. Owners usually are aware of common agents, such as insecticides and rodenticides, but may have difficulty identifying a source of lead poisoning and may be reluctant to admit a source of drug intoxication.

The clinical signs may be sufficient for the clinician to establish a presumptive diagnosis (for example, intoxication from strychnine and organophosphates). Other agents, such as lead and drugs, may require laboratory confirmation (Tables 16–21 through 16–24).

Toxicants Causing Seizures. The most common sign of poisoning in small animals is seizures (see Table 16–21). The animal may present with

Text continued on page 359

TABLE 16–12
A. Viral Diseases of the CNS of Dogs and Cats

Disease	Cause	Incidence	Clinical Signs and Pathology	Course and Prognosis	Diagnostic Tests	Treatment	Prevention
Canine distemper	Morbillivirus	Common; dogs	Young dogs: systemic illness; respiratory, gastrointestinal, and CNS signs; cerebellum, cerebellar peduncles, optic nerves and tracts, and spinal cord commonly affected; CNS signs may occur early or weeks to months after systemic illness	Acute to subacute, progressive; poor prognosis if CNS signs	History, EEG, CSF (increased lymphocytes, increased protein, especially IgG), CSF antibody, tissue fluorescent antibody (FA), ophthalmoscopy	Supportive: antibacterial agents, anticonvulsants	Vaccine
		Common; dogs	Mature dogs: similar to above or may have CNS disease without systemic illness; may start with focal signs (spinal cord, cerebellum) and progress to involve other areas	Subacute to chronic, progressive; poor prognosis if CNS signs	See above	See above	Vaccine
"Old dog" encephalitis	Morbillivirus	Uncommon but not rare; dogs	Mature to older dogs: chronic distemper encephalitis; Cerebral signs at onset	Chronic; poor prognosis	History, EEG, ophthalmoscopy, CSF often normal, CSF antibody	Supportive	Vaccine
Rabies	Rhabdovirus	Variable; all mammals	Initially behavioral changes; rapid progression to either furious or dumb form; atypical variants may be seen, especially in large animals *Furious:* restlessness, wandering, biting anything encountered, convulsions *Dumb:* progressive paralysis, pharyngeal and hypoglossal paralysis, respiratory paralysis	Acute, progresses to death in 3–8 days from onset	Necropsy: FA of brain, mouse inoculation. Dermal tissue FA is possible.	None	Vaccine
Pseudorabies (Aujeszky's disease)	Herpesvirus	Rare except in swine May affect all mammals	May be subclinical in swine Other animals: early excitement, progresses rapidly to coma and death. Intense pruritus and self-mutilation, especially at portal of entry. Contact with swine in history.	Peracute, progression to death in 1–2 days usually	History, signs, necropsy (FA)	None	None available except vaccine for swine
Infectious canine hepatitis	Canine adenovirus type I	Rare CNS; dogs	Affects vascular endothelium, potentially causing signs of CNS disease; primarily liver, kidney and respiratory signs; hepatic encephalopathy terminally	Acute to chronic	Signs, clinical laboratory profile (liver)	Supportive	Vaccine

Table continued on following page

TABLE 16–12
A. Viral Diseases of the CNS of Dogs and Cats *Continued*

Disease	Cause	Incidence	Clinical Signs and Pathology	Course and Prognosis	Diagnostic Tests	Treatment	Prevention
Feline infectious peritonitis	Coronavirus	Relatively common; cats	Two forms: *wet* (diffuse, fibrinous peritonitis) and *dry* (disseminated pyogranulomatous lesions in viscera, CNS, and eye); dry form may have only CNS signs, which may be focal in onset; meningeal involvement is common	Slowly progressive; eventually fatal	Signs, clinical laboratory profile (WBC, neutrophils, plasma protein >8 g/dl), increased globulin, ocular lesions, CSF (increased protein, increased cells, neutrophils or mixed), antibody titer	Supportive: immune suppression, glucocorticoids, antibiotics	None
Postvaccinal rabies	Inadequately attenuated virus in vaccines	Rare; most common in cats	Progressive ascending paralysis to diffuse meningoencephalomyelitis	Acute onset, rapid progression; poor prognosis	History, necropsy	None	Use proper vaccine
Postvaccinal canine distemper	Inadequately attenuated virus in vaccine	Rare; usually young dogs	Usually occurs 1–2 wk after vaccination; behavioral changes common; ataxia, depression, seizures; brain stem lesions predominate	Acute; poor prognosis	History, necropsy	None	None
Canine herpesvirus	Canine herpesvirus	Sporadic; neonates and young puppies	In utero or early exposure; multisystemic signs, depression, diarrhea, rhinitis, loss of consciousness, opisthotonus, seizures; may have residual neurologic deficits if they survive	Acute, progressive; frequently fatal	History, signs, virus isolation, histopathology	Supportive	Administer colostrum and hyperimmune serum in high-incidence kennels
Feline panleukopenia	Parvovirus	Sporadic; neonatal cats	CNS affected primarily in prenatal or neonatal; cerebellar damage common in prenatal (see Chap. 9).	Present at birth, nonprogressive	History, age, signs, necropsy	None	Vaccine
Feline leukemia virus	Retrovirus	Common; cats	CNS affected in some cases; epidural lymphoma causes spinal cord signs; diffuse brain disease may be present; systemic involvement usually apparent; immunosuppression may allow other infections	Chronic, progressive; usually fatal	History, signs, CBC, cytology of aspirates or CSF; extradural spinal masses should be considered likely for lymphoma	Combination chemotherapy	Vaccine
Feline paramyxovirus	Paramyxovirus	Unusual; cats	Signs similar to canine distemper encephalitis; demyelination, myoclonus reported	Chronic progressive	Virus isolation	None	None

TABLE 16–12 *Continued*
B. Viral Diseases of the CNS of Horses and Food Animals

Disease	Cause	Incidence	Clinical Signs and Pathology	Course and Prognosis	Diagnostic Tests	Treatment	Prevention
Encephalomyelitis	Togavirus	Variable; horses, dogs	Depression, fever, anorexia, lack of coordination, pacing, circling; primarily cerebral signs	Acute, progressive; recovery variable; may be permanent brain damage	History, CSF, serology, virus isolation	Supportive	Vaccine, horses
Enteroviral encephalomyelitis	Enterovirus	Variable; swine	Pelvic limb ataxia and paresis, paralysis, seizures	Acute, progressive; recovery or progression to death in 1–3 wk	History, virus isolation, serology	Supportive	Vaccine, swine
Equine herpesvirus (rhinopneumonitis)	Herpesvirus type 1	Variable; horses	Upper respiratory infection; ataxia, cauda equina signs, tetraplegia or paraplegia	Acute, progressive; fair to good prognosis	History, signs, CSF (xanthochromia, increased protein, few cells), serology, viral isolation	Supportive, corticosteroids	Vaccine
Scrapie	"Slow" virus	Sporadic; sheep >2 yr old	Pruritus, cerebellar ataxia, death; neuronal and spongiform degeneration of brain	Chronic, progressive; always fatal	History and signs, histopathology	None	None
Visna, maedi	Lentivirus	Variable; sheep >2 yr old	Ataxia, pelvic limb paresis, progressive to tetraparesis	Chronic, progressive; usually fatal	History, signs, CSF (increased cells, lymphocytes), histopathology, virus isolation, circulating antibody	None	None
Malignant catarrhal fever	Herpesvirus	Sporadic; adult cattle	Depression, blindness, pacing, seizures, death; nasal and ocular discharge	Acute, progressive; usually fatal	History and signs, histopathology	None	None
Hemagglutinating encephalomyelitis virus	Corona virus	Young swine	Depression, ataxia, tremors, seizures, and hyperesthesia	Acute CNS form, others more chronic	Serology and virus isolation	None	None
Pseudorabies (Aujeszky's disease)	Herpesvirus	Rare except in swine May affect all mammals	May be subclinical in swine Other animals: early excitement, progresses rapidly to coma and death; intense pruritus and self-mutilation, especially at portal of entry; contact with swine in history	Peracute, progression to death in 1–2 days usually	History, signs, necropsy (FA)	None	None available except vaccine for swine

Table continued on following page

TABLE 16–12 *Continued*
B. Viral Diseases of the CNS of Horses and Food Animals *Continued*

Disease	*Cause*	*Incidence*	*Clinical Signs and Pathology*	*Course and Prognosis*	*Diagnostic Tests*	*Treatment*	*Prevention*
Porcine paramyxovirus	Paramyxovirus	Rare; nursing pigs	Depression, ataxia, seizures, weakness, tremor, blindness; panophthalmitis common.	Acute, progressive; usually fatal	History and signs	None	None
Bovine spongiform encephalopathy	Possibly scrapie virus	Primarily Holstein-Friesian cattle in U.K.	Behavioral disorders, gait and postural abnormalities, hyperreactive to stimuli, aggressive	Chronic, progressive; usually fatal	Signs, histopathology, mouse inoculation	None	None
Equine infectious anemia	Retrovirus	Rare CNS; horses	Behavioral changes, blindness, ataxia, weakness	Chronic, progressive	Serology	Supportive	None
Caprine arthritis-encephalomyelitis	Retrovirus	Sporadic; young goats	Arthritis, ataxia and paresis, affects pelvic limbs first and progresses to all four limbs; some have cerebellar brain stem, or cranial nerve signs.	Acute to chronic, progressive; frequently fatal	History, signs, CSF, serology	Supportive	None
Infectious bovine rhinotracheitis	Bovine herpesvirus type 1	Rare; young calves	Depression, ataxia, blindness, tremor, seizures	Acute, progressive; fatal	Other animals with upper respiratory disease, serology, virus isolation	Supportive	Vaccine
Louping ill	Flavivirus	Primarily sheep in Great Britain	Ataxia of head and trunk, leaping gait	Acute, progressive; about 50% fatal	Presence of ticks, serology, virus isolation	Supportive	Vaccine

TABLE 16–13 Bacterial Diseases of the CNS

Disease	*Cause*	*Incidence*	*Clinical Signs and Pathology*	*Course and Prognosis*	*Diagnostic Tests*	*Treatment*
Meningitis	*Staphylococcus, Pasteurella,* others	Variable, but generally uncommon	Generalized or localized (especially cervical) hyperesthesia; degree of illness variable; temperature and WBC count may be normal	Usually acute onset, but may be chronic; prognosis good with early treatment	CSF (protein often >200 mg/dl, increased cells, primarily neutrophils), culture and sensitivity testing	Antibiotics according to sensitivity: ampicillin, trimethoprim, chloramphenicol
Meningoencephalomyelitis	As in meningitis	Uncommon	As in meningitis, plus signs of brain or spinal cord disease; often includes blindness, seizures, ataxia, cranial nerve deficits	Usually acute: prognosis good with early treatment, but neurologic deficits are common	Same as meningitis; EEG may indicate encephalitis	Same as for meningitis: seizures – diazepam, phenobarbital; acute cerebral edema – mannitol
Abscess	As in meningitis	Rare	May have focal signs or focal signs plus signs of meningitis or meningoencephalitis	May be chronic; progression may be rapid once signs are obvious	Same as in meningoencephalitis	Same as for meningoencephalitis
Vertebral osteomyelitis, diskospondylitis (see Chap. 7)	*Staphylococcus, Brucella canis,* others	Moderately frequent in dogs	Pain, usually focal; may have spinal cord compression; usually clinically ill, often over weeks to months	Chronic, may become acute when spinal cord is compressed	Radiography, myelography, *Brucella* serology	Antibiotics, preferably bactericidal, curettage, decompression if spinal cord is compressed

Table continued on following page

TABLE 16–13 Bacterial Diseases of the CNS *Continued*

Disease	*Cause*	*Incidence*	*Clinical Signs and Pathology*	*Course and Prognosis*	*Diagnostic Tests*	*Treatment*
Tetanus (see Chap. 11)	*Clostridium tetani*	Rare except in horses	Extensor rigidity of all limbs, often with opisthotonos; contraction of facial muscles, prolapsed nictitating membrane; usually an infected wound	Acute onset, often lasts 1–2 wk, animals may die; prognosis fair if treated	Signs, history, isolation of organism from wound	Penicillin, tetanus antitoxin, tranquilizers, or muscle relaxants; quiet environment; treat wound, nursing
Botulism (see Chap. 8)	*Clostridium botulinum*	Sporadic	LMN-type paralysis, often beginning in pelvic limbs, progressing to tetraparesis in less than 24 hours; caused by toxin blocking neuromuscular junction	Acute onset, lasts about 2 wk; good prognosis unless respiratory paralysis is present early	Serum, fecal analysis, history, EMG and nerve conduction velocity	Enemas and laxatives early, supportive care, antitoxin usually not effective
Thromboembolic meningoencephalitis	*Hemophilus somnus*	Cattle, primarily young in feedlot	Fever, depression, blindness, lack of coordination, cranial nerve signs, seizures	Acute progressive; fair prognosis with early treatment	History, CSF (increased protein, increased neutrophils), culture	Antibiotics, vaccine available
Listeriosis	*Listeria monocytogenes*	Sporadic in ruminants	Depression, asymmetric ataxia and paresis, cranial nerve signs, central vestibular signs	Acute progressive in sheep and goats, more chronic in cattle; poor prognosis if CNS signs are present	History, signs, CSF (increased protein, increased mononuclear cells), histopathology, fluorescent antibody, isolation of organism	Antibiotics (penicillin, sulfonamides, tetracyclines) for 2–4 wk

TABLE 16–14 Mycotic Diseases of the CNS

Disease	Cause	Incidence	Clinical Signs and Pathology	Course and Prognosis	Diagnostic Tests	Treatment
Cryptococcosis	*Cryptococcus neoformans*	Low; primarily in eastern and midwestern U.S. but reported throughout U.S.	Nose and sinuses usually are infected, with extension to brain; ocular lesions and blindness common; CNS involvement common	Chronic; poor prognosis	Smears and culture of exudate, serum titers, CSF (increased protein, increased cells, neutrophils and mononuclear cells, possibly organisms)	Amphotericin B, 5-fluorocytosine, ketoconazole, itraconazole
Blastomycosis	*Blastomyces dermatitidis*	Low; primarily in eastern and midwestern U.S.	Rarely involves CNS; pyogranulomatous encephalitis or single or multifocal granulomas are seen; frequently involves lungs, skin, and eyes	Chronic; poor prognosis	See Cryptococcosis	Amphotericin B, 5-fluorocytosine, ketoconazole, itraconazole
Histoplasmosis	*Histoplasma capsulatum*	Low, primarily in central U.S.	CNS involvement uncommon; involves reticuloendothelial cells of most viscera	Chronic; poor prognosis	See Cryptococcosis	Amphotericin B, 5-fluorocytosine, ketoconazole, itraconazole
Coccidioidomycosis	*Coccidioides immitis*	Can be relatively common in endemic areas of southwestern U.S.	CNS involvement uncommon; pulmonary infection common	Chronic; poor prognosis	See Cryptococcosis	Amphotericin B, 5-fluorocytosine, ketoconazole, itraconazole
Nocardiosis	*Nocardia* species	Low throughout U.S.	Systemic disease, signs similar to canine distemper, respiratory or cutaneous forms; CNS abscesses and vertebral osteomyelitis reported	Chronic; poor prognosis	Smears, cultures, CSF (increased protein, increased cells, neutrophils)	Penicillin, sulfonamides, trimethoprim
Actinomycosis	*Actinomyces* species	Low throughout U.S.	Similar to nocardiosis	Chronic; poor prognosis	Similar to nocardiosis	Penicillin, clindamycin, erythromycin, lincomycin
Paecilomycosis	*Paecilomyces* spp.	Rare	Disseminated form of diskospondylitis	Chronic; poor prognosis	Culture, biopsy	None
Aspergillosis	*Aspergillus* spp.	Primarily in large animals	Encephalitis can develop following immunosuppression or guttural pouch infection	Chronic; poor prognosis	Culture, CSF	Amphotericin B, 5-fluorocytosine, ketoconazole, itraconazole
Phaeomycosis	*Cladosporium* spp.	Rare	Encephalitis with granulomas have been reported in dogs and cats	Chronic; poor prognosis	Culture, biopsy	Amphotericin B, 5-fluorocytosine, ketoconazole, itraconazole Unknown efficacy

TABLE 16–15 Protozoal Diseases of the CNS

Disease	*Cause*	*Incidence*	*Clinical Signs and Pathology*	*Course and Prognosis*	*Diagnostic Tests*	*Treatment*
Toxoplasmosis	*Toxoplasma gondii*	Common infection but infrequent clinical problem	Clinical manifestations usually associated with another disease or immunosuppression; CNS, eyes, lungs, gastrointestinal tract and skeletal muscles often affected	Chronic; fair to poor prognosis	Serum titer, oocysts in stool, biopsy, CSF (increased protein, increased cells, mononuclear and neutrophils)	Sulfonamides, pyrimethamine, clindamycin
Neosporosis	*Neospora caninum*	Unknown frequency, cases of toxoplasmosis reported in past were sometimes *Neospora;* reported in dogs, cats, and cattle	Similar to toxoplasmosis; ascending paralysis of limbs with extension of the pelvic limbs is frequent	Chronic progressive; fair to poor prognosis	CSF, biopsy, isolation of organism	Sulfonamides, pyrimethamine, clindamycin are probably effective if given early
Babesiosis	*Babesia* spp.	Rare in U.S.	Parasite of RBC; rarely causes CNS disease, primarily infarction and hemorrhage; more severe with other infections, such as *Ehrlichia*	Acute to chronic; poor prognosis	Peripheral blood smears	Diminazene, phenamidine, or imidocarb

Encephalitozoonosis	*Encephalitozoon cuniculi*	Rare; primarily affects dogs <2 mo. old	Acute encephalitis, ataxia, tremors, behavioral changes	Acute; poor prognosis	Serum titers, culture, histopathology	None
Trypanosomiasis	*Trypanosoma cruzi*	Rare in U.S.	Parasite of RBC; rarely causes CNS disease	Chronic, fair prognosis with treatment	Peripheral blood smears	Nifurtimox
Equine protozoal myeloencephalitis	*Sarcocystis neurona*	Fairly common in horses	Systemic, multifocal, involving almost any part of the nervous system: commonly spinal cord, cauda equina, and cranial nerve signs are seen	Chronic, progressive; usually poor prognosis; treatment may be effective	Rule out other causes, CSF (sometimes increased protein, increased cells, mononuclears)	Pyrimethamine, trimethoprim-sulfonamide
Coccidiosis	Several species	Common enteric, rare CNS, several species of animals affected	Enteric coccidiosis is reported to cause CNS signs in some cases; *Sarcocystis* spp. may cause myopathy	Variable	Fecal identification, organism in muscle biopsy or necropsy	Sulfonamides, amprolium
Hepatozoonosis	*Hepatozoon canis*	Rare; dogs	Muscle pain and gait abnormalities may be seen	Chronic; poor prognosis	Biopsy	Possibly sulfonamides, pyrimethamine Efficacy not known

TABLE 16–16 Rickettsial and Chlamydial Diseases of the CNS

Disease	Cause	Incidence	Clinical Signs and Pathology	Course and Prognosis	Diagnostic Tests	Treatment
Rocky Mountain spotted fever	*Rickettsia rickettsii*	Fairly common in endemic areas of U.S.; dogs	Meningitis, ataxia, other CNS signs; can look like canine distemper	Acute; good prognosis with treatment	History of ticks, signs, thrombocytopenia, serum titer	Tetracycline, chloramphenicol
Ehrlichiosis	*Ehrlichia canis*	Rarely CNS signs in dogs	Meningitis, encephalitis	Acute to chronic; good prognosis if treated early	Pancytopenia, thrombocytopenia, serum titer	Tetracycline, chloramphenicol
Salmon poisoning	*Neorickettsia helminthoeca*	Rare, Pacific Northwest of U.S.	Depression and convulsions terminally; paresis of pelvic limbs less common; nonsuppurative meningoencephalitis	Acute; fair to good prognosis if treated early	History of eating salmon, fluke eggs in feces	Tetracycline, chloramphenicol
Sporadic bovine encephalomyelitis (Buss disease)	*Chlamydia psittaci*	Sporadic, young cattle	Respiratory disease, polyarthritis, diffuse cerebral signs	Acute progressive; mortality approximately 50%	History, signs, CSF (increased protein, increased mononuclear cells), serology	Tetracycline, tylosin

TABLE 16–17 Parasitic Diseases of the CNS

Disease	Cause	Incidence	Clinical Signs and Pathology	Course and Prognosis	Diagnostic Tests	Treatment
Dirofilariasis	*Dirofilaria immitis*, microfilaria or aberrant adult	Rare, areas with heartworm disease	CNS signs rare; microfilaria or migrating adult heartworms may cause infarction; seizures and other cerebral signs	Acute onset; prognosis poor	Knott test to confirm heartworm disease, CSF (increased eosinophils suggestive), impossible to prove ante mortem	None proved
Larva migrans	*Toxacara canis* and other species	Rare	Granulomas in brain or spinal cord from migrating larvae; signs related to location of lesion	Acute or chronic; prognosis depends on severity of signs	None, necropsy	None
Cuterebra	*Cuterebra* spp.	Rare	CNS signs depend on location of lesion	Acute to chronic; poor prognosis	None, necropsy	None
Coenurosis	*Coenurus* spp.	Rare; most often reported in sheep	CNS signs depend on location of lesion	Acute to chronic; prognosis poor	None, sheep have softening of skull that can be palpated or seen on radiographs	Surgical removal in sheep

TABLE 16–18 Immune-Mediated Diseases of the CNS

Disease	Cause	Incidence	Clinical Signs and Pathology	Course and Prognosis	Diagnostic Tests	Treatment
Coonhound paralysis (see Chap. 8)	Probable immune reaction to transmissible agent in raccoon saliva or environment	Fairly high in some areas; dogs	Ascending LMN paralysis; may last approximately 6 wk; ventral roots and peripheral nerves have segmental demyelination and some axon loss	Acute onset, lasts approximately 6 wk; good prognosis with good nursing	History, EMG, NCV	Supportive
Postvaccinal rabies	CNS tissues in vaccine	Rare—these vaccines no longer are used	Ascending paralysis; demyelination from immune reaction to myelin in brain-origin vaccines	Acute onset, progressive; poor prognosis	None	None

TABLE 16–19 Unclassified Inflammatory Diseases of the CNS

Disease	*Cause*	*Incidence*	*Clinical Signs and Pathology*	*Course and Prognosis*	*Diagnostic Tests*	*Treatment*
Granulomatous meningoencephalomyelitis (inflammatory reticulosis)	Unknown, probably immune-mediated	Relatively common; dogs	Nonsuppurative inflammation of brain or spinal cord and meninges; may be disseminated, focal, or multifocal; neoplastic forms are usually called reticulosis; signs depend on the location of the predominant lesions	Chronic progressive, poor prognosis	CSF (increased cells of a mixed population), histopathology	Corticosteroid therapy may prolong the course
Feline polioencephalomyelitis	Unknown	Rare; cats	Paresis, especially of the pelvic limbs, tremor, hyperesthesia; spinal cord neurons and white matter predominantly affected; brain lesions are scattered	Chronic progressive, poor prognosis	Some cats have leukopenia and nonregenerative anemia. Histopathology	None
Pug encephalitis	Unknown, possibly immune-mediated	Rare; pugs	Seizures, cerebral, vestibular, and cranial nerve signs; mononuclear inflammatory changes in cerebrum, brain stem, and meninges	Chronic progressive, poor prognosis	Breed, CSF (increased mononuclear cells), histopathology	None
Corticosteroid-responsive meningitis	Unknown, probably immune-mediated	Uncommon; usually large-breed dogs	Hyperesthesia, especially cervical, anorexia, muscular rigidity, and fever common	Acute; fair to good prognosis with therapy	CSF (increased protein and cells, especially neutrophils), neutrophilia in blood also	Corticosteroids, may be needed for several months
Pyogranulomatous meningoencephalomyelitis	Unknown, probably immune-mediated	Uncommon; reported in pointer dogs only	Hyperesthesia, especially cervical, atrophy of cervical muscles, rigidity, some incoordination are seen; both brain and spinal cord affected, worse in cervical spinal cord; mixed mononuclear and polymorphonuclear infiltrations in meninges and parenchyma	Acute progressive; poor prognosis	Breed, CSF (increased neutrophils), histopathology	None; some remission with antibiotics

TABLE 16–20 Common Toxicants

Use	Toxicant	Primary Effect
Pesticides	Chlorinated hydrocarbons	CNS stimulation
	Organophosphates	Binding of acetylcholinesterase
	Carbamates	Binding of acetylcholinesterase
	Pyrethrins	Blocking of nerve conduction and GABA inhibition
	Metaldehyde	CNS stimulation
	Arsenic	GI irritation
Rodenticides	Strychnine	Blocking of inhibitory interneurons
	Thallium	GI irritation, CNS stimulation, peripheral neuropathy, skin lesions
	α-Naphthyl thiourea (ANTU)	GI irritation, pulmonary edema, depression, coma
	Sodium fluoroacetate (1080)	CNS stimulation
	Warfarin	Anticoagulation
	Zinc phosphide	GI irritation, depression
	Phosphorus	GI irritation, CNS stimulation, coma
	Cholecalciferol	CNS depression, cardiac depression
	Bromethalin	Acute – CNS stimulation; chronic – CNS depression
Herbicides and fungicides	Numerous	GI irritation, CNS depression, some are stimulants
Heavy metals	Lead (see Arsenic and Thallium, above)	GI irritation, CNS stimulation or depression
Drugs	Narcotics	CNS depression
	Amphetamines	CNS stimulation
	Barbiturates	CNS depression
	Tranquilizers	CNS depression
	Aspirin	GI irritation, coma
	Marijuana	Abnormal behavior, depression
	Anthelmintics	GI irritation, CNS stimulation
	Ivermectin	Depression, tremors, ataxia, coma
Garbage	Staphylococcal toxin	GI irritation, CNS stimulation
	Botulinus toxin	LMN paralysis
Poisonous plants	Various	Various
Antifreeze	Ethylene glycol	GI irritation, CNS stimulation, renal failure
Detergents and disinfectants	Hexachlorophene	CNS stimulation or depression, tremors
	Phenols	GI irritation, CNS degeneration
Animal origin	Snake bite	Necrotizing wound, shock, CNS depression
	Toad (*Bufo* spp.)	Digitoxin-like action, CNS stimulation
	Lizards	GI irritation, CNS stimulation or depression
	Tick paralysis (*Dermacentor* spp., *Ixodes* in Australia)	LMN paralysis

continuous or closely spaced convulsions (e.g., from organophosphates or strychnine) or with a history of intermittent seizures (e.g., from lead). Animals in status epilepticus must be treated immediately, or they will die (see Chap. 14).

The tetany produced by strychnine is easily differentiated from the seizures produced by the other agents in this group. In spite of the severe muscle spasms, the animal is conscious. Tetany caused by strychnine may be confused with hypocalcemic tetany that is seen in lactating animals of all species or with tetanus. IV calcium provides immediate relief in cases of hypocalcemia. Tetanus is much slower in onset than is strychnine poisoning and generally causes a more continuous contraction of the muscles. Seizures from other agents produce clonus (alternating flexion and extension).

Organophosphates may be distinguished from organochlorines by their profound effect on the autonomic nervous system, including profuse salivation, constricted pupils, and diarrhea. Organochlorines frequently produce fine muscle fasciculations, even between seizures. Pyrethrins and pyrethroids are being used more frequently and may cause seizures. The seizure may be preceded by tremors, ataxia, salivation and other signs. Ingestion of products containing caffeine and other methylxanthines, including chocolate, may also cause seizures. Metaldehyde, a common snail bait, can cause continuous seizures.[64]

TABLE 16–21 Common Toxicants Causing Seizures

Toxicants	*Diagnosis*	*Management*	*Prognosis*
Organochlorines	Exposure; muscle fasciculations common; laboratory confirmation difficult	Removal of toxicant – washing, gastric lavage; sedation or anesthesia with barbiturates	Poor with seizures
Organophosphates and carbamates	Exposure; salivation, diarrhea, constricted pupils, muscle weakness; blood cholinesterase level decreased; tissue analysis poor	Removal of toxicant; atropine; pralidoxime chloride (2-PAM) (not for carbamates)	Good if treated early
Pyrethrins	Exposure; tremor, salivation, ataxia, seizures; analysis of tissues	Removal of toxicant; sedation	Good if treated early
Strychnine	Exposure; tetany without loss of consciousness, increased by stimulation or noise; laboratory analysis of stomach contents, urine, tissues	Removal of toxicant – gastric lavage or emesis; sedation – barbiturates; respiratory support if needed	Good if treated early
Bromethalin	Exposure; high dose – excitement, tremor, seizures; low dose – tremor, depression, ataxia	Removal of toxicant – activated charcoal; corticosteroids, mannitol	Fair if treated vigorously for several days
Sodium fluoroacetate (1080)	Exposure; seizures are clonic and severe; laboratory confirmation difficult	Removal of toxicant; sedation – barbiturates	Poor with seizures
Thallium	Exposure; GI signs, seizures only in severe poisonings; laboratory analysis of urine and tissues	Removal of toxicant; dithenylthiocarbazone (Dithion) early, ferric ferrocyanide (Prussian blue) late	Poor with seizures, fair with other signs, good with treatment
Lead	Exposure (may be difficult to document); chronic intoxication may cause intermittent seizures, behavioral change, tremor, GI signs; blood lead level >0.4 ppm; basophilic stippling, nucleated RBC, with no anemia	Removal of toxicant; calcium EDTA	Good with treatment
Staphylococcal toxin	Exposure to garbage; severe GI signs; isolation of toxins and testing in laboratory animals	Removal of toxicant; sedation	Poor with seizures; animals usually die rapidly
Toad (*Bufo* spp.); reported only in southern Florida	Exposure; severe buccal irritation	Wash mouth; sedation – anesthesia	Fair if treated within 15–30 min, otherwise poor
Amphetamines	Exposure to prescription or "street" drugs; hyperactivity, dilated pupils; analysis of urine	Removal of toxicant; sedation or anesthesia – barbiturates	Good if treated early
Metaldehyde	Exposure to snail bait; tremor, ataxia, salivation; seizures are tonic, similar to strychnine, but not changing with stimuli; laboratory analysis of stomach contents	Removal of toxicant; sedation or anesthesia; support respiration	Fair if treated early
Caffeine and other methylxanthines	Ataxia, tachycardia, seizures, coma; laboratory analysis of stomach contents or tissues	Removal of toxicant; sedation, fluids	Fair with treatment
Zinc phosphide	Exposure to rodenticide; behavioral changes, hysteria followed by seizures; GI irritation; analysis of stomach contents and tissues	Removal of toxicant; oral and intravenous bicarbonate; sedation – barbiturates	Poor

CNS signs of lead intoxication are seen most often in cases of chronic exposure.[65–68] The seizures are intermittent. The differential diagnosis of recurrent seizure disorders was discussed in Chapter 14. A laboratory analysis of the blood for evidence of lead is diagnostic. If the blood lead values are in the high normal range and lead poisoning is suspected, treatment followed by measurement of urine lead levels is diagnostic.

The other intoxicants causing seizures are seen infrequently.

Toxicants Causing Behavioral Change, Depression, or Coma. Depression or coma may be seen with almost any poison in the terminal stages. Drugs such as narcotics, barbiturates, and tranquilizers are the most frequent cause of depression or coma as the primary problem and may also cause behavioral changes in smaller doses (see Table 16–22). Some other agents, such as chlor-

TABLE 16–22 Common Toxicants Causing Behavior Changes, CNS Depression, or Coma

Toxicants	Diagnosis	Management	Prognosis
Drugs—narcotics, barbiturates, tranquilizers, marijuana	Degree of depression depends on dose; source of pharmaceuticals or "street" drugs; laboratory analysis of blood or urine	Removal of toxicant, narcotic antagonists, diuresis, support respiration	Good with treatment
α-Naphthyl thiourea (ANTU)	Exposure; pulmonary edema; depression and coma terminal; laboratory analysis of stomach contents and tissues	Removal of toxicant, treatment of pulmonary edema	Poor
Ethylene glycol	Exposure; GI irritation, renal failure; oxalate crystals in urine	IV ethanol (30%) with sodium bicarbonate IV; alternative for dogs—4-methylpyrazole	Poor if coma, fair to good if treated early
Cholecalciferol	Exposure; depression, weakness, cardiac depression, renal failure	Removal of intoxicant; IV saline diuresis, furosemide, corticosteroids	Fair with treatment
Many poisons produce coma terminally			

TABLE 16–23 Common Toxicants Causing Tremor, Ataxia, or Paresis

Toxicants	Diagnosis	Management	Prognosis
Hexachlorophene	Exposure; usually young, nursing animal; large dose causes GI irritation, severe depression; chronic exposure causes cerebellar signs and CNS edema	Removal of toxicant, supportive care; treatment for cerebral edema	Fair; may be residual effects
Lead	Chronic lead poisoning may produce cerebellar signs and dementia (see Table 16–21)	See Table 16–21	Good
Organophosphates	Chronic low doses (flea collars, dips) may produce tremor and weakness (see Table 16–21)	See Table 16–21	Good
Organochlorines	Low-dose exposure may produce weakness and muscle fasciculation (see Table 16–21)	See Table 16–21	Fair to good
Tranquilizers	Ataxia common with tranquilizers (see Table 16–21)	None needed	Good
Marijuana	Behavioral changes and ataxia common	Removal of toxicant	Good
Ergot alkaloids	Cattle and other herbivores grazing on Dallis grass or ryegrass; ataxia, uncoordinated gait	Removal from pasture	Good
Nitro-bearing plants, e.g., *Astragalus* spp. locoweed	Cattle, sheep and horses; ataxia, weakness or hyperexcitability, death	Removal from pasture	Fair in ruminants; may be permanent CNS damage
Yellow star thistle	Horses have an acute onset of rigidity of muscles of mastication and involuntary movement of the lips; ataxia, circling, and pacing may occur; lesions are necrosis of the globus pallidus and substantia nigra	No treatment known	Poor

TABLE 16–24 Common Toxicants Causing LMN Signs

Toxicants	Diagnosis	Management	Prognosis
Botulinus toxin	Exposure to contaminated food, carrion, and so forth; ascending LMN paralysis (see Chap. 8)	See Chapter 8	Good
Tick paralysis (*Dermacentor* spp., *Ixodes* species in Australia)	Presence of ticks; ascending LMN paralysis (see Chap. 8)	Removal of ticks (see Chap. 8)	Good, except *Ixodes* in Australia
Drug reaction (nitrofurantoins, doxorubicin, vinblastine)	Exposure; rare in animals	Removal of source	Fair
Cyanide (from *Sorghum* species grass)	Cauda equina syndrome with dysuria, flaccid anus and tail, prolapsed penis; may progress to paraplegia; usually occurs in horses	Removal from pasture; no treatment available	May improve after removal from source; residual deficits common
Organophosphates	Chronic exposure may cause LMN signs; axonopathy affecting pelvic limbs first	Removal of source; atropine and pralidoxime if acute signs present; no treatment for peripheral neuropathy	Fair to poor
Heavy metals (lead, arsenic, mercury, thallium)	Chronic exposure, rare in animals (see Table 16–21)	See Table 16–21	See Table 16–21
Industrial chemicals (acrylamide, carbon disulfide, polychlorinated	Not reported in animals; presumably could cause distal axonop-	Removal from source	Unknown

TABLE 16–25 Examples of Several Plant (and Fungal) Toxicoses of Domestic Herbivores That Can Result in Syndromes Characterized by Neurologic Signs

Plant	*Species Affected*	*Neurologic Signs*	*Pathophysiology*	*Neural Lesions*	*Treatment*	*Prognosis*
Ryegrass	Sheep, cattle, horses	Ataxia, tremor, tetany	Pentrem and fumi tremorgen mycotoxins from *Penicillium* spp.	Secondary Purkinje cell degeneration	Diazepam	Good
Phalaris spp.	Sheep, cattle	Ataxia, tremor, weakness, seizures	Dimethyltryptamine alkaloids act as monoamine oxidase inhibitors	Neuronal pigmentation (indole melanins)	?Diazepam	Bad
Paspallum, Dallis grass	Cattle, sheep	Ataxia, tremor	*Claviceps paspalli* ergot alkaloids probably neurotoxic	None	—	Good
Swainsona spp.	Sheep, cattle, horses	Weight loss, ataxia, aggressiveness	Indolizidine alkaloid (swainsonine) induces α-mannosidosis	Neuroaxonal dystrophy, neurovisceral storage products	—	Fair to very good
Locoweeds	Sheep, cattle, horses	Weight loss, ataxia, aggressiveness	Indolizidine alkaloid (swainsonine) induces α-mannosidosis	Neuroaxonal dystrophy, neurovisceral storage products	Reserpine	Fair to good
Sorghum spp.	Horses, cattle, sheep	Ataxia, bladder paralysis	Possibly HCN or lathyrogenic toxins	Neuronal fiber degeneration, spinal cord	—	Poor to fair
Solanum esuriale	Sheep	Exercise intolerance, weakness, arched back (humpyback)	Unknown (suspected toxin in *S. esuriale*)	Spinal cord fiber degeneration; myopathy	—	Bad
Solanum fastigiatum, S. dimidiatum, S. kwebense	Cattle	Cerebellar ataxia, "cerebellar seizures"	Suspected induction of gangliosidosis	Purkinje cell vacuolation and degeneration	—	Poor
Cycad palms	Cattle, goats, horses	Ataxia, recumbency	Possibly toxic glycosides, cycasin and macrozamin	Spinal cord fiber degeneration	—	Bad

Melochia pyramidata	Cattle	Ataxia, recumbency	Unknown	Spinal and nerve fiber degeneration	—	Bad
Tribulus terrestris	Sheep	Asymmetric pelvic limb weakness	Possibly neuromuscular process	None	—	Bad
Karwinskia humboldana	Goats	Hypermetria, weakness	Unknown	Peripheral neuropathy, central neuroaxonal dystrophy, myopathy	—	Bad
Nardoo fern, *Marsilea drummondi*	Sheep	Depression, blindness, convulsions	Probably a thiaminase	Polioencephalomalacia	Thiamine	Good if early
Birdsville indigo, *Indigofera linnaei*	Horses	Weight loss, ataxia, weakness	Arginine antagonist alkaloids; indospicine, canavine	None	Arginine-rich feeds (gelatin, lucerne)	Good
Mexican fireweed, *Kochia scoparia*	Cattle	Blindness (nephrosis, hepatitis)	Saponins, alkaloids, oxalates; possibly thiaminase	Polioencephalomalacia	—	Poor
Buckeye, *Aesculus* spp.	Cattle	Staggering, convulsions	Glycosides and alkaloids described	Unknown	—	Fair
Helichrysum argyrosphaerum	Sheep, cattle	Peripheral blindness, nystagmus, weakness	Unknown	Patchy status spongiosus, white matter	—	Fair for life, bad for vision
Yellow star thistle, *Centaurea solstitialis*	Horses	Depression, pacing, dystonia of muscles of prehension, mastication, and deglutition	Unknown	Nigropallidal encephalomalacia	Tube feed	Poor, starve

Modified with permission from Kornegay JN, Mayhew IG: Metabolic, toxic, and nutritional diseases of the nervous system. In Oliver JE, Hoerlein BF, Mayhew IG (eds): Veterinary Neurology. Philadelphia, WB Saunders, 1987.

pyrifos and lead, may also cause behavioral changes in chronic intoxication.[69,70] The diagnosis may be easy if the source is known (such as in cases of accidental overdosing with an anticonvulsant or of an animal that ate a bottle of the owner's tranquilizers). Reports of animals that have ingested "street" drugs are increasing, and the owner is usually reluctant to admit the source of the intoxication in these cases. A laboratory analysis of blood or urine may be necessary to confirm the diagnosis.

Toxicants Causing Tremors, Ataxia, and Paresis. Chronic organophosphate poisoning from the use of flea collars and topical or systemic insecticides frequently causes signs that are suggestive of cerebellar disease or muscle weakness (see Table 16–23). The finding of weakness is not consistent with pure cerebellar disease, so when both are present, poisoning must be considered.[71] Chronic lead poisoning also may cause tremor and ataxia (see Chap. 11).

Hexachlorophene toxicity has been seen in puppies with signs of tremor and ataxia.[72–74] Severe depression may follow. The usual source has been repeated washing of the bitch's mammary glands with a soap containing hexachlorophene. Bathing young dogs or cats of any age in hexachlorophene soap also has produced the syndrome. Hexachlorophene is rarely available now.

Metaldehyde poisoning, which produces tremor and ataxia progressing to depression and coma, is seen frequently in areas in which the substance is used for snail bait.

Numerous plant toxicities cause tremor and ataxia (Table 16–25).

Toxicants Causing LMN Signs. Botulism and tick paralysis cause a generalized LMN paralysis by blockade of the neuromuscular junction (see Table 16–24). These conditions are discussed in Chapter 8.

Some drugs (such as the nitrofurans and anticonvulsants) and some chronic toxicities (such as lead, organophosphate, and arsenic poisoning) may produce peripheral neuropathies. Other signs usually predominate, however.

Treatment

Removal of the toxic substance is the most important part of the treatment for many toxicities. Agents that have entered the animal's system through the skin, such as insecticides, should be removed by thorough washing and rinsing. Ingested agents may be removed by inducing emesis, performing gastric lavage, or administering laxatives or enemas. Diuresis may be useful in promoting excretion when absorption has occurred. Activated charcoal is an effective adsorbing agent.[75]

Status epilepticus is a life-threatening emergency and must be treated accordingly (see Chap. 14).

Specific treatments for the various toxicities are outlined in Tables 16–21 through 16–25. The reader should consult the references for details.[45,62,63,76]

CASE HISTORIES

The cases involve the same disorders as were covered in the chapter—systemic and multifocal diseases. However, because this is the last chapter, other entities might be included to test the reader's aptitude in making a neurologic diagnosis.

Case History 16A

Signalment

Canine, German shepherd, male, 10 months old.

History

Vaccinations were given on schedule. The dog had a "cold" 6 weeks ago that lasted for 1 week. One week ago the owner noticed a lack of coordination and falling to the left side. Yesterday the dog developed a head tilt to the left side.

Physical Examination

No abnormalities are found.

Neurologic Examination*

A. Observation
 1. Mental status: Depressed.
 2. Posture: Head tilt to left.
 3. Gait: Ataxia. The dog stumbles on the left thoracic limb at times.
B. Palpation: Normal.
C. Postural Reactions

Left	Reactions	Right
	Proprioceptive positioning	
+1	PL	+2
+1	TL	+2
+1	Hopping, PL	+2
+1	Hopping, TL	+2
+1	Extensor postural thrust	+2
0 to +1	Hemistand-hemiwalk	+2

* *Key*: 0 = absent, +1 = decreased, +2 = normal, +3 = exaggerated, +4 = very exaggerated or clonus, PL = pelvic limb, TL = thoracic limb, NE = not evaluated.

	Placing, tactile	
+1	PL	+2
+1	TL	+2
	Placing, visual	
+1	TL	+2

D. Spinal Reflexes

Left	Reflex	Right
	Spinal Segment	
+3	Quadriceps L4–L6	+2
+2	Extensor carpi radialis C7–T1	+2
+2	Flexion, PL L5–S1	+2
+2	Flexion, TL C6–T1	+2
0	Crossed extensor	0
+2	Perineal S1–S2	+2

E. Cranial Nerves

Left	Nerve + Function	Right
+2	CN II vision menace	+2
+2	CN II, III pupil size	+2
+2	Stim. left eye	+2
+2	Stim. right eye	+2
NE	CN II fundus	NE
+2	CN III, IV, VI Strabismus	+2
Changes direction	Nystagmus	Changes direction
+2	CN V sensation	+2
+2	CN V mastication	+2
+2	CN VII facial muscles	+2
+2	Palpebral	+2
+2	CN IX, X swallowing	+2
+2	CN XII tongue	+2

F. Sensation: Location
 Hyperesthesia: The dog resents palpation of the neck.
 Superficial pain: +2.
 Deep pain: +2.

Complete sections G and H before reviewing Case Summary.

G. Assessment (Anatomic diagnosis and estimation of prognosis)

H. Plan (Diagnostic)

Rule-outs *Procedure*

1.
2.
3.
4.

Case History 16B

Signalment

Yorkshire terrier litter: two female puppies, one male puppy, 4 weeks old.

History

Second litter of a 3-year-old bitch. The sire is different from that of the first litter. The bitch was the only dog in the household. One week ago the puppies were observed shaking. The condition progressed to coarse muscular twitching. The puppies are still nursing. The bitch is in good health and has had all immunizations. No vaccinations were given during pregnancy.

Physical Examination

Normal.

*Neurologic Examination**

A. Observation
 1. Mental status: Alert.
 2. Posture: Generalized tremor, worse when the puppies are active, usually stops when they are at rest.
 3. Gait: Dysmetria.

B. Palpation: Normal.

C. Postural Reactions: All present, but dysmetric.

D. Spinal Reflexes: All normal

E. Cranial Nerves: All normal

F. Sensation: Location
 Hyperesthesia: No.
 Superficial pain: +2.
 Deep pain: +2.

Complete sections G and H before reviewing Case Summary.

G. Assessment (Anatomic diagnosis and estimation of prognosis)

H. Plan (Diagnostic)

Rule-outs *Procedure*

1.
2.
3.
4.

Case History 16C

Signalment

Canine, Doberman pinscher, male, 3 years old.

* *Key*: 0 = absent, +1 = decreased, +2 = normal, +3 = exaggerated, +4 = very exaggerated or clonus, PL = pelvic limb, TL = thoracic limb, NE = not evaluated.

History

Intermittent lameness for several weeks.

Physical Examination

Neurologic Examination

A. Observation
  1. Mental status: Alert.
  2. Posture: Normal.
  3. Gait: The dog walks gingerly, as if he does not want to bear weight. Slight sway of pelvis.
B. Palpation
C. Postural Reactions: All normal, although resents manipulation.
D. Spinal Reflexes: All normal.
E. Cranial Nerves: All normal.
F. Sensation: Location
  Hyperesthesia
  Superficial pain
  Deep pain

Complete sections G and H before reviewing Case Summary.

G. Assessment (Anatomic diagnosis and estimation of prognosis)
H. Plan (Diagnostic)

  Rule-outs *Procedure*
  1.
  2.
  3.
  4.

Case History 16D

Signalment

English pointer, male, 6 years old.

History

The dog has been depressed and ataxic for 1 week. His appetite is poor. Vaccinations are current.

Physical Examination

The dog is depressed and thin.

*Neurologic Examination**

A. Observation
  1. Mental status: Alert.
  2. Posture: Normal.
  3. Gait: Slight truncal ataxia.
B. Palpation: Normal.
C. Postural Reactions

Left	Reactions	Right
	Proprioceptive positioning	
+2	PL	+2
+2	TL	+2
+2	Wheelbarrowing	+2
+1	Hopping, PL	+1
+1	Hopping, TL	+1
+2	Extensor postural thrust	+2
+2	Hemistand-hemiwalk	+2
	Placing, tactile	
+2	PL	+2
+2	TL	+2
	Placing, visual	
+2	TL	+2

D. Spinal Reflexes: All normal.
E. Cranial Nerves: All normal.
F. Sensation: Location
  Hyperesthesia: Resists turning of neck.
  Superficial pain: +2.
  Deep pain: +2.

Complete sections G and H before reviewing Case Summary.

G. Assessment (Anatomic diagnosis and estimation of prognosis)
H. Plan (Diagnostic)

  Rule-outs *Procedure*
  1.
  2.
  3.
  4.

* *Key*: 0 = absent, +1 = decreased, +2 = normal, +3 = exaggerated, +4 = very exaggerated or clonus, PL = pelvic limb, TL = thoracic limb, NE = not evaluated.

Case History 16E

Signalment

Canine, cairn terrier, male, 4 months old.

History

The dog is one of a litter of four; the others are normal. At 9 weeks he had a wide-based gait that gradually progressed to a swaying of the pelvis and a stumbling on the pelvic limbs. An examination by another veterinarian was otherwise negative. Now there is pelvic limb paresis.

Physical Examination

Normal.

*Neurologic Examination**

A. Observation
  1. Mental status: Alert.
  2. Posture: The dog cannot stand. Tremor of head, trunk, and limbs when the dog is active.

* *Key*: 0 = absent, +1 = decreased, +2 = normal, +3 = exaggerated, +4 = very exaggerated or clonus, PL = pelvic limb, TL = thoracic limb, NE = not evaluated.

3. Gait: The dog pulls around with the thoracic limbs. Some voluntary movements of the pelvic limbs, primarily hip flexion, are present.

B. Palpation: Normal.
C. Postural Reactions

Left	Reactions	Right
0	Proprioceptive positioning PL	0
+1	TL	+1
+1	Wheelbarrowing	+1
0	Hopping, PL	0
+1	Hopping, TL	+1
0	Extensor postural thrust	0
NE	Hemistand-hemiwalk	NE
0	Placing, tactile PL	0
+1	Placing, visual TL	+2

D. Spinal Reflexes: All normal.
E. Cranial Nerves: All normal.
F. Sensation: Location
Hyperesthesia: No.
Superficial pain: +2.
Deep pain: +2.

Complete sections G and H before reviewing Case Summary.

G. Assessment (Anatomic diagnosis and estimation of prognosis)
H. Plan (Diagnostic)

Rule-outs	*Procedure*
1.	
2.	
3.	
4.	

Assessment 16A

The dog has ataxia and hemiparesis from central vestibular disease on the left side (see Chap. 9 for a review of localization). The only finding not explained by a single lesion is the suggestion of hyperesthesia along the cervical vertebral column. The disease has a moderately acute onset and is progressive. In a young dog, the most common cause of an acute progressive disease is inflammation. The hyperesthesia suggests meningitis. The history of a respiratory problem several weeks ago should not be ignored. An alternative cause might be neoplasia, but this condition is much less likely. The primary question is the kind of infection: viral, bacterial, fungal, rickettsial, or protozoal. Canine distemper must be considered despite the apparent focal neurologic deficit. Focal brain stem disease and meningitis could also be bacterial (abscess plus subarachnoid involvement). Rickettsial diseases are possible if the dog was from an endemic area.

Localization. Left brain stem, vestibular nuclei, meninges.

Rule-outs. Inflammation: viral (distemper), bacterial, or other.

How does a clinician differentiate these types of infection?

If the examiner starts with simple, noninvasive methods, fundic and otoscopic examinations might reveal chorioretinitis from distemper, or a middle ear infection that has progressed medially. The results of both examinations are normal, however. Laboratory data might be of value but are frequently normal when either of our choices are present, as they are in this case. Rickettsial diseases frequently cause a thrombocytopenia, which was not found. EEG might be useful if there is also cerebral disease, but it would not really differentiate viral from bacterial inflammations. The best test is an examination of the CSF. In this case, a cisternal sample produced the following results:

Protein	65 mg/dl
RBCs	2/cu cm
WBCs	12/cu cm
Differential	All lymphocytes

These findings are indicative of a viral infection. A bacterial infection usually would cause more protein and more cells to be present, and the cells would be predominantly neutrophils. A fluorescent antibody examination of blood, conjunctival scrapings, or cells in the CSF might be used to confirm the diagnosis of distemper.

The dog was placed on chloramphenicol. The day following hospitalization, head tremors were observed, indicating involvement of the cerebellum. On the third day the dog started to have generalized seizures. The owners requested euthanasia. Necropsy confirmed the diagnosis of distemper encephalomyelitis.

Assessment 16B

The signs are compatible with cerebellar disease. Cerebellar hypoplasia or in utero damage to the cerebellum must be considered; however, toxic products also can produce cerebellar signs. The progressive nature of the syndrome suggests something other than a congenital defect, which is usually static with some improvement as compensation occurs. Other progressive diseases, such as storage diseases, are degenerative. None have been reported in the Yorkshire terrier.

Localization. Cerebellum.

Rule-outs.

1. toxic disorders,
2. degenerative diseases, and
3. cerebellar hypoplasia.

Further questioning of the owners revealed that they did not believe there were any toxic products available, because they had small children and were very careful. They were specifically asked to describe their management routine of the bitch and the puppies. They said that they were extremely careful and in fact washed the bitch's mammary glands every day because she went outside and got dirty. They were using a hexachlorophene soap to wash the bitch. They were instructed to wash her with a mild soap, rinse thoroughly, and discontinue cleaning the mammary glands. The pups gradually improved until they were normal, approximately 4 weeks later.

Diagnosis. Hexachlorophene toxicity.

Assessment 16C

A normal neurologic examination in the case of a gait abnormality should prompt consideration of a musculoskeletal disease. Although the history and the breed predilection suggest cervical spondylopathy or cervical disk disease, the neurologic examination does not. A vital portion of the examination—sensation—was left out. Palpation of the head and spine was normal, but the dog experienced pain on palpation of the long bones of the limbs. A radiographic examination confirmed the diagnosis of panosteitis.

It is very important to differentiate musculoskeletal problems from neurologic diseases. Dogs with musculoskeletal problems and no neurologic disease will have a normal neurologic examination. Severe hip dysplasia will not cause a proprioceptive deficit. Conversely, if a deficit is found on the neurologic examination, it almost never can be explained by musculoskeletal disease.

Assessment 16D

The neurologic findings are not localizing. Depression and slowing of the hopping reactions could be indicative of generalized disease not affecting the CNS, or of a mild CNS disease. Resistance to manipulation of the neck and the strong panniculus reaction may be indicative of pain. Deep palpation along the vertebral column elicits strong guarding reactions of the paraspinal muscles. Absolute evidence of pain cannot be demonstrated, but the breed must be considered. Hunting dogs are often very stoic. Systemic disease must be considered, with meningitis included as a strong possibility. Laboratory data are needed in order to rule out the former, and CSF analysis to rule out the latter.

Rule-outs.

1. systemic disease or
2. meningitis, possibly with mild encephalomyelitis.

Laboratory examination. The results of a blood chemistry profile and a urinalysis are normal.

WBCs	31,000/cu mm
Neutrophils	24,500
Bands	240
Lymphocytes	6,260
CSF Protein	235 mg/dl
RBCs:	5/cu mm
WBCs	2,435/cu mm
Neutrophils	94%
Mononuclear cells	6%

Blood and CSF cultures were submitted.

The findings are indicative of a bacterial meningitis, probably with septicemia. IV ampicillin therapy was started pending the results of the cultures. The dog improved in 48 hours. Blood cultures were negative, but CSF cultures revealed *Staphylococcus aureus,* which was sensitive to ampicillin. IV therapy was continued for 4 days, followed by ampicillin PO for 3 weeks. The dog recovered completely. The source of the infection was not found.

Assessment 16E

The head tremor suggests cerebellar disease. The paresis is caused by either brain stem or spinal cord dysfunction. There are no other signs of brain stem disease. The progression from pelvic limb paresis to tetraparesis can be seen with cervical spinal cord lesions or with progressive generalized myelopathy. The progression from spinal cord signs to cerebellar signs should suggest multifocal or systemic disease. The disorder is chronic and progressive in a young dog. These characteristics should prompt consideration of the inherited degenerative diseases. The next step is to review which diseases might be present in cairn terriers. Globoid cell leukodystrophy, a demyelinating disease, has been reported in this breed. The rule-outs might also include viral diseases, such as distemper. Lead toxicity should be considered, although paresis is unusual with this condition.

Localization. Cerebellum, spinal cord.

Rule-outs.

1. degenerative disease (globoid cell leukodystrophy),
2. inflammation (viral), or
3. toxicity (lead).

Laboratory examination. The hemanalysis, serum chemistry profile, and urinalysis are normal.

CSF	
Protein	95 mg/dl
Cells	
RBCs	4/cu mm
WBCs	2/cu mm
Blood lead level	0.02 ppm

The blood lead level is normal. The CSF content is indicative of a degenerative process without active inflammation (increased protein level, normal cell counts). This finding does not rule out viral diseases of the CNS, especially canine distemper, because the active inflammatory process may have been present several weeks earlier. Globoid cells may be seen in the CSF in some cases, but their absence is not significant. A biopsy of the peripheral nerve may reveal the pathologic changes characteristic of globoid cell leukodystrophy. The owners elected euthanasia, since all of the possible diseases had a very poor prognosis. No significant lesions were found on gross necropsy. Histopathology confirmed the diagnosis of globoid cell leukodystrophy.

REFERENCES

1. Baker HJ, Reynolds GD, Walkley S U, et al: The gangliosidoses: Comparative features and research applications. Vet Pathol 16:635–649, 1979.
2. Kornegay JN: Congenital and degenerative diseases of the central nervous system. In Kornegay JN (ed): Neurologic Disorders. New York, Churchill Livingstone, 1986, pp 109–129.
3. Braund KG: Degenerative and developmental diseases. In Oliver JE, Hoerlein BF, Mayhew IG: Veterinary Neurology. Philadelphia, WB Saunders, 1987, pp 185–215.
4. de Lahunta A: Abiotrophy in domestic animals: A review. Can J Vet Res 54:65–76, 1990.
5. Hardy RM: Pathophysiolgy of hepatic encephalopathy. Semin Vet Med Surg 5:100–106, 1990.
6. Bunch SE: Hepatic encephalopathy. Prog Vet Neurol 2: 287–296, 1992.
7. Center SA, Magne ML: Historical, physical examination, and clinicopathologic features of portosystemic vascular anomalies in the dog and cat. Semin Vet Med Surg 5:83–93, 1990.
8. Center SA: Liver function tests in the diagnosis of portosystemic vascular anomalies. Semin Vet Med Surg 5: 94–99, 1990.
9. Tyler JW: Hepatoencephalopathy: Part II. Pathophysiology and treatment. Comp Cont Educ Pract Vet 12: 1260–1270, 1990.
10. Taboada J: Medical management of animals with portosystemic shunts. Semin Vet Med Surg 5:107–119, 1990.
11. Johnson C, Armstrong P, Hauptman J: Congenital portosystemic shunts in dogs: 46 cases (1979–1986). J Am Vet Med Assoc 191:1478–1483, 1987.
12. Matushek KJ, Bjorling D, Mathews K: Generalized motor seizures after portosystemic shunt ligation in dogs: Five cases (1981–1988). J Am Vet Med Assoc 196:2014–2017, 1990.
13. Lorenz MD, Cornelius LM: Small Animal Medical Diagnosis. Philadelphia, JB Lippincott, 1987.
14. Lorenz MD, Cornelius LM, Ferguson DC: Small Animal Medical Therapeutics. Philadelphia, JB Lippincott, 1992.
15. Kelly M, Hill J: Canine myxedema stupor and coma. Comp Cont Educ Pract Vet 6:1049–1057, 1984.
16. Kelly MJ: Canine myxedema stupor and coma. In Kirk RW (ed): Current Veterinary Therapy X. Small Animal Practice. Philadelphia, WB Saunders, 1989, pp 998–999.
17. Jaggy A: Neurologic manifestations of hypothyroidism to dogs. In: Proceedings of the Eighth Annual Veterinary Medical Forum, Washington, DC, 1990, pp 1037–1040.
18. Spier SJ, Carlson GP, Holliday TA, et al: Hyperkalemic periodic paralysis in horses. J Am Vet Med Assoc 197: 1009–1017, 1990.
19. Dyer DR: Hypoglycemia: A common metabolic manifestation of cancer. Vet Med 87:40–47, 1992.
20. Vandevelde M: Brain tumors in domestic animals: An overview. In: Proceedings of a Conference on Brain Tumors in Man and Animals, Research Triangle Park, NC, 1984.
21. Hayes HM, Priester WA, Pendergrass TW: Occurrence of nervous-tissue tumors in cattle, horses, cats and dogs. Int J Cancer 15:39–47, 1975.
22. Luginbuhl H, Fankhauser R, McGrath JT: Spontaneous neoplasms of the nervous system in animals. Prog Neurol Surg 2:85–164, 1968.
23. LeCouteur RA: Brain tumors of dogs and cats: Diagnosis and management. Vet Med Rep 2:332–342, 1990.
24. Braund KG: Neoplasia. In Oliver JE, Hoerlein BF, Mayhew IG: Veterinary Neurology. Philadelphia, WB Saunders, 1987, pp 278–284.
25. LeCouteur RA: Tumors of the nervous system. In Withrow SJ, MacEwen EG (eds): Clinical Veterinary Oncology. Philadelphia, JB Lippincott, 1989, pp 325–350.
26. Summers BA, de Lahunta A, McEntee M, et al: A novel intradural extramedullary spinal cord tumor in young dogs. Acta Neuropathol 75:402–410, 1988.
27. Ribas JL: Thoracolumbar spinal cord blastoma: A unique tumor of young dogs. J Vet Intern Med 4:127, 1990.
28. Palmer AC, Malinowski W, Barnett KC: Clinical signs including papilloedema associated with brain tumors in twenty-one dogs. J Small Anim Pract 15:359–386, 1974.
29. Palmer AC: Tumours of the central nervous system. Proc R Soc Med 69:49–51, 1976.
30. Davidson MG, Nasisse MP, Breitschwerdt EB, et al: Acute blindness associated with intracranial tumors in dogs and cats: Eight cases (1984–1989). J Am Vet Med Assoc 199:755–758, 1991.
31. Kornegay JN: Imaging brain neoplasms: Computed tomography and magnetic resonance imaging. Vet Med Rep 2:372–390, 1990.
32. Bailey C, Higgins R: Characteristics of cisternal cerebrospinal fluid associated with primary brain tumors in the dog: A retrospective study. J Am Vet Med Assoc 188:414–417, 1986.
33. Wheeler SJ: Spinal tumours in cats. Vet Annu 29:270–277, 1989.
34. Fingeroth JM, Prata RG, Patnaik A: Spinal meningiomas in dogs: 13 cases (1972–1987). J Am Vet Med Assoc 191:720–726, 1987.
35. Bradley RL, Withrow SJ, Snyder SP: Nerve sheath tumors in the dog. J Am Anim Hosp Assoc 18:915–921, 1982.
36. Bundza A, Dukes T, Stead R: Peripheral nerve sheath neoplasms in Canadian slaughter cattle. Can Vet J 27: 268–271, 1986.
37. Wheeler S, Jones C, Wright J: The diagnosis of brachial plexus disorders in dogs: A review of twenty-two cases. J Small Anim Pract 27:147–157, 1986.
38. Chrisman CL: Electromyography in the localization of spinal cord and nerve root neoplasia in dogs and cats. J Am Vet Med Assoc 166:1074–1079, 1975.
39. Karkkainen M, Mero M, Nummi P, et al: Low field magnetic resonance imaging of the canine central nervous system. Vet Radiol 32:71–74, 1991.
40. Kornegay JN: Central nervous system neoplasia. In Kornegay JN (ed): Neurologic Disorders. New York, Churchill Livingstone, 1986, pp 79–108.
41. Turrel J, Fike J, LeCouteur R, et al: Radiotherapy of brain tumors in dogs. J Am Vet Med Assoc 184:82–86, 1984.
42. Ingram M, Jacques DB, Freshwater DB, et al: Adoptive immunotherapy of brain tumors in dogs. Vet Med Rep 2:398–402, 1990.
43. Heidner GL, Kornegay JN, Page RL, et al: Analysis of

survival in a retrospective study of 86 dogs with brain tumors. J Vet Intern Med 5:219–226, 1991.
44. Frier H, Gorgacz E, Hall R, et al: Formation and absorption of cerebrospinal fluid in adult goats with hypo- and hypervitaminosis A. Am J Vet Res 35:45–55, 1974.
45. Kornegay JN, Mayhew IG: Metabolic, toxic, and nutritional diseases of the nervous system. In Oliver JE, Hoerlein BF, Mayhew IG: Veterinary Neurology. Philadelphia, WB Saunders, 1987, pp 255–277.
46. Niebauer GW: Transsphenoidal hypophysectomy in the dog: A new technique. Vet Surg 17:296–303, 1988.
47. van Donkersgoed J, Clark EG: Blindness caused by hypovitaminosis A in feedlot cattle. Can Vet J 29:925–927, 1988.
48. Anderson WI, Rebhun WC, de Lahunta A, et al: The ophthalmic and neuro-ophthalmic effects of a vitamin A deficiency in young steers. Vet Med 86:1143–1148, 1991.
49. Mayhew I, Brown C, Stowe H, et al: Equine degenerative myeloencephalopathy: A vitamin E deficiency that may be familial. J Vet Intern Med 1:45–50, 1987.
50. Dill SG, Kallfelz FA, de Lahunta A, et al: Serum vitamin E and blood glutathione peroxidase values of horses with degenerative myeloencephalopathy. Am J Vet Res 50:166–168, 1989.
51. Anderson WI, Morrow LA: Thiamine deficiency encephalopathy with concurrent myocardial degeneration and polyradiculoneuropathy in a cat. Cornell Vet 77:251–257, 1987.
52. Houston DM, Hulland TJ: Thiamine deficiency in a team of sled dogs. Can Vet J 29:383–385, 1988.
53. Rammell C, Hill J: A review of thiamine deficiency and its diagnosis, especially in ruminants. NZ Vet J 34:202–204, 1987.
54. Read DH, Harrington DD: Experimentally induced thiamine deficiency in beagle dogs: Pathologic changes of the central nervous system. Am J Vet Res 47:2281–2289, 1986.
55. Mayhew IG: Large Animal Neurology: A Handbook for Veterinary Clinicians. Philadelphia, Lea & Febiger, 1989.
56. Thomas WB, Sorjonen DC: Diagnostic findings in confirmed CNS distemper viral infections. In: Proceedings of the Eighth Annual Veterinary Medical Forum, Washington, DC, 1990, pp 109–112.
57. Greene CE: Infectious diseases affecting the nervous system. In Kornegay JN (ed): Neurologic Disorders. New York, Churchill Livingstone, 1986, pp 57–77.
58. Braund KG: Granulomatous meningoencephalomyelitis. In Kirk RW (ed): Current Veterinary Therapy X. Small Animal Practice. Philadelphia, WB Saunders, 1989, pp 854–857.
59. Braund KG, Brewer BD, Mayhew IG: Inflammatory, infectious, immune, parasitic, and vascular diseases. In Oliver JE, Hoerlein BF, Mayhew IG (eds): Veterinary Neurology. Philadelphia, WB Saunders, 1987, pp 216–254.
60. Fenner W: Meningitis. In Kirk RW (ed): Current Veterinary Therapy IX. Small Animal Practice. Philadelphia, WB Saunders, 1986, pp 814–818.
61. Timoney JF, Gillespie JH, Scott FW, et al: Hagan and Bruner's Microbiology and Infectious Diseases of Domestic Animals. Ithaca, Comstock Publishing Associates, 1988.
62. Osweiler GD, Carson TL, Buck WB, et al: Clinical and Diagnostic Veterinary Toxicology, 3rd ed. Dubuque, IA, Kendall/Hunt Publishing Co, 1985.
63. Grauer GF, Hjelle JJ: Section 16. Toxicology. In Morgan RV (ed): Handbook of Small Animal Practice. New York, Churchill Livingstone, 1988, pp 1081–1128.
64. Dorman DC: Toxins that induce seizures in small animals. In: Proceedings of the Eighth Annual Veterinary Medical Forum, Washington, DC, 1990, pp 361–364.
65. Bratton GR, and Kowalczyk DF: Lead poisoning. In Kirk RW (ed): Current Veterinary Therapy X. Small Animal Practice. Philadelphia, WB Saunders, 1989, pp 152–158.
66. Dollahite JW, Younger RL, Crookshank HR, et al: Chronic lead poisoning in horses. Am J Vet Res 39: 961–964, 1978.
67. Zook BC, Carpenter JL, Leeds EB: Lead poisoning in dogs. J Am Vet Med Assoc 155:1329–1342, 1969.
68. Knecht CD, Crabtree J, Katherman A: Clinical, clinicopathologic, and electroencephalographic features of lead poisoning in dogs. J Am Vet Med Assoc 175:196–201, 1979.
69. Nicholls TJ, Handson PD: Behavioural change associated with chronic lead poisoning in working dogs. Vet Rec 112:607, 1983.
70. Jaggy A, Oliver JE: Chlorpyrifos toxicosis in two cats. J Vet Intern Med 4:135–139, 1990.
71. Farrow BRH: Tremor syndromes in dogs. In: Proceedings of the Sixth Annual Veterinary Medical Forum, Washington, DC, 1988, pp 57–60.
72. Bath ML: Hexachlorophene toxicity in dogs. J Small Anim Pract 19:241–244, 1978.
73. Scott DW, Bolton GR, Lorenz MD: Hexachlorophene toxicosis in dogs. J Am Vet Med Assoc 162:947–949, 1973.
74. Thompson J, Senior D, Pinson D, et al: Neurotoxicosis associated with the use of hexachlorophene in a cat. J Am Vet Med Assoc 190:1311–1312, 1987.
75. Dorman DC: Initial management of toxicoses. In: Proceedings of the Eighth Annual Veterinary Medical Forum, Washington, DC, 1990, pp 419–422.
76. Hamir A, Sullivan N, Handson P, et al: A comparison of calcium disodium ethylene diamine tetra-acetate (Ca EDTA) by oral and subcutaneous routes as a treatment of lead poisoning in dogs. J Small Anim Pract 27:39–43, 1986.
77. Shell LG, Potthoff A, Carithers R, et al: Neuronal-visceral GM1 gangliosidosis in Portuguese water dogs. J Vet Intern Med 3:1–7, 1989.
78. Baker HJ, Mole JA, Lindsey JR, et al: Animal models of human ganglioside storage diseases. Fed Proc 35: 1193–1201, 1976.
79. Read DH, Harrington DD, Keenan TW, et al: Neuronal-visceral GM1 gangliosidosis in a dog with β-galactosidase deficiency. Science 194:442–445, 1976.
80. Donnelly WJC, Sheahan BJ, Rogers TA: GM1 gangliosidosis in Friesian calves. J Pathol 111:173–179, 1973.
81. Baker HJ, Lindsey JR, McKann GM, et al: Neuronal GM1 gangliosidosis in a Siamese cat with β-galactosidase deficiency. Science 174:838–839, 1971.
82. Cummings JF, Wood PA, Walkley SU, et al: GM2 gangliosidosis in a Japanese spaniel. Acta Neuropathol 67:247–253, 1985.
83. Singer HS, Cork LC: Canine GM2 gangliosidosis: Morphological and biochemical analysis. Vet Pathol 26: 114–120, 1989.
84. Cork LC, Munnell JF, Lorenz MD: The pathology of feline GM2 gangliosidosis. Am J Pathol 90:723–734, 1978.
85. Cork LC, Munnell JF, Lorenz MD, et al: GM2 ganglioside lysosomal storage disease in cats with B-hexosaminidase deficiency. Science 196:1014–1017, 1977.
86. Read WK, Bridges CH: Neuronal lipodystrophy: occurrence in an inbred strain of cattle. Pathol Vet 6:235–243, 1969.
87. Hartley WJ, Blakemore WF: Neurovisceral glucocerebroside storage (Gaucher's disease) in a dog. Vet Pathol 10:191–201, 1973.

88. Cuddon PA, Higgins RJ, Duncan ID: Feline Niemann-Pick disease associated polyneuropathy. In: Proceedings of the Sixth Annual Veterinary Medical Forum, Washington, DC, 1988, p 726.
89. Baker H, Wood P, Wenger D, et al: Sphingomyelin lipidosis in a cat. Vet Pathol 24:386–391, 1987.
90. Bundza A, Lowden JA, Charlton KM: Niemann-Pick disease in a poodle dog. Vet Pathol 16:530–538, 1979.
91. Chrisp CE, Ringle DH, Abrams GD, et al: Lipid storage disease in a Siamese cat. J Am Vet Med Assoc 156:616–622, 1970.
92. Johnson KH: Globoid leukodystrophy in the cat. J Am Vet Med Assoc 157:2057–2067, 1970.
93. Selcer ES, Selcer RR: Globoid cell leukodystrophy in two West Highland white terriers and one Pomeranian. Comp Cont Educ Pract Vet 6:621–624, 1984.
94. Luttgen PJ, Braund KG, Storts RW: Globoid cell leukodystrophy in a basset hound. J Small Anim Pract 24: 153–160, 1983.
95. Zaki F, Kay WJ: Globoid cell leukodystrophy in a miniature poodle. J Am Vet Med Assoc 163:248–250, 1973.
96. Pritchard DH, Napthine DV, Sinclair AJ: Globoid cell leukodystrophy in polled Dorset sheep. Vet Pathol 17: 399–405, 1980.
97. Johnson GR, Oliver JE, Selcer R: Globoid cell leukodystrophy in a beagle. J Am Vet Med Assoc 167:380–384, 1975.
98. Fletcher TF: Electroencephalographic features of leukodystrophic disease in the dog. J Am Vet Med Assoc 157:190–198, 1970.
99. Fletcher TF, Kurtz HJ, Low DG: Globoid cell leukodystrophy (Krabbe type) in the dog. J Am Vet Med Assoc 149:165–172, 1966.
100. Fatzer R: Leukodystrophische Ershrankungen im Gehirn junger Katzen. Schweiz Arch Tierheilkd 117:641–648, 1975.
101. Hegreberg GA, Thuline HC, Francis BH: Morphologic changes in feline leukodystrophy. Fed Proc 30:341, 1971.
102. Cowell KR, Jezyk PF, Haskins ME, et al: Mucopolysaccharidosis in a cat. J Am Vet Med Assoc 169:334–339, 1976.
103. Haskins ME, Jezyk PF, Desnick RJ, et al: Animal models of mucopolysaccharidosis. In: Desnick RJ, Patterson DF, and Scarpelli DG (eds). Animal Models of Inherited Metabolic Diseases. New York, Alan R Liss, 1982, pp 177–201.
104. Haskins ME, Aguirre GD, Jezyk PF, et al: The pathology of the feline model of mucopolysaccharidosis VI. Am J Pathol 101:657–674, 1980.
105. Shull RM, Helman RG, Spellacy E, et al: Morphologic and biochemical studies of canine mucopolysaccharidosis I. Am J Pathol 114:487–495, 1984.
106. Haskins ME, Aguirre GD, Jezyk PF, et al: The pathology of the feline model of mucopolysaccharidosis I. Am J Pathol 112:27–36, 1983.
107. Shull RM, Munger RJ, Spellacy E, et al: Animal model of human disease: Canine alpha-L-Iduronidase deficiency—A model of mucopolysaccharidosis I. Am J Pathol 109:244–248, 1982.
108. Hegreberg GA, Padget GA: Inherited progressive epilepsy of the dog with comparisons to Lafora's disease of man. Fed Proc 35:1202–1205, 1976.
109. Cusick PK, Cameron AM, Parker AJ: Canine neuronal glycoproteinosis: Lafora's disease in the dog. J Am Anim Hosp Assoc 12:518–521, 1976.
110. Cummings JF, Wood PA, de Lahunta A, et al: The clinical and pathologic heterogeneity of feline alpha-mannosidosis. J Vet Intern Med 2:163–170, 1988.
111. Maenhout T, Kint JA, Dacremont G, et al: Mannosidosis in a litter of Persian cats. Vet Rec 122:351–354, 1988.
112. Blakemore W: A case of mannosidosis in the cat: Clinical and histopathological findings. J Small Anim Pract 27:447–455, 1986.
113. Embury DH, Jerrett IV: Mannosidosis in Galloway calves. Vet Pathol 22:548–551, 1985.
114. Vandevelde M, Fankhauser R, Bichsel P, et al: Hereditary neurovisceral mannosidosis with associated mannosidase deficiency in a family of Persian cats. Acta Neuropathol 58:64–68, 1982.
115. Shapiro JL, Rostkowski C, Little PB, et al: Caprine B-mannosidosis in kids from an Ontario herd. Can Vet J 26:155–158, 1985.
116. Healy PJ, Seaman JT, Gardner IA, et al: B-mannosidase deficiency in Anglo Nubian goats. Aust Vet J 57:504–507, 1981.
117. Fyfe JC, Giger U, van Winkle T, et al: Familial glycogen storage disease type IV (GSD IV) in Norwegian forest cats (NWFC). J Vet Intern Med 4:127, 1990.
118. Harvey JW, Mays MBC, Gropp KE, et al: Polysaccharide storage myopathy in canine phosphofructokinase deficiency (type VII glycogen storage disease). Vet Pathol 27:1–8, 1990.
119. Walvoort HC, VanNes JJ, Stokhof AA, et al: Canine glycogen storage disease type II: A clinical study of four affected Lapland dogs. J Am Anim Hosp Assoc 20:279–286, 1984.
120. O'Sullivan BM, Healy PJ, Fraser IR, et al: Generalised glycogenosis in Brahman cattle. Aust Vet J 57:227–229, 1981.
121. Manktelow CD, Hartley WJ: Generalized glycogen storage disease in sheep. J Comp Pathol 85:139–145, 1975.
122. McHowell J, Dorling PR, Cook RD, et al: Infantile and late onset form of generalised glycogenosis type II in cattle. J Pathol 134:266–277, 1981.
123. Mostafa IE: A case of glycogenic cardiomegaly in a dog. Acta Vet Scand 11:197–208, 1970.
124. Sandstrom B, Westman J, Ockerman PA: Glycogenosis of the central nervous system in the cat. Acta Neuropathol 14:194–200, 1969.
125. Jolly RD, Hartley WJ: Storage diseases of domestic animals. Aust Vet J 43:1–8, 1977.
126. Herrtage ME: Canine fucosidosis. Vet Annu 28:223–227, 1988.
127. Taylor R, Farrow B, Healy P: Canine fucosidosis: Clinical findings. J Small Anim Pract 28:291–300, 1987.
128. Kelly WR, Clague AE, Barns RJ, et al: Canine-L-fucosidosis: A storage disease of Springer spaniels. Acta Neuropathol 60:9–13, 1983.
129. Taylor RM, Farrow BRH: Ceroid-lipofuscinosis in border collie dogs. Acta Neuropathol 75:627–631, 1988.
130. Harper PAW, Walker KH, Healy PJ, et al: Neurovisceral ceroid-lipofuscinosis in blind Devon cattle. Acta Neuropathol 75:632–636, 1988.
131. Cho D, Leipold H, Rudolph R: Neuronal ceroidosis (ceroid-lipofuscinosis) in a blue heeler dog. Acta Neuropathol 69:161–164, 1986.
132. Nimmo Wilkie JS, Hudson EB: Neuronal and generalized ceroid-lipofuscinosis in a cocker spaniel. Vet Pathol 19:623–628, 1982.
133. Vandevelde M, Fatzer R: Neuronal ceroid-lipofuscinosis in older dachshunds. Vet Pathol 17:686–692, 1980.
134. Koppang N: Canine ceroid-lipofuscinosis in English setters. J Small Anim Pract 10:639–644, 1970.
135. Armstrong D, Koppang N, Jolly R: Ceroid-lipofuscinosis. Comp Pathol Bull 12:2–4, 1980.
136. Appleby EC, Longstaffe JA, Bell FR: Ceroid lipofuscinosis in two Saluki dogs. J Comp Pathol 92:375–380, 1982.
137. Hoover D, Little P, Cole W: Neuronal ceroid-lipofuscinosis in a mature dog. Vet Pathol 21:359–361, 1984.

138. Fiske RA, Storts RW: Neuronal ceroid-lipofuscinosis in Nubian goats. Vet Pathol 25:171–173, 1988.
139. Green P, Little P: Neuronal ceroid-lipofuscin storage in Siamese cats. Can J Comp Med 38:207–212, 1974.
140. Mayhew I, Jolly R: Ovine ceroid lipofuscinosis. Proc ACVIM Forum 11:57–59, 1986.
141. Reece RL, MacWhirter P: Neuronal ceroid lipofuscinosis in a lovebird. Vet Rec 122:187, 1988.
142. Sisk DB, Levesque DC, Wood PA, et al: Clinical and pathologic features of ceroid lipofuscinosis in two Australian cattle dogs. J Am Vet Med Assoc 197:361–364, 1990.
143. Cummings JF, de Lahunta A, Riis RC, et al: Neuropathologic changes in a young adult Tibetan terrier with subclinical neuronal ceroid-lipofuscinosis. Prog Vet Neurol 1:301–309, 1990.
144. Shell L, Jortner B, Leib M: Familial moter neuron disease in Rottweiler dogs: Neuropathologic studies. Vet Pathol 24:135–139, 1987.
145. Shell L, Jortner B, Leib M: Spinal muscular atrophy in two Rottweiler littermates. J Am Vet Med Assoc 190: 878–880, 1987.
146. Cummings JF, George C, de Lahunta A, et al: Focal spinal muscular atrophy in two German shepherd pups. Acta Neuropathol 79:113–116, 1989.
147. Cork LC, Griffin JW, Munnell JF, et al: Hereditary canine spinal muscular atrophy. J Neuropathol Exp Neurol 38: 209–221, 1979.
148. Inada S, Sakamoto H, Haruta K, et al: A clinical study on hereditary progressive neurogenic muscular atrophy in pointer dogs. Jpn J Vet Sci 40:539–547, 1978.
149. Sandefeldt E, Cummings JF, de Lahunta A, et al: Hereditary neuronal abiotrophy in the Swedish Lapland dog. Cornell Vet 63:1–71, 1973.
150. Lancaster M, Gill I, Hooper P: Progressive paresis in Angora goats. Aust Vet J 64:123, 1987.
151. Palmer AC, Blakmore WF: A progressive neuronopathy in the young cairn terrier. J Small Anim Pract 30:101–106, 1989.
152. Jaggy A, Vandevelde M: Multisystem neuronal degeneration in cocker spaniels. J Vet Intern Med 2:117–120, 1988.
153. Cummings JF, de Lahunta A, Moore JJ: Multisystemic chromatolytic neuronal degeneration in a cairn terrier pup. Cornell Vet 78:301–314, 1988.
154. Hartley WJ, Palmer AC: Ataxia in Jack Russell terriers. Acta Neuropathol 26:71–74, 1973.
155. Carmichael S, Griffiths IR, Harvey MJA: Familial cerebellar ataxia with hydrocephalus in bull mastiffs. Vet Rec 112:354–358, 1983.
156. Matthews NS, de Lahunta A: Degenerative myelopathy in an adult miniature poodle. J Am Vet Med Assoc 186: 1213–1214, 1985.
157. Waxman FJ, Clemmons RM, Johnson G, et al: Progressive myelopathy in older German shepherd dogs: I. Depressed response to thymus-dependent mitogens. J Immunol 124:1209–1215, 1980.
158. Averill DR: Degenerative myelopathy in the aging German shepherd dog. J Am Vet Med Assoc 162:1045–1051, 1973.
159. Griffiths IR, Duncan ID: Chronic degenerative radiculomyelopathy in the dog. J Small Anim Pract 16:461–471, 1975.
160. Aitchison S, Westfall J, Leipold H, et al: Ultrastructural alterations of motor cortex synaptic junctions in Brown Swiss cattle with weaver syndrome. Am J Vet Res 46:1733–1736, 1985.
161. Baird JD, Sarmiento UM, Basrur PK: Bovine progressive degenerative myeloencephalopathy (weaver syndrome) in brown swiss cattle in Canada: A literature review and case report. Can Vet J 29:370–377, 1988.
162. Gamble DA, Chrisman CL: A leukoencephalomyelopathy of Rottweiler dogs. Vet Pathol 21:274–280, 1984.
163. Zachary JF, O'Brien DP: Spongy degeneration of the central nervous system in two canine littermates. Vet Pathol 22:561–571, 1985.
164. Luttgen PJ, Storts RW: Central nervous system status spongiosus. Proc ACVIM Forum, San Diego, 1987, p 841.
165. Cockrell BY, Herigstad RR, Flo GJ, et al: Myelomalacia in Afghan hounds. J Am Vet Med Assoc 162:362–365, 1973.
166. Kelly DF, Gaskell CJ: Spongy degeneration of the central nervous system in kittens. Acta Neuropathol 35: 151–158, 1976.
167. Harper P, Dennis JA, Healy P, et al: Maple syrup urine disease in calves: A clinical, pathological and biochemical study. Aust Vet J 66:46–49, 1989.
168. Clark RG, Hartley WJ, Burgess GS, et al: Suspected neuroaxonal dystrophy in collie sheep dogs. NZ Vet J 30:102–103, 1982.
169. Cork LC, Troncoso JC, Price DL, et al: Canine neuronaxonal dystrophy. J Neuropathol Exp Neurol 42:286–296, 1983.
170. Chrisman CL, Cork LC, Gamble DA: Neuroaxonal dystrophy of Rottweiler dogs. J Am Vet Med Assoc 184: 464–467, 1984.
171. Blakemore W, Palmer A: Nervous disease in the chihuahua characterised by axonal swellings. Vet Rec 117: 498–499, 1985.
172. Duncan ID, Griffiths IR: Canine giant axonal neuropathy: Some aspects of its clinical, pathological and comparative features. J Small Anim Pract 22:491–501, 1981.
173. Duncan ID, Griffiths IR: Canine giant axonal neuropathy. Vet Rec 101:438–441, 1977.
174. Griffiths IR: Progressive axonopathy: An inherited neuropathy of boxer dogs. 1. Further studies of the clinical and electrophysiological features. J Small Anim Pract 26:381–392, 1985.
175. Griffiths IR, Duncan ID, Barker J: A progressive axonopathy of boxer dogs affecting the central and peripheral nervous system. J Small Anim Pract 21:29–43, 1980.
176. Woodard JC, Collins GH, Hessler JR: Feline hereditary neuroaxonal dystrophy. Am J Pathol 74:551–560, 1974.
177. Nuttall WO: Ovine neuroaxonal dystrophy in New Zealand. NZ Vet J 36:5–7, 1988.
178. Beech J, Haskind M: Genetic studies of neuroaxonal dystrophy in the morgan. Am J Vet Res 48:109–113, 1987.
179. Beech J: Neuroaxonal dystrophy of the accessory cuneate nucleus in horses. Vet Pathol 21:384–393, 1984.
180. de Lahunta A, Shively GN: Neurofibrillary accumulation in a puppy. Cornell Vet 65:240–247, 1975.
181. Vandevelde M, Greene C, Hoff E: Lower motor neuron disease with accumulation of neurofilaments in a cat. Vet Pathol 13:428–435, 1976.
182. Higgins RJ, Rings DM, Fenner WR, et al: Spontaneous lower motor neuron disease with neurofibrillary accumulation in young pigs. Acta Neuropathol 59:288–294, 1983.
183. Rousseaux CG, Klavano GG, Johnson ES, et al: Shaker calf syndrome: A newly recognized inherited neurodegenerative disorder of horned Hereford calves. Vet Pathol 22:104–111, 1985.
184. Cork LC, Troncoso JC, Price DL: Canine inherited ataxia. Ann Neurol 9:492–499, 1981.
185. de Lahunta A, Fenner WR, Indrieri RJ, et al: Hereditary cerebellar cortical abiotrophy in the Gordon setter. J Am Vet Med Assoc 177:538–541, 1980.
186. Montgomery D, Storts R: Hereditary striatonigral and

cerebello-olivary degeneration of the Kerry blue terrier: II. Ultrastructural lesions in the caudate nucleus and cerebellar cortex. J Neuropathol Exp Neurol 43: 263–275, 1984.

187. Montgomery D, Storts R: Hereditary striatonigral and cerebello-olivary degeneration of the Kerry blue terrier. Vet Pathol 20:143–159, 1983.

188. de Lahunta A, Averill DR: Hereditary cerebellar cortical and extrapyramidal nuclear abiotrophy in Kerry blue terriers. J Am Vet Med Assoc 168:1119–1124, 1976.

189. Steinberg S, Troncoso J, Cork L, et al: Clinical features of inherited cerebellar degeneration in Gordon setters. J Am Vet Med Assoc 179:886–890, 1981.

190. de Lahunta A: Comparative cerebellar disease in domestic animals. Comp Cont Educ Pract Vet 2:8–19, 1980.

191. de Lahunta A: Veterinary Neuroanatomy and Clinical Neurology, 2nd ed. WB Saunders, Philadelphia, 1983.

192. LeCouteur RA, Kornegay JN, Higgins RJ: Late onset progressive cerebellar degeneration of Brittany spaniel dogs. In: Proceedings of the Sixth Annual Veterinary Medical Forum, Washington, DC, 1988, pp 657–658.

193. Chrisman CL, Spencer CP, Crane SW, et al: Late-onset cerebellar degeneration in a dog. J Am Vet Med Assoc 182:717–720, 1983.

194. Haskins ME, Jezyk PF, Desnick RJ, et al: Mucopolysaccharidosis in a domestic short-haired cat: A disease distinct from that seen in the Siamese cat. J Am Vet Med Assoc 175:384–387, 1979.

195. Barlow R: Genetic cerebellar disorders in cattle. In: Rose FC, Behan PO (eds): Animal Models of Neurological Disease. Kent, Great Britain, Pitman Medical, 1980, pp 294–305.

196. Barlow R: Morphogenesis of cerebellar lesions in bovine familial convulsions and ataxia. Vet Pathol 18: 151–162, 1981.

197. White ME, Whitlock RH, de Lahunta A: A cerebellar abiotrophy of calves. Cornell Vet 65:476–491, 1975.

198. Terlecki S, Richardson C, Bradley R, et al: A congenital disease of lambs clinically similar to 'inherited cerebellar cortical atrophy' (daft lamb disease). Br Vet J 134:299–308, 1978.

199. Harper P, Duncan D, Plant J, et al: Cerebellar abiotrophy and segmental axonopathy: Two syndromes of progressive ataxia of Merino sheep. Aust Vet J 63:18–21, 1986.

200. Kidd A, Done J, Wrathall A, et al: A new genetically-determined congenital nervous disorder in pigs. Br Vet J 142:275–285, 1986.

201. Sorjonen D, Cox N, Kwapien R: Myeloencephalopathy with eosinophilic refractile bodies (Rosenthal fibers) in a Scottish terrier. J Am Vet Med Assoc 190:1004–1006, 1987.

202. Cooper BJ, de Lahunta Alexander, Cummings JF, et al: Canine inherited hypertrophic neuropathy: Clinical and electrodiagnostic studies. Am J Vet Res 45:1172–1177, 1984.

203. Cooper B, Duncan I, Cummings J, et al: Defective Schwann cell function in canine inherited hypertrophic neuropathy. Acta Neuropathol 63:51–56, 1984.

204. Cummings JF, de Lahunta A, Braund KG, et al: Animal model of human disease: Hereditary sensory neuropathy: Nociceptive loss and acral mutilation in pointer dogs: Canine hereditary sensory neuropathy. Am J Pathol 112:136–138, 1983.

205. Cummings JF, de Lahunta A, Winn SS: Acral mutilation and nociceptive loss in English pointer dogs. Acta Neuropathol 53:119–127, 1981.

206. Duncan ID, Griffiths IR, Munz M: The pathology of a sensory neuropathy affecting long haired dachshund dogs. Acta Neuropathol 58:141–151, 1982.

207. Chrisman CL: Distal polyneuropathy of doberman pinschers. In: Proceedings of the Third Annual Medical Forum, ACVIM, San Diego, 1985.

Appendix

Bovine Diseases

Breed	Disease	Chapter	Inherited*	References
Aberdeen Angus	Cerebellar degeneration	9		1
Aberdeen Angus	Cerebellar hypoplasia	9	?	2
Aberdeen Angus	Epilepsy	14	Y	3
Aberdeen Angus	Mannosidosis	16	Y	4–6
Angus-Shorthorn	Hypomyelination	11	Y	7, 8
Ayrshire	Cerebellar degeneration	9	Y	9, 10
Ayrshire	Cerebellar hypoplasia	9		10
Ayrshire ×	Atlanto-occipital malformation	8		11
Beefmaster	Ceroid lipofuscinosis	16		12
Beefmaster	Neuronal Lipodystrophy	16	Y	6
Brahman	Glycogenosis	16	Y	13
Brahman	Narcolepsy-cataplexy	14		14
Brown Swiss	Cerebellar degeneration	9		15
Brown Swiss	Degenerative myeloencephalopathy	8	?	15–17
Brown Swiss	Epilepsy	14	Y	18
Charolais	Cerebellar hypoplasia	9		19
Charolais	Demyelination	8, 16	Y	6, 20–23
Charolais	Cerebellar degeneration and epilepsy	14		6
Charolais	Myelodysplasia	7	Y	24, 25
Charolais ×	Atlanto-occipital malformation	8		11
Devon	Atlanto-occipital malformation	8		26
Devon	Ceroid lipofuscinosis	16		12, 27
Galloway	Mannosidosis	16		28
Guernsey	Narcolepsy-cataplexy	14		29
Hereford	Cerebellar degeneration	9	Y	30
Hereford	Cerebellar hypoplasia	9	Y	6, 30, 31
Hereford	Ceroid lipofuscinosis	16		6
Hereford	Epilepsy	14		32
Hereford	Hydrocephalus	13	Y	33–35
Hereford	Hypomyelination	11		8, 36
Hereford	Neuronal degeneration	8	Y	37, 38
Hereford	Spinocerebellar degeneration	16		37
Holstein Friesian	Atlanto-occipital malformation	8		39, 40
Holstein Friesian	Atlantoaxial luxation	8	?	39
Holstein Friesian	Cerebellar brain stem malformation	14		41
Holstein Friesian	Cerebellar degeneration	9	Y	6, 30, 42
Holstein Friesian	Cerebellar hypoplasia	9		43
Holstein Friesian	Gangliosidosis GM_1	16	Y	4, 44–46, 47
Holstein Friesian	Spinal dysraphism	7		48

Bovine Diseases *Continued*

Breed	Disease	Chapter	Inherited*	References
Holstein Friesian	Spinal dysraphism	7		48
Holstein Friesian	Spongiform degeneration	13		49
Jersey	Cerebellar degeneration	9		6
Jersey	Hypomyelination	11	Y	8, 50
Limousin	Epilepsy	14		6
Limousin ×	Neuronal degeneration	16	Y	51, 52
Murray Grey	Demyelination	8, 16	Y	53, 54
Murray Grey	Mannosidosis	16	Y	5
Norwegian Red poll	Pelvic limb paralysis	7	Y	52
Polled Hereford	Congenital myoclonus (neuraxial edema)	16	Y	55–59
Polled Hereford	Neuronal degeneration	16	Y	60
Red Danish	Paralysis		Y	61
Salers	β-Mannosidosis	16	Y	62, 63
Shorthorn	Cerebellar degeneration	9, 16	Y	6
Shorthorn	Cerebellar hypoplasia	9	Y	6, 30, 64, 65
Shorthorn	Glycogenosis	16	Y	6, 66, 67
Shorthorn	Hydrocephalus	13	Y	33, 34, 68
Shorthorn	Hypomyelination	11	Y	8, 36
Shorthorn	Retinal dysplasia	12	Y	69
Simmental	Neuronal degeneration	16	Y	51, 52
Swedish Red	Epilepsy	14		70
Various	Arthrogryposis	8		71
Various	Cerebellar brain stem malformation	14		72
Various	Myelodysplasia	7		73, 74
Various	Neurofibromatosis	16		75

* Y = yes, ? = suspected.

Canine Diseases

Breed	Diseases	Chapter	Inherited*	References
Afghan hound	Myelopathy	7	Y	76–79
Afghan hound	Retinal degeneration	12	Y	69
Airedale terrier	Cerebellar hypoplasia	9		80–82
Airedale terrier	Cerebellar degeneration	9	Y	30
Airedale terrier	Congenital myasthenia gravis	8	Y	83
Akita	Cerebellar degeneration	9, 16		30
Akita	Congenital vestibular disease	9	?	84
Alaskan Malamute	Retinal degeneration	12	Y	69
Australian cattle dog	Ceroid lipofuscinosis	16	Y	85
Australian heeler	Deafness	10	Y	86
Australian shepherd	Chorioretinal dysplasia	12	Y	69
Australian shepherd	Deafness	10	Y	86, 87
Basenji	Coloboma	12	Y	69
Basset hound	Cervical malformation	8	?	88–90
Basset hound	Globoid cell leukodystrophy	16	?	91
Basset hound	Glycoproteinosis	14	?	92
Beagle	Agenesis vermis cerebellum	9	?	93
Beagle	Cerebellar degeneration	9	Y	30, 84
Beagle	Congenital vestibular disease	9		94, 95
Beagle	Epilepsy	14	Y	81, 96–105
Beagle	Gangliosidosis GM_1	16	Y	45, 46, 106
Beagle	Globoid cell leukodystrophy	16	?	107
Beagle	Glycoproteinosis	14	?	92, 96, 97, 108
Beagle	Retinal degeneration	12	Y	69
Beagle	Retinal dysplasia	12		69
Bedlington terriers	Retinal dysplasia	12	Y	69, 81, 109
Bern running dog	Cerebellar degeneration	9	Y	30
Bernese mountain dog	Aggression			110
Bernese mountain dog	Cerebellar degeneration	9	Y	84
Bernese mountain dog	Hypomyelination	11		111
Bernese mountain dog	Malignant histiocytosis	16		112
Blue heeler	Ceroid lipofuscinosis	16		113, 114
Blue tick hound	Globoid cell leukodystrophy	16	Y	81, 115
Border collie	Cerebellar degeneration	9	Y	116
Border collie	Ceroid lipofuscinosis	16	Y	84, 117, 118

Table continued on following page

Canine Diseases *Continued*

Breed	Diseases	Chapter	Inherited*	References
Border collie	Deafness	10		87
Border collie	Retinal degeneration	12	Y	69, 81, 109
Border collie	Sensory neuropathy	15		119
Borzoi	Cervical vertebral malformation	8		120
Boston terrier	Deafness	10	Y	86
Boston terrier	Gliomas	16	?	75, 121, 122
Boston terrier	Hemivertebrae	7	Y	81, 123, 124
Boston terrier	Hydrocephalus	13	P	125, 126
Boston terrier	Myelodysplasia	7	Y	123
Boston terrier	Pituitary tumors	16	?	75
Bouvier des Flandres	Laryngeal paralysis	10	Y	127, 128
Boxer	Ependymoma	16		75
Boxer	Glioma	16	?	75, 121, 122
Boxer	Pituitary tumors	16	?	75
Boxer	Progressive axonopathy	8	Y	129, 130
Briard	Retinal degeneration	12	Y	69, 109
Brittany spaniel	Cerebellar degeneration	9		131
Brittany spaniel	Neurogenic muscular atrophy	8	Y	132, 133
Brittany spaniel	Retinal dysplasia	12		69
Bull mastiff	Cerebellar and neuronal degeneration	9	Y	134
Bull mastiff	Cervical vertebral malformation	8		135
Bull terrier	Cerebellar hypoplasia	9		136
Bull terrier	Deafness	10	Y	81, 87, 137, 138
Bull terrier	Hyperkinesis	11		139
Cairn terrier	Cerebellar degeneration	9		8
Cairn terrier	Globoid cell leukodystrophy	16	Y	81, 140–144
Cairn terrier	Hydrocephalus	13	P	126
Cairn terrier	Neuronal degeneration	8		145, 146
Cardigan corgi	Retinal degeneration	12	Y	69, 81
Cavalier King Charles Spaniel	Muscular hypertonicity, Scotty cramp	8	Y	147–149
Chesapeake Bay retriever	Retinal degeneration	12		69
Chihuahua	Ceroid lipofuscinosis	16	Y	12
Chihuahua	Hydrocephalus	13	P	81, 126, 150
Chihuahua	Neuroaxonal dystrophy	8		151
Chondrodystrophic breeds	Intervertebral disk disease	7	?	152–158
Chow chow	Cerebellar hypoplasia	9	?	30, 159, 160
Chow chow	Hypomyelination	11	Y	161–164
Chow chow	Myotonia	11	Y	165–171
Clumber spaniel	Cerebellar degeneration	16		30
Cocker spaniel	Aggression			110, 172
Cocker spaniel	Cerebellar degeneration	9, 16		8
Cocker spaniel	Ceroid lipofuscinosis	16	Y	173
Cocker spaniel	Congenital vestibular disease	9	?	84, 94
Cocker spaniel	Deafness	10	?	86
Cocker spaniel	Esophageal hypomotility		Y	174, 175
Cocker spaniel	Facial paralysis	10	?	176, 177
Cocker spaniel	Hydrocephalus	13	P	81
Cocker spaniel	Retinal degeneration	12	Y	69, 81, 109
Cocker spaniel	Retinal dysplasia	12	Y	69, 109
Cocker spaniel	Neuronal degeneration	8		178
Collie	Cerebellar degeneration	9	Y	30, 179, 180
Collie	Chorioretinal dysplasia	12	Y	69
Collie	Collie eye syndrome	12	Y	
Collie	Deafness	10	Y	181
Collie	Dermatomyositis	8	Y	167, 182–187
Collie	Myelodysplasia	7		188
Collie	Neuroaxonal dystrophy	8	Y	180
Collie	Neuronal degeneration	8		189
Collie	Retinal degeneration	12	Y	109
Dachshund	Cerebellar hypoplasia	9		136
Dachshund	Ceroid lipofuscinosis	16	Y	190
Dachshund	Epilepsy	14	Y	191
Dachshund	Esophageal hypomotility			174, 175
Dachshund, long-haired	Ceroid lipofuscinosis	16	Y	192
Dachshund, long-haired	Sensory neuropathy	15	Y	193, 194
Dachshund, miniature, long-haired	Retinal degeneration	12	Y	69, 109

Canine Diseases *Continued*

Breed	Diseases	Chapter	Inherited*	References
Dalmation	Deafness	10	Y	81, 86, 87, 137, 138, 181, 195–200
Dalmation	Globoid cell leukodystrophy	16		81
Dalmation	Hyperkinesis	11	?	201
Dalmation	Hypomyelination	11	Y	202
Dalmation	Leukodystrophy	16	Y	203
Dalmation	Myelodysplasia	7	?	204
Doberman pinscher	Aggression			205
Doberman pinscher	Cervical vertebral malformation	8	?	88–90, 206–212
Doberman pinscher	Congenital vestibular disease	9	?	84, 94, 95
Doberman pinscher	Deafness	10		213
Doberman pinscher	Distal polyneuropathy	8		214
Doberman pinscher	Hemivertebra	7		215
Doberman pinscher	Narcolepsy-cataplexy	14	Y	216–220
Doberman pinscher	Sensory neuropathy	15		221
Dolichocephalic breeds	Meningioma	16		75, 222
English bulldog	Deafness	10	?	86
English bulldog	Hemivertebrae	7	Y	81, 123, 124
English bulldog	Hydrocephalus	13	P	81, 125, 126
English bulldog	Myelodysplasia	7	Y	81, 188, 223–225
English bulldog	Vertebral canal stenosis	7		226
English pointer	Hyperkinesis	11	Y	227–229
English pointer	Sensory neuropathy	15	Y	81, 194, 230–232
English setter	Ceroid lipofuscinosis	16	Y	233–237
English setter	Deafness	10	Y	86, 238
English springer spaniel	Gangliosidosis GM_1	16	Y	239
English springer spaniel	Phosphofructokinase deficiency myopathy	8	Y	240, 241
English springer spaniel	Polymyopathy, dyserythropoiesis	8	P	242
Finnish harrier	Cerebellar degeneration	9	Y	30, 243
Foxhound	Deafness	10	Y	81, 137, 244
Fox terrier	Congenital myasthenia gravis	8	Y	167, 245, 246
Fox terrier	Deafness	10		81
Fox terrier	Spinocerebellar degeneration	16	?	81
French bulldog	Hemivertebra	7		81, 123
German shepherd	Aggression		?	205
German shepherd	Congenital vestibular disease	9	?	84, 94, 95, 247
German shepherd	Degenerative myelopathy	7	?	248–257
German shepherd	Esophageal hypomotility		?	174, 175, 258–260
German shepherd	Giant axonal neuropathy	8	Y	261–265
German shepherd	Lumbosacral malformation	7	?	266–268
German shepherd	Myelodysplasia	7		269
German shepherd	Epilepsy	14	Y	81, 98, 270
German shorthaired pointer	Gangliosidosis GM_2	16	Y	4, 44–46, 271
German shorthaired pointer	Hemivertebra	7		272
Golden retriever	Muscular dystrophy	8	Y	167, 273–276
Golden retriever	Myotonia	11	?	166
Golden retriever	Retinal degeneration	12	Y	69, 81
Golden retriever	Sensory neuropathy	15		277
Gordon setter	Cerebellar degeneration	9	Y	30, 278–281
Gordon setter	Retinal degeneration	12	Y	69, 81, 109
Great Dane	Cerebellar degeneration	9, 16		8
Great Dane	Cervical vertebral malformation	8	?	27, 88–90, 206–212, 282–284
Great Dane	Esophageal hypomotility		?	175, 258, 285, 286
Great Dane	Retinal dysplasia	12		69
Great Dane crossbreeds	Neuronal degeneration	8	Y	287
Greyhound	Esophageal hypomotility			260
Greyhound	Retinal degeneration	12	Y	69
Horak's	Epilepsy	14	Y	98, 288
Irish setter	Cerebellar degeneration	9	Y	30, 84
Irish setter	Cerebellar hypoplasia	9	?	30
Irish setter	Esophageal hypomotility		?	286
Irish setter	Lissencephaly	14	?	30
Irish setter	Quadriplegia and amblyopia	8	Y	30, 81

Table continued on following page

Canine Diseases *Continued*

Breed	Diseases	Chapter	Inherited*	References
Irish setter	Retinal degeneration	12	Y	69, 81, 109
Irish terrier	Muscular dystrophy	8	Y	167, 289
Jack Russell terrier	Congenital myasthenia gravis	8	Y	167, 290, 291
Jack Russell terrier	Spinocerebellar degeneration	16	Y	81, 292
Japanese retriever	Ceroid lipofuscinosis	16		293
Japanese spaniel	Gangliosidosis GM_2	16		294
Keeshond	Epilepsy	14	Y	81, 98, 295
Kerry blue terrier	Cerebellar degeneration	9	Y	30
Kerry blue terrier	Striatonigral olivocerebellar degeneration	9		296–298
Labrador retriever	Retinal degeneration	12	Y	69, 81, 109
Labrador retriever	Retinal dysplasia	12	Y	69, 81, 109
Labrador retriever	Cerebellar hypoplasia	9		136
Labrador retriever	Cerebellar degeneration	9	P	299
Labrador retriever	Muscular dystrophy	8	Y	166, 300–306
Labrador retriever	Narcolepsy-cataplexy	14	Y	216, 218–220, 307, 308
Labrador retriever	Reflex myoclonus	11	?	309
Labrador retriever	Spongiform (myelin) degeneration	13		310, 311
Lapland dog	Glycogenosis	16	Y	312, 313
Lapland dog	Neuronal degeneration	8	Y	81, 314, 315
Lhaso apso	Hydrocephalus	13	P	126, 316, 317
Lhaso apso	Lissencephaly	14	?	318, 319
Lurcher	Hypomyelination	11	?	162, 164, 320
Maltese	Hydrocephalus	13	P	126, 321, 322
Miniature pinscher	Retinal degeneration	12	Y	69
Miniature schnauzer	Esophageal hypomotility		Y	174, 175, 323, 324
Mix	Cerebellar brain stem malformation	14		72
Mix	GM_2 gangliosidosis	16		325
Mix	Mucopolysaccharidosis	16	Y	326
Newfoundland	Esophageal hypomotility		Y	175, 327
Norwegian dunkerhound	Deafness	10	Y	137
Norwegian elkhound	Retinal degeneration	12	Y	69, 81
Old English sheepdog	Deafness	10	Y	86, 328
Pekingese	Hydrocephalus	13	P	126
Plott hound	Mucopolysaccharidosis	16	Y	326, 329
Pointer	Neurogenic muscular atrophy	8	Y	330–332
Pointer	Retinal degeneration	12		69
Pomeranian	Globoid cell leukodystrophy	16		333
Pomeranian	Hydrocephalus	13	P	126
Poodle	Agenesis vermis cerebellum	9	?	334
Poodle	Cerebellar hypoplasia	9	?	334, 335
Poodle	Demyelination	8	?	336
Poodle	Globoid cell leukodystrophy	16	Y	81, 337
Poodle	Glycoproteinosis	14	?	92
Poodle	Sphingomyelin lipidosis	16	Y	338
Poodle, miniature, toy	Retinal degeneration	12	Y	69, 81, 109
Portuguese water dog	GM_1 gangliosidosis	16		339
Pug	Esophageal hypomotility			259
Pug	Hemivertebra	7		123
Pug	Hydrocephalus	13	P	126, 317
Pyrenean mountain dog	Demyelination	8		340
Red Bone coonhound	Retinal degeneration	12	Y	69
Rottweiler	Leukoencephalomyelopathy	16	Y	341, 342
Rottweiler	Neuroaxonal dystrophy	8	Y	342–345
Rottweiler	Neuronal degeneration	8		346–348
Rottweiler	Retinal dysplasia	12		69, 109
Rottweiler	Spinal dysraphism	7		349
Saluki	Ceroid lipofuscinosis	16	Y	350
Saluki	Retinal degeneration	12	Y	69
Saluki	Spongiform degeneration	13		351
Samoyed	Cerebellar degeneration	9	Y	30, 84
Samoyed	Hypomyelination	11		162, 164, 352
Samoyed	Retinal degeneration	12	Y	69
Samoyed	Spongiform degeneration	13	?	353
Scottish terrier	Deafness	10		81
Scottish terrier	Myeloencephalopathy	8		354
Scottish terrier	Scotty cramp	11	Y	81, 355–362

Canine Diseases *Continued*

Breed	Diseases	Chapter	Inherited*	References
Sealyham terrier	Retinal dysplasia	12	Y	69, 81, 109
Shetland sheepdog	Dermatomyositis	8		167, 363
Shetland sheepdog	Retinal degeneration	12	Y	69
Shetland sheepdogs	Chorioretinal dysplasia	12	Y	69
Shropshire terrier	Deafness	10		87
Siberian husky	Cerebellar hypoplasia	9		364
Siberian husky	Degenerative myelopathy	7		365
Siberian husky	Laryngeal paralysis	10	Y	366
Siberian husky	Sensory neuropathy	15		221
Silky terrier	Agenesis vermis cerebellum	9		93
Silky terrier	Glucocerebrosidosis	16	Y	367, 368
Silky terrier	Spongiform degeneration	13	?	369
Springer spaniel	Aggression		?	110, 205
Springer spaniel	Congenital myasthenia gravis	8	Y	167, 370
Springer spaniel	Fucosidosis	16	Y	371–377
Springer spaniel	Hypomyelination	11	Y	162, 164, 378
Springer spaniel	Retinal degeneration	12	Y	69, 379, 380
Springer spaniel	Retinal dysplasia	12	Y	69, 109
Terrier cross	Ceroid lipofuscinosis	16		381
Tervuren shepherd	Epilepsy	14	Y	81, 98, 382
Tibetan mastiff	Hypertrophic neuropathy	8	Y	383–386
Tibetan spaniel	Retinal degeneration	12	Y	109
Tibetan terrier	Retinal degeneration	12	Y	69, 109, 387
Toy breeds	Atlantoaxial luxation	8	?	81, 388–392
Toy breeds	Hydrocephalus	13	P	126
Toy breeds	Occipital dysplasia	9	?	393, 394
Toy poodle	Hydrocephalus	13	P	322
Various	Cartilaginous exostoses	7		395–398
West Highland white terrier	Globoid cell leukodystrophy	16	Y	81, 142–144, 333, 399
Weimaraner	Cerebellar hypoplasia	9		136
Weimaraner	Hypomyelination	11		162, 164, 400–402
Weimaraner	Spinal dysraphism	7	Y	81, 403–408
Whippet	Sensory neuropathy	15		221
Wire-haired fox terrier	Lissencephaly	14	?	30
Wire-haired fox terrier	Cerebellar hypoplasia	9	?	30
Wire-haired fox terrier	Esophageal hypomotility		Y	174, 175, 258, 260, 286, 409
Yorkshire terrier	Hydrocephalus	13	P	126
Yorkshire terrier	Retinal dysplasia	12		69

* Y = yes, P = probable, ? = suspected.

Caprine Diseases

Breed	Disease	Chapter	Inherited*	References
Goats	Myotonia	11	Y	300, 410, 411
Nubian	Mannosidosis	16	Y	412–414
Angora	Atlantoaxial luxation	8		415
Nubian	Ceroid lipofuscinosis	16	Y	416, 417

* Y = yes.

Equine Diseases

Breed	Disease	Chapter	Inherited*	References
Appaloosa	Myeloencephalopathy	8, 16		418
Appaloosa	Night blindness	12	?	
Appaloosa	Retinal degeneration, nyctalopia	12	Y	69
Arabian	Atlanto-occipital malformation	8	Y	419–421
Arabian	Cerebellar degeneration	9	Y	30, 422–424
Arabian	Cerebellar dysplasia	9		422, 423
Arabian foals	Epilepsy	14	?	425
Donkey	Myeloencephalopathy	8		426
Gotland pony	Cerebellar degeneration	9	Y	30, 427
Horses	Atlanto-occipital malformation	8		419, 428, 429
Horses	Cartilaginous exostoses	7		430, 431
Horses	Cervical vertebral malformation	8	?	419, 421, 432–436
Horses	Degenerative myeloencephalopathy	8	?	418, 426, 437, 438
Horses	Myotonia	11	?	439
Morgan	Myeloencephalopathy	8		418
Morgan	Neuroaxonal dystrophy	8		440, 441
Oldberg	Cerebellar degeneration	9, 16		51
Przewalskii	Myeloencephalopathy	8		418
Shetland ponies	Narcolepsy-cataplexy	14	?	421
Standardbred	Muscular dystrophy	8	Y	442
Standardbred	Myeloencephalopathy	8		418
Suffolk draft horses	Narcolepsy-cataplexy	14	?	421
Thoroughbred	Cerebellar dysplasia	9		443
Thoroughbred	Cervical vertebral malformation	8	?	419, 421, 435, 444–447
Thoroughbred (and others)	Laryngeal paralysis	10	?	448–460
Various	Neonatal maladjustment syndrome	13		461
Welsh pony	Myeloencephalopathy	8		426
Zebra	Cervical vertebral malformation	8		462
Zebra	Degenerative myeloencephalopathy	8	?	418

* Y = yes, ? = suspected.

Feline Diseases

Breed	Disease	Chapter	Inherited*	References
Abyssinian	Glucocerebrosidosis	16	Y	463, 464
Abyssinian	Retinal degeneration	12	Y	109
Abyssinian	Retinal dysplasia	12	Y	109
Balinese	Sphingomyelin lipidosis	16		465
Burmese	Congenital vestibular disease	9	?	84, 94, 95
Burmese	Encephalocele	13	Y	466, 467
Cats (white, blue eyes)	Deafness	10	Y	196, 468–475
Domestic	Atlanto-occipital-axial malformation	8		476
Domestic	Cartilaginous exostoses	7		475
Domestic	Cerebellar degeneration	9, 16		30
Domestic	Cerebellar hypoplasia	9		477, 475, 478, 479
Domestic	Degenerative myelopathy	7		480
Domestic	Gangliosidosis GM_1	16	Y	4, 44–46
Domestic	Gangliosidosis GM_2	16	Y	45, 46, 481, 482
Domestic	Globoid cell leukodystrophy	16	Y	4, 483
Domestic	Glycogenosis	16	Y	4, 484
Domestic	Laryngeal paralysis	10		485–487
Domestic	Leukodystrophy	16	Y	488, 489
Domestic	Lissencephaly	14		490
Domestic	Mannosidosis	16	Y	491, 492
Domestic	Meningioma	16	?	75, 121, 493–495
Domestic	Mucopolysaccharidosis	16	Y	496, 497
Domestic	Neuroaxonal dystrophy	8	Y	498
Domestic	Neuronal degeneration	8	Y	499
Domestic	Olivopontocerebellar degeneration	9		30
Domestic	Retinal degeneration	12		69
Domestic	Sphingomyelin lipidosis	16	Y	500, 501
Egyptian Mau	Spongiform (myelin) degeneration	13	Y	502
Himalayan	Esophageal hypomotility	0		503

Feline Diseases *Continued*

Breed	Disease	Chapter	Inherited*	References
Korat	Gangliosidosis GM_1	16	Y	44–46
Korat	Laryngeal paralysis	10		486
Manx	Myelodysplasia	7	Y	123, 504–507
Norwegian Forest	Glycogenosis	16	Y	508
Persian	Laryngeal paralysis	10		486
Persian	Mannosidosis	16	Y	509–511
Siamese	Ceroid lipofuscinosis	16	Y	512
Siamese	Congenital vestibular disease	9	?	84, 94, 95
Siamese	Esophageal hypomotility	0	?	175
Siamese	Gangliosidosis GM_1	16	Y	44–46, 77
Siamese	Hydrocephalus	13	Y	475
Siamese	Mucopolysaccharidosis	16	Y	513–519
Siamese	Neuroaxonal dystrophy	16		498
Siamese	Optic pathway anomaly	12	Y	69
Siamese	Sphingomyelin lipidosis	16	Y	520, 521
Siamese	Strabismus	12		475

* Y = yes, ? = suspected.

Ovine Diseases

Breed	Disease	Chapter	Inherited*	References
Border Leicester	Cerebellar degeneration	9		522
Coopworth	Neuroaxonal dystrophy	8	Y	523
Corriedale	Cerebellar degeneration	9	Y	30
Corriedale	Glycogenosis	16	Y	524
Merino	Agenesis vermis cerebellum	9		93
Merino	Anencephaly	13		525
Merino	Cerebellar degeneration	9		526
Merino	Muscular dystrophy	8	Y	527–529
Merino	Neuroaxonal dystrophy	8		526
Polled Dorset	Globoid cell leukodystrophy	16	Y	530
Rambouillet	Ceroid lipofuscinosis	16	Y	531
Sheep	Arthrogryposis	8		532, 533
Sheep	Atlantoaxial luxation	8		534
Sheep	Cerebellar hypoplasia	9		532
Sheep	Glucocerebrosidosis	16	Y	24
Sheep	Hydrocephalus	13		532
Sheep	Hypomyelination	11		532
Sheep	Myelodysplasia	7		532
South Hampshire	Ceroid lipofuscinosis	16	Y	12
Suffolk	Congenital myopathy	8	Y	527, 535
Suffolk	GM_1 gangliosidosis	16	Y	536
Suffolk	Neuroaxonal dystrophy	8	Y	523, 537
Welsh Mountain	Cerebellar degeneration	9	Y	30
Various	Agenesis vermis cerebellum	9		532
Various	Cerebellar brain stem malformation	14		72, 532

* Y = yes.

Porcine Diseases

Breed	Disease	Chapter	Inherited*	References
British Saddleback	Hypomyelination	11	Y	538
Landrace	Hypomyelination	11	Y	538–540
Landrace	Malignant hyperthermia	16	Y	541–545
Pietrain	Malignant hyperthermia	16	Y	541
Pietrain	Myopathy, hypertrophy	8	Y	546
Poland China	Malignant hyperthermia	16	Y	541, 545
Saddleback—large white	Cerebellar degeneration	9		547
Swine	Encephalocele	13		548
Swine	Glucocerebrosidosis	16	?	24
Swine	Hydrocephalus	13		540
Swine	Lissencephaly	14		548
Yorkshire	Cerebellar degeneration	9	Y	30
Yorkshire	Gangliosidosis GM_2	16	Y	44–46, 549
Yorkshire	Neuronal degeneration	8	?	550

* Y = yes, ? = suspected.

REFERENCES

1. Barlow R: Morphogenesis of cerebellar lesions in bovine familial convulsions and ataxia. Vet Pathol 18:151–162, 1981.
2. Edmonds L, Crenshaw D, Selby LA: Micrognathia and cerebellar hypoplasia in an Aberdeen Angus herd. J Hered 64:62–64, 1973.
3. Barlow RM, Linklater KA, Young GB: Familial convulsions and ataxia in Angus calves. Vet Rec 83:60–65, 1968.
4. Jolly RD, Hartley WJ: Storage diseases of domestic animals. Aust Vet J 43:1–8, 1977.
5. Healy PJ, Cole AE: Heterozygotes for mannosidosis in Angus and Murray grey cattle. Aust Vet J 52:385–386, 1976.
6. Barlow R: Genetic cerebellar disorders in cattle. In: Rose FC, Behan PO (eds): Animal Models of Neurological Disease. Kent, Great Britain, Pitman Medical Ltd, 1980, pp 294–305.
7. Young S: Hypomyelinogenesis congenita (cerebellar ataxia) in Angus-shorthorn calves. Cornell Vet 52:84–93, 1962.
8. Braund KG: Degenerative and developmental diseases. In: Oliver JE, Hoerlein BF, Mayhew IG (eds): Veterinary Neurology. Philadelphia, WB Saunders, 1987, pp 185–215.
9. Jennings A, Summer G: Cortical cerebellar disease in an Ayrshire. Vet Rec 63:60, 1951.
10. Howell J, Ritchie H: Cerebellar malformations in two Ayrshire calves. Pathol Vet 3:159–168, 1966.
11. Boyd J, McNeil P: Atlanto-occipital fusion and ataxia in the calf. Vet Rec 120:34–37, 1987.
12. Mayhew I, Jolly R: Ovine ceroid lipofuscinosis. In: Proceedings of an ACVIM Forum, 1986, pp 57–59.
13. O'Sullivan BM, Healy PJ, Fraser IR, et al: Generalised glycogenosis in Brahman cattle. Aust Vet J 57:227–229, 1981.
14. Strain GM, Olcott BM, Archer RM, et al: Narcolepsy in a Brahman bull. J Am Vet Med Assoc 185:538–541, 1984.
15. Aitchison S, Westfall J, Leipold H, et al: Ultrastructural alterations of motor cortex synaptic junctions in Brown Swiss cattle with weaver syndrome. Am J Vet Res 46:1733–1736, 1985.
16. Baird JD, Sarmiento UM, Basrur PK: Bovine progressive degenerative myeloencephalopathy ("weaver syndrome") in Brown Swiss cattle in Canada: A literature review and case report. Can Vet J 29:370–377, 1988.
17. Stuart LD, Leipold HW: Lesions in bovine progressive degenerative myeloencephalopathy ("weaver") of Brown Swiss cattle. Vet Pathol 22:13–23, 1985.
18. Atkeson FW, Ibsen HL, Eldridge E: Inheritance of an epileptic type character in Brown Swiss cattle. J Hered 34:45, 1944.
19. Cho DY, Leipold HW: Cerebellar cortical atrophy in a Charolais calf. Vet Pathol 15:264–266, 1978.
20. Palmer AC, Blakemore WF, Barlow RM, et al: Progressive ataxia of Charolais cattle associated with a myelin disorder. Vet Rec 91:592–594, 1972.
21. Montgomery D, Mayer J: Progressive ataxia of Charolais cattle. Southwest Vet 37:247–250, 1986.
22. Cordy D: Progressive ataxia of Charolais cattle: An oligodendroglial dysplasia. Vet Pathol 23:78–80, 1986.
23. Zickeer SC, Kasari TR, Scruggs DW, et al: Progressive ataxia in a Charolais bull. J Am Vet Med Assoc 192:1590–1592, 1988.
24. Done JT: Developmental disorders on the nervous system in animals. Adv Vet Sci Comp Med 21:69–114, 1977.
25. Leipold HW, Cates WF, Radostits OM, et al: Spinal dysraphism, arthrogryposis and cleft palate in newborn Charolais calves. Can Vet J 10:268–273, 1969.
26. McCoy D, Simpson R, Olcott B, et al: Stabilization of atlantoaxial subluxation secondary to atlantooccipital malformation in a Devon calf. Cornell Vet 76:277–286, 1986.
27. Harper PAW, Walker KH, Healey PJ, et al: Neurovisceral ceroid-lipofuscinosis in blind Devon cattle. Acta Neuropathol 75:632–636, 1988.
28. Embury DH, Jerrett IV: Mannosidosis in Galloway calves. Vet Pathol 22:548–551, 1985.
29. Palmer AC, Smith GF, Turner S: Cataplexy in a Guernsey bull. Vet Rec 106:421, 1980.
30. de Lahunta A: Comparative cerebellar disease in domestic animals. Comp Cont Educ Pract Vet 8:8–19, 1980.
31. O'Sullivan BM, McPhee CP: Cerebellar hypoplasia of genetic origin in calves. Aust Vet J 51:469–471, 1975.
32. Strain GM, Olcott BM, Turk MA: Diagnosis of primary generalized epilepsy in a cow. J Am Vet Med Assoc 191:833–836, 1987.
33. Greene HJ, Leipold HW, Hibbs CM: Bovine congenital defects: Variations of internal hydrocephalus. Cornell Vet 64:596–616, 1974.
34. Leech RW, Haugse CN, Christoferson LA: Congenital hydrocephalus. Am J Pathol 92:567–570, 1978.
35. Axthelm MK, Leipold HW, Phillips RM: Congenital internal hydrocephalus in polled hereford cattle. Vet Med Small Anim Clin 76:567–570, 1981.
36. Hulland TJ: Cerebellar ataxia in calves. Can J Comp Med 21:72–76, 1957.
37. Rousseaux CG, Klavano GG, Johnson ES, et al: "Shaker" calf syndrome: A newly recognized inherited neurodegenerative disorder of horned Hereford calves. Vet Pathol 22:104–111, 1985.
38. Rousseaux CG, Klavano GG, Johnson ES, et al: A newly recognized neurodegenerative disorder of horned Hereford calves. Can Vet J 24:296–297, 1983.
39. Watson AG, Wilson JH, Cooley AJ, et al: Occipito-atlanto-axial malformation with atlanto-axial subluxation in an ataxic calf. J Am Vet Med Assoc 187:740–742, 1985.
40. Leipold HW, Strafuss A, Blauch B, et al: Congenital defect of the atlantoocipital joint in a Holstein-Friesian calf. Cornell Vet 62:646–672, 1972.
41. Hiraga T, Abe M: Two calves of Arnold-Chiari malformation and their craniums. Jpn J Vet Sci 49:651–656, 1987.
42. White ME, Whitlock RH, de Lahunta A: A cerebellar abiotrophy of calves. Cornell Vet 65:476–491, 1975.
43. Umemura T, Sato H, Goryo M, et al: Histopathology of congenital and perinatal cerbellar anomalies in twelve calves. Jpn J Vet Sci 49:95–104, 1987.
44. Baker HJ, Mole JA, Lindsey JR, et al: Animal models of human ganglioside storage diseases. Fed Proc 35:1193–1201, 1976.
45. Baker HJ, Walkley SU, Rattazi MC, et al: Feline gangliosidoses as models of human lysosomal storage diseases. In: Desnick RJ, Patterson DF, and Scarpelli DG (eds). Animal Models of Inherited Metabolic Diseases. New York, Alan R. Liss, 1982.
46. Baker HJ, Reynolds GD, Walkley SU, et al: The gangliosidoses: Comparative features and research applications. Vet Pathol 16:635–649, 1979.
47. Donnelly WJC, Sheahan BJ, Rogers TA: GM1 gangliosidosis in Friesian calves. J Pathol 111:173–179, 1973.
48. Henninger RW, Sigler RE: Spinal dysraphism in a calf. Comp Cont Educ Pract Vet 5:5488–5491, 1983.
49. Wells G, Scott A, Johnson C, et al: A novel progressive spongiform encephalopathy in cattle. Vet Rec 121: 419–420, 1987.

50. Saunders LZ, Sweet JD, Martin SM, et al: Hereditary congenital ataxia in Jersey calves. Cornell Vet 42:559–591, 1952.
51. Mayhew IG: Large Animal Neurology: A Handbook for Veterinary Clinicians. Philadelphia, Lea & Febiger, 1989.
52. de Lahunta A: Abiotrophy in domestic animals: A review. Can J Vet Res 54:65–76, 1990.
53. Richards R, Edwards J: A progressive spinal myelinopathy in beef cattle. Vet Pathol 23:35–41, 1986.
54. Edwards JR, Richards RB, Carrick MJ: Inherited progressive spinal myelinopathy in Murray Grey cattle. Aust Vet J 65:108–109, 1988.
55. Healy P, Harper P, Dennis J: Diagnosis of neuraxial oedema in calves. Aust Vet J 63:95–96, 1986.
56. Duffell S: Neuraxial oedema of Hereford calves with and without hypomyelinogenesis. Vet Rec 117:95–98, 1986.
57. Donaldson C, Mason R: Hereditary neuraxial oedema in a Poll Hereford herd. Aust Vet J 61:188–189, 1984.
58. Healy PJ, Harper PAW, Bowler JK: Prenatal occurrence and mode of inheritance of neuraxial oedema in Poll Hereford calves. Res Vet Sci 38:96–98, 1985.
59. Gundlach AL, Dodd PR, Grabara CSG, et al: Deficit of spinal cord glycine/strychnine receptors in inherited myoclonus of poll Hereford calves. Science 241:1807–1810, 1988.
60. Harper P, Dennis JA, Healy P, et al: Maple syrup urine disease in calves: A clinical, pathological and biochemical study. Aust Vet J 66:46–49, 1989.
61. Innes JRM, Saunders LA: Comparative Neuropathology. New York, Academic Press, 1962.
62. Abbitt B, Jones MZ, Kasari TR, et al: β-Mannosidosis in twelve Salers calves. J Am Vet Med Assoc 198:109–113, 1991.
63. Jolly RD, Thompson KG, Bayliss SL, et al: β-Mannosidosis in a Salers calf: A new storage disease of cattle. NZ Vet J 38:102–105, 1990.
64. Swan R, Taylor E: Cerebellar hypoplasia in beef shorthorn calves. Aust Vet J 59:95–96, 1982.
65. O'Sullivan B, McPhee C: Cerebellar hypoplasia of genetic origin in calves. Aust Vet J 51:469–471, 1975.
66. Richards RB, Edwards JR, Cook RD, et al: Bovine generalized glycogenosis. Neuropathol Appl Neurobiol 3:45–56, 1977.
67. McHowell J, Dorling PR, Cook RD, et al: Infantile and late onset form of generalized glycogenosis type II in cattle. J Pathol 134:266–277, 1981.
68. Greene HJ, Saperstein G, Schalles R, et al: Internal hydrocephalus and retinal dysplasia in shorthorn cattle. Ir Vet 32:65–69, 1978.
69. Slatter D: Fundamentals of Veterinary Ophthalmology. Philadelphia, WB Saunders, 1981.
70. Chrisman CL: Epilepsy and seizures. In Howard JL (ed): Current Veterinary Therapy: Food Animal Practice. Philadelphia, WB Saunders, 1981, pp 1082–1083.
71. Russell RG, Oteruelo FT: Ultrastructural abnormalities of muscle and neuromuscular junction differentiation in a bovine congenital neuromuscular disease. Acta Neuropathol 62:112–120, 1983.
72. Van den Akker S: Arnold-Chiari malformation in animals. Acta Neuropathol (Suppl) 1:39–44, 1962.
73. Boyd JS: Unusual case of spina bifida in a Friesian cross calf. Vet Rec 116:203–205, 1985.
74. Wasserman C: Myelodysplasia in a calf. Mod Vet Pract 67:879–883, 1986.
75. Luginbuhl H, Fankhauser R, McGrath JT: Spontaneous neoplasms of the nervous system in animals. Prog Neurol Surg 2:85–164, 1968.
76. Averill DR, Bronson RT: Inherited necrotizing myelopathy of Afghan hounds. J Neuropathol Exp Neurol 36:734–747, 1977.
77. Baker HJ, Lindsey JR, McKann GM, et al: Neuronal GM1 gangliosidosis in a Siamese cat with β-galactosidase deficiency. Science 174:838–839, 1971.
78. Cockrell BY, Herigstad RR, Flo GJ, et al: Myelomalacia in Afghan hounds. J Am Vet Med Assoc 162:362–365, 1973.
79. Cummings JF, de Lahunta A: Hereditary myelopathy of Afghan hounds: A myelinolytic disease. Acta Neuropathol 42:173–181, 1978.
80. Cordy DR, Snelbaker HA: Cerebellar hypoplasia and degeneration in a family of Airedale dogs. J Neuropathol Exp Neurol 11:324–328, 1952.
81. Erickson F, Leipold HW, McKinley J: Congenital defects in dogs: Part 2. Canine Pract 14:51–61, 1977.
82. Dow RW: Partial agenesis of the cerebellum in dogs. J Comp Neurol 72:569–586, 1940.
83. Duncan ID, Griffiths I: Neuromuscular diseases. In Kornegay JN (ed): Neurologic Disorders. New York, Churchill Livingstone, 1986, pp 169–195.
84. de Lahunta A: Veterinary Neuroanatomy and Clinical Neurology, 2nd ed. Philadelphia, WB Saunders, 1983.
85. Sisk DB, Levesque DC, Wood PA, et al: Clinical and pathologic features of ceroid lipofuscinosis in two Australian cattle dogs. J Am Vet Med Assoc 197:361–364, 1990.
86. Hayes HM, Wilson GP, Fenner WR, et al: Canine congenital deafness: Epidemiologic study of 272 cases. J Am Anim Hosp Assoc 17:473, 1981.
87. Igarashi M, Alford B, Cohn A, et al: Inner ear anomalies in dogs. Ann Otol 81:249–255, 1972.
88. Shores A: Canine cervical vertebral malformation/malarticulation syndrome. Comp Cont Educ Pract Vet 6:326–333, 1984.
89. Wright F, Rest JR, Palmer AC: Ataxia of the Great Dane caused by stenosis of the cervical vertebral canal: Comparison with similar conditions in the basset hound, Doberman pinscher, ridgeback and the thoroughbred horse. Vet Rec 92:1–6, 1973.
90. Denny H, Gibbs C, Gaskell C: Cervical spondylopathy in the dog: A review of thirty-five cases. J Small Anim Pract 18:117–132, 1977.
91. Luttgen PJ, Braund KG, Storts RW: Globoid cell leukodystrophy in a basset hound. J Small Anim Pract 24:153–160, 1983.
92. Cusick PK, Cameron AM, Parker AJ: Canine neuronal glycoproteinosis: Lafora's disease in the dog. J Am Anim Hosp Assoc 12:518–521, 1976.
93. Pass DA, Howell JM, Thompson RR: Cerebellar malformation in two dogs and a sheep. Vet Pathol 18:405–407, 1981.
94. Lane SB: Vestibular disease in companion animals. Pedigree Forum 6:11–16, 1987.
95. Chrisman CL: Disorders of the vestibular system. Comp Cont Educ Pract Vet 1:744–757, 1979.
96. Hegreberg GA, Padget GA: Inherited progressive epilepsy of the dog with comparisons to Lafora's disease of man. Fed Proc 35:1202–1205, 1976.
97. Edmonds HL, Hegreberg GA, van Gelder NM, et al: Spontaneous convulsions in beagle dogs. Fed Proc 39:2424–2428, 1979.
98. Holliday TA: Epilepsy in animals. In: Frey H-H, Janz D (eds): Handbook of Experimental Pharmacology, vol 74, pp 55–76. Berlin, Springer-Verlag, 1985.
99. Biefelt SW, Redman HC, Broadhurst JJ: Sire and sex-related differences in rates of epileptiform seizures in a purebred beagle dog colony. Am J Vet Res 32:2039–2048, 1971.
100. Montgomery DL, Lee AC: Brain damage in the epileptic beagle dog. Vet Pathol 20:160–169, 1983.

101. Edmonds HL Jr, Hegreberg GA, VanGelder NM, et al: Spontaneous convulsions in beagle dogs. Fed Proc 38:2424–2428, 1979.
102. Redman HC, Wilson GL, Hogan JE: Effect of chlorpromazine combined with intermittent light stimulation on the electroencephalogram and clinical response of the beagle dog. Am J Vet Res 34:929–936, 1973.
103. Redman HC, Weir JE: Detection of naturally occurring neurologic disorders of beagle dogs by electroencephalography. Am J Vet Res 30:2075–2082, 1969.
104. Redman HC, Hogan JE, Wilson GL: Effect of intermittent light stimulation singly and combined with pentylenetetrazol on the electroencephalogram and clinical response of the beagle dog. Am J Vet Res 33:677–685, 1972.
105. Wiederholt WC: Electrophysiologic analysis of epileptic beagles. Neurology 24:149–155, 1974.
106. Read DH, Harrington DD, Keenan TW, et al: Neuronal-visceral GM1 gangliosidosis in a dog with β-galactosidase deficiency. Science 194:442–445, 1976.
107. Johnson GR, Oliver JE, Selcer R: Globoid cell leukodystrophy in a beagle. J Am Vet Med Assoc 167:380–384, 1975.
108. Tomchick T: Familial Lafora's disease in the beagle dog. Fed Proc 32:8–21, 1973.
109. Barnett KC: Inherited eye disease in the dog and cat. J Small Anim Pract 29:462–475, 1988.
110. Voith VL: Diagnosis and treatment of aggressive behavior problems in dogs. In: Proceedings of the 47th Annual Meeting of the AAHA, 1980, pp 35–38.
111. Palmer A, Blakemore W, Wallace M, et al: Recognition of 'trembler', a hypomyelination condition in the Bernese mountain dog. Vet Rec 120:609–612, 1987.
112. Rosin A, Moore P, Dubielzig R: Malignant histiocytosis in Bernese mountain dogs. J Am Vet Med Assoc 188:1041–1046, 1986.
113. Cho D, Leipold H, Rudolph R: Neuronal ceroidosis (ceroid-lipofuscinosis) in a blue heeler dog. Acta Neuropathol 69:161–164, 1986.
114. Wood PA, Sisk DB, Styer E, et al: Animal model: Ceroidosis (ceroid-lipofuscinosis) in Australian cattle dogs. Am J Med Genet 26:891–898, 1987.
115. Boysen BG, Tryphonas L, Harries NW: Globoid cell leukodystrophy in the bluetick hounds dog: I. Clinical manifestations. Can Vet J 15:303–308, 1974.
116. Gill JM, Hewland ML: Cerebellar degeneration in the border collie. NZ Vet J 8:170, 1980.
117. Taylor RM, Farrow BRH: Ceroid-lipofuscinosis in border collie dogs. Acta Neuropathol 75:627–631, 1988.
118. Studdert VP, Mitten RW: Clinical features of ceroid lipofuscinosis in border collies. Aust Vet J 68:137–140, 1991.
119. Wheeler SJ: Sensory neuropathy in a border collie puppy. J Small Anim Pract 28:281–289, 1987.
120. Jaggy A, Gaillard C, Lang J, et al: Hereditary cervical spondylopathy (wobbler syndrome) in the Borzoi dog. J Am Anim Hosp Assoc 24:453–460, 1988.
121. Hayes KC, Schiefer B: Primary tumors in the CNS of carnivores. Pathol Vet 6:94–116, 1969.
122. Hayes HM, Priester WA, Pendergrass TW: Occurrence of nervous-tissue tumors in cattle, horses, cats and dogs. Int J Cancer 15:39–47, 1975.
123. Bailey CS: An embryological approach to the clinical significance of congenital vertebral and spinal cord abnormalities. J Am Anim Hosp Assoc 11:426–434, 1975.
124. Morgan JP: Congenital anomalies of the vertebral column of the dog: A study of the incidence and significance based on a radiographic and morphometric study. J Am Vet Radiol Soc 9:21–29, 1968.
125. de Lahunta A, Cummings JF: The clinical and electroencephalographic features of hydrocephalus in three dogs. J Am Vet Med Assoc 146:954–964, 1965.
126. Selby L, Hayes H, Becker S: Epizootiologic features of canine hydrocephalus. Am J Vet Res 40:411–413, 1979.
127. Venker-van Haagen AJ, Bouw J, Hartman W: Hereditary transmission of laryngeal paralysis in young Bouviers. J Am Anim Hosp Assoc 17:75–76, 1981.
128. Venker-van Haagen AJ, Hartman W, Goedegebuure SA: Spontaneous laryngeal paralysis in young Bouviers. J Am Anim Hosp Assoc 14:714–720, 1978.
129. Griffiths I: Progressive axonopathy of boxer dogs. In: Proceedings of an ACVIM Forum, San Diego, 1987, pp 866–868.
130. Griffiths IR, Duncan ID, Barker J: A progressive axonopathy of boxer dogs affecting the central and peripheral nervous system. J Small Anim Pract 21:29–43, 1980.
131. LeCouteur RA, Kornegay JN, Higgins RJ: Late onset progressive cerebellar degeneration of Brittany spaniel dogs. In: Proceedings of the Sixth Annual Veterinary Medical Forum, Washington, DC, 1988, pp 657–658.
132. Cork LC, Griffin JW, Munnell JF, et al: Hereditary canine spinal muscular atrophy. J Neuropathol Exp Neurol 38:209–221, 1979.
133. Lorenz MD, Cork LC, Griffin JW, et al: Hereditary muscular atrophy in Brittany spaniels: Clinical manifestations. J Am Vet Med Assoc 175:833–839, 1979.
134. Carmichael S, Griffiths IR, Harvey MJA: Familial cerebellar ataxia with hydrocephalus in bull mastiffs. Vet Rec 112:354–358, 1983.
135. Raffe M, Knecht C: Cervical vertebral malformation in bull mastiffs. J Am Anim Hosp Assoc 14:593–594, 1978.
136. Kornegay J: Cerebellar vermian hypoplasia in dogs. Vet Pathol 23:374–379, 1986.
137. Hudson W, Ruben R: Hereditary deafness in the Dalmatian dog. Arch Otol 75:213–219, 1962.
138. Anderson H, Henricson B, Lundquist P, et al: Genetic hearing impairment in the Dalmatian dog. Acta Otolaryngol Suppl 232:1–34, 1968.
139. Brown S, Crowell-Davis S, Malcolm T, et al: Naloxone-responsive compulsive tail chasing in a dog. J Am Vet Med Assoc 190:884–886, 1987.
140. Kurtz HJ, Fletcher TF: The peripheral neuropathy of canine globoid-cell leukodystrophy (Krabbe-type). Acta Neuropathol 16:226–232, 1970.
141. Howell JM: Globoid cell leucodystrophy in two dogs. J Small Anim Pract 12:633–642, 1971.
142. Fletcher TF, Kurtz HJ, Low DG: Globoid cell leukodystrophy (Krabbe type) in the dog. J Am Vet Med Assoc 149:165–172, 1966.
143. McGrath JT, Schutta H, Yaseen A, et al: A morphologic and biochemical study of canine globoid cell leukodystrophy. J Neuropathol Exp Neurol 28:171, 1969.
144. Suzuki Y, Austin J, Armstrong D, et al: Studies in globoid leukodystrophy: Enzymatic and lipid findings in the canine form. Exp Neurol 29:65–75, 1970.
145. Palmer AC, Blakemore WF: Progressive neuronopathy in the cairn terrier. Vet Rec 123:39, 1988.
146. Cummings JF, de Lahunta A, Moore JJ: Multisystemic chromatolytic neuronal degeneration in a cairn terrier pup. Cornell Vet 78:301–314, 1988.
147. Wright J, Brownlie S, Smyth J, et al: Muscle hypertonicity in the Cavalier King Charles spaniel: Myopathic features. Vet Rec 118:511–512, 1986.
148. Jones BR, Johnstone AC: An unusual myopathy in a dog. NZ Vet J 30:119–121, 1982.
149. Herrtage ME, Palmer AC: Episodic falling in the Cavalier King Charles spaniel. Vet Rec 112:458–459, 1983.
150. Few AB: The diagnosis and surgical treatment of ca-

nine hydrocephalus. J Am Vet Med Assoc 149:286–293, 1966.

151. Blakemore W, Palmer A: Nervous disease in the chihuahua characterised by axonal swellings. Vet Rec 117:498–499, 1985.
152. Hansen HJ: A pathologic-anatomical study on disk degeneration in the dog. Acta Orthop Scand, 1952.
153. Ghosh P, Taylor T, Barund K, et al: A comparative chemical and histochemical study of the chondrodystrophoid and nonchondrodystrophoid canine intervertebral disc. Vet Pathol 13:414–427, 1976.
154. Priester W: Canine intervertebral disc disease: Occurrence by age, breed, and sex among 8,117 cases. Theriogenology 6:293–303, 1976.
155. Brown N, Helphrey M, Prata R: Thoracolumbar disk disease in the dog: A retrospective analysis of 187 cases. J Am Anim Hosp Assoc 13:665–672, 1977.
156. Hoerlein B: Comparative disk disease: Man and dog. J Am Anim Hosp Assoc 15:535–545, 1979.
157. Hoerlein B: Intervertebral disc protrusions in the dog: I. Incidence and pathological lesions. Am J Vet Res 51:260–283, 1953.
158. Braund KG: Intervertebral disk disease. In: Kornegay JN (ed): Neurologic Disorders. New York, Churchill Livingstone, 1986, pp 21–39.
159. Knecht CD, Lamar CH, Schaible R, et al: Cerebellar hypoplasia in chow chows. J Am Anim Hosp Assoc 15:51, 1979.
160. Knecht C, Lamar C, Schaible R, et al: Cerebellar hypoplasia in chow chows. J Am Anim Hosp Assoc 15:51–53, 1979.
161. Vandevelde M, Braund KG, Walker T, et al: Dysmyelination of the central nervous system in the chow-chow dog. Acta Neuropathol 42:211–215, 1978.
162. Duncan I: Congenital tremor and abnormalities of myelination. In: Proceedings of an ACVIM Forum, San Diego, 1987, pp 869–872.
163. Vandevelde M, Braund K, Luttgen PJ, et al: Dysmyelination in chow chow dogs: Further studies in older dogs. Acta Neuropathol 55:81–87, 1981.
164. Duncan I: Abnormalities of myelination of the central nervous system associated with congenital tremor. J Vet Intern Med 1:10–23, 1987.
165. Shores A, Redding RW, Braund KG, et al: Myotonia congenita in a chow chow pup. J Am Vet Med Assoc 188:532–533, 1986.
166. Braund KG: Identifying degenerative and developmental myopathies. Vet Med 81:713–718, 1986.
167. Shelton G, Cardinet H: Pathophysiologic basis of canine muscle disorders. J Vet Intern Med 1:36–44, 1987.
168. Farrow BRH: Canine myotonia. In: Proceedings of the Sixth Annual Veterinary Medical Forum, Washington, DC, 1988, pp 64–66.
169. Nafe LA, Shires P: Myotonia in the dog. In: Proceedings of an ACVIM Forum, 1984, 191–192.
170. Jones BR, Anderson LJ, Barnes GRG, et al: Myotonia in related chow chow dogs. NZ Vet J 25:217–220, 1977.
171. Farrow BRH, Malik R: Hereditary myotonia in the chow chow. J Small Anim Pract 22:451–465, 1981.
172. Mugford RA: Aggressive behavior in the English cocker spaniel. Vet Ann 24:310–314, 1984.
173. Nimmo Wilkie JS, Hudson EB: Neuronal and generalized ceroid-lipofuscinosis in a cocker spaniel. Vet Pathol 19:623–628, 1982.
174. Clifford DH, Malek R: Diseases of the canine esophagus due to prenatal influence. Am J Dig Dis 14:578–602, 1969.
175. Clifford DH: Esophageal achalasia. Comp Pathol Bull 10(4):2–3, 1978.
176. Kern TJ, Erb HN: Facial neuropathy in dogs and cats: 95 cases (1975–1985). J Am Vet Med Assoc 191:1604–1609, 1987.
177. Braund KG, Luttgen PJ, Sorjonen DC, et al: Idiopathic facial paralysis in the dog. Vet Rec 105:297–299, 1979.
178. Jaggy A, Vandevelde M: Multisystem neuronal degeneration in cocker spaniels. J Vet Intern Med 2:117–120, 1988.
179. Hartley WJ, Barker JSF, Wanner RA, et al: Inherited cerebellar degeneration in the rough coated collie. Aust Vet Pract 8:79–85, 1978.
180. Clark RG, Hartley WJ, Burgess GS, et al: Suspected neuroaxonal dystrophy in collie sheep dogs. NZ Vet J 30:102–103, 1982.
181. Lurie M: The membranous labyrinth in the congenitally deaf collie and dalmatian dog. Laryngoscope 58:279–287, 1948.
182. Hargis AM, Haupt KH, Hegreberg GA, et al: Familial canine dermatomyositis. Am J Pathol 116:234–244, 1984.
183. Haupt KH, Prieur DJ, Moore MP, et al: Familial canine dermatomyositis: Clinical, electrodiagnostic, and genetic studies. Am J Vet Res 46:1861–1869, 1985.
184. Hargis A, Prieur D, Haupt K, et al: Postmortem findings in four litters of dogs with familial canine dermatomyositis. Am J Pathol 123:480–496, 1986.
185. Hargis A, Prieur D, Haupt K, et al: Prospective study of familial canine dermatomyositis. Am J Pathol 123:465–479, 1986.
186. Hargis AM, Haupt KH, Prieur DJ, et al: Dermatomyositis: Familial canine dermatomyositis. Am J Pathol 120:323–235, 1985.
187. Kunkle GA, Chrisman CL, Gross TL, et al: Dermatomyositis in collie dogs. Comp Cont Educ Pract Vet 7:185–192, 1985.
188. Wilson JW, Kurtz HJ, Leipold HW, et al: Spina bifida in the dog. Vet Pathol 16:165–179, 1979.
189. de Lahunta A, Shively GN: Neurofibrillary accumulation in a puppy. Cornell Vet 65:240–247, 1975.
190. Cummings JF, de Lahunta A: An adult case of canine neuronal ceroid-lipofuscinosis. Acta Neuropathol 39:43–51, 1977.
191. Holliday TA, Cunningham JG, Gutnick MJ: Comparative clinical and electroencephalographic studies of canine epilepsy. Epilepsia 11:281–292, 1971.
192. Vandevelde M, Fatzer R: Neuronal ceroid-lipofuscinosis in older dachshunds. Vet Pathol 17:686–692, 1980.
193. Duncan ID, Griffiths IR, Munz M: The pathology of a sensory neuropathy affecting long haired dachshund dogs. Acta Neruopathol 58:141–151, 1982.
194. Braund KG: Identifying degenerative peripheral neuropathies in pets. Vet Med 88:352–380, 1987.
195. Johnsson L, Hawkins J, Muraski A, et al: Vascular anatomy and pathology of the cochlea in Dalmatian dogs. In Darin de Lorenzo AJ (ed): Vascular Disorders and Hearing Defects. University Park, Md, University Park Press, 1973, pp 249–295.
196. Suga F, Hattler K: Physiological and histopathological correlates of hereditary deafness in animals. Laryngoscope 80:80–104, 1970.
197. Marshall A: Use of brain stem auditory-evoked response to evaluate deafness in a group of Dalmatian dogs. J Am Vet Med Assoc 188:718–722, 1986.
198. Ferrara ML, Halnan CRE: Congenital brain defects in the deaf Dalmatian. Vet Rec 112:344–346, 1983.
199. Mair IWS: Hereditary deafness in the Dalmatian dog. Arch Otol 212:1–14, 1976.
200. Branis M, Burda H: Inner ear structure in the deaf and normally hearing Dalmatian dog. J Comp Pathol 95:295–299, 1985.

201. Woods CB: Hyperkinetic episodes in two Dalmatians. J Am Anim Hosp Assoc 13:255–257, 1977.
202. Greene CE, Vandevelde M, Hoff EJ: Congenital cerebrospinal hypomyelinogenesis in a pup. J Am Vet Med Assoc 171:534–536, 1977.
203. Bjerkas I: Hereditary "cavitating" leukodystrophy in Dalmatian dogs. Acta Neuropathol 40:163–169, 1977.
204. Neufeld JL, Little PB: Spinal dysraphism in a Dalmatian dog. Can Vet J 15:335–336, 1974.
205. Houpt KA: Aggression in dogs. Comp Cont Educ Pract Vet 1:123–128, 1979.
206. Seim H: Ventral decompression and stabilization for the treatment of caudal cervical spondylomyelopathy in the dog. In: Proceedings of an ACVIM Forum, San Diego, 1987, pp 624–631.
207. Lyman R: Continuous dorsal laminectomy for treatment of Doberman pinschers with caudal cervical vertebral instability and malformation. In: Proceedings of an ACVIM Forum, San Diego, 1987, pp 303–308.
208. Seim H, Withrow S: Pathophysiology and diagnosis of caudal cervical spondylo-myelopathy with emphasis on the Doberman pinscher. J Am Anim Hosp Assoc 18:241–251, 1982.
209. Read R, Robins G, Carlisle C: Caudal cervical spondylo-myelopathy (wobbler syndrome) in the dog: A review of thirty cases. J Small Anim Pract 24:605–621, 1983.
210. Trotter E, de Lahunta A, Geary J, et al: Caudal cervical vertebral malformation-malarticulation in Great Danes and Doberman pinschers. J Am Vet Med Assoc 168:917–930, 1976.
211. Mason T: Cervical vertebral instability (wobbler syndrome) in the dog. Vet Rec 104:142–145, 1979.
212. Raffe M, Knecht C: Cervical vertebral malformation: A review of 36 cases. J Am Anim Hosp Assoc 16:881–883, 1980.
213. Wilkes M, Palmer A: Congenital deafness in Dobermans. Vet Rec 118:218, 1986.
214. Chrisman CL: Distal polyneuropathy of Doberman pinschers. In: Proceedings of the Third Annual Medical Forum, ACVIM, San Diego, 1985.
215. Leyland A: Ataxia in a Doberman pinscher. Vet Rec 116:414–415, 1985.
216. Baker TL, Mitler MM, Foutz AS, et al: Diagnosis and treatment of narcolepsy in animals. In Kirk RW (ed): Current Veterinary Therapy VIII. Small Animal Practice. Philadelphia, WB Saunders, 1983.
217. Bowersox S, Kilduff K, Zeller-DeAmicis L, et al: Brain dopamine receptor levels elevated in canine narcolepsy. Brain Res 402:44–48, 1987.
218. Kaitin KI, Kilduff TS, Dement WC: Evidence for excessive sleepiness in canine narcoleptics. Electroencephalogr Clin Neurophysiol 65:447–454, 1986.
219. Foutz AS, Mitler MM, Dement WC: Narcolepsy. Vet Clin North Am 10:65–80, 1980.
220. Bakr TL, Foutz AS, McNerney V, et al: Canine model of narcolepsy: Genetic and developmental determinants. Exp Neurol 75:729–742, 1982.
221. Wouda W, Vandevelde M, Oettli P, et al: Sensory neuronopathy in dogs: A study of four cases. J Comp Pathol 93:437–450, 1983.
222. Patnaik A, Kay W, Hurvitz A: Intracranial meningioma: A comparative pathologic study of 28 dogs. Vet Pathol 23:369–373, 1986.
223. Parker AJ, Park RD, Byerly CS, et al: Spina bifida with protrusion of spinal cord tissue in a dog. J Am Vet Med Assoc 163:158–160, 1973.
224. Parker AJ, Byerly CS: Meningomyelocoele in a dog. Vet Pathol 10:266–273, 1973.
225. Kornegay JN: Congenital and degenerative diseases of the central nervous system. In Kornegay JN: Neurologic Disorders. New York, Churchill Livingstone, 1986, pp 109–129.
226. Knecht C, Blevins W, Raffe M: Stenosis of the thoracic spinal canal in English bulldogs. J Am Anim Hosp Assoc 15:182–183, 1979.
227. Klein E, Marangos PJ, Montgomery P, et al: Adenosine receptor alterations in nervous pointer dogs: A preliminary report. Clin Neuropharmacol 10:4622–4469, 1987.
228. Murphree OD, Dykman RA: Litter patterns in the offspring of nervous and stable dogs: I. Behavioral tests. J Nerv Ment Dis 141:321–332, 1965.
229. Dykman RA, Murphree OD, Ackerman PT: Litter patterns in the offspring of nervous and stable dogs: II. Autonomic and motor conditioning. J Nerv Ment Dis 141:419–431, 1966.
230. Cummings JF, de Lahunta A, Simpson ST, et al. Reduced substance P-like immunoreactivity in hereditary sensory neuropathy of pointer dogs. Acta Neuropathol 63:33–40, 1984.
231. Cummings JF, de Lahunta A, Braund KG, et al: Animal model of human disease: Hereditary sensory neuropathy: Nociceptive loss and acral mutilation in pointer dogs: Canine hereditary sensory neuropathy. Am J Pathol 112:136–138, 1983.
232. Cummings JF, de Lahunta A, Winn SS: Acral mutilation and nociceptive loss in English pointer dogs. Acta Neuropathol 53:119–127, 1981.
233. Koppang N: Canine ceroid-lipofuscinosis in English setters. J Small Anim Pract 10:639–644, 1970.
234. Watson B, Watson G: Electroretinograms in English setters with neuronal ceroid lipofuscinosis. Invest Ophthalmol Vis Sci 19:87–90, 1980.
235. Armstrong D, Koppang N, Jolly R: Ceroid-lipofuscinosis. Comp Pathol Bull 12:2–4, 1980.
236. Armstrong D, Koppang N, Nilsson S: Canine hereditary ceroid lipofuscinosis. Eur Neurol 21:147–156, 1982.
237. Jasty V, Kowalski RL, Fonseca EH, et al: An unusual case of generalized ceroid-lipofuscinosis in a cynomolgus monkey. Vet Pathol 21:46–50, 1984.
238. Sims MH, Shull-Selcer E: Electrodiagnostic evaluation of deafness in two English setter littermates. J Am Vet Med Assoc 187:398–404, 1985.
239. Alroy J, Orgad U, Ucci AA, et al: Neurovisceral and skeletal Gm1-gangliosidosis in dogs with β-galactosidase deficiency. Science 229:470–472, 1985.
240. Giger U, Argov Z: Metabolic myopathy in phosphofructokinase deficient English springer spaniels. In: Proceedings of an ACVIM Forum, San Diego, 1987, p 912.
241. Giger U, Roudebush P: Inherited phosphofructokinase deficiency in English springer spaniels causes hemolytic disorder with hemolytic crises. In: Proceedings of an ACVIM Forum, San Diego, 1987, pp 700–702.
242. Holland CT, Canfield PJ, Watson ADJ, et al: Dyserythropoiesis, polymyopathy, and cardiac disease in three related English springer spaniels. J Vet Intern Med 5:151–159, 1991.
243. Tontitila P, Lindberg LA: ETT Fall av cerebellar ataxi hos finsk stovare. Svoman Elainlaakarilehti 77:135, 1971.
244. Adams EW: Hereditary deafness in a family of foxhounds. J Am Vet Med Assoc 128:302–303, 1956.
245. Jenkins WL, Van Dyk E, McDonald CB: Myasthenia gravis in a fox terrier litter. J S Afr Vet Assoc 47:59–62, 1976.
246. Miller LM, Lennon VA, Lambert EH, et al: Congenital myasthenia gravis in 13 smooth fox terriers. J Am Vet Med Assoc 182:694–697, 1983.
247. Lee M: Congenital vestibular disease in a German shepherd dog. Vet Rec 113:571, 1983.

248. Braund KG, Vandevelde M: German shepherd dog myelopathy: A morphologic and morphometric study. Am J Vet Res 39:1309–1315, 1978.
249. Williams DA, Sharp NJH, Batt RM: Enteropathy associated with degenerative myelopathy in German shepherd dogs. In: Scientific Proceedings of the American College of Veterinarian Internal Medicine, 1983.
250. Waxman FJ, Clemmons RM, Johnson G, et al: Progressive myelopathy in older German shepherd dogs: I. Depressed response to thymus-dependent mitogens. J Immunol 124:1209–1215, 1980.
251. Waxman FJ, Clemmons RM, Hinrichs DJ: Progressive myelopathy in older German shepherd dogs: II. Presence of circulating suppressor cells. J Immunol 124: 1216–1222, 1980.
252. Averill DR: Degenerative myelopathy in the aging German shepherd dog. J Am Vet Med Assoc 162:1045–1051, 1973.
253. Griffiths IR, Duncan ID: Chronic degnerative radiculomyelopathy in the dog. J Small Anim Pract 16:461–471, 1975.
254. Braund KG: Hip dysplasia and degenerative myelopathy: Making the distinction in dogs. Vet Med 82:82–89, 1987.
255. Clemmons RM: Degenerative myelopathy. In Kirk RW (ed): Current Veterinary Therapy X. Small Animal Practice. Philadelphia, WB Saunders, 1989, pp 830–833.
256. Williams DA, Prymak C, Baughan J: Tocopherol (vitamin E) status in canine degenerative myelopathy. In: Proceedings of the Third Annual Medical Forum, ACVIM, San Diego, 1985.
257. Amanai H: Leukomyelodegeneration in two aged German shepherd littermates: Patho-morphological observations. Jpn J Vet Res 35:121, 1987.
258. Clifford DH, Pirsch JG: Myenteric ganglial cells in dogs with and without hereditary achalasia of the esophagus. Am J Vet Res 32:615–619, 1971.
259. Boudrieau RJ, Rogers WA: Megaesophagus in the dog: A review of 50 cases. J Am Anim Hosp Assoc 21:33–40, 1985.
260. Clifford DH, Gyorkey F: Myenteric ganglial cells in dogs with and without achalasia of the esophagus. J Am Vet Med Assoc 150:205–211, 1967.
261. Duncan ID, Griffiths IR: Canine giant axonal neuropathy. Vet Rec 101:438–441, 1977.
262. Duncan ID, Griffiths IR: Peripheral nervous system in a case of canine giant axonal neuropathy. Neuropathol Appl Neurobiol 5:25–39, 1979.
263. Duncan ID, Griffiths IR: Canine giant axonal neuropathy: Some aspects of its clinical, pathological and comparative features. J Small Anim Pract 22:491–501, 1981.
264. Griffiths IR, Duncan ID, McCulloch M, et al: Further studies of the central nervous system in canine giant axonal neuropathy. Neuropathol Appl Neurobiol 6:421–432, 1980.
265. Julien JP, Mushynski WE, Duncan I, et al: Giant axonal neuropathy: Neurofilaments isolated from diseased dogs have a normal polypeptide composition. Exp Neurol 72:619–627, 1981.
266. Jaggy A, Lang J, Schawalder P: Cauda equina-syndrom beim Hund. Schweiz Arch Tierheilk 129:171–192, 1987.
267. Oliver J, Selcer R, Simpson S: Cauda equina compression from lumbosacral malarticulation and malformation in the dog. J Am Vet Med Assoc 173:207–214, 1978.
268. Lenehan T: Canine cauda equina syndrome. Comp Cont Educ Pract Vet 5:941–951, 1983.
269. Clayton HM, Boyd JS: Spina bifida in a German shepherd puppy. Vet Rec 112:13–15, 1983.
270. Falco MJ, Barker J, Wallace ME: The genetics of epilepsy in the British Alsatian. J Small Anim Pract 15:685–692, 1974.
271. Karbe E: Animal model of human disease: GM2-gangliosidosis (amaurotic idiocies) types I, II, and III. Animal model: Canine GM2-gangliosidosis. Am J Pathol 71:151–154, 1973.
272. Kramer JW, Schiffer SP, Sande RD, et al: Characterization of heritable thoracic hemivertebra of the German shorthaired pointer. J Am Vet Med Assoc 181:814–815, 1982.
273. Kornegay JN: Golden retriever myopathy. In: Proceedings of an ACVIM Forum, Washington, DC, 1984, pp 193–196.
274. Kornegay JN: Golden retriever myopathy. In Kirk RW (ed): Current Veterinary Therapy IX. Small Animal Practice. Philadelphia, WB Saunders, 1986, 792–794.
275. Kornegay JN: Golden retreiver muscular dystrophy. In: Proceedings of the Sixth Annual Veterinarians Medical Forum, Washington, DC, 1988, pp 470–471.
276. Valentine B, Cooper B, Cummings J, et al: Progressive muscular dystrophy in a golden retriever dog: Light microscope and ultrastructural features at 4 and 8 months. Acta Neuropathol 71:301–310, 1986.
277. Steiss JE, et al: Sensory neuropathy in a dog. J Am Vet Med Assoc 190:205–208, 1987.
278. Cork LC, Troncoso JC, Price DL: Canine inherited ataxia. Ann Neurol 9:492–499, 1981.
279. de Lahunta A, Fenner WR, Indrieri RJ, et al: Hereditary cerebellar cortical abiotrophy in the Gordon setter. J Am Vet Med Assoc 177:538–541, 1980.
280. Steinberg S, Troncoso J, Cork L, et al: Clinical features of inherited cerebellar degeneration in Gordon setters. J Am Vet Med Assoc 179:886–890, 1981.
281. Troncoso JC, Cork LC, Price DL: Canine inherited ataxia: Ultrastructural observations. J Neuropathol Exp Neurol 44:165–175, 1985.
282. Hedhammer A, Wu FM, Krook L, et al: Overnutrition and skeletal disease: An experimental study in growing great Dane dogs. Cornell Vet (Suppl 5) 64:1–60, 1974.
283. Olsson S, Stavenhorn M, Hoppe F: Dynamic compression of the cervical spinal cord: A myelographic and pathologic investigation in Great Dane dogs. Acta Vet Scand 23:65–78, 1982.
284. Wright F, Rest J, Palmer A: Ataxia of the Great Dane caused by stenosis of the cervical vertebral canal: Comparison with similar conditions in the basset hound, Doberman pinscher, ridgeback and the thoroughbred horse. Vet Rec 92:1–6, 1973.
285. Strombeck DR, Troya L: Evaluation of lower motor neuron function in two dogs with megaesophagus. J Am Vet Med Assoc 169:411–414, 1976.
286. Strombeck DR: Pathophysiology of esophageal motility disorders in the dog and cat. Vet Clin North Am 8:229–244, 1978.
287. Stockard C: An hereditary lethal factor for localized motor and preganglionic neurons. Am J Anat 59:1–53, 1936.
288. Cunningham JG, Farnbach GC: Inheritance and idiopathic canine epilepsy. J Am Anim Hosp Assoc 24:421–424, 1988.
289. Wentink GH, van der Linde-Sipman JS, Meijer AEF, et al: Myopathy with a possible recessive X-linked inheritance in a litter of Irish terriers. Vet Pathol 9:328–349, 1972.
290. Palmer AC, Goodyear JV: Congenital myasthenia in the Jack Russell terrier. Vet Rec 103:433–434, 1978.
291. Wilkes MK, MeKerrell R, Patterson R, et al: Ultrastructure of motor endplates in canine congenital myasthenia gravis. J Comp Pathol 97:247–256, 1987.
292. Hartley WJ, Palmer AC: Ataxia in Jack Russell terriers. Acta Neuropathol 26:71–74, 1973.

293. Umemura T, Sato H, Goryo M, et al: Generalized lipofuscinosis in a dog. Jpn J Vet Sci 47:673–677, 1985.
294. Cummings JF, Wood PA, Walkley SU, et al: GM2 gangliosidosis in a Japanese spaniel. Acta Neuropathol 67:247–253, 1985.
295. Wallace ME: Keeshonds: A genetic study of epilepsy and EEG readings. J Small Anim Pract 16:1–10, 1975.
296. de Lahunta A, Averill DR: Hereditary cerebellar cortical and extrapyramidal nuclear abiotrophy in Kerry blue terriers. J Am Vet Med Assoc 168:1119–1124, 1976.
297. Montgomery D, Storts R: Hereditary striatonigral and cerebello-olivary degeneration of the Kerry blue terrier. Vet Pathol 20:143–159, 1983.
298. Montgomery D, Storts R: Hereditary striatonigral and cerebello-olivary degeneration of the Kerry blue terrier: II. Ultrastructural lesions in the caudate nucleus and cerebellar cortex. J Neuropathol Exp Neurol 43:263–275, 1984.
299. Perille AL, Baer K, Joseph RJ, et al: Postnatal cerebellar cortical degeneration in Labrador retriever puppies. Can Vet J 32:619–621, 1991.
300. Atkinson JB, LeQuire VS: Myotonia congenita. Comp Pathol Bull 17:3–4, 1985.
301. McKerrell RE, Braund KG: In Kirk RW (ed): Current Veterinary Therapy X. Small Animal Practice. Philadelphia, WB Saunders, 1989, pp 820–821.
302. Moore M, Reed S, Hegreberg G, et al: Electromyographic evaluation of adult Labrador retrievers with type-II muscle fiber deficiency. Am J Vet Res 48:1332–1336, 1987.
303. Braund KG: Labrador retriever myopathy. In: Proceedings of the Sixth Annual Veterinary Medical Forum, Washington, DC, 1988, pp 85–87.
304. McKerrell R, Braund K: Hereditary myopathy in Labrador retrievers: Clinical variations. J Small Anim Pract 28:479–489, 1987.
305. McKerrell R, Braund K: Hereditary myopathy in Labrador retrievers: A morphologic study. Vet Pathol 23:411–417, 1986.
306. Amann JF, Laughlin MH, Korthuis RJ: Muscle hemodynamics in hereditary myopathy of Labrador retrievers. Am J Vet Res 49:1127–1130, 1988.
307. Shores A, Redding R: Narcoleptic hypersomnia syndrome responsive to protriptyline in a Labrador retriever. J Am Anim Hosp Assoc 23:455–458, 1987.
308. Katherman AE: A comparative review of canine and human narcolepsy. Comp Cont Educ Pract Vet 2:818–822, 1980.
309. Fox JG, Averill DR, Hallett M, et al: Familial reflex myoclonus in Labrador retrievers. Am J Vet Res 45:2367–2370, 1984.
310. O'Brien DP, Zachary JF: Clinical features of spongy degeneration of the central nervous system in two Labrador retriever littermates. J Am Vet Med Assoc 186:1207–1210, 1985.
311. Zachary JF, O'Brien DP: Spongy degeneration of the central nervous system in two canine littermates. Vet Pathol 22:561–571, 1985.
312. Walvoort HC, VanNes JJ, Stokhof AA, et al: Canine glycogen storage disease type II: A clinical study of four affected Lapland dogs. J Am Anim Hosp Assoc 20:279–286, 1984.
313. Mostafa IE: A case of glycogenic cardiomegaly in a dog. Acta Vet Scand 11:197–208, 1970.
314. Sandefeldt E, Cummings JF, de Lahunta A, et al: Hereditary neuronal abiotrophy in the Swedish Lapland dog. Cornell Vet 63:1–71, 1973.
315. Sandefeldt E, Cummings JF, de Lahunta A, et al: Hereditary neuronal abiotrophy in Swedish Lapland dogs. Am J Pathol 82:649–652, 1976.
316. Schmahl W, Kaiser E: Hydrocephalus, syringomyelia, and spinal cord angiodysgenesis in a Lhasa-apso dog. Vet Pathol 21:252–254, 1984.
317. Sahar A, Hochwald GM, Kay WJ, et al: Spontaneous canine hydrocephalus: Cerebrospinal fluid dynamics: J Neurol Neurosurg Psychiatry 34:308–315, 1971.
318. Greene CE, Vandevelde M, Braund K: Lissencephaly in two Lhasa Apso dogs. J Am Vet Med Assoc 169:405–410, 1976.
319. Zaki FA: Lissencephaly in Lhasa Apso dogs. J Am Vet Med Assoc 169:1165–1168, 1976.
320. Mayhew IG, Blakemore WF, Palmer AC, et al: Tremor syndromes and hypomyelination in Lurcher pups. J Small Anim Pract 25:551–559, 1984.
321. Simpson ST: Hydrocephalus in the Maltese dog: Electroencephalographic and C.T. correlations. In: Proceedings of an ACVIM Forum, Washington, DC, 1986, vol 11, pp 29–33.
322. Simpson ST, Steiss JE, Reed RB, et al: Hydrocephalus. In: Proceedings of an ACVIM Forum, San Diego, 1987, pp 834–838.
323. Cox VS, Wallace LJ, Anderson VE, et al: Hereditary esophageal dysfunction in the miniature schnauzer dog. Am J Vet Res 41:326–330, 1980.
324. Clifford DH, Waddell ED, Patterson DR, et al: Management of esophageal achalasia in miniature schnauzers. J Am Vet Med Assoc 161:1012–1020, 1972.
325. Rotmistrovsky RA, Alcaraz A, Cummings JC, et al: GM_2 gangliosidosis in a mixed-breed dog. Prog Vet Neurol 2:203–208, 1991.
326. Shull RM, Helman RG, Spellacy E, et al: Morphologic and biochemical studies of canine mucopolysaccharidosis I. Am J Pathol 114:487–495, 1984.
327. Schwartz A, Ravin CE, Greenspan RH, et al: Congenital neuromuscular esophageal disease in a litter of Newfoundland puppies. J Am Vet Radiol Soc 17:101–105, 1976.
328. Coulter DB: A dog with a partial merle coat, white iris, and bilaterally impaired hearing. Calif Vet 12:9–11, 1982.
329. Shull RM, Munger RJ, Spellacy E, et al: Animal model of human disease: Canine alpha-L-Iduronidase deficiency—A model of mucopolysaccharidosis I. Am J Pathol 109:244–248, 1982.
330. Inada S, Yamauchi C, Igata A, et al: Canine storage disease characterized by hereditary progressive neurogenic muscular atrophy: Breeding experiments and clinical manifestation. Am J Vet Res 47:2294–2299, 1986.
331. Inada S, Sakamoto H, Haruta K, et al: A clinical study on hereditary progressive neurogenic muscular atrophy in pointer dogs. Jpn J Vet Sci 40:539–547, 1978.
332. Izumo S, Ikuta F, Igata A, et al: Morphological study on the hereditary neurogenic amyotrophic dogs: Accumulation of lipid compound-like structures in the lower motor neuron. Acta Neuropathol 61:270–276, 1983.
333. Selcer ES, Selcer RR: Globoid cell leukodystrophy in two West Highland white terriers and one pomeranian. Comp Cont Educ Pract Vet 6:621–624, 1984.
334. Oliver JE, Geary JC: Cerebellar anomalies: Two cases. Vet Med Small Anim Clin 60:697, 1965.
335. Kay WJ, Budzilovich, GN: Cerebellar hypoplasia and agenesis in the dog. J Neuropathol Exp Neurology 29:156, 1970.
336. Matthews NS, de Lahunta A: Degenerative myelopathy in an adult miniature poodle. J Am Vet Med Assoc 186:1213–1214, 1985.
337. Zaki F, Kay WJ: Globoid cell leukodystrophy in a miniature poodle. J Am Vet Med Assoc 163:248–250, 1973.

338. Bundza A, Lowden JA, Charlton KM: Niemann-Pick disease in a poodle dog. Vet Pathol 16:530–538, 1979.
339. Shell LG, Potthoff AD, Carithers R, et al: Neuronal-visceral GM1 gangliosidosis in Portuguese water dogs. In: Proceedings of the Sixth Annual Veterinary Medical Forum, Washington, DC, 1988, pp 360–363.
340. Wright JA, Brownlie S: Progressive ataxia in a Pyrenean mountain dog. Vet Rec 116:410–411, 1985.
341. Gamble DA, Chrisman CL: A leukoencephalomyelopathy of Rottweiler dogs. Vet Pathol 21:274–280, 1984.
342. Chrisman C: Neuroaxonal dystrophy and leukoencephalomyelopathy of Rottweiler dogs. In Kirk RW (ed): Current Veterinary Therapy IX. Small Animal Practice. Philadelphia, WB Saunders, 1986, pp 805–806.
343. Chrisman CL, Cork LC, Gamble DA: Neuroaxonal dystrophy of Rottweiler dogs. J Am Vet Med Assoc 184:464–467, 1984.
344. Cork LC, Troncoso JC, Price DL, et al: Canine neuronaxonal dystrophy. J Neuropathol Exp Neurol 42:286–296, 1983.
345. Evans MG, Mullaney TP, Lowrie CT: Neuroaxonal dystrophy in a Rottweiler pup. J Am Vet Med Assoc 192:1560–1562, 1988.
346. Shell L, Jortner B, Leib M: Familial motor neuron disease in Rottweiler dogs: Neuropathologic studies. Vet Pathol 24:135–139, 1987.
347. Shell L, Jortner B, Leib M: Spinal muscular atrophy in two Rottweiler littermates. J Am Vet Med Assoc 190:878–880, 1987.
348. Shell LG: Spinal muscular atrophy in Rottweiler pups. In: Proceedings of the Sixth Annual Veterinary Medical Forum, Washington, DC, 1988, pp 404–405.
349. Shell LG, Carrig CB, Sponenberg DP, et al: Spinal dysraphism, hemivertebra, and stenosis of the spinal canal in a Rottweiler puppy. J Am Anim Hosp Assoc 24:341–344, 1988.
350. Appleby EC, Longstaffe JA, Bell FR: Ceroid lipofuscinosis in two Saluki dogs. J Comp Pathol 92:375–380, 1982.
351. Luttgen PJ, Storts RW: Central nervous system status spongiosus. In: Proceedings of the ACVIM Forum, San Diego, 1987, p 841.
352. Cummings J, Summers B, de Lahunta A, et al: Tremors in Samoyed pups with oligodendrocyte deficiencies and hypomyelination. Acta Neuropathol 71:267–277, 1986.
353. Mason RW, Hartley WJ, Randall M: Spongiform degeneration of the white matter in a Samoyed pup. Aust Vet Pract 9:11–13, 1979.
354. Sorjonen D, Cox N, Kwapien R: Myeloencephalopathy with eosinophilic refractile bodies (Rosenthal fibers) in a Scottish terrier. J Am Vet Med Assoc 190:1004–1006, 1987.
355. Meyers KM, Lund JE, Padgett G, et al: Hyperkinetic episodes in Scottish terrier dogs. J Am Vet Med Assoc 155:129–133, 1969.
356. Robert DD, Hitt ME: Methionine as a possible inducer of Scotty cramp. Canine Pract 13:29–31, 1986.
357. Meyers KM, Dickson WM, Lund JE, et al: Muscular hypertonicity. Arch Neurol 25:61–67, 1971.
358. Meyers KM, Schaub RG: The relationship of serotonin to a motor disorder of Scottish terrier dogs. Life Sci 14:1895–1906, 1974.
359. Meyers KM, Padgett GA, Dickson WM: The genetic basis of a kinetic disorder of Scottish terrier dogs. J Hered 61:189–192, 1970.
360. Meyers KM, Dickson WM, Schaub RG: Serotonin involvement in a motor disorder of Scottish terrier dogs. Life Sci 13:1261–1274, 1973.
361. Andersson B, Andersson M: On the etiology of "Scotty cramp" and "splay"—two motoring disorders common in the Scottish terrier breed. Acta Vet Scand 23:550–558, 1982.
362. Clemmons RM, Peters RI, Meyers KM: Scotty cramp: A review of cause, characteristics, diagnosis and treatment. Comp Cont Educ Pract Vet 2:385–390, 1980.
363. Hargis A, Prieur D, Haupt K, et al: Post-mortem findings in a Shetland sheepdog with dermatomyositis. Vet Pathol 23:509–511, 1986.
364. Harari J, Miller D, Padgett G, et al: Cerebellar agenesis in two canine littermates. J Am Vet Med Assoc 182:622–623, 1983.
365. Bichsel P, Vandevelde M: Degenerative myelopathy in a family of Siberian husky dogs. J Am Vet Med Assoc 183:998–1000, 1983.
366. Reinke JD, Suter PF: Laryngeal paralysis in a dog. J Am Vet Med Assoc 172:714–716, 1978.
367. Hartley WJ, Blakemore WF: Neurovisceral glucocerebroside storage (Gaucher's disease) in a dog. Vet Pathol 10:191–201, 1973.
368. Van De Water N, Jolly R, Farrow B: Canine Gaucher disease: The enzymatic defect. Aust J Exp Biol Med Sci 57:551–554, 1979.
369. Richards RB, Kakulas BA: Spongiform leukencephalopathy associated with congenital myoclonia syndrome in the dog. J Comp Pathol 88:317–320, 1978.
370. Johnson RP, Watson ADJ, Smith J, et al: Myasthenia in Springer spaniel littermates. J Small Anim Pract 16:641–647, 1975.
371. Taylor R, Farrow B, Healy P: Canine fucosidosis: Clinical findings. J Small Anim Pract 28:291–300, 1987.
372. Abraham D, Blakemore W, Deli A, et al: The enzymic defect and storage products in canine fucosidosis. Biochem J 221:25–33, 1984.
373. Alroy J, Ucci AA, Warren CD: Human and canine fucosidosis: A comparative histochemistry study. Acta Neuropathol 67:265–271, 1985.
374. Hartley WJ, Canfield PJ, Donnelly TM: A suspected new canine storage disease. Acta Neuropathol 56:225–232, 1982.
375. Kelly WR, Clague AE, Barns RJ, et al: Canine α-L-fucosidosis: A storage disease of Springer spaniels. Acta Neuropathol 60:9–13, 1983.
376. Littlewood JD, Herrtage ME, Palmer AC: Neuronal storage disease in English springer spaniels. Vet Rec 112:86, 1983.
377. Keller CB, Lamarre J: Inherited lysosomal storage disease in an English springer spaniel. J Am Vet Med Assoc 200:194–195, 1992.
378. Griffiths IR, Duncan ID, McCulloch M, et al: Shaking pups: A disorder of central myelination in the spaniel dog. Part I. Clinical, genetic, and light microscopical observations. J Neurol Sci 50:423–433, 1981.
379. Slatter D: Fundamentals of Veterinary Ophthalmology. Philadelphia, WB Saunders, 1981.
380. Erickson F, Leipold HW, McKinley J: Congenital defects in dogs—part 2. Canine Pract 14:51–61, 1977.
381. Hoover D, Little P, Cole W: Neuronal ceroid-lipofuscinosis in a mature dog. Vet Pathol 21:359–361, 1984.
382. Van der Velden A: Fits in Tervuren shepherd dogs: A presumed hereditary trait. J Small Anim Pract 9:63–70, 1968.
383. Cummings J, Cooper BJ, de Lahunta A, et al: Canine inherited hypertrophic neuropathy. Acta Neuropathol 53:137–143, 1981.
384. Cooper BJ, Duncan I, Cummings J, et al: Defective Schwann cell function in canine inherited hypertrophic neuropathy. Acta Neuropathol 63:51–56, 1984.
385. Cooper BJ, de Lahunta A, Cummings JF, et al: Canine

inherited hypertrophic neuropathy: Clinical and electrodiagnostic studies. Am J Vet Res 45:1172–1177, 1984.
386. Cummings J, de Lahunta A: Hypertrophic neuropathy in a dog. Acta Neuropathol 20:325–336, 1974.
387. Millichamp NJ, Curtis R, Barnett KC: Progressive retinal atrophy in Tibetan terriers. J Am Vet Med Assoc 192:769–776, 1988.
388. Geary JC, Oliver JE, Hoerlein BF: Atlanto-axial subluxation in the canine. J Small Anim Pract 8:577–582, 1967.
389. Oliver JE, Lewis RE: Lesions of the atlas and axis in dogs. J Am Anim Hosp Assoc 9:304–313, 1973.
390. Ladds P, Guffy M, Blauch B, et al: Congenital odontoid process separation in two dogs. J Small Anim Pract 12:463–471, 1970.
391. Cook JR, Oliver JE: Atlantoaxial luxation in the dog. Comp Cont Educ Pract Vet 3:242–252, 1981.
392. Downey RS: An unusual cause of tetraplegia in a dog. Can Vet J 8:216–217, 1967.
393. Bardens JW: Congenital malformations of the foramen magnum in dogs. Southwest Vet 18:295–298, 1965.
394. Parker AJ, Park RD: Occipital dysplasia in the dog. J Am Anim Hosp Assoc 10:520–525, 1974.
395. Gee B, Doige C: Multiple cartilaginous exostoses in a litter of dogs. J Am Vet Med Assoc 156:53–59, 1970.
396. Bichsel P, Lang J, Vandevelde M, et al: Solitary cartilaginous exostoses associated with spinal cord compression in three large-breed dogs. J Am Anim Hosp Assoc 21:619–622, 1985.
397. Doige C: Multiple cartilaginous exostoses in dogs. Vet Pathol 24:276–278, 1987.
398. Acton CE: Spinal cord compression in young dogs due to cartilagenous exostosis. Calif Vet 41:7–26, 1987.
399. Vicini DS, Wheaton LG, Zachary JF, et al: Peripheral nerve biopsy for diagnosis of globoid cell leukodystrophy in a dog. J Am Vet Med Assoc 192:1087–1090, 1988.
400. Kornegay JN: Dysmyelinogenesis in dogs. In: Proceedings of the Third Annual Medical Forum, ACVIM, San Diego, 1985.
401. Kornegay J: Hypomyelination in Weimaraner dogs. Acta Neuropathol 72:394–401, 1987.
402. Comont PSV, Palmer AC, Williams AE: Weakness associated with myelopathy in a Weimaraner puppy. J Small Anim Pract 29:367–372, 1988.
403. McGrath JT: Spinal dysraphism in the dog. Pathol Vet Suppl 2:1–36, 1965.
404. Gieb LW, Bistner SI: Spinal cord dysraphism in a dog. J Am Vet Med Assoc 150:618–620, 1967.
405. Engel HN, Draper DD: Comparative prenatal development of the spinal cord in normal and dysraphic dogs: Embryonic stage. Am J Vet Res 43:1729–1734, 1982.
406. Engel HN, Draper DD: Comparative prenatal development of the spinal cord in normal and dysraphic dogs: Fetal stage. Am J Vet Res 43:1735–1743, 1982.
407. Botelho SY, Sheldon A, Mcgrath JT, et al: Electromyography in dogs with congenital spinal cord lesions. Am J Vet Res 28:205–212, 1967.
408. Confer AW, Ward BC: Spinal dysraphism: A congenital myelodysplasia in the Weimaraner. J Am Vet Med Assoc 160:1423–1426, 1972.
409. Osborne CA, Clifford DH, Jessen C: Hereditary esophageal achalasia in dogs. J Am Vet Med Assoc 151:572–581, 1967.
410. Bryant SH: Altered membrane potentials in myotonia. In Bolis L, Hoffman JF, Leaf A (eds): Membranes and Diseases. New York, Raven Press, 1976, pp 197–206.
411 Bryant SH: Myotonia in the goat. Ann NY Acad Sci 317:314–325, 1979.
412. Healy P, Sewell C: The use of plasma β-mannosidase activity for the detection of goats heterozygous for β-mannosidosis. Aust Vet J 62:286–287, 1985.
413. Fankhauser R: Hydrocephalus Studien. Schweiz Arch Tierheilkd 101:407–416, 1959.
414. Healy PJ, Seaman JT, Gardner IA, et al: β-Mannosidase deficiency in Anglo Nubian goats. Aust Vet J 57:504–507, 1981.
415. Robinson WF, Chapman HM, Grandage J, et al: Atlanto-axial malarticulation in Angora goats. Aust Vet J 58:105–107, 1982.
416. Luttgen PJ, Storts RW: Ceroid-lipofuscinosis in Nubian goats. In: Proceedings of an ACVIM Forum, San Diego, 1987, p 843.
417. Fiske RA, Storts RW: Neuronal ceroid-lipofuscinosis in Nubian goats. Vet Pathol 25:171–173, 1988.
418. Mayhew J, Brown C, Trapp A: Equine degenerative myeloencephalopathy. In: Proceedings of an ACVIM Forum, Washington, DC, 1986, pp 19–25.
419. Mayhew IG, de Lahunta A, Whitlock RH, et al: Spinal cord disease in the horse. Cornell Vet (Suppl 6) 68:1–207, 1978.
420. Watson AG, Mayhew IG: Familial congenital occipitoatlantoaxial malformation (OAAM) in the Arabian horse. Spine 11:334–339, 1986.
421. Smith JM, DeBowes RM, Cox JH: Central nervous system disease in adult horses: Part II. Differential diagnosis. Comp Cont Educ Pract Vet 9:771–780, 1987.
422. Duncan I: Congenital tremor and abnormalities of myelination. In: Proceedings of the Fifth Annual Veterinarians Medical Forum, 1987, pp 869–873.
423. Fraser H: Two dissimilar types of cerebellar disorder in the horse. Vet Rec 78:608–612, 1966.
424. Palmer AC, Blakemore WF, Cook WR, et al: Cerebellar hypoplasia and degeneration in the young Arab horse. Clinical and neuropathological features. Vet Rec 93:62–66, 1973.
425. Mayhew I: Seizures disorders. In Robinson NE (ed): Current Therapy in Equine Medicine. Philadelphia, WB Saunders, 1983, pp 344–349.
426. Scarratt WK, Saunders GK, Sponenberg DP, et al: Degenerative myelopathy in two equids. J Equine Vet Sci 5:139–141, 1985.
427. Bjorck G, Everz KE, Hansen HJ, et al: Congenital cerebellar ataxia in the Gotland pony breed. Zentralbl Veterinarmed 20:341–354, 1973.
428. Mayhew IG, Watson AG, Heissan JA: Congenital occipitoatlantoaxial malformation in the horse. Equine Vet J 10:103–113, 1978.
429. Wilson WD, Hughes SJ, Ghoshal NG, et al: Occipitatlantoaxial malformation in two non-Arabian horses. J Am Vet Med Assoc 187:36–40, 1985.
430. Shupe JL, Leone NC, Gardner EJ, et al: Hereditary multiple exostoses. Am J Pathol 104:285–288, 1981.
431. Maciulis A, Bunch T, Shupe J, et al: High resolution chromosome banding analysis of horses with hereditary multiple exostosis. J Equine Vet Sci 5:284–286, 1985.
432. Powers B, Stashak T, Nixon A, et al: Pathology of the vertebral column of horses with cervical static stenosis. Vet Pathol 23:392–399, 1986.
433. Alitalo I, Karkkainen M: Osteochondrotic changes in the vertebrae of four ataxic horses suffering from cervical vertebral malformation. Nord Vet Med 35:468–474, 1983.
434. Wagner P, Bagby G, Grant B, et al: Surgical stabilization of the equine cervical spine. Vet Surg 8:7–12, 1979.
435. Steel J, Whittem J, Hutchins D: Equine sensory ataxia ("wobbles"): Clinical and pathological observations in Australian cases. Aust Vet J 35:442–449, 1959.

436. Wagner P, Grant B, Bagby G, et al: Evaluation of cervical spinal fusion as a treatment in the equine "wobbler" syndrome. Vet Surg 8:84–88, 1979.
437. Mayhew I, Brown C, Stowe H, et al: Equine degenerative myeloencephalopathy: A vitamin E deficiency that may be familial. J Vet Intern Med 1:45–50, 1987.
438. Mayhew IG, de Lahunta A, Whitlock RH, et al: Equine degenerative myeloencephalopathy. J Am Vet Med Assoc 170:195–201, 1977.
439. Steinberg S, Bothelo S: Myotonia in a horse. Science 137:979, 1962.
440. Beech J: Neuroaxonal dystrophy of the accessory cuneate nucleus in horses. Vet Pathol 21:384–393, 1984.
441. Beech J, Haskind M: Genetic studies of neuroaxonal dystrophy in the Morgan. Am J Vet Res 48:109–113, 1987.
442. Roneus B: Glutathione peroxidase and selenium in the blood of healthy horses and foals affected by muscular dystrophy. Nord Vet Med 34:350–353, 1982.
443. Poss M, Young S: Dysplastic disease of the cerebellum of an adult horse. Acta Neuropathol 75:209–211, 1987.
444. Grant B, Wagner P, Bayly W, et al: Surgical treatment of multiple level cord compression in the horse. Equine Pract 7:19–24, 1985.
445. Rooney J: Equine incoordination: I. Gross morphology. Cornell Vet 53:411–422, 1963.
446. Fraser H, Palmer A: Equine inco-ordination and wobbler disease of young horses. Vet Rec 80:338–355, 1967.
447. Falco M, Whitwell K, Palmer A: An investigation into the genetics of 'wobbler disease' in thoroughbred horses in Britain. Equine Vet J 8:165–169, 1967.
448. Duncan I: Some aspects of the neuropathy of equine laryngeal hemiplegia. In: Proceedings of an ACVIM Forum, San Diego, 1987, pp 863–865.
449. Cole CR: Changes in the equine larynx associated with laryngeal hemiplegia. Am J Vet Res 7:69–77, 1946.
450. Duncan ID, Griffiths IR, McQueen A, et al: The pathology of equine laryngeal hemiplegia. Acta Neuropathol 27:337–348, 1974.
451. Hillidge C: Interpretation of laryngeal function tests in the horse. Vet Rec 118:535–536, 1986.
452. Cahill JI, Goulder B: The pathogenesis of equine laryngeal hemiplegia: A review. NZ Vet J 35:82–90, 1987.
453. Tulleners EP, Harrison IW, Raker CW: Management of arytenoid chondropathy and failed laryngoplasty in horses: 75 cases (1879–1985). J Am Vet Med Assoc 192:670–675, 1988.
454. Cahill JI, Goulden B: Equine laryngeal hemiplegia: Part II. An electron microscopic study of peripheral nerve. NZ Vet J 34:170–175, 1986.
455. Cahill JI, Goulden B: Equine laryngeal hemiplegia: Part I. A light microscopic study of peripheral nerves. NZ Vet J 34:161–169, 1986.
456. Cahill J, Goulden B: Equine laryngeal hemiplegia: Part V. Central nervous system pathology. NZ Vet J 34:191–193, 1986.
457. Cahill J, Goulden B: Equine laryngeal hemiplegia: Part IV. Muscle pathology. NZ Vet J 34:186–190, 1986.
458. Cahill J, Goulden BE: Equine laryngeal hemiplegia: Part III. A teased fibre study of peripheral nerves. NZ Vet J 34:181–185, 1986.
459. Baker GJ: Larynegeal hemiplegia in the horse. Comp Cont Educ Pract Vet 5:S61–S67, 1983.
460. Koch C: Diseases of the larynx and pharynx of the horse. Comp Cont Educ Pract Vet 2:573–480, 1980.
461. Vaala W: Diagnosis and treatment of prematurity and neonatal maladjustment syndrome in newborn foals. Comp Cont Educ Pract Vet 8:211–226, 1986.
462. Montali R, Bush M, Sauer R, et al: Spinal ataxia in zebras: Comparison with the wobbler syndrome of horses. Vet Pathol 11:68–78, 1974.
463. Van den Berg P, Baker M, Lange A: A suspected lysosomal storage disease in Abyssinian cats: Part I. Genetic, clinical and clinical pathological aspects. J S Afr Vet Assoc 48:195–199, 1977.
464. Lange AL, Brown JMM, Maree CC: Biochemical studies on a lysosomal storage disease in Abyssianian cats. Onderstepoort J Vet Res 50:149–155, 1983.
465. Baker H, Wood P, Wenger D, et al: Sphingomyelin lipidosis in a cat. Vet Pathol 24:386–391, 1987.
466. Sponenberg DP, Graf-Webster E: Hereditary meningoencephalocele in Burmese cats. J Hered 77:60, 1986.
467. Zook B, Sostaric BR, Draper DJ, et al: Encephalocele and other congenital craniofacial anomalies in Burmese cats. Vet Med Small Anim Clin 78:695–701, 1983.
468. Rebillard M, Rebillard G, Pujol R: Variability of the hereditary deafness in the white cat: I. Physiology. Hear Res 5:179–187, 1981.
469. Rebillard M, Pujol R, Rebillard G: Variability of the hereditary deafness in the white cat: II. Histology. Hear Res 5:189–200, 1981.
470. Elverland HH, Mair IWS: Hereditary deafness in the cat. Acta Otolaryngol 90:360–369, 1980.
471. Faith RE, Woodard JC: Waardenburg's syndrome. Comp Pathol Bull 5:3–4, 1973.
472. Coulter DB, Martin CL, Alvarado TP: A cat with white fur and one blue eye. Calif Vet 34:11–14, 1980.
473. Delack JB: Hereditary deafness in the white cat. Comp Cont Educ Pract Vet 6:609–616, 1984.
474. Creel D, Conlee JW, Parks TN: Auditory brainstem anomalies in albino cats: I. Evoked potential studies. Brain Res 260:1–9, 1983.
475. Saperstein G, Harris S, Leipold HW: Congenital defects in domestic cats. Feline Pract 6:18–41, 1976.
476. Watson AG, Hall MA, de Lahunta A: Congenital occipitoatlantoaxial malformation in a cat. Comp Cont Educ Pract Vet 7:245–254, 1985.
477. Carpenter M, Harter D: A study of congenital feline cerebellar malformations: An anatomic and physiologic evaluation of agenetic defects. J Comp Neurol 105:51–94, 1956.
478. Csiza C, de Lahunta A, Scott F, et al: Spontaneous feline ataxia. Cornell Vet 62:300–322, 1972.
479. Herndon R, Margolis G, Kilham L: The synaptic organization of the malformed cerebellum induced by perinatal infection with the feline panleukopenia virus (PLV). J Neuropathol Exp Neurol 30:196–205, 1971.
480. Mesfin GM, Kusewitt D, Parker A: Degenerative myelopathy in a cat. J Am Vet Med Assoc 176:62–64, 1980.
481. Cork LC, Munnell JF, Lorenz MD: The pathology of feline GM_2 gangliosidosis. Am J Pathol 90:723–734, 1978.
482. Cork LC, Munnell JF, Lorenz MD, et al: GM_2 ganglioside lysosomal storage disease in cats with β-hexosaminidase deficiency. Science 196:1014–1017, 1977.
483. Johnson KH: Globoid leukodystrophy in the cat. J Am Vet Med Assoc 157:2057–2067, 1970.
484. Sandstrom B, Westman J, Ockerman PA: Glycogenosis of the central nervous system in the cat. Acta Neuropathol 14:194–200, 1969.
485. Cribb A: Laryngeal paralysis in a mature cat. Can Vet J 27:27, 1986.
486. White R, Littlewood J, Herrtage M, et al: Outcome of surgery for laryngeal paralysis in four cats. Vet Rec 117:103–104, 1986.
487. Hardie EM, Kolata RJ, Stone EA, et al: Laryngeal paralysis in three cats. J Am Vet Med Assoc 179:879–882, 1981.
488. Fatzer R: Leukodystrophische Erschrankungen im Gehirn junger Katzen. Schweiz Arch Tierheilikd 117:641–648, 1975.

489. Hegreberg GA, Thuline HC, Francis BH: Morphologic changes in feline leukodystrophy. Fed Proc 30:341, 1971.
490. Oliver JE, Hoerlein BF, Mayhew IG: Veterinary Neurology. Philadelphia, WB Saunders, 1987.
491. Blakemore W: A case of mannosidosis in the cat: Clinical and histopathological findings. J Small Anim Pract 27:447–455, 1986.
492. Walkley SU, Blakemore WF, Purpura DP: Alterations in neuron morphology in feline mannosidosis. Acta Neuropathol 53:75–79, 1981.
493. Braund KG, Ribas JL: Meningiomas of the central nervous system in dogs and cats. In: Proceedings of an ACVIM Forum, Washington, DC, 1986, pp 35–41.
494. Lawson DC, Burk RL, Prata RG: Cerebral meningioma in the cat: Diagnosis and surgical treatment of ten cases. J Am Anim Hosp Assoc 20:333–342, 1984.
495. Braund K, Ribas J: Central nervous system meningiomas. Comp Cont Educ Pract Vet 8:241–248, 1986.
496. Haskins ME, Jezyk PF, Desnick RJ, et al: Mucopolysaccharidosis in a domestic short-haired cat: A disease distinct from that seen in the Siamese cat. J Am Vet Med Assoc 175:384–387, 1979.
497. Haskins ME, Aguirre GD, Jezyk PF, et al: The pathology of the feline model of mucopolysaccharidosis: I. Am J Pathol 112:27–36, 1983.
498. Woodard JC, Collins GH, Hessler JR: Feline hereditary neuroaxonal dystrophy. Am J Pathol 74:551–560, 1974.
499. Vandevelde M, Greene C, Hoff E: Lower motor neuron disease with accumulation of neurofilaments in a cat. Vet Pathol 13:428–435, 1976.
500. Percy DH, Jortner BS: Feline lipidosis. Arch Pathol 92:136–143, 1971.
501. Cuddon PA, Higgins RJ, Duncan ID: Feline Niemann-Pick disease associated polyneuropathy. In: Proceedings of the Sixth Annual Veterinary Medical Forum, Washington, DC, 1988, p 726.
502. Kelly DF, Gaskell CJ: spongy degeneration of the central nervous system in kittens. Acta Neuropathol 35:151–158, 1976.
503. Clifford DH, Soifer FK, Wilson CF, et al: Congenital achalasia of the esophagus in four cats of common ancestry. J Am Vet Med Assoc 158:1554–1560, 1971.
504. Davidson AP: Congenital disorders of the Manx cat. Southwest Vet 37:115–119, 1986.
505. Kitchen H, Murray RE, Cockrell BY: Animal model for human disease, spina bifida, sacral dysgenesis and myelocele. Am J Pathol 68:203–206, 1972.
506. Hall JA, Fettman MJ, Ingram JT: Sodium chloride depletion in a cat with fistulated meningomyelocele. J Am Vet Med Assoc 192:1445–1448, 1988.
507. Leipold HW, Huston K, Blauch B, et al: Congenital defects of the caudal vertebral column and spinal cord in Manx cats. J Am Vet Med Assoc 164:520–523, 1974.
508. Fyfe JC, Giger U, van Winkle T, et al: Familial glycogen storage disease type IV (GSD IV) in Norwegian forest cats (NWFC). J Vet Intern Med 4:127, 1990.
509. Maenhout T, Kint JA, Dacremont G, et al: Mannosidosis in a litter of Persian cats. Vet Rec 122:351–354, 1988.
510. Jezyk PF, Haskins ME, Newman LR: Alpha-mannosidosis in a Persian cat. J Am Vet Med Assoc 189:1483–1485, 1986.
511. Vandevelde M, Fankhauser R, Bichsel P, et al: Hereditary neurovisceral mannosidosis with associated mannosidase deficiency in a family of Persian cats. Acta Neuropathol 58:64–68, 1982.
512. Green P, Little P: Neuronal ceroid-lipofuscin storage in Siamese cats. Can J Comp Med 38:207–212, 1974.
513. Cowell KR, Jezyk PF, Haskins ME, et al: Mucopolysaccharidosis in a cat. J Am Vet Med Assoc 169:334–339, 1976.
514. Langweiler M, Haskins, ME, Jezyk PF: Mucopolysaccharidosis in a litter of cats. J Am Anim Hosp Assoc 14:748–751, 1978.
515. Haskins ME, Bingel SA, Northington JW, et al: Spinal compression and hindlimb paresis in cats with mucopolysaccharidosis: VI. J Am Vet Med Assoc. 182:983–985, 1983.
516. Breton L, Guerin P, Morin M: A case of mucopolysaccharidosis VI in a cat. J Am Anim Hosp Assoc 19:891–896, 1983.
517. Jezyk P, Haskins M, Patterson DF: Mucopolysaccharidosis in a cat with arylsulfatase B deficiency: A model of Maroteaux-Lamy syndrome. Science 198:834–836, 1977.
518. Haskins ME, Aguirre GD, Jezyk PF, et al: The pathology of the feline model of mucopolysaccharidosis VI. Am J Pathol 101:657–674, 1980.
519. Haskins ME, Jezyk PF, Desnick RJ, et al: Animal model of human disease mucopolysaccharidosis VI Maroteaux-Lamy syndrome arylsulfatase β-deficient mucopolysaccharidosis in the Siamese cat. Am J Pathol 105:191–193, 1981.
520. Chrisp CE, Ringle DH, Abrams GD, et al: Lipid storage disease in a Siamese cat. J Am Vet Med Assoc 156:616–622, 1970.
521. Snyder S, Kingston R, Wenger D: Animal model of human disease: Niemann-Pick disease. Sphingomyelinosis of Siamese cats. Am J Pathol 108:252–254, 1982.
522. Terlecki S, Richardson C, Bradley R, et al: A congenital disease of lambs clinically similar to 'inherited cerebellar cortical atrophy' (Daft lamb disease). Br Vet J 134:299–308, 1978.
523. Nuttall WO: Ovine neuroaxonal dystrophy in New Zealand. NZ Vet J 36:5–7, 1988.
524. Manktelow CD, Hartley WJ: Generalized glycogen storage disease in sheep. J Comp Pathol 85:139–145, 1975.
525. Dennis SM, Leipold HW: Anencephaly in sheep. Cornell Vet 62:273–281, 1972.
526. Harper P, Duncan D, Plant J, et al: Cerebellar abiotrophy and segmental axonopathy: Two syndromes of progressive ataxia of Merino sheep. Aust Vet J 63:18–21, 1986.
527. McGavin: Progressive ovine muscular dystrophy. Comp Pathol Bull 6:3–4, 1974.
528. Richards R, Passmore I, Bretag A, et al: Ovine congenital progressive muscular dystrophy: Clinical syndrome and distribution of lesions. Aust Vet J 63:396–401, 1986.
529. Richards RB, Lewer RP, Passmore IK, et al: Ovine congenital progressive muscular dystrophy: Mode of inheritance. Aust Vet J 65:93–94, 1988.
530. Pritchard DH, Napthine DV, Sinclair AJ: Globoid cell leukodystrophy in polled Dorset sheep. Vet Pathol 17:399–405, 1980.
531. Woods PR: Neuronal ceroid-lipofuscinosis in Rambouillet sheep. In: Proceedings of the Ninth Annual Veterinary Medical Forum, New Orleans, 1991, pp 551–553.
532. Saperstein G, Leipold HW, Dennis SM: Congenital defects in sheep. J Am Vet Med Assoc 167:314–322, 1974.
533. Whittington RJ, Glastonbury JRW, Plant JW, et al: Congenital hydranencephaly and arthrogryposis of Corriedale sheep. Aust Vet J 65:124–127, 1988.
534. Parish S, Gavin P, Knowles D: Quadriplegia associated with cervical deformity in a lamb. Vet Rec 114:196, 1984.
535. Nisbet DI, Renwick CC: Congenital myopathy in lambs. J Comp Pathol 71:177, 1961.
536. Prieur DJ, Ahern-Rindell AJ, Murnane RD: Animal

model of human disease: Ovine GM-1 gangliosidosis. Am J Pathol 139:1511–1513, 1991.

537. Cordy DR, Richards WPC, Bradford GE: Systemic neuroaxonal dystrophy in Suffolk sheep. Acta Neuropathol 8:133–140, 1967.
538. Done J: The congenital tremor syndrome in pigs. Vet Ann 16:98–102, 1975.
539. Foulkes JA: Myelin and dysmyelination in domestic animals. Vet Bull 8:441–450, 1974.
540. Done JT: Congenital nervous diseases of pigs: A review. Lab Animal 2:207–217, 1968.
541. Chambers J, Hall RR: Porcine malignant hyperthermia (porcine stress syndrome). Comp Cont Educ Pract Vet 9:F317–F322, 1987.
542. Eikelenboom G, Minkema D: Prediction of pale, soft and exudative muscle with a non-lethal test for the halothane-induced porcine malignant hyperthermia syndrome. Neth J Vet Sci 99:421–426, 1974.
543. Lucke JN, Hall GM, Lister D: Malignant hyperthermia in the pig and the role of stress. Ann NY Acad Sci 317:326–337, 1979.
544. Sybesma W, Eikelenboom G: Malignant hyperthermia in pigs. Neth J Vet Sci 2:155–160, 1969.
545. Steiss JE, Bowen JM, Williams CH: Electromyographic evaluation of malignant hyperthermia-susceptible pigs. Am J Vet Res 42:1173–1176, 1981.
546. Wells GAH, Pinsent PJN, Todd JN: A progressive, familial myopathy of the Pietrain pig: The clinical syndrome. Vet Rec 106:556–558, 1980.
547. Kidd A, Done J, Wrathall A, et al: A new genetically-determined congenital nervous disorder in pigs. Br Vet J 142:275–285, 1986.
548. Vogt D, Ellersieck M, Deutsch W, et al: Congenital meningocele-encephalocele in an experimental swine herd. Am J Vet Res 47:188–191, 1986.
549. Read WK, Bridges CH: Cerebrospinal lipodystrophy in swine. Pathol Vet 5:67–74, 1968.
550. Higgins, RJ, Rings DM, Fenner WR, et al: Spontaneous lower motor neuron disease with neurofibrillary accumulation in young pigs. Acta Neuropathol 59:288–294, 1983.

Index

Note: Page numbers followed by f refer to illustrations; page numbers followed by t refer to tables.